Essentials of Small Animal Anesthesia and Analgesia

Second Edition

Essentials of Small Animal Anesthesia and Analgesia

Second Edition

Edited by

Kurt A. Grimm
William J. Tranquilli
Leigh A. Lamont

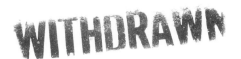

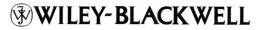

WILEY-BLACKWELL

A John Wiley & Sons, Inc., Publication

Wiley-Blackwell is an imprint of John Wiley & Sons, formed by the merger of Wiley's global Scientific, Technical and Medical business with Blackwell Publishing.

Registered office: John Wiley & Sons Ltd, The Atrium, Southern Gate, Chichester, West Sussex, PO19 8SQ, UK

Editorial offices: 2121 State Avenue, Ames, Iowa 50014-8300, USA
The Atrium, Southern Gate, Chichester, West Sussex, PO19 8SQ, UK
9600 Garsington Road, Oxford, OX4 2DQ, UK

For details of our global editorial offices, for customer services and for information about how to apply for permission to reuse the copyright material in this book please see our website at www.wiley.com/wiley-blackwell.

Library of Congress Cataloging-in-Publication Data
Essentials of small animal anesthesia and analgesia. – 2nd ed. / editors, Kurt A. Grimm, William J. Tranquilli, Leigh A. Lamont.
        p. ; cm.
    "Companion to the recently published Lumb and Jones' Veterinary Anesthesia and Analgesia, 4th edition"–Pref.
    Includes bibliographical references and index.
    ISBN-13: 978-0-8138-1236-6 (pbk. : alk. paper)
    ISBN-10: 0-8138-1236-4
  1. Veterinary anesthesia–Handbooks, manuals, etc. 2. Analgesia–Handbooks, manuals, etc.
3. Pets–Surgery–Handbooks, manuals, etc. I. Grimm, Kurt A. II. Tranquilli, William J. III. Lamont, Leigh A. IV. Lumb & Jones' veterinary anesthesia and analgesia.
    [DNLM: 1. Analgesia–veterinary. 2. Anesthesia–veterinary. SF 914]
    SF914.E77 2011
    636.089′7–dc23

                                                                    2011017805

A catalogue record for this book is available from the British Library.

Set in 10 on 12.5 pt Times Roman by Toppan Best-set Premedia Limited
Printed and bound in Singapore by Markono Print Media Pte Ltd

1 2011

Contents

This book has a companion website providing review questions, illustrations, and videos only available online at www.wiley.com/go/grimm.

Contributors

The following authors contributed new material to this book:

Jennifer G. Adams, DVM, ACVIM(LA), ACVA
1341 Buford Carey Road
Hull, Georgia 30646

Stuart Clark-Price, DVM, MS, DACVIM-LA, DACVA
University of Illinois Veterinary Teaching Hospital
Urbana, IL 61802

Fernando Garcia, DVM, MS, DACVA
Department of Small Animal Clinical Sciences
College of Veterinary Medicine
Michigan State University
East Lansing, MI 48824-1314

Stephen A. Greene, DVM, MS, DACVA
Department of Veterinary Clinical Sciences
College of Veterinary Medicine
Washington State University
Pullman, WA 99164-6610

Tamara L. Grubb, DVM, MS, DACVA
Department of Veterinary Clinical Sciences
College of Veterinary Medicine
Washington State University
Pullman, WA 99164

Craig Mosley, DVM, MSc, DACVA
Canada West Veterinary Specialists and Critical Care Hospital
Vancouver, Canada V5M 4Y3

Contributors

This book was distilled and revised from material contributed to *Lumb and Jones' Veterinary Anesthesia and Analgesia, Fourth Edition* by the following authors:*

Richard M. Bednarski, DVM, MS, DACVA
Department of Veterinary Clinical Sciences
College of Veterinary Medicine
Ohio State University
Columbus, OH 43210

Keith R. Branson, DVM, MS, DACVA
Department of Medicine and Surgery
College of Veterinary Medicine
University of Missouri
Columbia, MO 65211

David B. Brunson, DVM, MS, DACVA
Department of Surgical Sciences
School of Veterinary Medicine
University of Wisconsin
Madison, WI 53711

Rachael E. Carpenter, DVM
Department of Veterinary Clinical Medicine
College of Veterinary Medicine
University of Illinois
Urbana, IL 61802

Gwendolyn L. Carroll, DVM, MS, DACVA
Department of Small Animal Clinical Sciences
College of Veterinary Medicine and Biomedical Sciences
Texas A&M University
College Station, TX 77843-4474

Janyce L. Cornick-Seahorn, DVM, MS, DACVA, DACVIM
Equine Veterinary Specialists
Georgetown, KY 40324

Helio S. A. de Morais, DVM, PhD, DACVIM
Department of Medical Sciences
School of Veterinary Medicine
University of Wisconsin
Madison, WI 53706

Dianne Dunning, DVM, MS, DACVS
College of Veterinary Medicine
North Carolina State University
Raleigh, NC 27606

A. Thomas Evans, DVM, MS, DACVA
Veterinary Clinical Center
Michigan State University
East Lansing, MI 48824

Anna D. Fails, DVM, PhD, DACVIM
Department of Biomedical Sciences
College of Veterinary Medicine and Biomedical Sciences
Colorado State University
Fort Collins, CO 80523

Paul A. Flecknell, VetMB, PhD, DECLAM, DECVA
Comparative Biology Centre
Newcastle University
Newcastle upon Tyne, UK NE2 4HH

* Note: Many author affiliations have changed since the fourth edition of *Lumb & Jones' Veterinary Anesthesia and Analgesia* was published.

James S. Gaynor, DVM, MS, DACVA
Animal Anesthesia and Pain Management Center
Colorado Springs, CO 80918

Elizabeth A. Giuliano, DVM, MS, DACVO
Department of Medicine and Surgery
College of Veterinary Medicine
University of Missouri–Columbia
Columbia, MO 65211

Maria Glowaski, DVM, DACVA
Department of Veterinary Clinical Sciences
College of Veterinary Medicine
Ohio State University
Columbus, OH 43210-1089

Stephen A. Greene, DVM, MS, DACVA
Department of Veterinary Clinical Sciences
College of Veterinary Medicine
Washington State University
Pullman, WA 99164-6610

Jennifer B. Grimm, DVM, MS, DACVR
Veterinary Specialist Services, PC
Conifer, CO 80433-0504

Kurt A. Grimm, DVM, PhD, DACVA, DACVP
Veterinary Specialist Services, PC
Conifer, CO 80433-0504

Marjorie E. Gross, DVM, MS, DACVA
Department of Clinical Medicine
College of Veterinary Medicine
Oklahoma State University
Stillwater, OK 74078-2005

Tamara L. Grubb, DVM, MS, DACVA
Pfizer Animal Health
Uniontown, WA 99179

Elizabeth M. Hardie, DVM, PhD, DACVS
Department of Clinical Sciences
College of Veterinary Medicine
North Carolina State University
Raleigh, NC 27606

Steve C. Haskins, DVM, MS, DACVA, DACVECC
Department of Surgical and Radiological Sciences
School of Veterinary Medicine
University of California
Davis, CA 95616

Peter W. Hellyer, DVM, MS, DACVA
College of Veterinary Medicine and Biomedical Sciences
Colorado State University
Fort Collins, CO 80523

Robert D. Keegan, DVM, DACVA
Department of Veterinary Clinical Sciences
College of Veterinary Medicine
Washington State University
Pullman, WA 99164

Carolyn L. Kerr, DVM, DVSc, PhD, DACVA
Department of Clinical Studies
Ontario Veterinary College
University of Guelph
Guelph, Canada N1G 2W1

Leigh A. Lamont, DVM, MS, DACVA
Department of Companion Animals
Atlantic Veterinary College
University of Prince Edward Island
Charlottetown, Canada C1A 4P3

Duncan X. Lascelles, BVSc, PhD, DECVS, DACVS
Department of Clinical Sciences
College of Veterinary Medicine
North Carolina State University
Raleigh, NC 27606

Kip A. Lemke, DVM, MS, DACVA
Department of Companion Animals
Atlantic Veterinary College
University of Prince Edward Island
Charlottetown, Canada C1A 4P3

Hui-Chu Lin, DVM, MS, DACVA
Department of Clinical Sciences
College of Veterinary Medicine
Auburn University
Auburn, AL 36849

Victoria M. Lukasik, DVM, DACVA
Southwest Veterinary Anesthesiology
Southern Arizona Veterinary Specialty
    Center
Tucson, AZ 85705

Khursheed R. Mama, DVM, DACVA
Department of Clinical Sciences
College of Veterinary Medicine and
    Biological Sciences
Colorado State University
Fort Collins, CO 80523-1620

Sandra Manfra Marretta, DVM,
    DAVDC
Department of Veterinary Clinical
    Medicine
College of Veterinary Medicine
University of Illinois
Urbana, IL 61802

Steven L. Marks, BVSc, MS, DACVIM
Department of Clinical Sciences
College of Veterinary Medicine
North Carolina State University
Raleigh, NC 27606

David D. Martin, DVM, DACVA
Veterinary Operations
Companion Animal Division
Pfizer Animal Health
New York, NY

Elizabeth A. Martinez, DVM,
    DACVA
Department of Small Animal Clinical
    Sciences
College of Veterinary Medicine and
    Biomedical Sciences
Texas A&M University
College Station, TX 77843-4474

Karol A. Mathews, DVM, DVSc,
    DACVECC
Department of Clinical Studies
Ontario Veterinary College
University of Guelph
Guelph, Canada N1G 2W1

Wayne N. McDonell, DVM, PhD,
    DACVA
Department of Clinical Studies
Ontario Veterinary College
University of Guelph
Guelph, Canada N1G 2W1

William W. Muir, DVM, PhD, DACVA,
    DACVECC
Department of Veterinary Clinical
    Sciences
College of Veterinary Medicine
Ohio State University
Columbus, Ohio 43210

Mark G. Papich, DVM, MS,
    DACVCD
Department of Molecular Biomedical
    Sciences
College of Veterinary Medicine
North Carolina State University
Raleigh, NC 27606

Glenn R. Pettifer, DVM, DVSc, DACVA
Veterinary Emergency Clinic and Referral
   Centre
Toronto, Canada M4W 3C7

Aleksandar Popovic, DVM, Cert LAS
Merck Frosst Centre for Therapeutic
   Research
Kirkland, Canada H9H 3I1

Marc R. Raffe, DVM, MS, DACVA,
   DACVECC
Department of Veterinary Clinical
   Medicine
College of Veterinary Medicine
University of Illinois
Urbana, IL 61802

Claire A. Richardson, BVM&S
Comparative Biology Centre
Newcastle University Medical School
Newcastle upon Tyne, UK NE2 4HH

Sheilah A. Robertson, BVM&S, PhD,
   DACVA
Department of Small Animal Clinical
   Sciences
College of Veterinary Medicine
University of Florida
Gainesville, FL 32610

David C. Seeler, DVM, MSc, DACVA
Department of Companion Animals
Atlantic Veterinary College
University of Prince Edward Island
Charlottetown, Canada, C1A 4P3

Roman T. Skarda, (*deceased*) DMV,
   PhD, DACVA, DECVA
Department of Veterinary Clinical
   Sciences
College of Veterinary Medicine
Ohio State University
Columbus, OH 43210-1089

Eugene P. Steffey, VMD, PhD, DACVA,
   DECVA
Department of Surgical and Radiological
   Sciences
School of Veterinary Medicine
University of California
Davis, CA 95616

William J. Tranquilli, DVM, MS,
   DACVA
Department of Veterinary Clinical
   Medicine
College of Veterinary Medicine
University of Illinois
Urbana, IL 61802

Deborah V. Wilson, BVSc, MS,
   DACVA
Department of Large Animal Clinical
   Sciences
College of Veterinary Medicine
Michigan State University
East Lansing, MI 48824

Preface

The *Essentials of Small Animal Veterinary Anesthesia and Analgesia, Second Edition* is the companion to the recently published *Lumb and Jones' Veterinary Anesthesia and Analgesia, Fourth Edition*. Its major purpose is to provide veterinary care providers and students with the essentials of anesthetic and analgesic pharmacology, physiology, and clinical case management for small animal patients. The editors have included clinically focused small animal content from chapters covering physiology, pharmacology, patient assessment, and monitoring originally published in *Lumb and Jones' Veterinary Anesthesia and Analgesia, Fourth Edition*. Readers may find it helpful to refer back to those chapters if they wish to delve deeper into subject matter or references not included in this *Essentials* book. Additionally, several authors contributed new chapters on the equipment and management of patients with specific conditions specifically for this book. Those chapters have detailed references included and provide different perspectives on clinical case management.

The editors wish to express our gratitude to all the authors who provided content for the original chapters in *Lumb and Jones Veterinary Anesthesia and Analgesia, Fourth Edition*, as well as the new authors making contributions to this book. Dr. Steven Greene deserves a special thank you for assisting us with the coordination and editing of the chapters on management of patients with specific conditions. We would also like to thank the professionals at Wiley-Blackwell and specifically Erica Judisch, Nancy Turner, and Susan Engelken for their assistance with this project. Finally, we can never thank our families enough for their patience, understanding, and love when our work takes us away from them.

Kurt A. Grimm
Leigh A. Lamont
William J. Tranquilli

Essentials of Small Animal Anesthesia and Analgesia

Second Edition

Chapter 1

Patient evaluation and risk management

*William W. Muir, Steve C. Haskins, and
Mark G. Papich*

Introduction

The purpose of anesthesia is to provide reversible unconsciousness, amnesia, analgesia, and immobility for invasive procedures. The administration of anesthetic drugs and the unconscious, recumbent, and immobile state, however, compromise patient homeostasis. Anesthetic crises are unpredictable and tend to be rapid in onset and devastating in nature. The purpose of monitoring is to achieve the goals while maximizing the safety of the anesthetic experience.

Preanesthetic evaluation

All body systems should be examined and any abnormalities identified. The physical examination and medical history will determine the extent to which laboratory tests and special procedures are necessary. In all but extreme emergencies, packed cell volume and plasma protein concentration should be routinely determined. Contingent on the medical history and physical examination, additional evaluations may include complete blood counts; urinalysis; blood chemistries to identify the status of kidney and liver function, blood gases, and pH; electrocardiography; clotting time and platelet counts; fecal and/or filarial examinations; and blood electrolyte determinations. Radiographic and/or ultrasonographic examination may also be indicated.

Following examination, the physical status of the patient should be classified as to its general state of health according to the American Society of Anesthesiologists (ASA) classification (Table 1.1). This mental exercise forces the anesthetist to evaluate the patient's condition and proves valuable in the proper selection of anesthetic drugs. Classification of overall health is an essential part of any anesthetic record system. The preliminary physical examination should be done in the owner's presence, if possible, so that a prognosis can be given personally. This allows the client to ask questions and enables the veterinarian to communicate the risks of anesthesia and allay any fears regarding management of the patient.

Essentials of Small Animal Anesthesia and Analgesia, Second Edition. Edited by Kurt A. Grimm,
William J. Tranquilli, Leigh A. Lamont.
© 2011 John Wiley & Sons, Inc. Published 2011 by John Wiley & Sons, Inc.

Table 1.1.   Classification of physical status[a]

Category	Physical status	Possible examples of this category
I	Normal healthy patients	No discernible disease; animals entered for ovariohysterectomy, ear trim, caudectomy, or castration
II	Patients with mild systemic disease	Skin tumor, fracture without shock, uncomplicated hernia, cryptorchidectomy, localized infection, or compensated cardiac disease
III	Patients with severe systemic disease	Fever, dehydration, anemia, cachexia, or moderate hypovolemia
IV	Patients with severe systemic disease that is a constant threat to life	Uremia, toxemia, severe dehydration and hypovolemia, anemia, cardiac decompensation, emaciation, or high fever
V	Moribund patients not expected to survive 1 day with or without operation	Extreme shock and dehydration, terminal malignancy or infection, or severe trauma

[a] This classification is the same as that adopted by the ASA.
Source: Muir W.W. 2007. Considerations for general anesthesia. In: *Lumb and Jones' Veterinary Anesthesia and Analgesia*, 4th ed. W.J. Tranquilli, J.C. Thurmon, and K.A. Grimm, eds. Ames, IA: Blackwell Publishing, p. 17.

Preanesthetic pain evaluation

The diagnosis and treatment of pain require an appreciation of its consequences, a fundamental understanding of the mechanisms responsible for its production, and a practical appreciation of the analgesic drugs that are available. Semiobjective and objective behavioral, numerical, and categorical methods have been developed for the characterization of pain and, among these, the visual analog scale (VAS) has become popular. Ideally, pain therapy should be directed toward the mechanisms responsible for its production (multimodal therapy), with consideration, when possible, of initiating therapy before pain is initiated (preemptive analgesia). The American Animal Hospital Association (AAHA) has developed standards for the assessment, diagnosis, and therapy of pain that should be adopted by all veterinarians (Table 1.2).

Preanesthetic stress evaluation

Both acute and chronic pain can produce stress. Untreated pain can initiate an extended and potentially destructive series of events characterized by neuroendocrine dysregulation, fatigue, dysphoria, myalgia, abnormal behavior, and altered physical performance. Even without a painful stimulus, environmental factors (loud noise, restraint, or a predator) can produce a state of anxiety or fear that sensitizes and amplifies the stress response. Distress, an exaggerated form of stress, is present when the biologic cost of stress negatively affects the biologic functions critical to survival. Pain, therefore, should be considered in terms of the stress response and the potential to develop distress.

Increased central sympathetic output causes increases in heart rate and arterial blood pressure, piloerection, and pupil dilatation. The secretion of catecholamines from the

Table 1.2. AAHA pain management standards (2003)

1. Pain assessment for all patients regardless of presenting complaint
2. Pain assessment using standardized scale/score and recorded in the medical record
3. Pain management is individualized for each patient
4. Practice utilizes preemptive pain management
5. Appropriate pain management is provided for the anticipated level of pain
6. Pain management is provided for the anticipated duration of pain
7. Patient is reassessed for pain throughout potentially painful procedure
8. Patients with persistent or recurring disease are evaluated to determine their pain management needs
9. Analgesic therapy is used as a tool to confirm the existence of a painful condition when pain is suspected but cannot be confirmed by objective methods
10. A written pain management protocol is utilized
11. When pain management is part of the therapeutic plan, the client is effectively educated

Sources: Muir W.W. 2007. Considerations for general anesthesia. In: *Lumb and Jones' Veterinary Anesthesia and Analgesia,* 4th ed. W.J. Tranquilli, J.C. Thurmon, and K.A. Grimm, eds. Ames, IA: Blackwell Publishing, p. 19, and the AAHA, Lakewood, CO.

adrenal medulla and spillover of norepinephrine released from postganglionic sympathetic nerve terminals augment these central effects. Ultimately, changes in an animal's behavior may be the most noninvasive and promising method to monitor the severity of an animal's pain and associated stress.

Patient preparation

Preanesthetic fasting

Too often, operations are undertaken with inadequate preparation of patients. With most types of general anesthesia, it is best to have patients off feed for 12 hours previously. Some species are adversely affected by fasting. Birds, neonates, and small mammals may become hypoglycemic within a few hours of starvation, and mobilization of glycogen stores may alter rates of drug metabolism and clearance. Induction of anesthesia in animals having a full stomach should be avoided, if at all possible, because of the hazards of aspiration.

Preanesthetic fluid therapy

In most species, water is offered up to the time that preanesthetic agents are administered. It should be remembered that many older animals have clinical or subclinical renal compromise. Although these animals remain compensated under ideal conditions, the stress of hospitalization, water deprivation, and anesthesia, even without surgery, may cause acute decompensation. Ideally, a mild state of diuresis should be established with intravenous fluids in nephritic patients prior to the administration of anesthetic drugs.

Dehydrated animals should be treated with fluids and appropriate alimentation prior to operation; fluid therapy should be continued as required. An attempt should be made to correlate the patient's electrolyte balance with the type of fluid that is administered. Anemia and hypovolemia, as determined clinically and hematologically, should be corrected by administration of whole blood or blood components and balanced electrolyte solutions. Patients in shock without blood loss or in a state of nutritional deficiency benefit by administration of plasma or plasma expanders. In any case, it is good anesthetic practice to administer intravenous fluids during anesthesia to help maintain adequate blood volume and urine production, and to provide an available route for drug administration.

Prophylactic antibiotic administration

Systemic administration of antibiotics preoperatively is a helpful prophylactic measure prior to major surgery or if contamination of the operative site is anticipated. Antibiotics are ideally given approximately 1 hour before anesthetic induction.

Oxygenation and ventilation

Several conditions may severely restrict effective oxygenation and ventilation. These include upper airway obstruction by masses or abscesses, pneumothorax, hemothorax, pyothorax, chylothorax, diaphragmatic hernia, and gastric distention. Affected animals are often in a marginal state of oxygenation. Oxygen administration by nasal catheter or mask is indicated if the patient will accept it. Intrapleural air or fluid should be removed by thoracocentisis prior to induction because the effective lung volume may be greatly reduced and severe respiratory embarrassment may occur on induction. Anesthetists should be prepared to carry out all phases of induction, intubation, and controlled ventilation in one continuous operation.

Heart disease

Decompensated heart disease is a relative contraindication for general anesthesia. If animals must be anesthetized, an attempt at stabilization through administration of appropriate inotropes, antiarrhythmic drugs, and diuretics should be made prior to anesthesia. If ascites is present, fluid may be aspirated to reduce excessive pressure on the diaphragm.

Hepatorenal disease

In cases of severe hepatic or renal insufficiency, the mode of anesthetic elimination should receive consideration, with inhalation anesthetics often preferred. Just prior to induction, it is desirable to encourage defecation and/or urination by giving animals access to a run or exercise pen.

Patient positioning

During anesthesia, patients should, if possible, be restrained in a normal physiological position. Compression of the chest, acute angulation of the neck, overextension or compression of the limbs, and compression of the posterior vena cava by large viscera can all lead to serious complications, which include hypoventilation, nerve and/or muscle damage, and impaired venous return.

Tilting anesthetized patients alters the amount of respiratory gases that can be accommodated in the chest (functional residual capacity [FRC]) by as much as 26%. In dogs subjected to hemorrhage, tilting them head-up (reverse Trendelenburg position) was detrimental, producing lowered blood pressure, hyperpnea, and depression of cardiac contractile force. When dogs were tilted head-down (Trendelenburg position), no circulatory improvement occurred. In most species, the head should be extended to provide a free airway and to prevent kinking of the endotracheal tube.

Selection of an anesthetic and analgesic drugs

The selection of an anesthetic is based on appraising several factors, including:

(1) The patient's species, breed, and age.
(2) The patient's physical status.
(3) The time required for the surgical (or other) procedure, its type and severity, and the surgeon's skill.
(4) Familiarity with the proposed anesthetic technique.
(5) Equipment and personnel available.

In general, veterinarians will have greatest success with drugs they have used most frequently and with which they are most familiar. The skills of administration and monitoring are developed only with experience; therefore, change from a familiar drug to a new one is usually accompanied by a temporary increase in anesthetic risk.

The length of time required to perform a surgical procedure and the amount of help available during this period often dictate the anesthetic that is used. Generally, shorter procedures are done with short-acting agents, such as propofol, alphaxalone-CD, and etomidate, or with combinations using dissociative, tranquilizing, and/or opioid drugs. Where longer anesthesia is required, inhalation or balanced anesthetic techniques are preferred.

Drug interactions

When providing anesthesia and analgesia to animals, veterinarians often administer combinations of drugs without fully appreciating the possible interactions that may and do occur. Many drug interactions, both beneficial (resulting in decreased anesthetic risk) and harmful (increasing anesthetic risk), are possible. Although most veterinarians view drug interactions as undesirable, modern anesthesia and analgesic practice emphasizes the use of drug interactions for the benefit of the patient (multimodal anesthesia or analgesia).

A distinction should be made between drug interactions that occur *in vitro* (such as in a syringe or vial) from those that occur *in vivo* (in patients). Veterinarians frequently mix drugs together (compound) in syringes, vials, or fluids before administration to animals.

In vitro reactions, also called pharmaceutical interactions, may form a drug precipitate or a toxic product or inactivate one of the drugs in the mixture. *In vivo* interactions are also possible, affecting the pharmacokinetics (absorption, distribution, or biotransformation) or the pharmacodynamics (mechanism of action) of the drugs and can result in enhanced or reduced pharmacological actions or increased incidence of adverse events.

Nomenclature

Commonly used terms to describe drug interactions are addition, antagonism, synergism, and potentiation. In purely pharmacological terms that have underlying theoretical implications, addition refers to simple additivity of fractional doses of two or more drugs, the fraction being expressed relative to the dose of each drug required to produce the same magnitude of response; that is, response to X amount of drug A = response to Y amount of drug B = response to 1/2XA + 1/2YB, 1/4XA + 3/4YB, and so on. Additivity is strong support for the assumption that drug A and drug B act via the same mechanism (e.g., on the same receptors). Confirmatory data are provided by *in vitro* receptor-binding assays. Minimum alveolar concentration (MAC) fractions for inhalational anesthetics are additive. All inhalants have similar mechanisms of action but do not appear to act on specific receptors.

Synergism refers to the situation where the response to fractional doses as described previously is greater than the response to the sum of the fractional doses (e.g., 1/2XA + 1/2YB produces more than the response to XA or YB).

Potentiation refers to the enhancement of action of one drug by a second drug that has no detectable action of its own.

Antagonism refers to the opposing action of one drug toward another. Antagonism may be competitive or noncompetitive. In competitive antagonism, the agonist and antagonist compete for the same receptor site. Noncompetitive antagonism occurs when the agonist and antagonist act via different receptors.

The way anesthetic drugs are usually used raises special considerations with regard to drug interactions. For example, (1) drugs that act rapidly are usually used; (2) responses to administered drugs are measured, often very precisely; (3) drug antagonism is often relied upon; and (4) doses or concentrations of drugs are usually titrated to effect. Minor increases or decreases in responses are usually of little consequence and are dealt with routinely.

Commonly used anesthetic drug interactions

Two or more different kinds of injectable neuroactive agents are frequently used to induce anesthesia with the goal of achieving a better quality of anesthesia with minimal side effects. Agents frequently have complementary effects on the brain, but one agent may also antagonize an undesirable effect of the other. Examples of such combinations are tiletamine and zolazepam (Telazol®) or ketamine and midazolam. Tiletamine and ketamine produce sedation, immobility, amnesia, and differential analgesia, but may also produce muscle rigidity and grand mal seizures. Zolazepam and midazolam produce sedation, reduce anxiety, and minimize the likelihood of inducing muscle rigidity and seizures.

To better manage the pain associated with surgical procedures, it is becoming increasingly common to combine the use of regionally administered analgesics and light general anesthesia (twilight anesthesia). An example of such an approach is to administer a local anesthetic alone or in combination with an opioid or an alpha$_2$ adrenergic agonist into the epidural space before or during general anesthesia. Benefits sought with this approach are reduction in the amount of general anesthetic required and the provision of preemptive analgesia. Reducing general anesthetic requirements decreases the potential of systemic side effects.

Interactions among opioid drugs

In recent years, there has been some confusion as to whether the administration of opioid agonists with opioid agonist/antagonists will produce an interaction that diminishes the analgesic effect of the combination. In theory, drugs such as butorphanol and nalbuphine have antagonistic properties on the μ receptor, so they should partially reverse some effects of μ-receptor agonists (e.g., morphine) when administered together. The clinical significance of this antagonism has been debated, however. In dogs, for example, although butorphanol reverses some respiratory depression and sedation produced by pure agonists, the analgesic efficacy may be preserved. Similarly, in dogs given butorphanol for postoperative pain associated with orthopedic surgery, there was no diminished efficacy with subsequent administration of oxymorphone. However, in another study, dogs that had not responded to butorphanol after shoulder arthrotomy responded to subsequent administration of oxymorphone, but the oxymorphone dose required to produce an adequate effect was higher than what would be required if oxymorphone was used alone, suggesting that some antagonism of analgesia may have been present. When butorphanol and oxymorphone have been administered together to cats, a greater efficacy has been reported than when either drug was used alone. These clinical observations, taken together, suggest that antagonism may indeed occur in some clinical patients, but in other patients, coadministration actually results in a synergistic analgesic effect. These divergent results from one individual to the next may be due to a variety of factors, including: (1) differences in the pain syndrome being treated, (2) species variation in response to opioids, (3) dosage ratios of the specific opioids being administered, and (4) variation in opioid efficacy between genders. For example, when looking at the first of these factors in humans, whether antagonism or synergism occurs with the coadministration of butorphanol and a pure opioid agonist appears to depend on whether somatic pain versus visceral pain is present. These types of studies have not been performed to date in common pet species.

Risk

Risk refers to uncertainty and the potential for adverse outcome as a result of anesthesia and surgery. It should be emphasized that physical status, anesthetic risk, and operative risk are different.

Major surgical procedures and complex procedures are associated with increased morbidity and mortality as compared with minor procedures. Involvement of major organs increases risk; central nervous system (CNS), cardiac, and pulmonary procedures have the highest risk, followed by the gastrointestinal tract, liver, kidney, reproductive organs, muscles, bone, and skin. Emergency procedures are more risky because of unstable or severely compromised homeostasis, decreased ability to prepare or stabilize the patient, and lack of preparation by the surgical and anesthetic team. Operating conditions refer to the physical facilities and equipment and support personnel available. The aggressiveness of the surgical team, experience with the procedure, and frequency of performance are also important. Lastly, the duration of the procedure and fatigue must be considered because patients cannot be operated on indefinitely. The incidence of morbidity and mortality increases with the duration of anesthesia and surgery. Thus, efficiency of the surgical team is important in reducing risk.

Anesthetic factors that can affect risk include the choice of anesthetic drugs to be used, the anesthetic technique, and the duration of anesthesia. The choice of anesthetic can adversely affect the outcome, but more commonly the agents are not so much at fault as the manner in which they are given. Experience of the anesthetist with the protocol is important to its safe administration. It is worth noting that human error remains the number one reason for anesthesia-related mishap and is a major contributor to anesthetic risk.

Several retrospective studies have reported a perioperative mortality rate of 20–189 per 10,000 patients administered anesthetics. Anesthesia reportedly contributed to 2.5–9.2 deaths per 10,000 patients (Table 1.3). Mortality rates were higher among patients

Table 1.3.　Complications in small animal anesthesia

Species	Number at risk	Number of anesthetic- and sedative-related fatalities	Risk of anesthetic-/ sedative-related death (%)	95% CI (%)
Dog	98,036	163	0.17	0.14–0.19
Cat	79,178	189	0.24	0.20–0.27
Rabbit	8209	114	1.39	1.14–1.64
Guinea pig	1288	49	3.80	2.76–4.85
Ferret	601	2	0.33	0.04–1.20[a]
Hamsters	246	9	3.66	1.69–6.83[a]
Chinchilla	334	11	3.29	1.38–5.21
Rat	398	8	2.01	0.87–3.92[a]
Other small mammals	232	4	1.72	0.47–4.36[a]
Budgerigar	49	8	16.33	7.32–29.66[a]
Parrot	127	5	3.94	1.29–8.95[a]
Other birds	284	5	1.76	0.57–4.06[a]
Reptiles	134	2	1.49	0.18–5.29[a]
Other	50	0	0	0–7.11[a]

[a] Exact 95% confidence interval (CI).
Source: Broadbelt D.C., Blissitt K.J., Hammond R.A., Neath P.J., Young L.E., Pfeiffer D.U., Wood J.L. 2008. The risk of death: the confidential enquiry into perioperative small animal fatalities. *Vet Anaesth Analg* **35**(5): 365–373. Epub May 5, 2008.

with poorer preoperative physical status and greater age where biologic reserves are limited, and among patients undergoing emergency procedures where preoperative planning and preparation are limited, but were still of notable frequency in young, healthy patients undergoing planned procedures (Table 1.4). Of the deaths, 1% occurred at premedication, 6–8% at induction, 30–46% intraoperatively, and 47–61% postoperatively (Table 1.5). Intraoperative causes of death included the primary disease process;

Table 1.4. Risks of anesthetic- and sedation-related death in healthy and sick dogs, cats, and rabbits

Species	Health status[a]	Number of anesthetic-related deaths	Estimated number of anesthetics	Risk of anesthetic- and sedation-related death (%)	95% CI (%)
Dog	Healthy	49	90,618	0.05	0.04–0.07
	Sick	99	7418	1.33	1.07–1.60
	Overall[b]	163	98,036	0.17	0.14–0.19
Cat	Healthy	81	72,473	0.11	0.09–0.14
	Sick	94	6705	1.40	1.12–1.68
	Overall[b]	189	79,178	0.24	0.20–0.27
Rabbit	Healthy	56	7652	0.73	0.54–0.93
	Sick	41	557	7.37	5.20–9.54
	Overall[b]	114	8209	1.39	1.14–1.64

[a] Healthy (ASA I and II) no/mild preoperative disease, sick (ASA III–V) severe preoperative disease.
[b] Overall risks include additional deaths for which insufficient information was available (including health status) to exclude them from being classified as anesthetic related.
Source: Broadbelt D.C., Blissitt K.J., Hammond R.A., Neath P.J., Young L.E., Pfeiffer D.U., Wood J.L. 2008. The risk of death: the confidential enquiry into perioperative small animal fatalities. *Vet Anaesth Analg* **35**(5): 365–373. Epub May 5, 2008.
CI, confidence interval.

Table 1.5. Timing of anesthetic- and sedation-related deaths in dogs, cats, and rabbits

Timing of death	Dogs (%)	Cats (%)	Rabbits (%)
After premedication	1 (1)	2 (1)	0
Induction of anesthesia	9 (6)	14 (8)	6 (6)
Maintenance of anesthesia	68 (46)	53 (30)	29 (30)
Postoperative death[a]	70 (47)	106 (61)	62 (64)
0–3 hours postoperative	31	66	26
3–6 hours postoperative	11	9	7
6–12 hours postoperative	12	7	13
12–24 hours postoperative	13	12	9
24–48 hours postoperative	3	10	3
Unknown time	0	2	4
Total	148 (100)	175 (100)	97 (100)

[a] Postoperative deaths were additionally categorized by time after anesthesia. The percent values are given within parentheses.
Source: Broadbelt D.C., Blissitt K.J., Hammond R.A., Neath P.J., Young L.E., Pfeiffer D.U., Wood J.L. 2008. The risk of death: the confidential enquiry into perioperative small animal fatalities. *Vet Anaesth Analg* **35**(5): 365–373. Epub May 5, 2008.

aspiration; hypovolemia and hypotension; hypoxia secondary to airway or endotracheal tube problems, or pneumothorax; misdosing of drugs; and hypothermia. Postoperative causes of death included the primary disease process, arrest during endotracheal tube suctioning, aspiration, pneumonia, and heart failure (Table 1.6).

Claims presented to the American Veterinary Medical Association Professional Liability Insurance Trust based on anesthetic, surgical, and medical incidents reflect changing trends in veterinary practice and owner concern for optimal patient care (Table 1.7). It should be noted that the percentage of anesthesia claims decreased by over 50% for both dogs and horses from 1982 to 2003, reflecting the increasing sophistication and safety of veterinary anesthesia during this period. For more recent data on

Table 1.6. Primary causes of death in dogs, cats, and rabbits

Cause of death	Dogs (%)	Cats (%)	Rabbits (%)
Cardiovascular cause	34 (23)	11 (6)	3 (3)
Respiratory causes	20 (13)	16 (9)	13 (13)
Either cardiovascular or respiratory	55 (37)	99 (57)	22 (23)
Neurological cause	7 (5)	8 (5)	2 (2)
Renal	1 (1)	6 (3)	0
Unknown	31 (21)	35 (20)	57 (59)
Total	148 (100)	175 (100)	97 (100)

Deaths are expressed as number of animals (percent of total). Only cases where a case–control questionnaire was received are included.
Source: Broadbelt D.C., Blissitt K.J., Hammond R.A., Neath P.J., Young L.E., Pfeiffer D.U., Wood J.L. 2008. The risk of death: the confidential enquiry into perioperative small animal fatalities. *Vet Anaesth Analg* **35**(5): 365–373. Epub May 5, 2008.

Table 1.7. Trends in claims involving anesthesia, surgery, and medicine presented to the American Veterinary Medical Association Professional Liability Insurance Trust (AVMA-PLIT)

Species	Total	Anesthesia (%)	Medical (%)	Surgical (%)
1976–1982				
Dogs	1225	13.1	44.4	42.5
Cats	216	6.5	47.7	45.8
Horses	542	13.8	44.5	41.7
Cattle	436	3.9	51.8	44.2
1999–2003				
Dogs	6892	5.1	41.8	40.7
Cats	2135	7.0	42.2	40.7
Horses	1521	4.5	42.3	37.2
Cattle	727	2.1	29.3	52.4
2005–November 30, 2010				
Dogs	9586	4.3	35.5	60.3
Cats	2571	6.0	38.3	55.7
Horses	994	4.9	37.3	57.8
Cattle	385	0.8	24.4	74.8

Source: Data courtesy of the AVMA-PLIT.

ANESTHETIC RECORD

PATIENT INFORMATION	Date:		Cage #:		Surgeon:
	Procedure(s):				Anesthetist:

Preanesthetic Values / Animal Status

	HR	RR	MM color	Temp	PCV	TP	Weight (kg / lb)	Hydration

Preanesthetic Drugs / Induction Drugs / Physical Status

Drug	Dose	Route	Time	Drug	Dose	Route	Time	1	2	3	4	5	E

PAIN Evaluation: No Pain I---I Worst Pain

Time		00	15	30	45	00	15	30	45	00	15	30	45

Anesthesia (Vaporizer Setting)

_ Isoflurane
_ Sevoflurane
_ Other

Vaporizer Setting: 5.0 / 4.0 / 3.0 / 2.5 / 2.0 / 1.5 / 1.0 / 0

O$_2$ Flow (L/min)

CODES

A Anesthesia — 200
O Surgery — 180
D Drape — 160
R Recovery — 140

SYMBOLS — 120

X Pulse — 100
o Respirations — 80
∨ Systolic — 60
∧ Diastolic — 40
- Mean — 30
* SpO$_2$ — 20
Δ PCO$_2$ — 10
τ Temp — 0

Fluids type_____ mL
Total fluids_____ Extubation Time _____ Sternal Time _____ Temperature _____ ≥98°F Time _____
Comments:

PAIN Evaluation Post-Op: No Pain I---I Worst Pain

Figure 1.1. Example of an anesthetic record.
Source: Muir W.W. 2007. Considerations for general anesthesia. In: *Lumb and Jones' Veterinary Anesthesia and Analgesia*, 4th ed. W.J. Tranquilli, J.C. Thurmon, and K.A. Grimm, eds. Ames, IA: Blackwell Publishing, p. 26.

anesthetic-related claims, the reader is referred to the American Veterinary Medical Association Liability Insurance Trust.

As long as anesthetics are administered, the hazard of death can never be eliminated completely; however, it can be minimized, particularly if one is willing to investigate and to learn from mistakes. Once an anesthetic fatality has occurred, the sequence of the perioperative events preceding the death should be reviewed, their significance should be evaluated, and a necropsy should be recommended to piece together its pathogenesis and etiology. Armed with this information, the practitioner can then take steps to prevent a recurrence.

Record keeping

The American College of Veterinary Anesthesiologists (ACVA) has recently updated its recommendations for anesthetic monitoring, with the intention of improving the care of veterinary patients. The ACVA recognizes that some of the methods may be impractical in certain clinical settings and that anesthetized patients can be monitored and managed without specialized equipment. The aspects of anesthetic management addressed by the ACVA guidelines that deserve careful attention include patient circulation, oxygenation, ventilation, record keeping, and personnel.

To obtain meaningful data concerning anesthesia, certain information must be collected. An individual record must be made for each animal anesthetized. Among the items that should be recorded in the anesthetic or patient record are:

(1) Patient identification, species, breed, age, gender, weight, and physical status of the animal.
(2) Surgical procedure or other reason for anesthesia.
(3) Preanesthetic agents given (dose, route, and time).
(4) Anesthetic agents used (dose, route, and time).
(5) Person administering anesthesia (veterinarian, technician, student, or lay personnel).
(6) Duration of anesthesia.
(7) Supportive measures.
(8) Difficulties encountered and methods of correction.

It is necessary that each step of anesthetic administration be recorded in an anesthetic record (Figure 1.1). Minimally, the pulse and respiratory rate should be monitored at 5-minute intervals and recorded at 10-minute intervals. Trends in these parameters thus become apparent before a patient's condition severely deteriorates, so that remedial steps may be taken.

Revised from "Considerations for General Anesthesia" by William W. Muir; "Monitoring Anesthetized Patients" by Steve C. Haskins; and "Drug Interactions" by Mark G. Papich in Lumb & Jones' Veterinary Anesthesia and Analgesia, Fourth Edition.

Chapter 2

Anesthetic physiology and pharmacology

William W. Muir, Wayne N. McDonell,
Carolyn L. Kerr, Kurt A. Grimm, Kip A. Lemke,
Keith R. Branson, Hui-Chu Lin, Eugene P. Steffey,
Khursheed R. Mama, Elizabeth A. Martinez, and
Robert D. Keegan

Cardiovascular anatomy and physiology

The uptake, distribution, and elimination of anesthetic drugs depend on blood flow. The cardiovascular system, which is composed of the heart, blood vessels, lymph vessels, and blood, is designed to supply a continuous flow of blood to all tissues of the body.

Heart

The heart is composed of four chambers: two thin-walled atria separated by an interatrial septum, and two thick-walled ventricles separated by an interventricular septum. The atria receive blood returning from the systemic circulation (right atrium [RA]) and pulmonary circulation (left atrium [LA]), and to a limited degree act as storage chambers. The ventricles, the major pumping chambers of the heart, are separated from the atria by the tricuspid valve on the right side and the mitral valve on the left side. The ventricles receive blood from their respective atria and eject it across semilunar valves (the pulmonic valve between the right ventricle [RV] and pulmonary artery and the aortic valve between the left ventricle [LV] and aorta) into the pulmonary circulation and systemic circulation, respectively.

Once the process of cardiac contraction is initiated, almost simultaneous contraction of the atria is followed by nearly synchronous contraction of the ventricles, which results in pressure differences between the atria, ventricles, and pulmonary and systemic circulations. Cardiac contraction produces differential pressure changes that are responsible for atrioventricular (AV) and semilunar valve opening and closing and the production of heart sounds. Chordae tendineae originating from papillary muscles located on the inner

Essentials of Small Animal Anesthesia and Analgesia, Second Edition. Edited by Kurt A. Grimm, William J. Tranquilli, Leigh A. Lamont.
© 2011 John Wiley & Sons, Inc. Published 2011 by John Wiley & Sons, Inc.

wall of the ventricular chambers are attached to the free edges of the AV valve leaflets and help to maintain valve competence and prevent regurgitation of blood into the atrium during ventricular contraction. Alteration in heart chamber geometry (e.g., stretch or hypertrophy) produced by changes in blood volume, deformation (pericardial tamponade), or disease can have profound effects on myocardial function, as do the effects produced by neurohumoral, metabolic, and pharmacological perturbations.

Blood vessels

The large and small vessels of the pulmonary and systemic circulations facilitate the delivery of blood to the exchange sites in the pulmonary and systemic capillary beds and return blood to the heart. The aorta and other large arteries compose the high-pressure portion of the systemic circulation and are relatively stiff compared to veins, possessing a high proportion of elastic tissue in comparison to smooth muscle and fibrous tissues. The flow of blood to peripheral tissues throughout the cardiac cycle (contraction–relaxation–rest) has been termed the Windkessel effect. The Windkessel effect is believed to be responsible for as much as 50% of peripheral blood flow in most species during normal heart rates (HRs). Tachyarrhythmias and vascular diseases (stiff nonelastic vessels) hamper the Windkessel effect and produce distinctive changes in the arterial pressure waveform. More distal larger arteries contain greater percentages of smooth muscle compared to elastic tissue and act as conduits for the transfer of blood under high pressure to tissues. The most distal small arteries, terminal arterioles, and arteriovenous anastomoses contain a predominance of smooth muscle, are highly innervated, and function as resistors that regulate the distribution of blood flow, aid in the regulation of systemic blood pressure (BP), and modulate tissue perfusion pressure. The capillaries are the functional exchange sites for oxygen, nutrients, electrolytes, cellular waste products, and other substances. Capillaries are of three different types: continuous (lung and muscle), fenestrated (kidney and intestine), and discontinuous (liver, spleen, and bone marrow).

Postcapillary venules are composed of an endothelial lining and fibrous tissue and function to collect blood from capillaries. Some venules act as postcapillary sphincters, and all venules merge into small veins. Small and larger veins contain increasing amounts of fibrous tissue in addition to smooth muscle and elastic tissue, although their walls are much thinner than comparably sized arteries. Many veins contain valves that act in conjunction with external compression (contracting muscles and pressure differences in the abdominal and thoracic cavities) to facilitate venous return of blood to the RA. The venous system also acts as a major blood reservoir. Indeed, 60–70% of the blood volume may be stored in the systemic venous vasculature during resting conditions (Figure 2.1).

Two additional structural components that are important during normal circulatory function are arteriovenous anastomoses and the lymphatic system. Arteriovenous anastomoses bypass capillary beds. They possess smooth muscle cells throughout their entire length and are located in most, if not all, tissue beds. Most arteriovenous anastomoses are believed to be important in regulating blood flow to highly vascular tissue (skin, feet, and hooves). Their role in maintaining normal homeostasis, however, is speculative other than for thermoregulation.

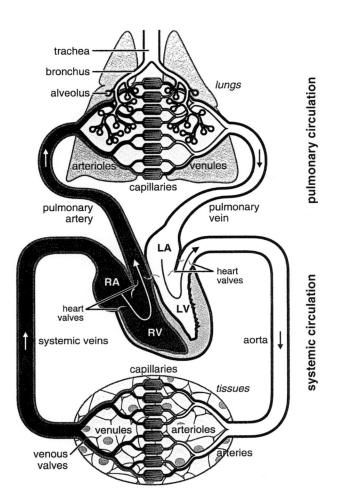

Figure 2.1. The cardiovascular system is comprised of the heart, blood, and two parallel circulations (pulmonary and systemic). *Pulmonary circulation*: The pulmonary artery carries blood from the right ventricle (RV) to the lungs, where carbon dioxide is eliminated and oxygen is taken up. Oxygenated blood returns to the left atrium (LA) via the pulmonary veins. *Systemic circulation*: Blood is pumped by the left ventricle (LV) into the aorta, which distributes blood to the peripheral tissues. Oxygen and nutrients are exchanged for carbon dioxide and other by-products of tissue metabolism in capillary beds, after which the blood is returned to the right atrium (RA) through the venules and large systemic veins.
Sources: Modified from Shepherd J.T., Vanhoutte P.M. 1979. *The Human Cardiovascular System; Facts and Concepts*, 1st ed. New York: Raven; and Muir W.W. 2007. Cardiovascular system. In: *Lumb and Jones' Veterinary Anesthesia and Analgesia*, 4th ed. W.J. Tranquilli, J.C. Thurmon, and K.A. Grimm, eds. Ames, IA: Blackwell Publishing, Ames, IA, p. 62.

The peripheral lymphatic system is not anatomically part of the blood circulatory system. Nevertheless, it is integrally involved in maintaining normal circulatory dynamics, especially interstitial fluid volume (approximately 10% of the capillary filtrate). Lymphatic capillaries collect interstitial fluid—lymph—which is eventually returned to the cranial vena cava and RA after passing through a series of lymph vessels, lymph nodes, and the thoracic duct. Lymph vessels have smooth muscle within their walls and contain valves similar to those in veins. Contraction of skeletal muscle (lymphatic pump) and lymph vessel smooth muscle, in conjunction with lymphatic valves, are responsible for lymph flow.

Blood

Blood is a suspension of red (erythrocytes) and white (leukocytes) blood cells and platelets (thrombocytes) in plasma. The most essential function of blood is to deliver oxygen to tissues. Oxygen is relatively insoluble in plasma (0.003 mL oxygen per 100 mL blood per 1 mm Hg partial pressure of oxygen [PO_2]; approximately 0.3 mL oxygen per 100 mL blood at $PO_2 = 100$ mm Hg). The erythrocytes transport much larger amounts of oxygen than can be carried in solution, and functionally the amount that can be carried depends on the amount of hemoglobin (Hb) in the erythrocytes. The affinity of Hb for oxygen depends on the partial pressure of carbon dioxide (PCO_2), pH, body temperature, the intraerythrocyte concentration of 2,3-diphosphoglycerate, and the chemical structure of Hb (Figure 2.2). Once the amount of deoxygenated Hb (unsaturated

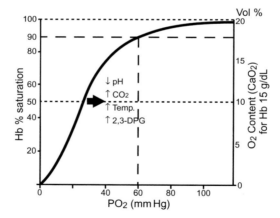

Figure 2.2.   The oxyhemoglobin dissociation curve illustrates the relationship between the blood partial pressure of oxygen (PO_2) and the saturation of hemoglobin (Hb) with oxygen (O_2). Note that this curve is shifted to the right (Hb has less affinity for O_2) by acidosis, increased body temperature, and the enzyme 2,3-diphosphoglycerate (2,3-DPG). This effect helps to unload O_2 from Hb in tissues and increases the Hb affinity for O_2 in the lungs. The total arterial oxygen content (CaO_2) is determined by the total blood Hb concentration, its percent saturation (%SaO_2), and the PaO_2.
Source: Muir W.W. 2007. Cardiovascular system. In: *Lumb and Jones' Veterinary Anesthesia and Analgesia*, 4th ed. W.J. Tranquilli, J.C. Thurmon, and K.A. Grimm, eds. Ames, IA: Blackwell Publishing, p. 64.

Hb) exceeds 5 g/100 mL of blood, the blood changes from a bright red to a purple-blue color (cyanosis). Some of the carbon dioxide produced by metabolizing tissues binds to deoxygenated Hb and is eliminated by the lungs during the Hb oxygenation process prior to the blood returning to the systemic circulation and the cycle repeating itself.

Maintaining adequate tissue oxygenation depends on oxygen uptake by the lungs, oxygen delivery (DO_2) to and oxygen extraction (OE) by tissues, and oxygen use by the metabolic machinery within cells. The factors that determine the supply of oxygen to tissues are Hb concentration, the affinity of Hb for oxygen (P_{50}), the saturation of Hb with oxygen (SaO_2), the arterial oxygen partial pressure (PaO_2), the cardiac output (CO), and the tissue oxygen consumption (VO_2). The Fick equation ($VO_2 = CO\,[CaO_2 - CvO_2]$) contains all the essential components of this relationship. Arterial blood oxygen content (CaO_2) is calculated by $CaO_2 = Hb \times 1.35 \times SaO_2 + (PaO_2 \times 0.003)$. Arterial blood (Hb = approximately 15 g/dL at packed cell volume [PCV] = 45%), for example, contains approximately 20–21 mL of oxygen/dL of blood when the $SaO_2 = 100\%$ and the $PaO_2 = 100$ mm Hg (room air). The venous blood oxygen content (CvO_2) is generally 14–15 mL/dL, yielding an OE ratio of 0.2–0.3 (20–30%). An increase in arterial blood lactate concentration is the cardinal sign of inadequate oxygen delivery to metabolizing tissues and suggests that oxygen consumption has become delivery dependent or that some defect in tissue OE or use has developed.

Pressure, resistance, and flow

In electric circuits, current flow (I) is determined by the electromotive force or voltage (E) and the resistance to current flow (R); according to Ohm's law:

$$I = E/R$$

The flow of fluids (Q) through nondistensible tubes depends on pressure (P) and the resistance to flow (R). Therefore, $Q = P/R$.

The resistance to blood flow is determined by blood viscosity (η) and the geometric factors of blood vessels (radius and length). The steady, nonpulsatile, laminar flow of Newtonian fluids (homogenous fluids in which viscosity does not change with flow velocity or vascular geometry), like water, saline, and, under physiological conditions, plasma, can be described by the Poiseuille–Hagen law, which states:

$$Q = (P_1 - P_2)r^4\pi/8L\eta; \ R = 8L\eta/r^4\pi,$$

where $P_1 - P_2$ is the pressure difference, r^4 is the radius to the fourth power, L is the length of the tube, η is the viscosity of the fluid, and $\pi/8$ is a constant of proportionality. The maintenance of laminar flow is a fundamental assumption of the resistance offered to steady-state fluid flow in the Poiseuille–Hagen equation.

The relationship between vessel (or chamber when describing the heart)-distending pressure, vessel diameter, vessel wall thickness, and vessel wall tension is described by Laplace's law:

$$P = 2Th/r \text{ or } T = Pr/2h,$$

where T is wall tension, P is developed pressure, r is the internal radius, and h is the wall thickness. This relationship is important because it relates pressure and vessel dimension to changes in developed tension, which is known to be an important determinant of ventricular–vascular coupling (afterload), myocardial work, and myocardial oxygen consumption.

Blood pressure

BP in arteries, whether measured directly or indirectly, is frequently assessed during anesthesia. Arterial BP measurement is one of the fastest and most informative means of assessing cardiovascular function and provides an accurate indication of drug effects, surgical events, and hemodynamic trends.

The factors that determine arterial BP are HR, stroke volume (SV), vascular resistance, arterial compliance, and blood volume. Mean arterial BP is a key component in determining tissue perfusion pressure and the adequacy of tissue blood flow. Perfusion pressures greater than 60 mm Hg are generally thought to be adequate for perfusion of tissues. Structures like the heart (coronary circulation), lungs (pulmonary circulation), kidneys (renal circulation), and the fetus (fetal circulation) contain special circulations where changes in perfusion pressure can have immediate effects on organ function. Clinically, arterial BP is generally measured as mean arterial pressure. When mean arterial BP cannot be directly assessed, it is estimated by this formula:

$$P_m = P_d + 1/3\,(P_s - P_d),$$

where P_m, P_s, and P_d are mean (m), systolic (s), and diastolic (d) BPs, respectively (Figure 2.3). Both P_s and P_d can be measured (estimated) indirectly using either Doppler or oscillometric techniques. Most drugs used to produce anesthesia decrease CO and peripheral vascular resistance. However, vasoconstricting drugs (e.g., alpha$_2$ adrenergic agonists) can increase peripheral vascular resistance and maintain BP in physiological ranges while dramatically decreasing CO and blood flow to certain tissues (e.g., skin and skeletal muscle) (Figure 2.4).

The arterial pulse pressure $(P_s - P_d)$ and pulse-pressure waveform analysis can provide valuable information regarding changes in vascular compliance and vessel tone. Generally, drugs (phenothiazines) or diseases (endotoxic shock) that produce marked arterial dilation increase vascular compliance, causing a rapid rise, short duration, and rapid fall in the arterial waveform while increasing the arterial pulse pressure. Situations that produce vasoconstriction decrease vascular compliance, producing a longer duration pulse waveform and a slower fall in the systolic BP to diastolic values. The pulse pressure may contain secondary and sometimes tertiary pressure waveforms, particularly if the measuring site is in a peripheral artery some distance from the heart.

Nervous, humoral, and local control

Regulation of the cardiovascular system is integrated through the combined effects of the central and peripheral nervous systems, the influence of circulating (humoral) vasoactive substances, and local tissue mediators that modulate vascular tone. These regulatory

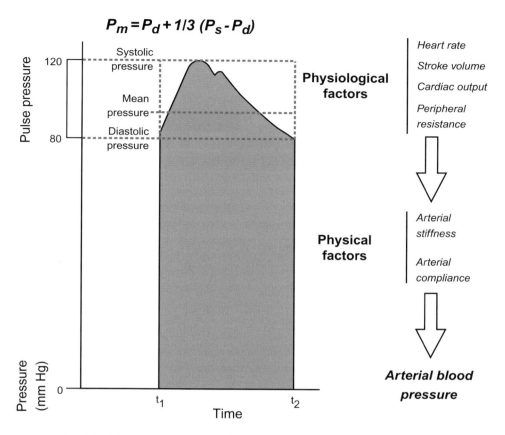

$$P_m = P_d + 1/3 \ (P_s - P_d)$$

Figure 2.3. Arterial BP is determined by both physiological and physical factors. The mean arterial pressure (P_m) represents the area under the arterial pressure curve divided by the duration of the cardiac cycle and can be estimated by adding one-third the difference between the systolic arterial pressure (P_s) and diastolic arterial pressure (P_d) to P_d. P_s minus P_d is the pulse pressure.
Sources: Modified from Berne R.M., Levey M.N. 1990. *Principles of Physiology*, 1st ed. St. Louis, MO: Mosby; and Muir W.W. 2007. Cardiovascular system. In: *Lumb and Jones' Veterinary Anesthesia and Analgesia*, 4th ed. W.J. Tranquilli, J.C. Thurmon, and K.A. Grimm, eds. Ames, IA: Blackwell Publishing, p. 92.

processes maintain blood flow at an appropriate level while distributing blood flow to meet the needs of tissue beds that have the greatest demand.

Cardiac electrophysiology

Normal cardiac electrical activity is essential for normal cardiac contractile function (excitation–contraction coupling). The cardiac cell membrane (sarcolemma) is a highly specialized lipid bilayer that contains protein-associated channels, pumps, enzymes, and exchangers in an architecturally sophisticated, yet fluid (reorganizable and movable), medium. Most drugs and many anesthetic drugs produce important direct and indirect

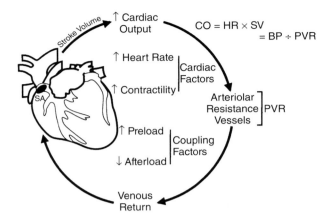

Figure 2.4.   CO is equal to heart rate (HR) times stroke volume (SV), or arterial blood pressure (BP) divided by peripheral vascular resistance (PVR). Increases in HR, cardiac contractility, and preload, and decreases in afterload can all increase CO. Preload and afterload are considered to be coupling factors because they depend on vascular resistance, capacitance, and compliance.
Source: Muir W.W. 2007. Cardiovascular system. In: *Lumb and Jones' Veterinary Anesthesia and Analgesia*, 4th ed. W.J. Tranquilli, J.C. Thurmon, and K.A. Grimm, eds. Ames, IA: Blackwell Publishing, p. 81.

effects on the cell membrane and intracellular organelles, ultimately altering cardiac excitation–contraction coupling (Figure 2.5).

   The cardiac pacemaker (sinoatrial or SA node) normally suppresses the automaticity of slower or subsidiary pacemakers (overdrive suppression), preventing more than one pacemaker from controlling HR. Initiation of an electric impulse in the SA node is followed by rapid electrochemical transmission of the impulse through the atria, giving rise to the P wave. Repolarization of the atria gives rise to the Ta wave, which is most obvious in large animals (horses and cattle), where the total atrial tissue mass is substantial enough to generate enough electromotive force to be electrocardiographically recognizable. Repolarization of the atria in smaller species (dogs and cats) and depolarization of the SA and AV nodes do not generate a large enough electric potential to be recorded at the body surface except in some cases of sinus tachycardia. Once the wave of depolarization reaches the AV node, conduction is slowed because of the AV node's low resting membrane potential. Increased parasympathetic tone can produce marked slowing of AV nodal conduction, leading to first-degree, second-degree, and, rarely, third-degree heart block. Many drugs used in anesthesia, including opioids, alpha$_2$ adrenergic agonists, and occasionally acepromazine, increase the parasympathetic tone, predisposing patients to heart block and bradyarrhythmias. The use of antimuscarinic drugs such as atropine and glycopyrrolate is generally effective therapy in these situations unless the block is caused by structural disease (e.g., inflammation, fibrosis, or calcification).

   Under normal conditions, conduction of the electric impulse through the AV node produces the PR or PQ interval of the electrocardiogram (ECG) and provides time for the atria to contract prior to activation and contraction of the ventricles. This delay is functionally important, particularly at faster HRs, because it enables atrial contraction to

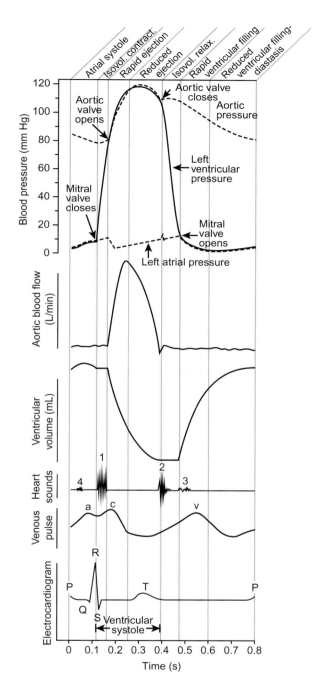

Figure 2.5. The cardiac cycle diagrammatically illustrates the relationship between mechanical, acoustical, and electrical events as a function of time. Isovol. contract., isovolumetric contraction; Isovol. relax, isovolumetric relaxation.
Sources: Modified from Berne R.M., Levey M.N. 1990. *Principles of Physiology*, 1st ed. St. Louis, MO: Mosby; and Muir W.W. 2007. Cardiovascular system. In: *Lumb and Jones' Veterinary Anesthesia and Analgesia*, 4th ed. W.J. Tranquilli, J.C. Thurmon, and K.A. Grimm, eds. Ames, IA: Blackwell Publishing, p. 78.

contribute to ventricular filling. Once the electric impulse has traversed the AV node it is rapidly transmitted to the ventricular muscle by specialized muscle cells commonly referred to as Purkinje fibers. Bundles of Purkinje cells—the right and left bundle branches—transmit the electric impulses to the ventricular septum and the right and left ventricular free walls, respectively. Their distribution accounts for differences in the pattern of the ECG (ventricular depolarization) among species. Purkinje fibers have much longer action potentials and refractory periods than do ventricular muscle cells, which normally prevents reentry of the electric impulse and reactivation of the ventricles.

The configuration and magnitude of the T wave vary considerably among species and are influenced by changes in HR, temperature, and the extracellular potassium concentration. Hyperkalemia, for example, produces an increase in membrane conductance to potassium. This shortens repolarization and produces T waves that are of large magnitude, generally spiked or pointed, and of short duration (short QT interval).

The interval beginning immediately after the S wave of the QRS complex (J point) and preceding the T wave is referred to as the ST segment and is important clinically. Elevation or depression of the ST segment (± 0.2 mV or greater) from the isoelectric line is usually an indication of myocardial hypoxia or ischemia, low CO, anemia, pericarditis, or cardiac contusion, and suggests the potential for arrhythmia development.

Determinants of performance and output

Clinically, M-mode and color-flow Doppler echocardiography are used to assess ventricular function. These techniques provide a dynamic temporal representation of cardiac function and, when coupled with hemodynamic computer software analysis systems, a pictorial and quantitative assessment of cardiac performance.

The oxygen requirements of tissues are met by the continuous adjustment of CO, which is the product of HR and SV:

$$CO = HR \times SV$$

SV is the amount of blood ejected from the ventricle during contraction and therefore represents the difference between the end-diastolic and end-systolic ventricular volumes.

Preload

Preload is usually explained in terms of the Frank–Starling relationship or as heterometric autoregulation: increases in myocardial fiber length (ventricular volume) increase the force of cardiac contraction and CO. Whether or not individual sarcomeres actually increase in length (stretch) with increases in ventricular volume is controversial. Because of the difficulty in accurately determining ventricular volume in the clinical setting, ventricular diameter, ventricular end-diastolic pressure, pulmonary capillary wedge pressure, and, occasionally, mean atrial pressure are used as estimates of preload. The substitution of pressure for volume, although common, must be done with the understanding that there are many instances (open-chest procedures and stiff or noncompliant hearts) when pressure does not accurately represent changes in ventricular volume and therefore is not an accurate index of preload.

Afterload

The term afterload is used throughout the basic and clinical cardiology literature to describe the force opposing ventricular ejection. One major reason for the great interest in this physiological determinant of cardiac function is its inverse relationship with SV and its direct correlation with myocardial oxygen consumption. Afterload changes continuously throughout ventricular ejection and is more accurately described by the tension (stress) developed in the left ventricular wall during ejection or as the arterial input impedance (Z_i). Ventricular wall stress or tension has traditionally been estimated from the Laplace relationship:

$$\text{tension (T)} = Pr / 2h$$

It is noteworthy that using this assessment of ventricular afterload assumes a spherical ventricular geometry.

The measurement of systemic vascular resistance (SVR) is used clinically as a measure of afterload and vascular tone because it is technically simple to obtain and intuitively easier to understand.

Inotropy

Cardiac contractility (inotropy) is the intrinsic ability of the heart to generate force. A decrease in cardiac contractility is a key factor in heart failure in patients with cardiac disease or following the administration of potent negative inotropic drugs (e.g., inhalant anesthetics). Ideal indexes of cardiac contractility should be independent of changes in HR, preload, afterload, and cardiac size—in other words, be load independent.

Lusitropy

A description of the relaxation phases following cardiac contraction is often omitted from textbooks of cardiovascular physiology, but is fundamentally important to an understanding of cardiac performance. Mechanical factors, loading factors, inotropic activity, HR, and asynchronicity (patterns of relaxation) are the major determinants of lusitropy.

Respiratory system physiology

Maintenance of adequate respiratory function is a requirement for successful anesthesia. Inadequate tissue oxygenation at a severe level may lead to acute death. Excessive elevations in arterial carbon dioxide (CO_2) tensions (arterial CO_2 partial pressure [$PaCO_2$]) or sustained moderate hypoxemia may produce some level of organ dysfunction, which contributes to a less than optimal anesthetic recovery.

During general anesthesia, there is always a tendency for arterial oxygen tensions (PaO_2) to be less than observed with the same species while conscious and breathing the same fraction of inspired oxygen concentration (FiO_2). There is also a tendency for $PaCO_2$ to be elevated above the conscious resting values if the anesthetized animal is breathing spontaneously, and for increases in airway resistance to occur unless an endotracheal tube is used. Some differences are seen, depending on the actual anesthetic regimen used, but the depth of anesthesia is often more of a factor.

Definitions

Respiration is the overall process whereby oxygen is supplied to and used by body cells and carbon dioxide is eliminated by means of partial pressure gradients. Ventilation is the movement of gas into and out of alveoli. The ventilatory requirement for homeostasis varies with the metabolic requirement of animals, and it thus varies with body size, level of activity, body temperature, and depth of anesthesia. Inadequate ventilation to meet the gas exchange requirements of metabolism is termed respiratory depression or hypoventilation. It is manifested clinically as an increase in $PaCO_2$ and a respiratory acidosis. When breathing high FiO_2, Hb saturation does not decrease unless hypoventilation is severe. Pulmonary ventilation is accomplished by thoracic cavity expansion and elastic contraction of the lungs. Several terms are used to describe the various types of breathing patterns that may be observed:

(1) Eupnea is ordinary quiet breathing.
(2) Dyspnea is labored breathing.
(3) Tachypnea is increased respiratory rate.
(4) Hyperpnea is fast and/or deep respiration, indicating "overrespiration."
(5) Polypnea is a rapid, shallow, panting type of respiration.
(6) Bradypnea is slow regular respiration.
(7) Hypopnea is slow and/or shallow breathing, possibly indicating "underrespiration."
(8) Apnea is transient (or longer) cessation of breathing.
(9) Cheyne–Stokes respirations increase in rate and depth, and then become slower, followed by a brief period of apnea.
(10) Biot's respirations are sequences of gasps, apnea, and several deep gasps.
(11) Kussmaul's respirations are regular deep respirations without pause.
(12) Apneustic respiration occurs when an animal holds an inspired breath at the end of an inhalation for a short period before exhaling. Apneustic breathing is commonly seen with dissociative anesthetic administration (e.g., ketamine or Telazol®).

To describe the events of pulmonary ventilation, air in the lungs has been subdivided into four different volumes and four different capacities (Figure 2.6). Only tidal volume (V_T) and functional residual capacity (FRC) can be measured in conscious uncooperative animals:

(1) V_T is the volume of air inspired or expired in one breath.
(2) Inspiratory reserve volume (IRV) is the volume of air that can be inspired over and above the normal V_T.
(3) Expiratory reserve volume (ERV) is the amount of air that can be expired by forceful expiration after a normal expiration.
(4) Residual volume (RV) is the air remaining in the lungs after the most forceful expiration.

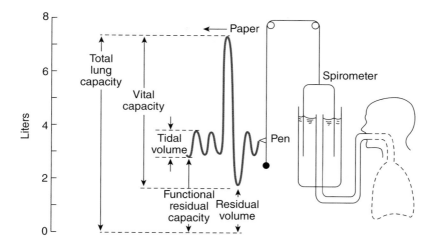

Figure 2.6. Lung volumes and capacities. TLC, FRC, and RV cannot be measured with spirometry. IRV, ERV, and IC are not included in the diagram.
Source: West J.B. 2001. Chronic obstructive pulmonary disease. In: *Pulmonary Physiology and Pathophysiology: An Integrated, Case-Based Approach*. Baltimore, MD: Lippincott Williams & Wilkins. Baltimore, p. 39.

Another term frequently used is the minute respiratory volume or minute ventilation (V_E). This is equal to V_T times the respiratory frequency (f). Occasionally, it is desirable to consider two or more of the aforementioned volumes together. Such combinations are termed pulmonary capacities:

(1) Inspiratory capacity (IC) is the V_T plus the IRV. This is the amount of air that can be inhaled starting after a normal expiration and distending the lungs to the maximum amount.
(2) FRC is the ERV plus the RV. This is the amount of air remaining in the lungs after a normal expiration. From a mechanical viewpoint, at FRC the inward "pull" of the lungs due to their elasticity equals the outward "pull" of the chest wall.
(3) Vital capacity (VC) is the IRV plus the V_T plus the ERV. This is the maximum amount of air that can be expelled from the lungs after first filling them to their maximum capacity.
(4) Total lung capacity (TLC) is the IRV plus the V_T plus the ERV plus the RV, or the maximum volume to which the lungs can be expanded with the greatest possible inspiratory effort (or by full inflation to 30-cm H_2O airway pressure when a patient is anesthetized).

Control of respiration

With the aid of the circulation, respiration maintains the oxygen, CO_2, and pH of the cell. Respiratory function is controlled by central respiratory centers, central and peripheral chemoreceptors, pulmonary reflexes, and nonrespiratory neural input. The central neural "controller" includes specialized groups of neurons located in the cerebrum, brain stem, and spinal cord that govern both voluntary and automatic ventilation through regulation of the activity of the respiratory muscles. The respiratory muscles, by contracting, expand the chest cavity and produce alveolar ventilation (V_A). Changes in V_A affect blood gas tensions and hydrogen ion concentration. Blood gas tensions and hydrogen ion concentrations are monitored by peripheral and central chemoreceptors that return signals to the central controller to provide necessary adjustments in V_A. Mechanoreceptors in the lungs and stretch receptors in the respiratory muscles monitor, respectively, the degree of expansion or stretch of the lungs and the "effort" of breathing, feeding back information to the central controller to alter the pattern of breathing. Adjustments also occur to accommodate nonrespiratory activities such as thermoregulation and vocalization.

Overall, this complex control system produces a combination of f and depth that is best suited for optimum ventilation with minimal effort for the particular species, and that adjusts oxygen supply and CO_2 elimination so as to maintain homeostasis (reflected by stable arterial blood gas levels) over a wide range of environmental and metabolic situations. Sedatives, analgesics, anesthetics, and the equipment used for inhalational anesthesia may profoundly alter respiration and the ability of an animal to maintain cellular homeostasis.

The important factor in pulmonary ventilation is the rate at which alveolar gas is exchanged with atmospheric air. This is not equal to the alveolar minute ventilation volume because a large portion of inspired air is used to fill the respiratory passages (anatomic dead space, V_{Danat}), rather than alveoli, and no significant gaseous exchange occurs in this air. The f and V_T determine the V_E. The "effective" volume, or portion of V_T that contributes to gas exchange, is the alveolar volume, usually referred to as minute V_A. Nonperfused alveoli do not contribute to gas exchange and constitute alveolar dead space (V_{DA}). Physiological dead space (V_D) includes V_{Danat} and V_{DA}, and is usually expressed as a minute value (V_D) along with V_A, or as a ratio of V_D/V_T (Figure 2.7).

Hypoxia refers to any state in which the PO_2 in the lungs, blood, and/or tissues is abnormally low, resulting in abnormal tissue metabolism and/or cellular damage. Hypoxemia refers to insufficient oxygenation of blood to meet the metabolic requirement. In spontaneously breathing animals, hypoxemia is characterized by PaO_2 levels lower than the normal for the species. Resting PaO_2 levels in domestic species generally range from 80 to 100 mm Hg in healthy, awake animals at sea level. Some clinicians consider a PaO_2 below 70 mm Hg (ca. 94% Hb saturation) as hypoxemia in animals at or near sea level, although the clinical significance of this degree of blood oxygen tension would vary depending on factors such as the health and age of an animal, Hb concentration, and the duration of low oxygen tension in relation to the rate of tissue metabolism (e.g., hypothermic patients would be at less risk).

Oxygen transport

Under normal conditions, oxygen is taken into the pulmonary alveoli and CO_2 is removed from them at a rate that is sufficient to maintain the composition of alveolar air at a

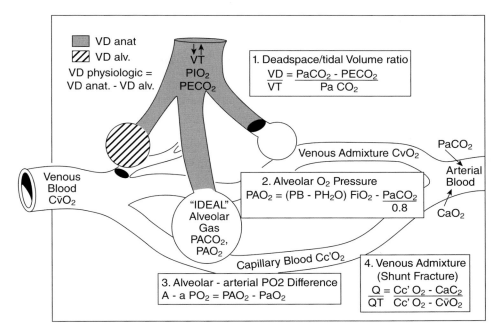

Figure 2.7. Schematic of uneven ventilation and blood flow. The alveolus on the left is ventilated, but not perfused, and thus is considered to be alveolar dead space, whereas the alveolus on the right is perfused, but not ventilated, and thus contributes to venous admixture or shunt flow. The center alveolus is perfused and ventilated equally and thus would have a V/Q ratio of 1.0. Relevant equations are shown, respectively, as Equations 1–4 for calculation of the dead space/V_T ratio, the alveolar partial pressure of oxygen (P_AO_2), the alveolar-to-arterial partial pressure of oxygen $P(A-a)O_2$ difference, and the venous admixture (Q/QT) fraction.
Source: Reproduced from Robinson NE. 1991. The respiratory system. In: *Equine Anesthesia: Monitoring and Emergency Therapy*. W.W. Muir and J.E. Hubbell, eds. St. Louis, MO: Mosby Year Book, pp. 7–38. With permission by Elsevier.

relatively constant concentration. In the lungs, gas is exchanged across both the alveolar and the capillary membranes. The total distance across which the exchange takes place is less than 1 μm; therefore, it occurs rapidly. Other than at high exercise levels, equilibrium almost develops between blood in the lungs and air in the alveolus, and the PO_2 in the pulmonary venous blood almost equals the PO_2 in the alveolus. While diffusion of oxygen across the alveolar-capillary space is a theoretical barrier to oxygenation, it is seldom a practical problem during veterinary anesthesia unless significant pulmonary edema or disease is present.

The normal average alveolar composition of respiratory gases in humans is listed below. At normal human body temperature, alveolar air is saturated with water vapor, which has a pressure of 48 mm Hg at 37°C. If the barometric pressure in the alveolus is 760 mm Hg (sea level), then the pressure due to dry air is 760 − 48 = 712 mm Hg. Knowing the composition of alveolar air, one can calculate the partial pressure of each gas in the alveolus:

$$O_2 = (760-48)\times0.14 = 100 \text{ mm Hg,}$$

$$CO_2 = (760-48)\times0.056 = 40 \text{ mm Hg,}$$

$$N_2 = (760-48)\times0.80 = 570 \text{ mm Hg}$$

The PO_2 in the lungs at sea level is thus approximately 100 mm Hg at 37–38°C. Under these conditions, 100 mL of plasma will hold 0.3 mL of oxygen in physical solution. Whole blood, under the same conditions, will hold 20 mL of oxygen, or about 60 times as much as plasma. CO_2 is similarly held by blood. Thus, it is apparent that oxygen and CO_2 in blood are transported largely in chemical combination, since both are carried by blood in much greater quantities than would occur if simple absorption took place. At complete saturation, each gram of Hb combines with 1.36–1.39 mL of oxygen. This is the total carrying capacity of Hb, or four oxygen molecules combined with each Hb molecule. The ability of Hb to combine with oxygen depends on the PO_2 in the surrounding environment. The degree to which it will become saturated at various PO_2 values varies considerably. It is adjusted so that, even when ventilation is inefficient or the supply of oxygen is sparse at higher altitudes, the degree of saturation still approaches 100%. For instance, although it is probably not fully saturated until it is exposed to a PO_2 of 250 mm Hg, Hb is approximately 94% saturated when the PO_2 is only 70 mm Hg.

Carbon dioxide transport

Arterial CO_2 levels are a function of both CO_2 elimination and production, and under normal circumstances $PaCO_2$ levels are maintained within narrow limits. During severe exercise, the production of CO_2 is increased enormously, whereas during anesthesia, production likely decreases. Elimination of CO_2 depends on pulmonary blood flow (CO) and V_A. Normally, the production of CO_2 parallels the oxygen consumption according to the respiratory quotient: $R = VCO_2/VO_2$. Although the value varies depending on the diet, usually R is 0.8 at steady state.

A CO_2 pressure gradient, opposite to that of oxygen and much smaller, exists from the tissues to the atmospheric air: tissues = 50 mm Hg (during exercise, this may be higher); venous blood = 46 mm Hg; alveolar air = 40 mm Hg; expired air = 32 mm Hg; atmospheric air = 0.3 mm Hg; and arterial blood = 40 mm Hg (equilibrium with alveolar air). Carbon dioxide is carried from the mitochondria to the alveoli in a number of forms. In the plasma, some CO_2 is transported in solution (5%), and some combines with water and forms carbonic acid, which in turn dissociates into bicarbonate and hydrogen ions (5%). Most (ca. 90%) of the CO_2 diffuses into the red cells, where it is either bound to Hb or transformed (reversibly) to bicarbonate and hydrogen ions through the action of the enzyme carbonic anhydrase. The formation of bicarbonate in the red blood cell is accompanied by the chloride shift (this accounts for approximately 63% of the total CO_2 transport). Just as the amount of oxygen transported by the blood depends on the PO_2 to which the blood is exposed, so is CO_2 transport likewise affected; however, the CO_2 dissociation curve is more or less linear. Thus, in contrast to the minimal effects on oxygen content, hyperventilation and hypoventilation may have marked effects on the CO_2 content of blood and tissues.

Normal control mechanisms

As important as the detailed information referred to earlier is in helping us understand the respiratory adaptations to high altitude, disease, and exercise for the successful management of clinical anesthesia, a much simplified understanding of the control of respiration will suffice. In conscious animals, V_E and V_A are primarily determined by central chemoreceptor responsiveness to $PaCO_2$ levels. The central chemoreceptors, located on the ventral surface of the medulla and bathed by cerebrospinal fluid (CSF), are exquisitely sensitive to changes in $PaCO_2$ levels because CO_2 is readily diffusible into CSF and the central chemoreceptor cell. The changes in $PaCO_2$ are probably ultimately detected as a change in the pH within the chemoreceptor cell. A fall in arterial pH will also stimulate respiration through the central and peripheral chemoreceptors, as seen with metabolic acidosis. The peripheral chemoreceptors, which are located in the carotid and aortic bodies, generally play a significant part in respiratory drive only when PaO_2 levels fall below 60 mm Hg.

The apneustic and pneumotaxic centers, and pulmonary and airway receptors, are primarily responsible for adjusting the balance between f and V_T to achieve a given level of V_A, usually in a way that minimizes the energy cost of breathing. Although the function of these receptors is generally not considered to be greatly influenced by the action of anesthetic and perianesthetic agents, they may play a part in some of the species differences we see in response to a particular drug or group of drugs.

Apneic threshold

The apneic threshold is the $PaCO_2$ level where spontaneous ventilatory effort ceases. A $PaCO_2$ reduction of 5–9 mm Hg from normal values through voluntary hyperventilation (a conscious human), or by artificial ventilation of sedated or anesthetized animals, produces apnea. The distance between the resting $PaCO_2$ level and the apnea threshold is relatively constant (i.e., 5–9 mm Hg), irrespective of the anesthetic depth. Veterinary anesthetists use the apneic threshold to control respiration (i.e., abolish spontaneous efforts) when putting an animal on a ventilator, or to temporarily provide for a quiet surgical field without having to resort to the use of muscle relaxant drugs.

Drug effect on control of ventilation

Anesthetics and some perianesthetic drugs alter the central and peripheral chemoreceptor response to CO_2 and oxygen in a dose-dependent manner. This has important clinical implications in terms of maintaining homeostasis during the perioperative period. There will also be a diminution in external signs in hypoxemic or hypercarbic anesthetized animals. Whereas unsedated animals usually demonstrate obvious tachypnea and an increase in V_T or respiratory effort in response to serious hypoxemia or hypercapnia, these external signs of an impending crisis may well be absent or greatly diminished in anesthetized animals.

Inhalants and injectable drugs

All of the general anesthetic agents in current use produce a dose-dependent decrease in the response to CO_2. With commonly used inhalant agents, the CO_2 response is almost flat at a minimum alveolar concentration (MAC) of 2.0. The reduced sensory input and central sensitivity to CO_2 produce a marked fall in V_A, usually through a dose-related fall in V_T, with f being reasonably well maintained. A proportional increase in V_D/V_T occurs because V_{Danat} is more or less constant. As a result of these changes, $PaCO_2$ levels increase as the anesthetic dose is increased when animals breathe spontaneously. In light anesthetic planes (e.g., MAC multiple of 1.2), $PaCO_2$ will generally remain moderately elevated, but stable, over many hours of anesthesia, whereas at higher concentrations $PaCO_2$ increases progressively over time. The degree of hypercarbia at equipotent doses of inhalant (and intravenous [IV]) anesthetic agents varies with the species and the degree of surgical stimulation.

Opioids

When given alone, opioids shift the CO_2 response curve to the right with little change in slope, except at very high doses. This means that the resting $PaCO_2$ level might be a little higher in an animal receiving a therapeutic dose of an opioid for premedication or postoperative recovery, but that the response to further CO_2 challenge (from metabolism, airway obstruction, etc.) will not be abolished. Clinically, when opioids are used at high doses as part of a balanced anesthetic regimen, there is an additive effect of the opioid depression of the respiratory center and the general anesthetic, and considerable hypercarbia or even apnea may be produced. At the doses commonly employed for routine opioid premedication or postoperative analgesia in veterinary practice, severe respiratory depression is very rarely seen; but mild/moderate depression is common.

Tranquilizers

The phenothiazine and benzodiazepine sedatives often reduce the respiratory rate, especially if an animal is somewhat excited prior to administration, but they do not appreciably alter arterial blood gas tensions.

Sedatives and hypnotics

The alpha$_2$ adrenoceptor agonists produce a more complicated effect on respiration. When used alone at sedative doses, the alpha$_2$ agonists exhibit little evidence of true respiratory depression in healthy dogs or cats. There may be a decrease in respiratory rate and perhaps a small increase in $PaCO_2$ levels, but PaO_2 levels are well maintained. The peripheral cyanosis that has been reported in up to one-third of dogs sedated with medetomidine is believed to be caused by the low blood flow through mucous membrane capillary beds and venous desaturation, rather than a fall in arterial Hb saturation.

It is important to appreciate, however, that the degree of respiratory depression produced by any alpha$_2$ agonist will be increased when the agonist is given along with other sedatives or anesthetic agents. A number of studies have clearly demonstrated that medetomidine produces elevated $PaCO_2$ levels and PaO_2 levels in the mildly hypoxic range (i.e., 60–70 mm Hg) when combined with opioids, propofol, or ketamine at clinical doses in healthy animals.

Ventilation–perfusion relationships during anesthesia

The onset of general anesthesia or a change in body position often produces lower PaO_2 levels than expected for the delivered concentration of inspired oxygen. This change can occur even without hypoventilation and during both spontaneous and controlled breathing. Lower PaO_2 is produced by altered ventilation/perfusion ratios within the lung. Much of what we know about this phenomenon of altered gas exchange is derived from studies of the human response to anesthesia, some experiments in dogs, and many studies on anesthetized horses. It is obvious when one looks at the collective results that there are important species differences, although the reason(s) for these differences are not always obvious.

Measurement of V/Q mismatch

When the barometric pressure, inspired oxygen concentration, $PaCO_2$, and respiratory quotient are known, the PAO_2 can be calculated by using one form of the alveolar air equation. The difference between this value and the PaO_2 (i.e., the alveolar-to-arterial gradient $[P(A - a)O_2]$) provides a convenient and practical measure of the relative efficiency of gas exchange. The measured $P(A - a)O_2$ value increases as FiO_2 goes up for any given V/Q situation, and it is imperative that the FiO_2 level be taken into account when comparisons are made. In practice, most $P(A - a)O_2$ determinations are made at oxygen concentrations of 21% or near 100%.

The amount of venous admixture or pulmonary shunt flow can be determined if mixed venous (pulmonary artery) and arterial blood oxygen contents are obtained along with a measurement of CO and calculated PaO_2. The terms venous admixture and shunt flow do not mean exactly the same thing, although they are often used interchangeably in the literature, which causes some confusion. Venous admixture refers to the degree of admixture of mixed venous blood with pulmonary end-capillary blood that would be required to produce the observed difference between the arterial and the end-capillary PO_2. The end-capillary PO_2 is assumed to equal the alveolar PO_2. Venous admixture is a calculated amount (i.e., a proportion of CO) and includes the PaO_2 lowering effect of low V/Q areas, blood flow past nonventilated areas, and true anatomical shunt flow (bronchial and thebesian venous blood flow). When the inspired oxygen level is high, blood passing low V/Q areas will be oxygenated, and the $P(A - a)O_2$ gradient and determination of venous admixture is a measure of the total blood flow not contributing to gas exchange, hence the term pulmonary shunt flow. Note that this flow includes both anatomical shunt flow and flow past nonventilated or collapsed alveoli. If one knows the inspired oxygen concentration and the PaO_2, and assumes that the arterial–venous oxygen difference is normal, an isoshunt diagram can be used to provide a convenient and reasonably accurate estimate of the magnitude of pulmonary shunt flow.

Clinical implications of altered respiration during anesthesia

In reasonably healthy dogs and cats, the $P(A - a)O_2$ gradient and the degree of venous admixture are less than in humans. Perhaps this is owing to the smaller lungs in these species or to the difference in the chest wall changes during anesthesia, or perhaps because there is excellent collateral pulmonary ventilation in these species. A high degree of collateral ventilation means that if an alveolus is not ventilated via the airway, it may well receive gas exchange through passages (pores of Kohn) leading to other alveoli that are ventilated. Despite the relatively favorable situation in regard to V/Q mismatch in these species, a minimum inspired oxygen level of 30–35% is still recommended. Obese, deeply anesthetized animals, animals with a distended abdomen (e.g., pregnancy or bowel obstruction), or those with pulmonary disease or space-occupying lesions of the thorax (tumor, pneumothorax, hemothorax, or diaphragmatic hernia) are particularly at risk. Oxygen supplementation is needed nearly as much in deeply sedated animals as in those receiving a general anesthetic (IV or inhalant). This is why simple maneuvers such as placing a face mask with oxygen on a high-risk patient before and during induction or use of a nasal oxygen catheter in the postoperative period are beneficial.

When 100% oxygen mixtures are used with the common inhalant anesthetics in dogs and cats free of serious cardiopulmonary disease, the arterial PaO_2 level is generally 450–525 mm Hg whether the animal is breathing spontaneously or being ventilated and irrespective of body position. With such high inspired oxygen levels, hypoxemia usually occurs only through disconnection of the animal from the anesthetic machine, or with faulty placement of the endotracheal tube, cardiac arrest, or apnea for over 5 minutes. Nevertheless, even with such high PaO_2 levels, tissue hypoxia can occur if Hb levels are low or circulation is inadequate (low CO). The decision to institute assisted or controlled intermittent positive pressure ventilation (IPPV) is generally made to prevent or treat hypercapnia, rather than to achieve oxygenation. Nearly all spontaneously breathing dogs and cats show some degree of hypoventilation and hypercapnia ($PaCO_2$ of 45–55 mm Hg).

Here are a few guidelines relative to the respiratory component of anesthesia for dogs and cats:

(1) Nearly all canine anesthetics are better done with an endotracheal tube in place, and in many situations cats should be intubated.
(2) Use at least 30–35% inspired oxygen in all anesthetized dogs and cats, even those on an injectable anesthetic mixture, or when deeply sedated.
(3) Hypoxemia is rare in spontaneously breathing dogs and cats if they are breathing an oxygen mixture approaching 100%.
(4) After a prolonged period of anesthesia in cats and smaller dogs, and with shorter anesthetics in larger dogs with deep chests, it is advisable to inflate the lungs to 30 cm H_2O of airway pressure (i.e., to "sigh" the lungs) periodically and at the end of anesthesia.
(5) Prolonged immobility and excessive fluid administration can lead to increased venous admixture and a fall in PaO_2, in addition to that produced by anesthesia per se.

Nervous system anatomy and physiology

Generally, the nervous system can be separated into central and peripheral divisions, although they are integrated and function together. The central division, composed of the brain and spinal cord, contains all of the important nuclei and is essential for integrating sensory and motor functions. The peripheral division is composed of nerves (including cranial nerves) and ganglia that connect the organs and tissues to the central nervous system (CNS).

Brain anatomy

The brain is divisible into five regions based on embryological development: telencephalon, diencephalon, mesencephalon, metencephalon, and myelencephalon. Grossly, it can be divided into the cerebrum and the brain stem. The cerebrum consists of telencephalic and diencephalic portions. The telencephalic portion can be further divided into the cerebral hemispheres and basal ganglia (also known as the basal nuclei). Together, the right and left hemispheres comprise the cerebral cortex, which is organized into an outer cortical layer of gray matter that contains a high density of nerve cell bodies and an inner medulla of white matter consisting mainly of myelinated nerve fibers. The cerebral cortex is where sensory, motor, and associational activity occurs.

The diencephalic portion of the cerebrum, which is located below and between the cerebral hemispheres, is the central area through which most of the information traveling into and out of the hemispheres must traverse. It consists of the thalamus, subthalamus, epithalamus, and hypothalamus, and is positioned between the telencephalon and the brain stem. The brain stem is comprised of the portion of the brain caudal to the telencephalon, excluding the cerebellum (e.g., the midbrain, pons, and medulla oblongata). The midbrain contains sensory and motor pathways, the nuclei of the third and fourth cranial nerves (oculomotor and trochlear), and two major motor nuclei: the red nucleus and the substantia nigra.

Cranial nerves

These consist of a peripheral segment, a nuclear center in the brain stem (except olfactory and optic nerves), and communicating connections with other parts of the brain. All 12 cranial nerves are paired. Functionally, cranial nerves can be divided into motor (efferent), sensory (afferent), and mixed. Sensory and motor cranial nerves are associated with at least one nuclei, and mixed cranial nerves are associated with at least two nuclei) (Figure 2.8).

Brain physiology

The energy consuming processes of the brain are divided into those of neuroprocessing and maintenance of cellular integrity. Oxygen requirements for the conscious, healthy canine brain are approximately 5.5 mL/100 g/min, with 60% needed for neuroprocessing and 40% for maintenance of brain cell integrity. If cardiovascular function is normal,

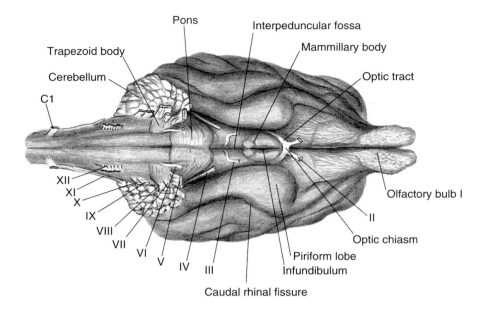

Figure 2.8.   Ventral view of the canine brain and cranial nerves.
Source: Jenkins TJ. 1978. *Functional Mammalian Neuroanatomy*, 2nd ed. Philadelphia, PA: Lea and Febiger.

Afferent nerves	Efferent nerves	Mixed nerves
I. Olfactory	III. Oculomotor	V. Trigeminal
II. Optic	IV. Trochlear	VII. Facial
VIII. Vestibulocochlear	VI. Abducens	IX. Glossopharyngeal
	XI. Spinal accessory	X. Vagus
	XII. Hypoglossal	

adequate oxygen delivery and normal electroencephalogram (EEG) function is expected with a PaO_2 of approximately 100 mm Hg and cerebral blood flow (CBF) of 50 mL/100 g/min. Irreversible cerebral tissue damage is likely when PaO_2 drops below 20–23 mm Hg and CBF below 10 mL/100 g/min. In humans, normal function of the awake brain requires approximately 3.5 mL O_2/100 g/min, or a total of about 50 mL/min extracted from an average normal CBF of 57 mL/100 g/min. In the awake state, most of the brain's cellular energy stores are depleted within 2–4 minutes after oxygen delivery is interrupted. During the anoxic period, cellular lactate concentrations can increase three- to fivefold. Anesthesia, hypothermia, or brain injury can alter cerebral metabolic requirements for oxygen ($CMRO_2$) and must be considered when interpreting the adequacy of monitored cardiopulmonary parameters during anesthesia.

Effects of anesthetics on brain physiology

Anesthetic management of patients requires that CBF be maintained at a level sufficient to meet the brain's metabolic demands. Autoregulation enables maintenance of a constant CBF over a wide range of systemic BPs. Autoregulation is not immediate; when systemic BP changes, it takes about 2 minutes for CBF to return to normal. There have been many studies on the effects of anesthetics on CBF and autoregulation, and the results have sometimes been confusing. All potent inhaled anesthetics tend to decrease cerebral metabolism and increase CBF and intracranial pressure (ICP), but vary in degree.

Spinal cord

Caudal to the medulla, the CNS continues as the spinal cord, which is contained in the spinal canal. The spinal cord is a complex collection of fibers organized into ascending and descending tracts, interneurons, neuron-supporting cells, blood vessels, and connective tissue. The cord is surrounded by the meninges, which support and protect it. From superficial to deep, they are the dura mater, arachnoid, and pia mater. In dogs, the cord and associated subarachnoid structures usually terminate at the level of L6–L7 and in cats, the cord terminates variably between L6 and the sacrum. Inadvertent subarachnoid administration of anesthetic or analgesic drugs is more likely in felines when the needle is inserted at the lumbosacral space.

The epidural space is not an empty cavitary space, but instead contains blood vessels, lymphatics, and epidural fat, and communicates with the paravertebral tissues via the intervertebral foramina. This communication may be interrupted in older animals by fibrous connective tissue and bony malformations associated with spinal arthritis, and in obese patients by fat. This is of clinical significance because epidural injection volumes are often reduced in older or obese animals to prevent excessive cranial spread of drugs.

The subarachnoid space is located between the arachnoidea and pia mater. The subarachnoid space contains CSF and is continuous between the cranial and vertebral segments. There is no direct communication between the epidural and subarachnoid spaces; however, drugs (especially lipophilic drugs) can diffuse across the arachnoidea and enter the CSF after epidural administration. The pia mater, which is one cell layer thick, lies directly on the brain and spinal cord. The pia probably does not present a significant barrier to drug diffusion. The meninges cover the dorsal and ventral spinal nerve roots until they fuse, at which point they merge with the spinal nerve and extend no farther peripherally.

CSF and ICP

Within the calvarium, CSF is found in both an internal (ventricular) system and an external (subarachnoid) system. The internal system consists of the bilaterally symmetrical lateral ventricles within the cerebral hemispheres, the third ventricle medially between the thalamus and hypothalamus, and the fourth ventricle lying beneath the cerebellum and within the medulla. CSF is produced by the choroid plexus, a fringelike fold of pia mater found on the floor of both lateral ventricles, in the fourth ventricle, and also by

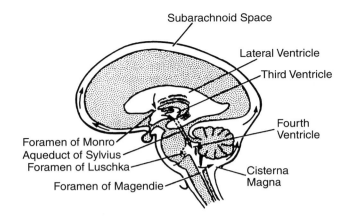

Figure 2.9.   Circulation of CSF in the human and subhuman primates. Nonprimate animals do not have the foramen of Magendie.
Source: Stoelting RK. 1991. *Pharmacology and Physiology in Anesthetic Practice*, 2nd ed. Philadelphia, PA: Lippincott.

the ependymal lining of the ventricles. CSF is formed from the blood by secretory and filtration processes. Fluid in the lateral ventricles empties into the third ventricle through the paired foramina of Monro. The third ventricle, in turn, empties into the fourth through the aqueduct of Sylvius. The central canal of the spinal cord is continuous with the fourth ventricle. The external or subarachnoid system overlies the brain and spinal cord. The bilateral foramina of Luschka enable fluid to pass between the ventricular and subarachnoid systems. In most primates, the unpaired foramen of Magendie is present and enables an additional connection between the fourth ventricle and the subarachnoid space. The foramen of Magendie is not found in most common veterinary species (Figure 2.9).

CSF is absorbed at the arachnoid villi located primarily in the subdural venous sinuses. The arachnoid villi are fingerlike projections of the arachnoidal membrane that penetrate the venous sinuses. Their endothelium is porous and highly permeable, allowing free passage of water, electrolytes, proteins, and even red blood cells.

CSF cushions the brain and spinal cord. CSF normal pressure is approximately 10 mm Hg but can fluctuate within a narrow range. The composition of the CSF remains different from plasma because of the blood–brain barrier. The barrier is as much an enzymatic and cellular transporter barrier as an anatomical separation. The concentration of sodium is equal to that of plasma, the concentration of chloride in the CSF is 15% greater, and the concentration of potassium and glucose is 40% and 30% less than in plasma, respectively. The specific gravity of CSF is 1.002–1.009. The pH of CSF is closely maintained at 7.32.

Carbon dioxide, but not hydrogen ions, readily crosses the blood–brain barrier. Bicarbonate ions are actively transported. As a result, the pH of CSF is rapidly altered by changes in $PaCO_2$ but not by changes in arterial pH. The pH of CSF, not the PCO_2 directly, is the major mechanism regulating ventilation in most mammals.

The skull forms a noncompliant chamber filled with brain parenchyma, blood, and CSF. An increase in volume of one component must be accompanied by a compensatory decrease in the others or the ICP will increase (Monro–Kellie hypothesis). Normal ICP is less than 15 mm Hg. As the ICP increases, blood flow to the brain will decrease unless an increase in mean arterial pressure occurs to maintain cerebral perfusion pressure (cerebral perfusion pressure = mean arterial pressure – ICP). Arterial BP should always be measured in animals suspected of having intracranial hypertension, because anesthetic-induced decreases in mean arterial BP can lead to catastrophic cerebral ischemia even though arterial BPs were maintained above acceptable levels for healthy animals (e.g., mean arterial pressure of 60 mm Hg). Increased cerebral or spinal fluid pressure produces a reflex increase in HR and BP (Cushing's response). It has been hypothesized that the increase in CSF pressure creates ischemia of neurons, and that this is the stimulus for increased sympathetic activity.

Drugs that reduce cerebral metabolic activity or CBF, osmotic diuretics, hypothermia, and mechanical normoventilation or hyperventilation may all be used to decrease ICP. It is imperative that anesthetic management focus on maintaining adequate cerebral perfusion pressure rather than on reducing CBF or ICP alone. Administration of analgesic drugs, especially opioids, must be carefully monitored in animals with intracranial disease, because of their potential to increase $PaCO_2$, which could lead to increased CBF and ICP. Ventilatory support may be required if respiratory depression occurs.

Spinal nerves

These supply efferent and afferent innervation to most of the body, with the exception of the head and viscera. They also form part of the autonomic nervous system, which controls homeostatic functions. Spinal nerves vary in number, depending on species. Nerves can be classified by their size and degree of myelination, which determine speed of impulse transmission. Large, heavily myelinated fibers have the highest conduction velocities, whereas small nonmyelinated fibers have lower conduction rates. The largest fibers, type A, are subclassified as A-alpha, A-beta, A-gamma, and A-delta fibers. A-alpha fibers innervate skeletal muscles and also subserve proprioception. A-beta fibers normally subserve innocuous touch and pressure, but can be involved in nervous system "windup" that can result in hyperalgesia and/or allodynia following chronic nociceptor stimulation. A-gamma fibers innervate the skeletal muscle spindles to maintain muscle tone. A-delta fibers subserve temperature, fast pain, and touch. Type B fibers are preganglionic autonomic fibers. Type C fibers are small nonmyelinated fibers responsible for postganglionic sympathetic innervation and transmission of visceral and slow pain, touch, and temperature sensations. Abnormal nociceptive C fiber activity causes many chronic pain syndromes best described in humans, with diabetic neuropathy and postherpetic neuralgia being two examples. Similar C-fiber dysfunction is likely in a variety of chronic pain conditions in other mammalian species.

After leaving the intervertebral foramen, each spinal nerve divides into dorsal and ventral branches. The dorsal branches generally supply the muscles and skin of the back, whereas the ventral branches supply the muscles and skin of the thorax, abdomen, and extremities. Branches from several spinal nerves may combine to form plexuses such as the brachial plexus or major nerves such as the sciatic nerve.

Autonomic nervous system

In contrast with the somatic nervous system supplying the striated muscles, the autonomic nervous system requires no conscious control. The autonomic nervous system is composed of the efferent and afferent nerves innervating the viscera, glands, and other tissues required for homeostasis and the fight-or-flight response. Its primary homeostatic role is control of circulation, breathing, excretion, and maintenance of body temperature. These regulatory functions are subject to modification by input from higher brain centers, especially as a result of reactions to the environment.

Visceral autonomic efferent pathways consist of two neurons rather than a single motor neuron as occurs in the somatic system. The cell body of the first neuron is in the brain stem or spinal cord. Its axon terminates on the cell body of the second neuron, located in an autonomic ganglion. The axon of the ganglion cell terminates in the effector cell.

Autonomic visceral afferents are primarily sensory neurons similar to those in somatic tissues, although they tend to have wider receptive areas, leading to less ability to discriminate the anatomic origin of the afferent signals. They elicit reflex responses in viscera and a feeling of fullness of hollow organs, such as the stomach, large intestine, and bladder. Afferent impulses contribute to feelings of well-being or malaise and transmit signals from nociceptors. Visceral pain afferents are associated with the sympathetic division.

The hypothalamus is the primary area of the brain that controls the autonomic nervous system. The autonomic system can be subdivided into the craniosacral or parasympathetic system and the thoracolumbar or sympathetic system. A characteristic of the autonomic nervous system is that both divisions are constantly active, resulting in a basal level of sympathetic and parasympathetic activity. Thus, each division can increase or decrease its effect at a given organ to regulate function more closely.

Neuron function

Axonal conduction

Nerve impulses are electrochemical currents that pass along the axon to the presynaptic membrane. From a pharmacological standpoint, there is an important distinction between electric conduction of a nerve impulse along an axon and chemical transmission of this signal across the synapse. Most general anesthetics have little effect on nerve conduction velocity.

Neuroregulators

These play a key role in communication among nerve cells and may be subdivided into two groups. Small molecule neurotransmitters are synthesized in the cytosol of the presynaptic terminal, absorbed into the transmitter vesicles, and released into the synaptic cleft in response to the arrival of an action potential at the nerve ending. Release of neurotransmitters is voltage dependent and requires calcium influx into the presynaptic terminal. Following its release, the transmitter binds with the postsynaptic receptor. The postjunctional membrane is excited by increased sodium conductance and inhibited when potassium or chloride conductance is enhanced. Some transmitters bind to receptors that activate enzymes, thus altering cellular function.

Neuropeptide modulators are synthesized in the neuronal cell body and transported to the nerve terminal by axonal streaming. They are released in response to an action potential, but in much smaller quantities than are the small molecule transmitters. The neuropeptides induce prolonged effects to amplify or dampen neuronal activity. They exert their effects through a variety of mechanisms, including prolonged closure of calcium channels, alteration of cellular metabolism, activation or inactivation of specific genes, and prolonged alteration in the numbers of excitatory or inhibitory receptors. Although usually only a single small molecule neurotransmitter is released by each type of neuron (Dale's law), the same neuron may release one or more neuropeptide modulators at the same time.

Sedative and anticholinergic pharmacology

Anticholinergic drugs

Anticholinergics are used perioperatively to manage bradycardia and AV block associated with surgical manipulation (oculovagal and viscerovagal reflexes) or with the administration of other anesthetic adjunctive drugs (e.g., alpha$_2$ agonists or opioids). Occasionally, they are also used to control excessive oral and airway secretions. Anticholinergics should not be administered perioperatively on an indiscriminate basis. Rather, the risks and benefits associated with the administration of different drugs should be assessed, and the safest drugs chosen for each patient.

Anticholinergics are often called parasympatholytic drugs because they block the effects of the parasympathetic nervous system on other body systems, especially the cardiovascular and gastrointestinal systems. Atropine and glycopyrrolate are the anticholinergics used most commonly in veterinary medicine. These two drugs do not block nicotinic cholinergic receptors and are more accurately classified as antimuscarinics. There are three major types of muscarinic receptors: M_1, M_2, and M_3. M_1 receptors are located on neurons in the CNS and on autonomic ganglia. M_2 receptors are located in the SA and AV nodes and in the atrial myocardium. M_3 receptors are located in secretory glands, vascular endothelium, and smooth muscle.

Atropine and glycopyrrolate are relatively nonselective muscarinic antagonists, but despite this lack of selectively the effectiveness of muscarinic blockade varies considerably from tissue to tissue. Salivary and bronchial glands are the most sensitive to muscarinic blockade. Cardiac tissues and smooth muscle are intermediate in sensitivity, and gastric parietal cells are the least sensitive to muscarinic blockade.

Anticholinergic administration routinely causes sinus tachycardia, which is problematic for many patients with cardiovascular disease. Tachycardia associated with administration of anticholinergics leads to an increase in myocardial work and a decrease in myocardial perfusion. Further, coadministration of anticholinergics and ketamine has been associated with the development of myocardial infarcts in, and the death of, young cats undergoing routine surgical procedures. At lower doses, a transient decrease in sinus rate and slowing of AV nodal conduction (AV blockade) can occur. This response appears to be due to blockade of presynaptic muscarinic receptors that normally inhibit acetylcholine (ACh) release. Once postsynaptic muscarinic blockade is established, this paradoxical increase in vagal tone usually resolves.

Anticholinergic administration also has dramatic effects on gastrointestinal function. At therapeutic doses, nonselective muscarinic antagonists like atropine and glycopyrrolate reduce lower esophageal sphincter tone and have little effect on gastric pH. These two factors increase the incidence of gastroesophageal reflux and esophagitis in anesthetized dogs. Perioperative administration of anticholinergics also reduces intestinal motility and can lead to gastrointestinal complications postoperatively.

Atropine

Chemically, atropine consists of two components (tropic acid and an organic base) that are bound by an ester linkage. Atropine has approximately the same affinity for all three major types of muscarinic receptors. Relative to other synthetic muscarinic antagonists, atropine is very selective for muscarinic receptors and has little effect on nicotinic receptors.

Pharmacokinetics and pharmacodynamics   Atropine is rapidly absorbed after intramuscular (IM) administration. Onset of cardiovascular effects occurs within 5 minutes, and peak effects occur within 10–20 minutes. After IV administration at a dose of 0.03 mg/kg, onset of cardiovascular effects occurs within 1 minute, peak effects occur within 5 minutes, and HR increases by 30–40% for approximately 30 minutes. The effects of atropine on other body systems subside within a few hours, but ocular effects can persist for 1–2 days. Atropine is rapidly eliminated from the blood after parenteral administration. Some of the drug is hydrolyzed to inactive metabolites (tropine and tropic acid), and some of it is excreted unchanged in the urine. Rabbits and some other species (cats and rats) have a plasma enzyme (atropine esterase) that accelerates metabolism and clearance of the drug.

At therapeutic doses, atropine administration produces limited effects on the CNS. A mild sedative effect may be observed, and the incidence of vomiting mediated by the vestibular system may be reduced. Blockade of the pupillary constrictor muscle and the ciliary muscle produces long-lasting mydriasis and cycloplegia, respectively. Lacrimal secretions are also reduced, which may contribute to corneal drying during anesthesia unless artificial tears are applied concurrently. Atropine should be used with discretion in animals with acute glaucoma because its mydriatic effect may impede drainage from the anterior chamber.

Airway smooth muscle and secretory glands also receive parasympathetic input from the vagus nerves. Blockade of M_3 receptors by therapeutic doses of atropine decreases airway secretions and increases airway diameter and anatomical dead space. In the past, atropine was given before administration of noxious inhaled anesthetics (ether) to reduce airway secretions and the potential for laryngospasm. Modern inhaled anesthetics do not cause the same degree of airway irritation, and routine preoperative administration of atropine for this reason is difficult to justify.

Clinical uses Atropine can be given subcutaneously (SC), IM, or IV, but the IM and IV routes are preferred because uptake from subcutaneous sites can be erratic in patients with altered hydration and peripheral circulation. Doses for dogs and cats range from 0.02 to 0.04 mg/kg. Atropine is also effective when given endotracheally or endobronchially to dogs for cardiopulmonary resuscitation.

Glycopyrrolate

Glycopyrrolate is a synthetic quaternary ammonium muscarinic antagonist. Like atropine, the drug consists of two components (mandelic acid and an organic base) bound together by an ester linkage. Glycopyrrolate is four times as potent as atropine and has approximately the same affinity for all three major types of muscarinic receptors. The drug's polar structure (quaternary amine) limits diffusion across lipid membranes and into the CNS and fetal circulation.

Pharmacokinetics and pharmacodynamics Absorption, metabolism, and elimination of glycopyrrolate are similar to that of atropine. Absorption is rapid after IM administration. Onset of cardiovascular effects occurs within 5 minutes, peak effects occur within 20 minutes, and HR remains elevated for approximately 1 hour. Glycopyrrolate is rapidly eliminated from the blood after parenteral administration, and most of the drug is excreted unchanged in the urine.

At therapeutic doses, glycopyrrolate produces few, if any, effects on the CNS. Unlike atropine administration, sedation is not observed, and recovery times are not prolonged. Administration of glycopyrrolate to conscious dogs with normal intraocular pressure does not alter pupil diameter and intraocular pressure, and intraoperative administration of glycopyrrolate to dogs with glaucoma and increased intraocular pressure appears to be safe.

Glycopyrrolate administration produces effects on the heart that are comparable to those of atropine. Studies in people suggest that glycopyrrolate produces less tachycardia than atropine, but the two drugs produce similar increases in HR when administered IV to sedated or anesthetized dogs. The typical response to IV or IM administration of therapeutic doses (5–10 μg/kg) of glycopyrrolate is an increase in sinus rate, acceleration of AV nodal conduction, and an increase in atrial contractility. At lower doses, a transient decrease in sinus rate and slowing of AV nodal conduction can occur. Glycopyrrolate can also be given intraoperatively to correct bradycardia.

Like atropine, glycopyrrolate affects the gastrointestinal system. Intestinal motility is reduced for at least 30 minutes in anesthetized dogs.

Clinical uses Glycopyrrolate is used perioperatively to prevent severe bradycardia caused by surgical manipulation (vagal reflexes) or by administration of other anesthetic drugs. Doses for dogs and cats range from 5 to 10 μg/kg.

Sedatives

Behavioral responses to different classes of sedatives vary considerably among species. The phenothiazines and alpha$_2$ agonists are effective sedatives in dogs and cats. Conversely, the benzodiazepines are effective sedatives in ferrets, rabbits, and birds but are not reliable sedatives in cats and young dogs.

Phenothiazines and butyrophenones

Phenothiazines and, to a lesser extent, butyrophenones produce a wide variety of behavioral, autonomic, and endocrine effects. The behavioral effects of these drugs are mediated primarily by blockade of dopamine receptors in the basal ganglia and limbic system. At therapeutic doses, phenothiazines and butyrophenones inhibit conditioned avoidance behavior and decrease spontaneous motor activity. At higher doses, extrapyramidal effects (tremor, rigidity, and catalepsy) can occur. These sedatives also have significant binding affinity for adrenergic and muscarinic receptors. For example, phenothiazines bind with great affinity to, and act as antagonists at, alpha$_1$ adrenergic receptors, which may result in hypotension that is typically associated with perioperative use of these drugs. Blockade of dopamine receptors in the chemoreceptor trigger zone of the medulla produces an antiemetic effect, and depletion of catecholamines in the thermoregulatory center of the hypothalamus leads to a loss of thermoregulatory control.

Acepromazine (a phenothiazine) is one of the most widely used sedatives in veterinary medicine. The chemical name of acepromazine is 2-acetyl-10-(3-dimethylaminopropyl) phenothiazine. Acepromazine is often given in combination with an opioid as a preanesthetic to facilitate the placement of IV catheters and to reduce the dose of injectable and inhalational anesthetics required to induce and maintain anesthesia. Acepromazine can also be given postoperatively to smooth recovery, provided that patients are hemodynamically stable and that pain has been managed effectively. IM doses for cats and small dogs range from 0.01 to 0.2 mg/kg, and those for larger dogs range from 0.01 to 0.05 mg/kg. Generally, doses less than 0.05 mg/kg are adequate for mild to moderate sedation in the pre- or postanesthetic period.

Alpha$_2$ adrenergic agonists

In most species, alpha$_2$ agonists produce reliable dose-dependent sedation, analgesia, and muscle relaxation that can be readily reversed by administration of selective antagonists. Xylazine has been used in both small and large animals for over three decades. In small animals, medetomidine, and more recently its purified isomer dexmedetomidine, have been used.

The alpha$_2$ receptors are located in tissues throughout the body, and norepinephrine is the endogenous ligand for these receptors. The alpha$_2$ receptors exist presynaptically and postsynaptically in neuronal and nonneuronal tissues, and extrasynaptically in the vascular endothelium and in platelets. Within the nervous system, alpha$_2$ receptors are located presynaptically on noradrenergic neurons (autoreceptors) and on nonnoradrenergic neurons (heteroceptors). The sedative and anxiolytic effects of alpha$_2$ agonists are mediated by activation of supraspinal autoreceptors or postsynaptic receptors located in the pons (locus ceruleus), and some of the analgesic effects are mediated by activation of heteroceptors located in the dorsal horn of the spinal cord. Supraspinal alpha$_2$ receptors located in the pons also play a prominent role in descending modulation of nociceptive input.

Three distinct alpha$_2$ receptor subtypes (A, B, and C) have been identified. The cellular response to activation of these receptor subtypes is mediated by several different molecular mechanisms.

Medetomidine and dexmedetomidine   Medetomidine, ($\pm$)-4-(1-[2,3-dimethylphenyl] ethyl)-1H-imidazole monohydrochloride is a racemic mixture of levo- and dextrorotory enantiomers. All or nearly all of the pharmacological action is due to the dextrorotory enantiomer, dexmedetomidine. Shortly after medetomidine was approved for use in dogs as a sedative–analgesic in North America, dexmedetomidine was approved for use in people as a postoperative sedative in the United States. As expected, dexmedetomidine is approximately twice as potent as the racemic mixture that is available for use in animals. In dogs and cats, both dexmedetomidine and medetomidine have a rapid onset of action and can be administered IV or IM. After IM administration, the drug is rapidly absorbed, and peak plasma concentrations are reached within 30 minutes. Elimination occurs mainly by biotransformation in the liver, and inactive metabolites are excreted in the urine.

Onset of sedation, analgesia, and muscle relaxation is rapid after IM administration of medetomidine to dogs and cats, and the intensity and duration of these effects depend on dose. When medetomidine is given IM to dogs at a dose of 30 μg/kg, significant sedation is apparent within 5 minutes and persists for 1–2 hours. Similarly, when medetomidine is given to cats at a dose of 50 μg/kg, significant sedation is apparent within 15 minutes and persists for 1–2 hours. At these doses, analgesia peaks within 30 minutes and persists for 1–2 hours.

Medetomidine administration decreases injectable and inhalational anesthetic requirements dramatically (by over 50% in dogs). Administration of medetomidine IM at doses of 10, 20, and 40 μg/kg decreases the amount of thiopental required for intubation to 7.0, 4.5, and 2.4 mg/kg, respectively. Similarly, administration of medetomidine IM at a dose of 20 μg/kg decreases the amount of propofol required for intubation to 1.8 mg/kg. Administration of medetomidine IM also reduces the dose of ketamine required to induce anesthesia in dogs and cats. Administration of medetomidine IV at a dose of 30 μg/kg decreased the MAC of isoflurane by 47%. Additionally, administration of medetomidine IM at a dose of 8 μg/kg consistently reduced the bispectral index value (an index of anesthetic depth) in dogs anesthetized with isoflurane (1.0, 1.5, and 2.0 MAC).

As with other alpha$_2$ agonists, medetomidine administration produces changes in commonly monitored cardiovascular parameters. Cardiovascular effects are best described in two phases: an initial peripheral phase characterized by vasoconstriction, increased BP, and reflex vagal bradycardia; and a subsequent central phase characterized by decreased sympathetic tone, sympathetically driven HR, and BP. Occasionally, AV blockade occurs secondary to the initial increase in BP and reflex (baroreceptor-mediated) increase in vagal tone. In conscious dogs, mean arterial pressure increases transiently, and HR and cardiac index decrease by approximately 60% after IV administration of medetomidine at doses ranging from 5 to 20 µg/kg. At these doses, changes in mean arterial pressure, central venous pressure, and vascular resistance are dose dependent, whereas changes in HR and cardiac index are not. In conscious cats, mean arterial pressure does not appear to change (perhaps related to higher baseline stress levels) and HR and cardiac index decrease by approximately 50% after IM administration of medetomidine at a dose of 20 µg/kg. In cats anesthetized with isoflurane (2%), mean arterial pressure increases from 77 to 122 mm Hg, HR decreases from 150 to 125 beats per minute, and mean arterial flow decreases from 578 to 325 mL/min, 20 minutes after the IM administration of medetomidine at a dose of 10 µg/kg.

In conscious animals, the decrease in CO is caused primarily by the decrease in HR and increase in vascular resistance, and not by a direct depression of myocardial contractility. Although CO decreases after medetomidine or dexmedetomidine administration, blood flow to the heart, brain, and kidneys is maintained by redistribution of flow from less vital organs and tissues. In patients with good cardiopulmonary reserve, the concurrent administration of an anticholinergic agent will prevent bradyarrhythmias while slightly improving CO at the expense of a rather large increase in myocardial work and O_2 consumption. Thus, the use of an anticholinergic preoperatively with alpha$_2$ agonists to prevent bradycardia and AV blockade continues to be somewhat controversial. The use of an anticholinergic has been recommended for the following reasons: First, even at low preanesthetic doses, significant bradycardia can occur if an anticholinergic is not administered concurrently. Second, the potential for severe vagotonic responses and profound bradycardia, secondary to surgical manipulation and administration of other anesthetic drugs (opioids), is higher during the perioperative period. Third, while the concurrent administration of anticholinergics with high doses of medetomidine can cause dramatic increases in vascular resistance and myocardial work, these increases can be minimized and are generally well tolerated by healthy patients given low doses of medetomidine prior to inhalant (vasodilatory) anesthesia.

Medetomidine administration has little effect on pulmonary function. Respiratory rate and V_E decrease after medetomidine administration, but this decrease in V_E appears to parallel a decrease in metabolic CO_2 production, and arterial blood gas values remain stable.

Medetomidine administration has significant effects on gastrointestinal function in animals. Vomiting occurs in 10% of dogs and over 50% of cats administered medetomidine IM at mean doses of 40 and 80 µg/kg, respectively. Vomiting dramatically increases intraocular pressure, which is a potential problem for some patients with ocular injury or disease. Medetomidine administration decreases gastrin release and intestinal and colonic motility in dogs. These effects are mediated by activation of visceral alpha$_2$ receptors and inhibition of ACh release.

Medetomidine administration has significant effects on renal and urogenital function in animals. In dogs, administration of medetomidine (10–20 µg/kg IV) decreases urine specific gravity and increases urine production for approximately 4 hours. Apparently, alpha$_2$ agonists interfere with the action of antidiuretic hormone on the renal tubules and collecting ducts, which increases the production of dilute urine.

Preoperative administration of alpha$_2$ agonists attenuates the stress response associated with surgical trauma. In dogs undergoing ovariohysterectomy, preoperative administration of medetomidine reduces catecholamine and cortisol concentrations postoperatively. Similarly, preoperative administration of medetomidine (20 μg/kg IM) attenuates perioperative increases in norepinephrine, epinephrine, and cortisol concentrations to a greater degree than does acepromazine. Administration of xylazine or medetomidine activates alpha$_2$ receptors on pancreatic beta cells and inhibits release of insulin for approximately 2 hours, resulting in an increase in plasma glucose concentrations.

As a general rule, medetomidine should not be administered to pediatric or geriatric animals, or to animals with significant neurological, cardiovascular, respiratory, hepatic, or renal disease. Once preanesthetic and anesthetic drugs are administered, patients should be monitored carefully throughout the perioperative period, with special attention being paid to HR and rhythm.

Xylazine   Although its mechanism of action was unknown at the time of its introduction into clinical practice, xylazine was the first alpha$_2$ agonist to be used by veterinarians. The drug was synthesized in West Germany in 1962 for use as an antihypertensive in people but was found to have potent sedative effects in animals. The chemical name for xylazine is 2(2,6-dimethylphenylamino)-4H-5,6-dihydro-1,3-thiazine hydrochloride. Initially, the drug was used as a sedative in cattle and other ruminants in Europe. In the early 1970s, reports of xylazine's utility as an anesthetic adjunct began appearing in American and European veterinary literature. These reports documented the effectiveness of xylazine in eliminating muscular hypertonicity in dogs and cats given ketamine, and in producing rapid, predictable sedation, analgesia, and muscle relaxation in horses and cattle after IV administration. It was also evident that there was tremendous variation in the dose of xylazine required to produce equivalent levels of sedation and analgesia in different species. In 1981, the sedative and analgesic effects of xylazine were definitively linked to the activation of central alpha$_2$ adrenergic receptors.

Most clinical studies show that the sedative and analgesic effects of xylazine are comparable in duration and do not support the "conventional wisdom" that the analgesic effect is significantly shorter than the sedative effect. Xylazine administration dramatically decreases injectable and inhalational anesthetic requirements in several species (similar to dexmedetomidine).

Alpha$_2$ adrenergic antagonists

Alpha$_2$ agonists are used to reverse the sedative and cardiovascular effects of alpha$_2$ agonists. Currently, three antagonists (tolazoline, yohimbine, and atipamezole) are available for use in animals, with only atipamezole recommended for reversal of medetomidine and dexmedetomidine in small animals.

In addition to reversing the sedative and cardiovascular effects of alpha$_2$ agonists, alpha$_2$ antagonists can produce significant side effects. If a relative overdose of an antagonist is administered, neurological (excitement and muscle tremors), cardiovascular (hypotension and tachycardia), and gastrointestinal (salivation and diarrhea) side effects can occur. Death has also been reported after rapid IV administration. The mechanism is likely due to the rapid reversal of vasoconstriction without sufficient time for the sympathetic nervous system to increase CO, resulting in severe hypotension.

Complete reversal of the sedative, analgesic, and cardiovascular effects of medetomidine is achieved when atipamezole is administered IM to dogs and cats at four to six times and two to four times the dose (based on micrograms given and not on volume) of medetomidine, respectively. Therefore, if the initial dose of medetomidine is 20 µg/kg for a dog, then atipamezole would be given IM at a dose of 100 µg/kg. Similarly, if the initial dose of medetomidine is 40 µg/kg for a cat, then atipamezole would be given IM at a dose of 120 µg/kg. In both of these examples, the dose of atipamezole may be reduced if more than 30 minutes has elapsed since medetomidine administration.

Benzodiazepine sedatives

Benzodiazepines produce most of their pharmacological effects by modulating gamma-aminobutyric acid (GABA)-mediated neurotransmission. GABA is the primary inhibitory neurotransmitter in the mammalian nervous system and cell membranes of most CNS neurons express GABA receptors. These receptors are also found outside the CNS in autonomic ganglia. Two main types of GABA receptors are involved in neuronal transmission: The $GABA_A$ receptor complex is a ligand-gated chloride channel that consists of a central pore surrounded by five glycoprotein subunits.

The benzodiazepine-binding site, as well as the binding sites for other injectable anesthetics (barbiturates, propofol, and etomidate), is located in the $GABA_A$ receptor complex. Benzodiazepines enhance binding between GABA and the $GABA_A$ receptor, and increase the frequency of channel opening. In contrast, barbiturates enhance intrinsic activity and increase the duration of channel opening. Both mechanisms increase chloride conductance and hyperpolarize the cell membrane, which reduces neuronal excitability. Benzodiazepines have no intrinsic agonist activity and cannot alter chloride conductance in the absence of GABA. This lack of intrinsic activity limits CNS depression and provides benzodiazepines with a much wider margin of safety than barbiturates.

Ligands that bind to benzodiazepine receptors are classified as agonists, inverse agonists, and antagonists. Agonists bind to benzodiazepine receptors and produce sedative, anxiolytic, muscle relaxant, and anticonvulsant effects in most animals. Inverse agonists bind to the same receptor and produce the opposite effects. Antagonists have high affinity for the benzodiazepine receptor and have little or no intrinsic activity. These ligands block or reverse the effects of both agonists and inverse agonists. Diazepam, midazolam, and zolazepam are the benzodiazepine agonists used most commonly in veterinary medicine. Diazepam and midazolam are used primarily as sedatives, muscle relaxants, and anticonvulsants. Zolazepam is available in combination with a dissociative anesthetic (tiletamine), which is approved for use as an anesthetic in dogs and cats in the United States.

Diazepam The chemical name for the diazepam is 7-chloro-1,3-dihydro-1-methyl-5-phenyl-2H-1,4-benzodiazepin-2-one. Diazepam is not soluble in water, and parenteral formulations contain 40% propylene glycol and 10% ethanol. The drug is also sensitive to light and adheres to plastic, so it should not be stored in plastic syringes for extended periods. Diazepam is used primarily as a muscle relaxant and as an anticonvulsant for dogs and cats.

Diazepam is highly lipid soluble and is rapidly distributed throughout the body. Approximately 90% of the drug is protein bound, and diazepam is metabolized by demethylation and hydroxylation to N-desmethyldiazepam (nordiazepam), 3-hydroxydiazepam, and oxazepam. Nordiazepam and oxazepam produce significant pharmacological effects at clinically relevant concentrations. In dogs, the elimination half-life of diazepam after administration of a relatively high dose (2 mg/kg IV) is 3.2 hours. Nordiazepam appears rapidly in plasma and quickly exceeds concentrations of diazepam, whereas oxazepam concentrations peak within 2 hours. The elimination half-lives of nordiazepam and oxazepam are 3.6 and 5.7 hours, respectively. In cats, the mean elimination half-life of diazepam after administration of relatively high doses (5, 10, and 20 mg/kg IV) is 5.5 hours. Approximately 50% of the diazepam dose is converted to nordiazepam, and the mean elimination half-life of the metabolite is 21 hours, which is approximately four times longer than the half-life of diazepam.

Diazepam does not sedate dogs reliably, and can cause excitement, dysphoria, and ataxia. In dogs, IV administration of diazepam (0.5 mg/kg) produces arousal and excitement. Diazepam administration can produce dysphoria and aggressive behavior in cats, and the drug should be used with this potential response in mind in this species. Because of these behavioral effects, diazepam alone has limited value as a sedative for dogs and cats.

Diazepam is not a reliable sedative, but is a good muscle relaxant and anticonvulsant in most species. In dogs, diazepam is commonly administered IV at a dose of 0.2–0.5 mg/kg immediately before induction of anesthesia with ketamine. Diazepam also can be administered prior to induction of anesthesia with thiopental, propofol, etomidate, or an opioid. Diazepam appears to be a more reliable sedative in older dogs and can be administered alone or in combination with an opioid to produce sedation in this subpopulation. Higher doses are often administered when diazepam is used as an anticonvulsant. In small animals, diazepam is administered IV at a dose of 0.5–1.0 mg/kg to control seizures. The parenteral formulation of diazepam is very irritating and potentially cardiotoxic, and should be administered by slow IV injection.

Midazolam Midazolam is a benzodiazepine with a fused imidazole ring that accounts for the water solubility of the drug at pH values below 4.0. The chemical name of midazolam is 8-chloro-6-(2-fluorophenyl)-1-methyl-4H-imidazo(1,5-a)(1,4)-benzodiazepine. The pH of the parenteral formulation is 3.5, and the drug is light sensitive like diazepam. At blood pH, midazolam changes its chemical configuration and becomes more lipid soluble, facilitating diffusion into tissues. Midazolam is almost completely (>90%) absorbed after IM injection, and peak plasma concentrations are reached within 15 minutes. The drug is also highly protein bound (>95%) and rapidly crosses the blood–brain barrier. Midazolam is hydroxylated in the liver, and glucuronide conjugates are excreted in the urine.

Midazolam is commonly given to enhance muscle relaxation and facilitate intubation in dogs and cats, and is coadministered with ketamine, etomidate, or propofol. Preanesthetic administration (0.1–0.2 mg/kg IV) reduces the induction dose of barbiturates and propofol and the concentration of isoflurane required to maintain anesthesia during surgery. Midazolam administration produces minimal effects on cardiopulmonary function in mammals and birds. Because midazolam has limited effects on cardiopulmonary function, the drug is an ideal sedative for many older or compromised animals. In dogs, midazolam is typically administered alone at doses of 0.2–0.4 mg/kg IM or in combination with opioids (butorphanol, hydromorphone, or oxymorphone) to induce sedative effects. It can be administered IV at doses of 0.1–0.2 mg/kg before induction of anesthesia with ketamine, thiopental, propofol, or etomidate.

Benzodiazepine antagonists

Antagonists have a strong affinity for the benzodiazepine receptor but have no intrinsic activity and are relatively free of side effects. Additionally, benzodiazepine antagonists cannot reverse the effects of anesthetic drugs (barbiturates) that bind to other sites on the $GABA_A$ receptor complex. Flumazenil is the only benzodiazepine antagonist currently available for clinical use. In animals, it is used primarily to reverse the sedative and muscle relaxant effects of diazepam and other benzodiazepines.

Flumazenil   Flumazenil is a highly selective, competitive benzodiazepine receptor antagonist. The chemical name of the drug is ethyl-8-fluro-5,6-dihydro-5-methyl-6-oxo-4H-imidazolo-(1,5-a)benzodiazepine-3-carboxylate. Limited pharmacokinetic data are available for animals. An elimination half-life of 0.4–1.3 hours has been reported for dogs. In people, midazolam and flumazenil have similar pharmacokinetic profiles, which makes flumazenil a suitable antagonist for midazolam. Flumazenil rapidly reverses the sedative and muscle relaxant effects of benzodiazepine agonists in animals. In dogs, flumazenil administration completely reverses the behavioral and muscle relaxant effects of an overdose of diazepam (2 mg/kg IV) or midazolam (1 mg/kg IV) within 5 minutes. In addition, flumazenil may reverse the anticonvulsant effects of benzodiazepine agonists. Although flumazenil has minimal intrinsic activity, administration of the antagonist could facilitate the development of seizures in predisposed animals. Flumazenil also appears to have minimal effects on cardiopulmonary function in animals. Currently, flumazenil is the only benzodiazepine antagonist used in veterinary medicine. In dogs, an overdose of diazepam (2.0 mg/kg IV) or midazolam (1.0 mg/kg IV) can be effectively antagonized with flumazenil at a dose of 0.08 mg/kg. These doses correspond to agonist/antagonist ratios of 26:1 and 13:1 for diazepam/flumazenil and midazolam/flumazenil, respectively.

Injectable anesthetic agents

Injectable anesthetic drugs are used to induce an unconscious or hypnotic state or are administered by repeated injection and continuous infusion to maintain the mental depression necessary for anesthesia. The search for new drugs and combinations with appropriate pharmacokinetic–pharmacodynamic profiles for use in domestic and wild animals is ongoing. In animals, unlike in people, a state approaching general anesthesia is not achievable with the use of opioids alone. Consequently, in veterinary anesthesia, opioids have been primarily used as analgesics perioperatively and as anesthetic adjuncts to induce a state of neuroleptanesthesia and are not employed alone as IV anesthetics.

Barbiturate drugs

The barbiturates have been classified into four groups according to duration of action: long, intermediate, short, and ultrashort. All of those used for clinical anesthesia fall in the short or ultrashort classification, whereas those used for sedation or control of convulsions are of long or intermediate action.

The principal effect of a barbiturate is depression of the CNS by interference with passage of impulses to the cerebral cortex. Barbiturates act directly on CNS neurons in a manner similar to that of the inhibitory transmitter GABA. At clinical drug concentrations, barbiturates have two mechanisms of action at $GABA_A$ receptors. At lower concentrations, barbiturates exert a GABA-mimetic effect by decreasing the rate of dissociation of GABA from the $GABA_A$ receptor. At increasing drug concentrations, barbiturates directly activate the chloride ion channel associated with the $GABA_A$ receptor. The GABA-mimetic effects of barbiturates are thought to produce their sedative hypnotic effects, whereas the direct chloride ion channel activation produces their anesthetic effects.

Barbiturates diffuse throughout the body, penetrating cell walls and crossing the placenta. The extent of ionization, lipid solubility (partition coefficient [PC]), and protein binding are the three most important factors in distribution and elimination of barbiturates.

Phenobarbital sodium

Phenobarbital is a long-acting barbiturate, and advantage has been taken of its prolonged action in treating various convulsive disorders. Phenobarbital is not used as an anesthetic agent. However, coadministration of some anesthetics metabolized by the same microsomal enzyme may result in shorter half-life and duration of action due to microsomal enzyme induction.

Pentobarbital sodium

The duration of surgical anesthesia with anesthetizing doses (ca. 30 mg/kg) of pentobarbital varies widely with individual animals, averaging about 30 minutes. Complete recovery usually occurs in 6–18 hours. Occasionally, animals, particularly cats, may not rouse for as long as 24–72 hours. Because of the longer recoveries and availability of more predictable shorter acting agents, pentobarbital is no longer used in North America to produce anesthesia in most small companion animals. It is, however, the main component of most injectable euthanasia solutions.

Methohexital sodium

This is an ultrashort-acting barbiturate that is unique in that it contains no sulfur atom. Its short duration owes more to redistribution than to rapid metabolism. The dose for dogs or cats is 6–10 mg/kg of body weight. Half of the estimated dose is injected IV at a rapid rate, followed by administration to effect. Surgical anesthesia for 5–15 minutes is obtained by an initial injection. More prolonged anesthesia can be maintained by intermittent administration or continuous drip. Recovery is quick and may be accompanied by muscular tremors and violent excitement, which detract from the usefulness of the drug. Even with preanesthetic sedation, the recovery period is characterized by muscle tremors and struggling. Dogs are usually ambulatory 30 minutes after administration ceases.

Thiopental sodium

Thiopental is the thio-analog of pentobarbital sodium, and differs only in that the number 2 carbon has a sulfur atom instead of an oxygen atom attached to it. Thiopental has an ultrashort action because it is rapidly redistributed (e.g., into muscle tissue) and becomes localized in body fat. As concentrations in the plasma, muscle, and viscera fall, the thiopental concentration in fat continues to rise. On the other hand, an appreciable amount is metabolized by the liver, and this contributes to the early rapid reduction of arterial thiopental concentration.

For rapid induction of anesthesia of short duration, the dose is 10–12 mg/kg. Should 10–20 minutes of surgical anesthesia be required, the dose range is 20–30 mg/kg. One-third of the estimated dose is injected rapidly within 15 seconds, and the remainder is administered slowly to effect. Additional doses may be administered to prolong anesthesia when required. Following large-dose administration, recovery (to standing) usually requires 1–1.5 hours. Large doses will saturate the tissues and cause a prolonged emergence. When induction is preceded by preanesthetic sedation, a dose range of 8–15 mg/kg is used (Figure 2.10).

Occasionally, animals may struggle during induction of barbiturate anesthesia, and some of the drug may be administered perivascularly. This should be avoided if at all possible because a tissue slough may develop. If it is suspected that barbiturate solution has been injected perivascularly, the area should be infiltrated with 1 or 2 mL of 2% lidocaine solution. Local anesthetics are effective for two reasons. First, they are vasodilators and prevent vasospasm in the area, and thus aid in dilution and absorption of the barbiturate. Second, they are broken down in an alkaline medium, and this reaction neutralizes the alkali (barbiturate). The use of hot packs or hydrotherapy may be beneficial, as is infiltration of the area with saline to dilute the barbiturate further. Additionally, systemic anti-inflammatory drugs may be of benefit.

Neurosteroids

This class of drugs was first evaluated as a combination of two steroids: alphaxalone and alphadolone acetate. The combination of the two steroids has an exceptionally high

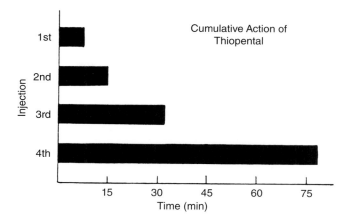

Figure 2.10. The average duration of anesthesia after successive hourly IV injections of equal doses of thiopental to dogs.
Sources: Adapted from data published in Wyngaarden J.N., Woods L.A., Ridley R., Seevers M.H. 1949. Anesthetic properties of sodium-5-allyl-5-(1-methylbutyl)-2-thiobarbiturate (Surital) and certain other thiobarbiturates in dogs. *J Pharmacol Exp Ther* **95**:322; and Branson K.R. 2007. Injectable and alternative anesthetic techniques. In: *Lumb and Jones' Veterinary Anesthesia and Analgesia*, 4th ed. W.J. Tranquilli, J.C. Thurmon, and K.A. Grimm, eds. Ames, IA: Blackwell Publishing, p. 284.

therapeutic index (30.6). It has little cumulative effect and the duration of anesthesia varies with species. A new neurosteroid product has been developed that is a 10 mg/mL solution of alphaxalone in 2-hydroxypropyl-ß-cyclodextrin (Alfaxan-CD; Jurox, Rutherford, Australia). This preparation does not appear to cause histamine release, which has been associated with the vehicle used in earlier neurosteroid preparations.

Etomidate

Etomidate appears to work in a fashion similar to that of propofol and the barbiturates in that it enhances the action of the inhibitory neurotransmitter GABA. Single injections produce relatively brief hypnosis. In dogs, doses of 1.5 and 3.0 mg/kg last 8 ± 5 and 21 ± 9 minutes, respectively. Etomidate is rapidly hydrolyzed in the liver and excreted in the urine. Induction and recovery are rapid, with a brief period of myoclonus early in the recovery period.

It was introduced in the United States as an induction agent for poor-risk human patients because it does not depress the cardiovascular and respiratory systems or release histamine. When used alone in dogs, it produces no change in HR, BP, or myocardial performance. Neonates born to mothers anesthetized with etomidate have minimal respiratory depression.

Etomidate inhibits adrenal steroidogenesis in dogs, suppressing the usual increase in plasma cortisol observed during surgery. A single induction dose of etomidate may depress adrenal function for up to 3 hours. However, the lack of a stress response to surgery does not have deleterious effects, and it has been argued that attenuation of metabolic and endocrine responses to surgery actually reduces morbidity and may make this unique action of etomidate beneficial to overall patient outcome. Attention has been given to the development of Addisonian crisis produced by etomidate-induced blockade of corticosteroid production during prolonged infusion to maintain sedation in intensive care patients. Consequently, long-term infusion is not recommended. Etomidate (2 mg/kg) can cause acute hemolysis. The mechanism of hemolysis appears to be propylene glycol, which causes a rapid osmolality increase that causes red cell rupture.

Etomidate is compatible with other common preanesthetic agents. Venous pain is common on injection in humans, and myoclonia may occur if premedication is not administered. Nausea and vomiting are troublesome, especially after the use of multiple doses, and can occur at recovery as well as induction. For the most part, these side effects can be prevented by adequate preanesthetic sedation. In summary, etomidate may be one of the better induction drugs in traumatized patients and those with severe myocardial disease, cardiovascular instability, cirrhosis, or intracranial lesions, or in patients requiring cesarean section surgery.

Propofol

Propofol (2,6-diisopropylphenol) is unrelated to barbiturates, euganols, or steroid anesthetics. Prior to 2010 it was marketed in the United States only as an aqueous emulsion containing 10 mg of propofol, 100 mg of soybean oil, 22.5 mg of glycerol, and 12 mg of egg lecithin/mL. Propofol emulsion can support microbial growth and endotoxin production. Because of the potential for iatrogenic sepsis, unused propofol remaining in an open ampule should be discarded and not be kept overnight for use the next day. Some formulations contain bacterial growth inhibitors to slow the growth rate of contaminants after a vial is opened, but these additives will not completely inhibit bacterial growth, so any unused propofol should still be discarded 6 hours after a vial or ampule is opened unless specifically labeled with a longer shelf life.

Rapid onset of action is caused by rapid uptake into the CNS. The short action and rapid smooth emergence result from rapid redistribution from the brain to other tissues and efficient elimination from plasma by metabolism. Propofol has a large volume of distribution, as would be expected from its lipophilic nature. It is metabolized primarily by conjugation, but propofol's rapid disappearance from plasma is greater than hepatic blood flow, suggesting extra hepatic sites of metabolism.

If administration is preceded by a preanesthetic such as morphine or dexmedetomidine, the induction dose of propofol can be decreased substantially. The dose for induction of anesthesia in nonpremedicated dogs ranges from 6 to 8 mg/kg IV, whereas the dose in sedated animals may be as low as 2–4 mg/kg IV. The continuous infusion rate for anesthetic maintenance ranges from 0.15 to 0.4 mg/kg/min. When using an intermittent bolus technique, doses of 0.5–2 mg/kg are administered as needed.

Propofol is a phenolic compound and, as such, can induce oxidative injury to feline red blood cells when administered repeatedly over several days. This toxicity is likely the result of the cat's reduced ability to conjugate phenol. Heinz bodies form, and clinical signs of anorexia, diarrhea, and malaise can result.

Dissociative anesthetics

The term dissociative anesthesia is used to describe an anesthetic state induced by drugs that interrupt ascending transmission from the parts of the brain responsible for unconscious and conscious functions, rather than by generalized depression of all brain centers, as seen with most other general anesthetics. Dissociative anesthesia is characterized by a cataleptoid state in which the eyes remain open with a slow nystagmic gaze. Varying degrees of hypertonus and purposeful or reflexive skeletal muscle movements often occur unrelated to surgical stimulation.

Analgesia produced by dissociative anesthetics occurs at subanesthetic doses. Elevated pain thresholds correlate with plasma ketamine concentrations of 0.1 µg/mL or greater. The degree of analgesia appears to be greater for somatic pain than for visceral pain. In cats, visceral analgesia induced by ketamine (2, 4, and 8 mg/kg, IV) is similar to that produced by butorphanol (0.1 mg/kg, IV). With increasing doses of ketamine, or when ketamine and butorphanol are administered simultaneously, visceral analgesia is not increased. At a high dose of ketamine (8 mg/kg), cats appear anesthetized but still respond to colonic nociceptor stimulation, suggesting limited visceral analgesia in cats and probably other species. Dissociative anesthetics appear to be more useful for anesthesia and postoperative analgesia related to integumentary and superficial musculoskeletal surgery.

N-methyl-D-aspartate (NMDA) receptors appear to be involved in hyperalgesic responses after peripheral tissue injury and inflammation, suggesting that ketamine (and possibly other dissociatives) would be effective at reducing hyperalgesia following tissue trauma. Local infiltration of ketamine may produce a brief period of local anesthetic effect. When administered simultaneously with bupivacaine, ketamine doubles the duration of analgesic and local anesthetic effects of bupivacaine. This peripheral analgesic effect of ketamine may be attributed to one or all of the following mechanisms: (1) blockade of sodium and potassium currents in peripheral nerves; (2) blockade of NMDA, a-amino-hydroxy-5-methyl-4-isoxazoleproprionic acid (AMPA), and kainate receptors on unmyelinated axons; and (3) blockade of glutamate effects on C-fiber free nerve endings.

Similar to systemic administration, epidural ketamine appears to produce profound somatic but poor visceral analgesia. Epidural administration produces a dose-dependent analgesic action.

Dissociative anesthetics induce significant increases in CBF, ICP, and CSF pressure as a result of cerebral vasodilation and elevated systemic BP. Dissociative anesthetics may not be contraindicated in all patients at risk for intracranial hypertension, particularly when administered in the presence of another anesthetic and/or when controlled ventilation is instituted. Nevertheless, administration of ketamine should be avoided in spontaneously breathing patients with suspected intracranial hypertension or disease until scientific evidence to the contrary emerges.

Abnormal behavior, which may progress to delirium, may occur during emergence from dissociative anesthesia. Depression of the inferior colliculus and medial geniculate nucleus leading to misperception of auditory and visual stimuli may be responsible for this reaction. Emergence reactions are characterized by ataxia, increased motor activity, hyperreflexia, sensitivity to touch, and sometimes violent recovery. These reactions usually disappear within several hours without recurrence.

The cardiovascular effects of dissociative anesthetics are characterized by indirect cardiovascular stimulation. Various effects on target organs include sympathomimetic effects mediated from within the CNS, inhibition of neuronal uptake of catecholamines by sympathetic nerve endings, direct vasodilation of vascular smooth muscle, and an inotropic effect on the myocardium. HR and arterial BP usually increase as a result of increased sympathetic efferent activity.

Ketamine has been shown to suppress activation of endotoxin-induced neuronal nuclear factor kB, which regulates the production of proinflammatory cytokines, including tumor necrosis factor alpha in human glioma cells *in vitro* and intact mouse brain cells *in vivo*. Therefore, in theory, ketamine may offer some neuroprotective effects during endotoxemia.

Dissociatives often cause increased salivation and respiratory tract secretions, which can be partially controlled by administration of an antimuscarinic (e.g., atropine). Laryngeal and pharyngeal reflexes are usually partially or fully maintained during dissociative anesthesia. Nevertheless, swallowing reflexes may be somewhat obtunded because most species can be intubated when anesthetized with ketamine. Careful airway management and/or endotracheal intubation should always be performed to prevent aspiration.

Clinical usage in dogs

Dissociatives can increase muscle tone and can induce spontaneous movement and rough recoveries, and occasionally convulsions, in dogs. To reduce these undesirable effects, dissociatives are often used in combination with adjunctive drugs. Benzodiazepines induce a central muscle relaxant effect that decreases the muscle hypertonus associated with ketamine. Zolazepam is combined with tiletamine in a fixed ratio in the proprietary mixture Telazol. This combination reduces the adverse effects of tiletamine when given alone, although the metabolism of zolazepam can vary among species and may result in a longer or shorter effect relative to tiletamine.

In dogs, IV continuous rate infusion of a low dose of ketamine (10 µg/kg/min) reduces the isoflurane MAC by 25%, whereas the continuous rate infusion of a combination of morphine (3.3 µg/kg/min), lidocaine (50 µg/kg/min), and ketamine (10 µg/kg/min) has reduced the isoflurane requirement by as much as 45%. Concurrent administration of either morphine–lidocaine or morphine–ketamine combinations reportedly reduces CNS hypersensitivity in people suffering inflammatory or neuropathic pain.

Clinical usage in cats

In cats, dissociatives have been used as primary anesthetic agents. Diazepam (0.3 mg/kg) is commonly mixed in the same syringe with ketamine (5.5 mg/kg) and given slowly IV for short-term anesthesia. This has proven to be a safe combination in cats with compromised cardiovascular function. Diazepam (0.22 mg/kg IV or 0.44 mg/kg IM) followed by ketamine (1–5 mg/kg IM) has also been used successfully in geriatric cats. Telazol has been used alone or in combination in cats. Zolazepam appears to be metabolized at a slower rate than tiletamine in this species, resulting in residual muscle relaxation and sedation, which often prolongs complete recovery. The use of oxymorphone, morphine, meperidine, and butorphanol has been assessed in combination with ketamine in cats.

Inhalation anesthetics

Inhalation anesthetics are used widely for the anesthetic management of animals. They are unique among the anesthetic drugs because they are administered, and in large part removed from the body, via the lungs. Their popularity arises in part because their pharmacokinetic characteristics favor predictable and rapid adjustment of anesthetic depth. In addition, a special apparatus is usually used to deliver the inhaled agents. This apparatus includes a source of oxygen (O_2) and a patient breathing circuit that, in turn, usually includes an endotracheal tube or face mask, a means of eliminating carbon dioxide (CO_2), and a compliant gas reservoir. These components help minimize patient morbidity or mortality because they facilitate lung ventilation and improved arterial oxygenation. In addition, inhalation anesthetics in gas samples can now be readily and affordably measured almost instantaneously. Measurement of inhalation anesthetic concentration enhances the precision and safety of anesthetic management beyond the extent commonly possible with injectable anesthetic agents.

Physiochemical characteristics

The chemical structure of inhalation anesthetics and their physical properties determine their actions and safety of administration. The physiochemical considerations given in Tables 2.1 and 2.2 determine and/or influence practical considerations of their clinical use. For example, they determine the form in which the agents are supplied by the manufacturer (i.e., as a gas or liquid) and account for the resistance of the anesthetic molecule to degradation by physical factors (e.g., heat and light) and substances it contacts during use (e.g., metal components of the anesthetic delivery apparatus and the CO_2 absorbents such as soda lime). The equipment necessary to deliver the agent safely to patients (e.g., vaporizer and breathing circuit) is influenced by some of these properties, as are the agent's uptake, distribution within, and elimination (including potential for metabolic breakdown) from the patient.

Chemical characteristics

All contemporary inhalation anesthetics are organic compounds except N_2O and xenon. Agents of current interest are further classified as either aliphatic (i.e., straight or branch chained) hydrocarbons or ethers (i.e., two organic radicals attached to an atom of oxygen; the general structure is ROR). In the continued search for a less reactive, more potent, nonflammable inhalation anesthetic, focus on halogenation (i.e., addition of fluorine, chlorine, or bromine; iodine is least useful) of these compounds has predominated.

Table 2.1. Some physical and chemical properties of inhalation anesthetics

Property	Desflurane	Enflurane	Halothane	Isoflurane	Methoxyflurane[a]	N$_2$O	Sevoflurane
Molecular weight (g)	168	185	197	185	165	44	200
Liquid specific gravity (20°C) (g/mL)	1.47	1.52	1.86	1.49	1.42	1.42	1.52
Boiling point (°C)	23.5	57	50	49	105	−89	59
Vapor pressure (mmHg)							
20°C	700[325]	172	243	240	23	—	160
24°C	804	207	288	286	28	—	183
mL vapor/mL liquid at 20°C	209.7	197.5	227	194.7	206.9	—	182.7
Preservative	None	None	Yes	None	Not available	None	Yes
Stability in:							
Soda lime	Yes	Yes	No	Yes	No	Yes	No
Ultraviolet light	Yes	Yes	No	Yes	No	Yes	?

Except for new citations where noted, references appear in the immediate past edition of this text and chapter.
[a] Methoxyflurane is no longer available.
Source: Steffey E.P., Mama K.R. 2007. Inhalation anesthetics. In: *Lumb and Jones' Veterinary Anesthesia and Analgesia*, 4th ed. W.J. Tranquilli, J.C. Thurmon, K.A. Grimm, eds. Ames, IA: Blackwell Publishing, p. 357.
N$_2$O, nitrous oxide.

Table 2.2. PCs (solvent/gas) of inhalation anesthetics at 37°C

Solvent	Desflurane	Enflurane	Halothane	Isoflurane	Methoxyflurane	N_2O	Sevoflurane
Water	—	0.78	0.82	0.62	4.50	0.47	0.60
Blood	0.42	2.00	2.54	1.46	15.00	0.47	0.68
Olive oil	18.70	96.00	224.00	91.00	970.00	1.40	47.00
Brain	1.30	2.70	1.90	1.60	20.00	0.50	1.70
Liver	1.30	3.70	2.10	1.80	29.00	0.38	1.80
Kidney	1.00	1.90	1.00	1.20	11.00	0.40	1.20
Muscle	2.00	2.20	3.40	2.90	16.00	0.54	3.10
Fat	27.00	83.00	51.00	45.00	902.00	1.08	48.00

Tissue samples are derived from human sources. Data are from sources referenced in the immediate past edition of this text and chapter.
Source: Steffey E.P., Mama K.R. 2007. Inhalation anesthetics. In: *Lumb and Jones' Veterinary Anesthesia and Analgesia*, 4th ed. W.J. Tranquilli, J.C. Thurmon, and K.A. Grimm, eds. Ames, IA: Blackwell Publishing, p. 359.
N_2O, nitrous oxide.

Physical characteristics

There is a constant interchange of respiratory gases (O_2 and CO_2) between cells and the external environment via blood. Inhalation anesthesia involves additional considerations whereby an anesthetic must be transferred under control from a container to sites of action in the CNS. Early in this process the agent is diluted to an appropriate amount (concentration) and supplied to the respiratory system in a gas mixture that contains at least enough O_2 to support life. The chain of events that ensues is influenced by many physical and chemical characteristics that can be quantitatively described.

The physical characteristics of importance to our understanding of the action of inhalation anesthetics can be conveniently divided into two general categories: those that determine the means by which the agents are administered and those that help determine their kinetics in the body. This information is applied in the clinical manipulation of anesthetic induction and recovery and in facilitating changes in anesthetic-induced CNS depression in a timely fashion.

Properties determining methods of administration A variety of physical and chemical properties determine the means by which inhalation anesthetics are administered. These include characteristics such as molecular weight, boiling point, liquid density (specific gravity), and vapor pressure. Inhalation anesthetics are either gases or vapors. In relation to inhalation anesthetics the term gas refers to an agent, such as N_2O, that exists in its gaseous form at room temperature and sea level pressure. The term vapor indicates the gaseous state of a substance that at ambient temperature and pressure is a liquid. With the exception of N_2O, all the contemporary anesthetics fall into this category. Desflurane is one of the volatile liquids that comes close to the transition stage and offers some unique considerations.

Whether inhalation agents are supplied as a gas or volatile liquid under ambient conditions, the same physical principles apply to each agent when it is in the gaseous state. Molecules move about haphazardly at high speeds and collide with each other or the walls of the containing vessel. The force of the bombardment is measurable and referred to as pressure. Relationships such as those described by Boyle's law (volume vs. pressure), Charles's law (volume vs. temperature), Gay-Lussac's law (temperature vs. pressure), and Dalton's Law of Partial Pressure (the total pressure of a mixture of gases is equal to the sum of the partial pressures of all of the gaseous substances present), among others, are important to our overall understanding of aspects of respiratory and anesthetic gases and vapors.

Quantities of inhalation anesthetic agent are usually characterized by one of three methods: pressure (i.e., in millimeters of mercury [mm Hg]), concentration (in volume percent [vol%]), or mass (in milligrams [mg] or grams [g]). The form most familiar to clinicians is that of concentration (e.g., X% of agent A in relation to the whole gas mixture). Modern monitoring equipment samples inspired and expired gases and provides concentration readings for inhalation anesthetics. Precision vaporizers used to control delivery of inhalation anesthetics are calibrated in percentage of agent, and effective doses are almost always reported in percentages.

Pressure is also an important way of describing inhalation anesthetics and is further discussed as a measure of anesthetic potency. A mixture of gases in a closed container will exert a pressure on the walls of the container. The individual pressure of each gas in a mixture of gases is referred to as its partial pressure.

Molecular weight and agent density are used in many calculations to convert from liquid to vapor volumes and mass. Briefly (and in simplified fashion), Avogadro's principle is that equal volumes of all gases under the same conditions of temperature and pressure contain the same number of molecules (6.0226×10^{23} [Avogadro's number] per gram molecular weight). Furthermore, under standard conditions the number of gas molecules in a gram molecular weight of a substance occupies 22.4 L. To compare properties of different substances of similar state, it is necessary to do so under comparable conditions; with respect to gases and liquids this usually means with reference to pressure and temperature. Physical scientists have arbitrarily selected standard conditions as being 0°C (273 K in absolute scale) and 760 mm Hg pressure (1 atmosphere at sea level). If conditions differ, appropriate temperature and/or pressure corrections must be applied to resultant data.

The weight of a given volume of liquid, gas, or vapor may be expressed in terms of its density or specific gravity. The density is an absolute value of mass (usually grams) per unit volume (for liquids, volume = 1 mL; for gases, 1 L at standard conditions). The specific gravity is a relative value, that is, the ratio of the weight of a unit volume of one substance to a similar volume of water in the case of liquids or air in the case of gases (or vapors) under similar conditions. The value of both air and water is 1. At least for clinical purposes, the value for density and specific gravity for an inhalation anesthetic is the same. Thus, for example, we can determine the volume of isoflurane gas (vapor) at 20°C from a milliliter of isoflurane liquid according to the scheme given in Figure 2.11. This type of calculation has practical applications.

Molecules of liquids are in constant random motion. Some of those in the surface layer gain sufficient velocity to overcome the attractive forces of neighboring molecules, and in escaping from the surface, enter the vapor phase. Molecules of a vapor exert a force per unit area or pressure in exactly the same manner as do molecules of a gas. The pressure (mm Hg) that the vapor molecules exert when the liquid and vapor phases are in

a. Isoflurane specific gravity = 1.49 g/mL, therefore:
   1 mL liquid isoflurane = 1 mL × 1.49 g/mL = 1.49 g

b. Since molecular weight of isoflurane = 185 g (from Table 2.1, then:
   1.49 g ÷ 185 g = 0.0081 mol of liquid

c. Since 1 mol of gas = 22.4 L, then:
   0.0081 mol × 22,400 mL/mol = 181.4 mL of isoflurane vapor at 0°C, 1 atm

d. But vapor is at 20°C not 0°C (i.e., 273 K),
   So, 181.4 × 293/273 = 194.7 mL vapor/mL liquid isoflurane at 20°C and at sea level pressure

   For substantial variation in ambient pressure, the final figure noted above would have to be further "corrected" by a factor of: 760/ambient barometric pressure

Figure 2.11. Example of calculations to determine the volume of isoflurane vapor at 20°C from 1 mL of isoflurane liquid.
Source: Steffey E.P., Mama K.R. 2007. Inhalation anesthetics. In *Lumb and Jones' Veterinary Anesthesia and Analgesia*, 4th ed. W.J. Tranquilli, J.C. Thurmon, and K.A. Grimm, eds. Ames, IA: Blackwell Publishing, p. 360.

equilibrium is known as the vapor pressure. Thus, the vapor pressure of an anesthetic is a measure of its ability to evaporate; that is, it is a measure of the tendency for molecules in the liquid state to enter the gaseous (vapor) phase. Herein lies a practical difference between substances classified as a gas or vapor: A gas can be administered over a range of concentrations from 0% to 100%, whereas the vapor has a ceiling that is dictated by its vapor pressure.

The saturated vapor concentration can be easily determined by relating the vapor pressure to the ambient pressure. For example, in the case of halothane, a maximal concentration of 32% halothane is possible under usual conditions (i.e., [244/760] × 100 = 32%, where 760 mm Hg is the barometric pressure at sea level). With other variables considered constant, the greater the vapor pressure, the greater is the concentration of the drug deliverable to a patient.

The barometric pressure also influences the final concentration of an agent. For example, in locations such as Denver, CO, where the altitude is about 5000 feet above sea level and the barometric pressure is only about 635 mm Hg, the saturated vapor concentration of halothane at 20°C is now (243/635) × 100 = 38.3%.

The boiling point of a liquid is defined as the temperature at which the vapor pressure of the liquid is equal to the atmospheric pressure. Customarily, the boiling temperature is stated at the standard atmospheric pressure of 760 mm Hg. The boiling point decreases with increasing altitude because the vapor pressure does not change, but the barometric pressure decreases. The boiling point of N_2O is −89°C at 1 atmosphere pressure at sea level. It is thus a gas under operating room conditions. Because of this, it is distributed for clinical purposes in steel tanks compressed to the liquid state at about 750 psi (pounds per square inch; 750/14.9 psi [1 atmosphere] = 50 atmospheres). As the N_2O gas is drawn from the tanks, liquid N_2O is vaporized, and the overriding gas pressure remains constant until no further liquid remains in the tank. At that point, only N_2O gas remains, and the gas pressure decreases from this point as remaining gas is vented from the tank. Consequently, the weight of the N_2O minus the weight of the tank, rather than the gas pressure within the tank, is a more accurate guide to the remaining amount of N_2O in the tank.

Desflurane possesses an interesting consideration because its boiling point is near room temperature. This characteristic accounted for an interesting engineering challenge in developing an administration device (i.e., a vaporizer) for routine use in the relatively constant environment of the operating room and limits further consideration of its use in all but a narrow range of circumstances commonly encountered in veterinary medical applications. For example, because of its low boiling point, even evaporative cooling has large influences on vapor pressure and thus the vapor concentration of gas mixtures delivered to patients.

Calculation of anesthetic concentration delivered by a vaporizer   The saturated vapor pressure of most volatile anesthetics is of such magnitude that the maximal concentration of anesthetic attainable at usual operating room conditions is above the range of concentrations that are commonly necessary for safe clinical anesthetic management. Therefore, some control of the delivered concentration is necessary and usually provided by a device known as a vaporizer. The purpose of the vaporizer is to dilute the vapor generated from the liquid anesthetic with O_2 (or an O_2 and N_2O mixture) to produce a more satisfactory inspired anesthetic concentration. This anesthetic dilution is usually accomplished by diverting the gas entering the vaporizer into two streams, one that enters the vaporizing chamber (anesthetic chamber volume: V_{anes}) and the other that bypasses the vaporizing chamber (dilution volume or $V_{dilution}$). If the vaporizer is efficient, the carrier gas passing through the vaporizing chamber becomes completely saturated to an anesthetic concentration (percent) reflected by (anesthetic agent vapor pressure/atmospheric pressure) $\times$ 100, at the vaporizer chamber temperature. The resultant anesthetic concentration then is decreased (diluted) downstream by the second gas stream to a "working" concentration. In modern, precision, agent-specific vaporizers no mental effort is required to set the dial; the manufacturers have precalibrated the vaporizer for accurate delivery of the dialed concentration.

To calculate the anesthetic concentration from the vaporizer, one must know the vapor pressure of the agent (at the temperature of use), the atmospheric pressure, the fresh gas flow entering the vaporizing chamber, and the diluent gas flow. Then:

% anesthetic = flow of anesthetic from the vaporizing chamber/total gas flow

More detail for interested readers is presented in Figure 2.12.

Properties influencing drug kinetics   Anesthetic gases and vapors dissolve in liquids and solids. The solubility of an anesthetic is a major characteristic of the agent and has important clinical ramifications. For example, anesthetic solubility in blood and body tissues is a primary factor in the rate of uptake and its distribution within the body. It is therefore a primary determinant of the speed of anesthetic induction and recovery. Solubility in lipid bears a strong relationship to anesthetic potency, and its tendency to

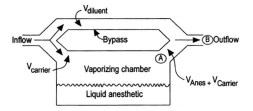

3

Steps:

1. The saturated *concentration* of anesthetic in the anesthetic vaporizing chamber and leaving it (ideally at A above) is calculated knowing the saturated vapor pressure (P_{VP}) (from Table 2.1) and barometric pressure (P_B).

For example:

$$\text{Halothane\%} = \frac{243}{760} \times 100 = 32.0\% \qquad (a)$$

2. The *volume* of anesthetic leaving the vaporizing chamber is the original volume of the carrier gas (O_2) entering the anesthetic vaporizing chamber ($V_{carrier}$) and the volume of anesthetic (V_{halo}) added to it.

$$\text{Halothane\%} - \frac{V_{halo}}{V_{carrier} + V_{halo}} \times 100. \qquad (b)$$

Halothane% is known from (a) above and $V_{carrier}$ is known from control of a flowmeter (e.g., a measured flow vaporizer) or via the design characteristics of a commercial, agent-specific, vaporizer that automatically "splits" the fresh gas flow from a single flow meter. In the first case, two gas flow controls are necessary, one for $V_{carrier}$ and one for a larger gas dilution flow ($V_{dilution}$). In either the case of manual or automatic fresh gas flow alteration, the equation is then solved for V_{halo} (expressed in mL of halothane vapor).

For example, if $V_{carrier} = 100$ mL O_2, then:

$$32\% = \frac{V_{halo}}{100 + V_{halo}} \times 100$$
$$3200 + 32V_{halo} = 100V_{halo}$$
$$3200 = 68V_{halo}$$
$$V_{halo} = 47.1 \text{ mL halothane vapor.}$$

3. V_{halo} is then contained in a total gas volume at B of

$$V_{total\ gas} = V_{halo} + V_{carrier} + V_{diluent} \qquad (c)$$

Where $V_{diluent}$ is set by the anesthetist using a second gas control (i.e., flowmeter; units here of mL/min) or by the vaporizer design and dial setting.

Then in our example for a $V_{diluent}$ of 1000 mL (in 1 minute)

$$V_{total} = 47.1 + 100 + 1000$$
$$= 1147 \text{ mL (rounded off)}$$

4. So the final halothane vapor concentration is determined by

$$\text{halothane \%} = \frac{V_{halo}}{V_{Total}} \times 100.$$

Again, in our example,

$$\text{halothane \%} = \frac{47.1}{1147} = 4.1\%.$$

Alternatively, with some basic algebraic work with equations given above, the same numbers can be applied to the resultant formula given below to arrive at the anesthetic concentration. The condensed formula is:

$$\text{Anesthetic concentration (\%)} = \frac{V_{carrier} \cdot P_{VP} \cdot 100}{V_{diluent} \cdot (P_B - P_{VP}) + (V_{carrier} \cdot P_B)}$$

Figure 2.12.   An anesthetic vaporizer to assist in illustrating the principles associated with the calculation of the vapor concentration of an inhalation anesthetic emerging from a vaporizer. Conditions associated with halothane delivery in San Francisco (i.e., sea level; barometric pressure = 760 mm Hg) at 20°C are used as an example of general principals. *Source*: Steffey E.P., Mama K.R. 2007. Inhalation anesthetics. In: *Lumb and Jones' Veterinary Anesthesia and Analgesia*, 4th ed. W.J. Tranquilli, J.C. Thurmon, and K.A. Grimm, eds. Ames, IA: Blackwell Publishing, p. 363.

dissolve in anesthetic delivery components such as rubber goods influences equipment selection and other aspects of anesthetic management.

Within the body there is a partition of anesthetic gases between blood and body tissues in accordance with Henry's law. This process can perhaps be better understood by visualizing a system composed of three compartments (e.g., gas, water, and oil) contained in a closed container. In such a system the gas overlies the oil, which in turn overlies the water. Because there is a passive gradient from the gas phase to the oil, gas molecules move into the oil compartment. This movement in turn develops a gradient for the gas molecules in oil relative to water. If gas is continually added above the oil, there will be a continual net movement of the gas molecules from the gas phase into both the oil and, in turn, the water. At a given temperature, when no more gas dissolves in the solvent, the solvent is said to be fully saturated. At this point the pressure of the gas molecules within the three compartments will be equal, but the amount (i.e., the number of molecules or volume of gas) partitioned between the two liquids will vary with the nature of the liquid and gas.

Finally, it is important to understand that the amount of gas that goes into solution depends on the temperature of the solvent. Less gas dissolves in a solvent as temperature increases, and more gas is taken up as solvent temperature decreases. The extent to which a gas will dissolve in a given solvent is usually expressed in terms of its solubility coefficient. With inhalation anesthetics, solubility is most commonly measured and expressed as a PC. Other measurements of solubility include the Bunsen and Ostwald solubility coefficients.

The PC is the concentration ratio of an anesthetic in the solvent and gas phases (e.g., blood and gas) or between two tissue solvents (e.g., brain and blood). It thus describes the capacity of a given solvent to dissolve the anesthetic gas; that is, how the anesthetic will partition itself between the gas and the liquid solvent phases after equilibrium has been reached. Remember, anesthetic gas movement occurs because of a partial pressure difference in the gas and liquid solvent phases, so when there is no longer any anesthetic partial pressure difference there is no longer any net movement of anesthetic, and equilibrium has been achieved.

Solvent–gas PCs are summarized in Table 2.2. The values noted in this table are for human tissues because these values are most widely available in the anesthesia literature. Regardless of the species, it is important to emphasize that many factors can alter anesthetic agent solubility. Perhaps the most notable after the nature of the solvent is temperature. Of all the PCs that have been described or are of interest, two are of particular importance in the practical understanding of anesthetic action. They are the blood–gas and the oil–gas solubility coefficients.

Blood–gas PCs provide a means for predicting the speed of anesthetic induction, recovery, and change of anesthetic depth. Assume, for example, that anesthetic A has a blood–gas PC value of 15. This means that the concentration of the anesthetic in blood will be 15 times greater at equilibrium than that in alveolar gas. Expressed differently, the same volume of blood, say 1 mL, will hold 15 times more of anesthetic A than 1 mL of alveolar gas despite an equal partial pressure. Alternatively, consider anesthetic B with a PC of 1.4. This PC indicates that, at equilibrium, the amount of anesthetic B is only 1.4 times greater in blood than it is in alveolar air. Comparing the PC of anesthetic A with that of anesthetic B indicates that anesthetic A is much more soluble in blood than B (nearly 11 times more soluble: 15/1.4). From this, and assuming other conditions are equal, anesthetic A will require a longer time of administration to attain a partial pressure in the body for a particular end point (say, anesthetic induction) than will anesthetic B. Also, since there is more of anesthetic A contained in blood and other body tissues under similar conditions, elimination (and therefore anesthetic recovery) will be prolonged when compared with anesthetic B.

Uptake and elimination of inhalation anesthetics

The aim in administering an inhalation anesthetic to a patient is to achieve an adequate partial pressure or tension of anesthetic (P_{anes}) in the CNS to cause a desired level of depression commensurate with the definition of general anesthesia. Anesthetic depth varies directly with P_{anes} in brain tissue. The rate of change of anesthetic depth is of obvious clinical importance and depends directly on the rate of change in anesthetic tensions in the various media in which it is contained before reaching the brain. Thus, knowledge of the factors that govern these relationships is of fundamental importance to skillful control of general inhalation anesthesia.

Inhalation anesthetics are unique among the classes of drugs that are used to produce general anesthesia because they are administered via the lungs. The pharmacokinetics of the inhaled anesthetics describe the rate of their uptake by blood from the lungs, distribution in the body, and eventual elimination by the lungs and other routes.

Anesthetic uptake

Inhalation anesthetics move down a series of partial pressure gradients from regions of higher tension to those of lower tension until equilibrium is established. Thus, on induction, the P_{anes} at its source in a vaporizer is high, as is dictated by the vapor pressure, and progressively decreases as anesthetic travels from vaporizer to patient breathing circuit, from circuit to lungs, from lungs to arterial blood, and, finally, from arterial blood to body tissues (e.g., the brain) (Figure 2.13). At this point it may be also helpful to recall that although the partial pressure of anesthetic is of primary importance, we frequently define clinical dose of an inhaled anesthetic in terms of concentration (C; i.e., vol%). As previously noted, this is because it is common practice for clinicians to regulate and/or measure respiratory and anesthetic gases in volume percent. In addition, in the gaseous phase, the relationship between the P_{anes} and the C_{anes} is a simple one:

P_{anes} = fractional anesthetic concentration × total ambient pressure

Anesthetic elimination

Recovery from inhalation anesthesia results from the elimination of anesthetic from the CNS. This requires a decrease in alveolar anesthetic partial pressure (concentration), which in turn fosters a decrease in arterial and then CNS anesthetic partial pressure.

Prominent factors accounting for recovery are the same as those for anesthetic induction. Therefore, factors such as V_A, CO, and especially agent solubility greatly influence recovery from inhalation anesthesia. Indeed, the graphic curves representing the washout of anesthetic from alveoli versus time are essentially inverses of the wash-in curves. That is, the washout of the less soluble anesthetics is high at first and then rapidly declines to a lower output level that continues to decrease but at a slower rate. The washout of more soluble agents is also high at first, but the magnitude of decrease in alveolar anesthetic concentration is less and decreases more gradually with time.

Biotransformation

Inhalation anesthetics are not chemically inert. They undergo varying degrees of metabolism primarily in the liver but also, to lesser degrees, in the lung, kidney, and intestinal tract. The importance of this is twofold. First, in a very limited way with older

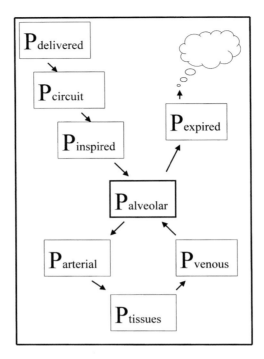

Figure 2.13. The flow pattern of inhalation anesthetic agents during anesthetic induction and recovery. Inhalation anesthesia may be viewed as the development of a series of partial pressure gradients. During induction there is a high anesthetic partial pressure in the vaporizer that decreases progressively as the flow of anesthetic gas moves from its source to the brain. Some of these gradients are easily manipulated by the anesthetist; others are not or are done so with difficulty.
Source: Steffey E.P., Mama K.R. 2007. Inhalation anesthetics. In: *Lumb and Jones' Veterinary Anesthesia and Analgesia*, 4th ed. W.J. Tranquilli, J.C. Thurmon, and K.A. Grimm, eds. Ames, IA: Blackwell Publishing, p. 365.

anesthetics, metabolism may facilitate anesthetic recovery. Second and more important is the potential for acute and chronic toxicities by intermediary or end metabolites of inhalation agents, especially on kidneys, liver, and reproductive organs.

The magnitude of metabolism of inhalation anesthetic agents is determined by a variety of factors, including the chemical structure, hepatic enzyme activity (cytochrome P-450 enzymes located in the endoplasmic reticulum of the hepatocyte), the blood concentration of the anesthetic, disease states, and genetic factors (i.e., some species and individuals are more active metabolizers of these drugs than are others, e.g., humans compared to rats).

Sevoflurane degrades *in vivo* to about the same extent as isoflurane and as indicated by transient postanesthetic increases in blood and urinary fluoride levels. The peak serum fluoride concentrations observed in people during and after sevoflurane anesthesia are low, and nephrotoxicity is not expected. Desflurane resists degradation *in vivo*. The increase in serum inorganic fluoride is much smaller than that found with isoflurane.

Anesthetic dose: The MAC

In 1963, Merkel and Eger described what has become the standard index of anesthetic potency for inhalation anesthetics: the MAC. The MAC is defined as the minimum alveolar concentration of an anesthetic at 1 atmosphere that produces immobility in 50% of subjects exposed to a supramaximal noxious stimulus. Thus, the MAC corresponds to the median effective dose (ED_{50}): Half of the subjects are anesthetized and half have not yet reached that "level." The dose that corresponds to the ED_{95} (95% of the individuals are anesthetized), at least in people, is 20–40% greater than the MAC. Anesthetic potency of an inhaled anesthetic is inversely related to the MAC (i.e., potency = 1/MAC). From information presented earlier, it also follows that the MAC is inversely related to the oil–gas PC. Thus, a very potent anesthetic like the formally available agent methoxyflurane, which has a high oil–gas PC, has a lower MAC, whereas an agent with a low oil–gas PC has a higher MAC.

A number of characteristics of the MAC deserve emphasis. First, the *A* in MAC represents alveolar concentration, not inspired or delivered (e.g., as from a vaporizer). This is important because the alveolar concentration is easily monitored with contemporary technology. Also, as we reviewed earlier, after sufficient time for equilibration (minutes), alveolar partial pressure will more closely approximate arterial and brain anesthetic partial pressures.

Second, the MAC is defined in terms of volume percent of 1 atmosphere and therefore represents an anesthetic partial pressure (P) at the anesthetic site of action; that is, remember,

$$P_x = (C/100) \cdot P_{bar},$$

where P_x stands for the partial pressure of the anesthetic in the gas mixture, C is the anesthetic concentration in volume percent, and P_{bar} is the barometric or total pressure of the gas mixture. Thus, although the concentration at the MAC for a given agent may vary depending on ambient pressure conditions (e.g., sea level vs. high altitude), the anesthetic partial pressure always remains the same. For example, the MAC for isoflurane in healthy dogs is reported as 1.63 vol%. The study reporting this value was conducted at near sea level conditions at Davis, CA (i.e., P_{bar} = 760 mm Hg). Based on the foregoing discussion, a MAC of 1.63 vol% represents an alveolar isoflurane partial pressure (P_{iso}) of 11.6 mm Hg. In comparison, for the same dog at Mexico City (elevation, 2240 m above sea level; P_{bar} = 584 mm Hg), the alveolar P_{iso} at the MAC is expected to be the same as determined at Davis (i.e., 11.6 mm Hg), whereas the MAC (i.e., the alveolar concentration) would be about 2.17 vol%.

Finally, it is important to note that the MAC is determined in healthy animals under laboratory conditions in the absence of other drugs and circumstances common to clinical use that may modify the requirements for anesthesia. General techniques for determining the MAC in animals are given elsewhere.

In a single species the variability in the MAC (response to a noxious stimulus) is generally small and not substantially influenced by gender, duration of anesthesia, variation in $PaCO_2$ (from 10 to 90 mm Hg), metabolic alkalosis or acidosis, variation in PaO_2

(from 40 to 500 mm Hg), moderate anemia, or moderate hypotension. Even between species the variability in the MAC for a given agent is usually not large.

In humans, the MAC for N_2O is 104%, making it the least potent of the inhalation anesthetics currently used in this species. Its potency in other species is less than half that in humans (i.e., around 200%). Because the N_2O MAC is above 100% it cannot be used by itself at 1 atmosphere pressure in any species and still provide adequate amounts of O_2. Consequently, and assuming that the MAC values for combinations of inhaled anesthetics are additive, N_2O is usually administered with another more potent inhalant agent to thereby reduce the concentration of the second agent necessary for anesthesia. However, because of the potency difference between animals and people, the amount of reduction differs in an important way. For example, administration of 60% N_2O with halothane reduces the amount of halothane needed to produce the MAC by about 55% in healthy people but reduces it only by about 20–30% in dogs.

Equipotent doses (i.e., equivalent concentrations of different anesthetics at the MAC) are useful for comparing effects of inhalation anesthetics on vital organs. In this regard anesthetic dose is commonly defined in terms of multiples of the MAC (i.e., 1.5 or 2.0 times the MAC or simply 1.5 MAC or 2.0 MAC). From the preceding discussion, therefore, the ED_{50} equals the MAC or 1.0 MAC and represents a light level of anesthesia (clearly inadequate in 50% of otherwise unmedicated, healthy animals). The ED_{95} is 1.2–1.4 MAC, and 2.0 MAC represents a deep level of anesthesia, in some cases even an anesthetic overdose. The concept of MAC multiples can be used to compare drug effects and contrast pharmacodynamics of multiple doses of a specific drug.

Actions and toxicity of the volatile anesthetics

All contemporary inhalation anesthetic agents in one way or another influence vital organ function. Some actions are inevitable and accompany the use of all agents, whereas other actions are a special or prominent feature of one or a number of the agents. In addition, dose–response relationships of inhalation anesthetics are not necessarily parallel. Differences in action, and especially undesirable action, of specific anesthetic agents form the basis for selecting one agent over another for a particular patient and/or procedure. Undesirable actions also provide primary impetus for development of new agents and/or anesthetic techniques.

CNS

Inhalation anesthetics affect the CNS in many ways. Mostly these agents are selected because they induce a reversible, dose-related state of CNS (somatic and motor) unresponsiveness to noxious stimulation: that is, a state of general anesthesia. Interestingly, although clinical anesthesia was introduced more than 150 years ago, the sites and mechanisms by which general anesthetics (including the inhalation anesthetics) cause unresponsiveness to surgical or other forms of noxious stimulation remain unknown. Traditionally, this summary state we refer to as general anesthesia was assumed to result from a focus in the brain. However, mounting evidence is causing a shift in thinking such that this state we know as general anesthesia is likely the collection of a number of end points that are distinct and site specific, and include supraspinal and spinal events.

Electroencephalographic effects   The electroencephalograph (EEG) is used to help identify pathological brain disorders and to predict the outcome of brain insults. Studies have also shown that general anesthesia alters EEG parameters, and we apply this knowledge to better understand anesthetic circumstances. In general, as the depth of anesthesia increases from awake states, the electrical activity of the cerebral cortex becomes desynchronized. With further increases in anesthetic concentration, a decrease in frequency and increased amplitude of the EEG waves occur. The wave amplitude increases to a peak (about 1 MAC), and then, with further dose increase, the amplitude progressively declines (burst suppression occurs at about 1.5 MAC; i.e., bursts of slow high-voltage activity separated by electrical silence) and eventually becomes flatline (predominance of electrical silence). With isoflurane, an isoelectric pattern occurs at about 2.0 MAC, whereas, on the other extreme, it is not seen with halothane until >3.5 MAC. The two newest volatile anesthetics—sevoflurane and desflurane—cause dose-related changes similar to those of isoflurane.

Cerebral metabolism   All volatile anesthetics decrease cerebral metabolic rate (CMR; cerebral O_2 consumption). The magnitude of decrease is least with halothane but similar with isoflurane, sevoflurane, and desflurane.

CBF   The volatile anesthetics cause no change or often an increase in CBF. The net effect is likely the sum of a tendency both to decrease CBF due to anesthetic-induced reductions in cerebral O_2 consumption, while increasing CBF due to vasodilation caused by direct anesthetic action on vascular smooth muscle. The rank order of CBF increase is generally regarded as halothane > enflurane, isoflurane, desflurane, and sevoflurane (all four being similar).

ICP   The inhalation anesthetics increase ICP, and this change parallels the CBF increase that similarly accompanies these agents. It is generally regarded across species lines that ICP increases can be decreased by hyperventilation and decreasing $PaCO_2$. Accordingly, use of hyperventilation is a common strategy in clinical situations in which even small elevations in ICP are of special concern.

Analgesia   A clinically desirable general anesthetic includes both hypnotic and analgesic actions. However, studies to differentiate hypnotic potency from analgesic potency within the anesthetic concentration range are, at the least, difficult to interpret. Studies of subanesthetic concentrations of inhalation anesthetics have been performed but with conflicting results. Some inhalation anesthetics have been reported to increase the response threshold to noxious stimulation compared with similar, but unmedicated, conditions (e.g., diethyl ether), whereas others (e.g., isoflurane and sevoflurane) do not change the threshold, and still others, like halothane, may decrease the threshold for response and contribute a heightened awareness to noxious stimulation (i.e., antianalgesia).

Respiratory system

Inhalation anesthetics depress respiratory system function. The volatile agents, in particular, decrease ventilation in a drug-specific and species-specific manner. Depending on conditions, including species of interest, some of the most commonly considered measures of breathing effectiveness—that is, f and V_T—may not be revealing or may even be misleading. In general, spontaneous ventilation progressively decreases as inhalation anesthetic dose is increased, because at low dose, V_T decreases more than f increases. As anesthetic dose is further increased, f also decreases. In otherwise unmedicated animals (as well as people) anesthetized with volatile agents, respiratory arrest occurs at 1.5–3.0 MAC. The overall decrease in V_E and the likely variable increase in dead-space ventilation reduce V_A. In addition, the normal stimulation of ventilation caused by increased $PaCO_2$ (or decreased PaO_2) is depressed by the inhalation anesthetics, presumably via the action of these agents directly on the medullary and peripheral (aortic and carotid body) chemoreceptors. Changes in perianesthetic PaO_2, other than what might be related to the magnitude of V_A, are not notably different among the various inhalation anesthetics in a given species.

Cardiovascular system

All of the volatile inhalation anesthetics cause dose-dependent and drug-specific changes in cardiovascular performance. The magnitude and sometimes direction of change may be influenced by other variables that often accompany general anesthesia. The mechanisms of cardiovascular effects are diverse but often include direct myocardial depression and a decrease in sympathoadrenal activity.

All of the volatile anesthetics decrease CO. The magnitude of change is dose related and depends on the agent. In general, among the contemporary agents in use with animals, halothane depresses CO the most. Desflurane in many ways is similar in cardiovascular action to isoflurane, whereas sevoflurane has characteristics resembling both halothane and isoflurane. All three of the newer volatile anesthetics tend to preserve CO at clinically useful concentrations. The decrease in CO is largely due to a decrease in SV as a result of dose-related depression in myocardial contractility.

The effect of inhalation anesthetics on HR is variable and depends on agent and species. For example, in humans, HR is not substantially altered with halothane anesthesia but is usually increased by isoflurane, desflurane, and sevoflurane. Compared with conditions in awake, calm dogs, HR is increased with the use of any of the four anesthetics listed. There is evidence to suggest that differences between agents in the degree of increase in HR in dogs are explained by differences in the vagolytic activity of the agents. In dogs, the HR usually remains constant over a range of clinically useful alveolar concentrations in the absence of other modifying factors (e.g., noxious stimulation). The distribution of blood flow to organs is altered during inhalation anesthesia.

Volatile anesthetics cause a dose-dependent decrease in arterial BP. In general the dose-related decrease in arterial BP is similar regardless of the species studied. In animals, the dose-related decrease in BP with all four of the contemporary agents is usually related, mostly to a decrease in SV. In some cases (agent and/or species) a decrease in peripheral vascular resistance may also play an important, but lesser, role. This common scenario in animals differs from results generally reported from studies with people anesthetized at least with isoflurane, sevoflurane, and desflurane, whereby pressure decreases primarily from a decrease in SVR.

Inhalation anesthetics may increase the automaticity of the myocardium and the likelihood of propagated impulses from ectopic sites, especially from within the ventricle. Although spontaneously derived dysrhythmias were most notable with earlier inhalation anesthetics (e.g., halothane), none of the three most recently introduced ether-derivative agents appear to predispose the heart to generated extrasystoles.

Drugs administered immediately before or in conjunction with inhalation anesthetics (preanesthetic medication, injectable anesthetic induction drugs, vasoactive and cardiotonic drugs, etc.) may influence cardiovascular function by altering the anesthetic requirement (i.e., the MAC and thereby increase or decrease anesthetic level) or by their own direct action on cardiovascular performance. Injectable drugs, such as acepromazine, alpha$_2$ agonists, thiobarbiturates, and dissociatives (e.g., ketamine), are frequently administered to animals as part of their anesthetic management. These drugs confound the primary effects of the inhalation anesthetics and may accentuate cardiovascular depression.

Effects on the kidneys

It is generally regarded that present-day volatile anesthetics produce similar mild, reversible, dose-related decreases in renal blood flow and glomerular filtration rate and that such changes largely reflect an anesthetic-induced decrease in CO. However, some studies show little or no change in these kidney-related parameters. As a consequence of the anesthetic-induced decrease in glomerular filtration, healthy anesthetized animals commonly produce a smaller volume of concentrated urine compared with when awake. An increase in serum urea nitrogen, creatinine, and inorganic phosphate may accompany especially prolonged anesthesia.

The reduction in renal function is highly influenced by an animal's state of hydration and hemodynamics during anesthesia. Accordingly, attendant IV fluid therapy and prevention of a marked reduction in renal blood flow will lessen or counteract the tendency for reduced renal function. In most cases, effects of inhalation anesthesia on renal function are rapidly reversed after anesthesia.

Among the inhalation anesthetics, methoxyflurane is the most nephrotoxic. Although it is no longer available for use in human or in animal patients, its actions are of pathophysiological interest and therefore is briefly reviewed here. Particularly in humans and in some strains of rats, the use of methoxyflurane caused renal failure that was characterized not by oliguria but by a large urine volume unresponsive to vasopressin. This was caused by the biotransformation of methoxyflurane and the large release of free fluoride ion that, in turn, directly damaged the renal tubules. With the possible exception of enflurane and sevoflurane, the breakdown of other inhalation anesthetics does not pose a risk of fluoride-induced nephrotoxicity. Biotransformation of enflurane and sevoflurane by humans following a moderate duration of anesthesia causes serum inorganic fluoride concentrations to increase even beyond the 50 µmol/L level, which is normally considered the nephrotoxic threshold in humans. However, clinical, histological, or biochemical evidence of injury related to increases in fluoride has only rarely been reported in human patients. The overriding consensus is that sevoflurane has little potential for nephrotoxicity caused by defluorination.

Two factors may explain the general lack of injury despite the body's ability to degrade sevoflurane. In 1977, Mazze et al. proposed that the area under the serum fluoride concentration-versus-time curve may be a more important determinant of nephrotoxicity than is peak serum fluoride concentration. Because sevoflurane is poorly soluble and is rapidly eliminated via the lungs, the duration of its availability for biotransformation is notably limited. More recently, Kharasch and coworkers proposed another consideration: Sevoflurane is primarily metabolized by the liver, whereas hepatic and renal sites are important for methoxyflurane breakdown. The relative lack of intrarenal anesthetic defluorination may markedly reduce its nephrotoxic potential.

Sevoflurane is degraded by CO_2 absorbents such as soda lime and Baralyme (Chemetron Medical Division, Allied Healthcare Products, St. Louis, MO). A nephrotoxic breakdown product, compound A, is produced. Compound A can cause renal injury and death in rats, and the concentration threshold for nephrotoxicity in rats is within the range of concentrations that may be found associated with the anesthetic management of human patients. Not surprisingly, compound A is formed in the rebreathing circuits used for animals in veterinary medical practice. The ultimate importance of *in vitro* sevoflurane degradation to the well-being of veterinary patients like dogs and cats remains to be established, but clinical impression is that the risk is relatively low.

Effects on the liver

Depression of hepatic function and hepatocellular damage may be caused by the action of volatile anesthetics. Effects may be mild and transient or permanent, and injury may be by direct or indirect action. A reduction in intrinsic hepatic clearance of drugs along with anesthetic-induced alteration of other pharmacokinetically important variables (e.g., reduced hepatic blood flow) fosters a delayed drug removal or an increase in plasma drug concentration during anesthesia.

All of the potent inhalation anesthetics can cause hepatocellular injury by reducing liver blood flow and oxygen delivery. However, available data suggest that, of the four contemporary volatile anesthetics, isoflurane is most likely to better maintain tissue O_2 supply and thereby is the agent least likely to produce liver injury even when administered for prolonged periods. The effects of the two newest agents, sevoflurane and desflurane, are nearly similar to isoflurane, whereas halothane produces the most striking adverse changes.

It now appears that halothane produces two types of hepatotoxicity in susceptible individuals. One is a mild, self-limiting postanesthetic form of hepatocellular destruction and associated increase in serum concentrations of liver enzymes. Signs of hepatotoxicity occur shortly after anesthetic exposure. The other is a rare, severe, often fatal hepatotoxicity with delayed onset and largely clinically limited to human patients (i.e., halothane hepatitis) and thought to be an immune-mediated toxicity.

Effects on skeletal muscle: Malignant hyperthermia

Malignant hyperthermia (MH) is a potentially life-threatening pharmacogenetic myopathy that is most commonly reported in susceptible human patients and swine (e.g., Landrace, Pietrain, or Poland China strains). However, reports of its occurrence in other species are available. All of the four contemporary volatile anesthetics can initiate MH, but halothane is the most potent triggering agent relative to other inhalation anesthetics. The syndrome is characterized by a rapid rise in body temperature that, if not treated quickly, causes death. Monitoring of temperature and CO_2 production is warranted in susceptible or suspected patients. Patients known to be susceptible to MH can be anesthetized safely. Avoiding the use of triggering agents and administering prophylactic dantrolene before anesthesia are effective in preventing the onset of MH.

Nitrous oxide-specific toxicities

Nitrous oxide was introduced into clinical practice more than 150 years ago. Since then, its use has formed the basis for more general anesthetic techniques in human patients than any other single inhalation agent. Its use became widespread because of its many desirable properties, including low blood solubility, limited cardiovascular and respiratory system depression, and apparently relatively minimal toxicity. Its use in the anesthetic management of animals became a natural extension of its use in people.

Despite its use, nitrous oxide is not the ideal anesthetic for people or animals. To derive the important benefits from the use of N_2O, it is usually administered in high inspired concentrations. However, as the concentration of N_2O is increased, there is a change in the proportion and partial pressure of the various other constituents of the inspired breath, notably O_2. Consequently, to avoid hypoxemia, 75% of the inspired breath is the highest concentration that can be administered safely under conditions at sea level. Use of N_2O at locations above sea level requires a lower N_2O concentration to ensure an adequate partial pressure of inspiratory O_2 (PiO_2). Nitrous oxide has less value in the anesthetic management of animals than in that of human patients because the anesthetic potency of N_2O in animals is only about half of that found for humans, thus, the value of N_2O in veterinary clinical practice is primarily as an anesthetic adjuvant.

Nitrous oxide's low blood solubility is responsible for a rapid onset of action. Although it does not have the potency to produce anesthesia, it may be used to speed induction of inhalation anesthesia as a result of its own (albeit limited) CNS effects and, as mentioned earlier, also by augmenting the uptake of a concurrently administered more potent volatile anesthetic such as halothane (the second gas effect). When a high concentration of N_2O is administered concurrently in a mixture with an inhalation agent (e.g., N_2O plus halothane), the alveolar concentration of the simultaneously administered anesthetic (halothane) increases more rapidly than when the "second" gas has been administered without N_2O. The second gas effect is the result of an increased inspiratory volume secondary to the large volume of N_2O taken up (remember, N_2O is used at high concentrations), and a concentrating effect on the second gas in a smaller volume (and thus increased gradient for transfer to blood) as a result of the uptake of the large volume of N_2O.

N_2O's effects on cardiovascular and respiratory function (other than reducing the inspired O_2 concentration) are small compared with other inhalation anesthetics. It does depress myocardial function directly, but its sympathetic stimulation properties counteract some of the direct depression (its own as well as that from accompanying volatile anesthetics). As a result of its sympathetic nervous system activation it may contribute to an increased incidence of cardiac arrhythmias. Overall, a conservative outlook regarding N_2O use relative to respiration and circulation is that significant concern is warranted only in patients with initially compromised function. As with any agent, its advantages and disadvantages should be weighed on an individual patient basis.

Nitrous oxide has little or no effect on liver and kidney function. Although there is evidence of N_2O-induced interference with the production of red and white blood cells by bone marrow, the risk of adverse outcomes to a patient exposed under most clinical veterinary circumstances is little or none. However, prolonged exposure to N_2O causes megaloblastic hematopoiesis and polyneuropathy. Seriously ill patients may have increased sensitivity to these toxicities. Problems result from N_2O-induced inactivation of the vitamin B_{12}-dependent enzyme methionine synthase, an enzyme that controls interrelations between vitamin B_{12} and folic acid metabolism. Although an occasional patient may develop signs suggestive of vitamin B_{12} and folic acid deficiency after an anesthetic technique that includes the use of N_2O, this is a rare event in human and animal patients.

Nitrous oxide is rapidly and mainly eliminated in the exhaled breath. The extent of biotransformation (to molecular nitrogen [N_2]) is very small and mainly by intestinal flora.

Transfer of nitrous oxide to closed gas spaces   Gas spaces exist or may exist in the body under a variety of conditions and to varying degrees. For example, gas is normally found in the stomach and intestines. The gut is a dynamic reservoir; the gas it contains is freely movable into and out of it according to the laws of diffusion. The gas in the gut originates from air swallowing, normal production of bacteria, chemical reactions, and diffusion from the blood. There is marked variability in both composition and volume of stomach and bowel gas (e.g., herbivore vs. carnivore). There are other natural air cavities, such as the air sinuses and the middle ear, and then there are circumstances in which air may be electively or inadvertently introduced as part of diagnostic or therapeutic actions (e.g., pneumoencephalogram, pneumocystogram, endoscopy, and vascular air emboli).

Potential problems associated with gas spaces arise when an animal breathing air is given a gas mixture containing N_2O. Nitrogen is the major component of air (80%) and of most gas spaces (methane, CO_2, and hydrogen are also found in variable quantities in the gut). When N_2O is introduced into the inspired breath, a reequilibration of gases in the gas space begins with N_2O quickly entering and N_2 slowly leaving. That is, because of its greater blood solubility, the volume of N_2O that can be transported to a closed gas space is many times the volume of N_2 that can be carried away. For example, the blood–gas PC for N_2O is 0.47, whereas that for N_2 is about 0.015. Thus, N_2O is more than 30 times more soluble in blood than is N_2 (0.47/0.015). The result of the net transfer of gas to the gas space can be manifested as an increase in volume, as with the gut, pneumothorax, or vascular air embolus; an increase in pressure (e.g., middle ear or pneumoencephalogram); or both (as the distending limits of the compliant space are reached). Usually air is used to inflate the cuff of an endotracheal tube. This cuff is another relatively compliant, enclosed air space. Nitrous oxide will similarly expand this gas space and may increase the pressure exerted on the tracheal wall.

Occupational exposure: Trace concentrations of inhalation anesthetics

Operating room personnel are often exposed to low concentrations of inhalation anesthetics. Ambient air is contaminated via vaporizer filling, known and unknown leaks in the patient breathing circuit, and careless spillage of liquid agent. Measurable amounts of anesthetic gases and vapors are present in operating-room air under a variety of conditions. Personnel inhale and, as shown by studies, retain these agents for some time. The slow rate of elimination of some vapors (especially the more blood-soluble agents like halothane) enables retained trace anesthetic quantities to accumulate from one day to the next.

Concern is raised because epidemiological studies of humans and laboratory studies of animals have suggested that chronic exposure to trace levels of anesthetics may constitute a health hazard. Of particular concern are reports that inhaled anesthetics possess mutagenic, carcinogenic, or teratogenic potential. Depending on the point in life at which exposure occurs, there is concern that these underlying mechanisms, in turn, may be responsible for an increased incidence of fetal death, spontaneous abortion, birth defects, or cancer in exposed workers. However, to date, no genotoxic effect of long-term or short-term exposure to inhaled anesthetics has been demonstrated in humans.

Although the data to date, especially regarding effects on human reproduction, remain equivocal, a firm cause-and-effect relationship between chronic exposure to trace levels of anesthetics and human health problems does not exist. Although the risk of long-term exposure to trace concentrations of anesthetics for those in operating room conditions appears minimal, current evidence is suggestive enough to cause concern and to encourage practices to reduce the contamination by anesthetics of operating room personnel. Indeed, exposure levels have been recommended by the government: 2.0 parts per million (ppm) for volatile agents and 25 ppm for N_2O. In this regard, inexpensive methods to reduce and control anesthetic exposure by operating room personnel are available and should be used.

Muscle relaxants and neuromuscular blockade

Muscle relaxants are anesthetic adjuncts administered to improve relaxation of skeletal muscles during surgical or diagnostic procedures. The term neuromuscular blocking agents (NMBAs) is a cumbersome, but descriptive, name that refers to this class of drugs producing their effect by actions at the neuromuscular junction. The more general term muscle relaxant refers to any drug that has relaxant properties and would include centrally acting agents such as benzodiazepines, $alpha_2$ adrenoceptor agonists, and guaifenesin. Although used frequently in human anesthesia and in some veterinary specialties such as ophthalmology, the use of NMBAs in general veterinary practice is limited.

Physiology of the neuromuscular junction

All NMBAs exert their effects at the neuromuscular junction, which forms the interface between the large myelinated motor nerve and the muscle that is supplied by that nerve. The neuromuscular junction itself may be divided into the prejunctional motor nerve ending, the synaptic cleft, and the postjunctional membrane of the skeletal muscle fiber. Present on the prejunctional and postjunctional areas of the neuromuscular junction are nicotinic receptors, which bind and respond to ACh or another suitable ligand. The prejunctional receptor is thought to be important in the synthesis and mobilization of ACh stores, but not for its release. There appear to be two types of postjunctional receptors: junctional and extrajunctional. The junctional receptors are found on the motor end plates of normal adult animals and are responsible for interacting with the released ACh, initiating muscle contraction. Antagonism of ACh at the junctional receptors is responsible for the relaxant effect seen when an NMBA is administered. The extrajunctional receptors are not present in high numbers on the skeletal muscle membranes of adult mammals, but are important because they are synthesized by muscles that are receiving a less than normal degree of motor nerve stimulation. Thus, their number may be increased following spinal cord injury or after a period of muscle disuse, such as when a limb is cast. They are also present in neonates. Extrajunctional receptors appear to be more responsive to depolarizing NMBAs such as succinylcholine and less responsive to nondepolarizing NMBAs such as atracurium. If the degree of neuromuscular deficit is severe, extrajunctional receptors may be more numerous and widely distributed over the muscle membrane. Such patients may have a more intense response to the actions of a depolarizing NMBA and a more profound release of intracellular potassium ions (K^+) with its concomitant adverse cardiac effects.

The prejunctional nerve endings synthesize and store a quantity of ACh in synaptic vesicles. During normal neuromuscular transmission, an action potential arrives at the prejunctional motor nerve ending, causing depolarization of the nerve terminal. ACh is rapidly hydrolyzed into choline and acetate by acetylcholinesterase. Thus, the muscle cell is depolarized by the end-plate potential created by the binding of ACh to the receptor and then is repolarized as the ACh is removed from the receptor and hydrolyzed.

Depolarizing and nondepolarizing drugs

Depolarizing and nondepolarizing neuromuscular junction-blocking drugs both have an affinity for, and bind to, nicotinic ACh receptors at the neuromuscular junction; however, their intrinsic activity at the receptor is very different. Nondepolarizing drugs bind to the receptor but do not activate it. Their onset of action is characterized by a progressive weakening of muscle contraction and, ultimately, flaccid paralysis. Depolarizing drugs also bind to the receptor and, similar to ACh, the receptor is stimulated, causing depolarization of the postjunctional membrane. Unlike ACh, succinylcholine and other depolarizing NMBAs are not susceptible to breakdown by acetylcholinesterase and thus the ion channel remains open and repolarization does not occur. The persistent state of depolarization associated with administration of depolarizing NMBAs causes inexcitability of the motor end plate and, as with nondepolarizing NMBA, flaccid paralysis results. In addition to the differing mechanism of action of depolarizing drugs, several other differences are clinically apparent when comparing depolarizing and nondepolarizing NMBAs.

Succinylcholine administration can cause muscle fasciculations immediately prior to the development of flaccid paralysis. Large doses, repeated administration, or administration of succinylcholine as an infusion causes the character of the block to change from the aforementioned classic depolarizing action (i.e., phase I block) to a phase II block, which resembles that of nondepolarizing drugs such as d-tubocurarine. Despite years of investigation into the genesis of phase II block, its mechanism is still not clearly understood.

Prolonged exposure of the cholinergic receptors to the agonist succinylcholine likely causes receptor desensitization, channel blockade, or a combination of both. Both receptor desensitization and channel blockade have properties that would mimic those of the nondepolarizing NMBAs and thus would change the mechanism and nature of the succinylcholine-induced block.

Individual neuromuscular blocking drugs

The NMBAs are quaternary ammonium compounds that mimic the quaternary nitrogen atom of ACh. They are attracted to the nicotinic receptors at the motor end plate, as well as to nicotinic receptors located in autonomic ganglia. Most NMBAs are positively charged, water-soluble compounds that have a limited volume of distribution and, in many cases, limited hepatic biotransformation. The low lipid solubility exhibited by the NMBAs limits drug transfer across membrane structures, including the placenta and blood–brain barrier. Hepatic metabolism and redistribution to sites other than the skeletal muscles are not major mechanisms in the termination of NMBA effects. An exception is vecuronium, where biliary excretion is important in its elimination from the body. Because of their water solubility, most NMBAs are excreted by glomerular filtration and are generally not reabsorbed by the renal tubules. The water-soluble nature of these drugs may also contribute to the observation that neonates may require relatively higher doses of NMBAs because neonates have a higher percentage of body water than do adults and typically higher apparent volumes of distribution for water-soluble drugs. Recommended doses of muscle relaxants used in common domesticated species are listed in Table 2.3.

Table 2.3.   Doses of commonly used NMBAs in some domestic species

Drug (mg/kg)	Dog	Cat	Horse
Succinylcholine	0.3–0.4	0.2	0.12–0.15
Pancuronium	0.07	0.06	0.12
Atracurium	0.15–0.2	0.15–0.25	0.07–0.15
Vecuronium	0.1–0.2	0.025–0.05	0.1
Pipecuronium	0.05	0.003	

Source: Martinez E.A., Keegan R.D. 2007. Muscle relaxants and neuromuscular blockade. In: *Lumb and Jones' Veterinary Anesthesia and Analgesia*, 4th ed. W.J. Tranquilli, J.C. Thurmon, and K.A. Grimm, eds. Ames, IA: Blackwell Publishing, p. 423.

Succinylcholine   This is currently the only depolarizing NMBA used in veterinary medicine. Structurally, the succinylcholine molecule is two ACh molecules joined end to end. This drug is rapidly hydrolyzed in plasma by pseudocholinesterase (plasma cholinesterase), so only a small fraction of the injected dose survives degradation in plasma to reach the site of action at the neuromuscular junction. Very little pseudocholinesterase is present in the synaptic cleft, so succinylcholine-induced paralysis is terminated by diffusion of the drug away from the neuromuscular junction and into the extracellular fluid. Paradoxically, the rapid degradation of succinylcholine in the plasma is in some way responsible for the rapid onset of effect achieved by the drug. Because of the rapid degradation by plasma pseudocholinesterase, comparatively large doses of succinylcholine may be administered without worry of an increased duration of effect. The higher the succinylcholine dose, the more rapid the onset of paralysis will be. This strategy does not apply when using nondepolarizing NMBAs, where a significant increase in the duration of action will follow increased dosages.

Pseudocholinesterase is synthesized in the liver, and production is decreased by liver disease, chronic anemia, malnutrition, burns, pregnancy, cytotoxic drugs, metoclopramide, and cholinesterase inhibitor drugs. Additionally, species differences in pseudocholinesterase activity may exist. A reduction in plasma cholinesterase activity can be expected to prolong the action of succinylcholine.

Pancuronium   Pancuronium was the first in a series of nondepolarizing NMBAs having a steroid nucleus. The drug has a dose-dependent onset of approximately 5 minutes and action ranging from 40 to 60 minutes in dogs. A large fraction of the drug is excreted by the kidney and the remainder is metabolized by the liver. In addition to having affinity for the nicotinic receptors at the neuromuscular junction, pancuronium can also inhibit cardiac muscarinic receptors, thus mildly to moderately increasing HR in some patients.

Atracurium   This is a short-acting nondepolarizing NMBA having a benzylisoquinoline structure similar to that of d-tubocurarine. The drug has a dose-dependent onset of action of approximately 5 minutes, and its action lasts approximately 30 minutes in dogs. Repeated doses do not tend to be cumulative, so neuromuscular blockade is sometimes maintained via continuous IV infusion. Atracurium is unique in that almost half of it is degraded by Hofmann elimination and nonspecific ester hydrolysis. The remaining fraction is degraded by as yet undefined routes, although evidence exists that its action is not prolonged in people in hepatic or renal failure. Hepatic metabolism and renal excretion are not necessary for termination of effect. Consequently, atracurium may be administered to patients with hepatic or renal insufficiency without significantly increasing its duration of action.

Hofmann elimination is a process of spontaneous molecular decomposition and appears to be pH and temperature dependent. It does not require enzymatic activity. Because Hofmann elimination may occur *ex vivo*, atracurium should be kept refrigerated and is supplied at a pH of 3.25–3.65. When injected intravenously, it spontaneously decomposes into laudanosine and a quaternary monoacrylate at physiological pH and temperature. The laudanosine metabolite is a known CNS stimulant and can induce seizures. Unlike atracurium, laudanosine is almost totally dependent on hepatic biotransformation for elimination; thus, laudanosine plasma concentrations may be elevated in patients who have hepatic insufficiency and are given atracurium for longer surgical procedures.

Ester hydrolysis of atracurium is accomplished by several plasma esterases unrelated to plasma cholinesterase. In contrast to succinylcholine metabolism, the duration of action of atracurium is not prolonged in the presence of cholinesterase inhibitors.

Many NMBAs having the benzylisoquinoline structure are associated with histamine release and a varying degree of hypotension. Newer drugs having the benzylisoquinoline structure, such as atracurium and mivacurium, require several times the effective dose for neuromuscular blockade before appreciable amounts of histamine are released. Although signs of histamine release, such as hypotension and tachycardia, are not usually observed when atracurium is administered, slow IV administration is always preferred.

Cisatracurium   Atracurium is a racemic mixture of 10 optical isomers. The 1R-cis, 1R9-cis isomer, or cisatracurium, comprises approximately 15% of racemic atracurium, is approximately four times more potent, and has much less potential for histamine release. For example, in cats, plasma histamine concentrations were unchanged when up to 60 times the effective dose of cisatracurium was administered. Cisatracurium has a similar onset time and duration of action to atracurium. Hofmann elimination metabolizes more than half the administered dose of cisatracurium, but, unlike with the racemic compound, ester hydrolysis does not occur. As with atracurium, Hofmann elimination causes laudanosine production. Since cisatracurium is approximately fourfold as potent as atracurium, the administered dose is correspondingly less, as is production of laudanosine.

Vecuronium   Introduced in the 1980s, this was one of the first NMBAs free of cardiovascular effects. This drug has a dose-dependent onset of action of approximately 5 minutes and an intermediate duration of action similar to that of atracurium: 30 minutes. As with atracurium, a cumulative effect with subsequent doses is not a prominent feature of this drug. Vecuronium is unstable when prepared in solution and is supplied as a lyophilized powder that is reconstituted with sterile water prior to injection. The powder does not need refrigeration and, once reconstituted, the solution is stable for 24 hours. Slightly more than half of the drug is metabolized by hepatic microsomal enzymes and excreted in the bile while a significant fraction undergoes renal elimination.

Rocuronium   This is a derivative of vecuronium, having approximately one-eighth the potency of the parent compound. Since vecuronium and rocuronium have similar molecular weights and rocuronium has lower potency, a higher injected dose of rocuronium places a greater number of molecules near the neuromuscular junction, translating into a more rapid onset of neuromuscular blockade. The rapid onset of effect of rocuronium makes the drug an attractive nondepolarizing alternative to succinylcholine for tracheal intubation. Its duration of action in dogs is similar to that of vecuronium and atracurium. Similar to vecuronium, rocuronium seems to be without cardiovascular effects and does not release histamine. The primary route of elimination is via the hepatic system while a small fraction is eliminated via the kidney.

Doxacurium   This is a very potent benzylisoquinoline NMBA with a long duration of action. Similar to other benzylisoquinoline NMBAs such as atracurium, doxacurium does not have vagolytic properties or cause ganglion blockade. Similar to cisatracurium, administration of clinical doses does not cause appreciable histamine release. Doxacurium appears to be minimally metabolized and is excreted unchanged into the bile and urine.

Mivacurium   This drug is a rapid-acting, short-duration NMBA marketed for use in humans for facilitating tracheal intubation at anesthetic induction. Similar to atracurium, mivacurium can induce histamine release if high doses are administered. Mivacurium is rapidly biotransformed by plasma pseudocholinesterase, and metabolites do not have appreciable neuromuscular blocking activity. Its dose-dependent duration of action differs between species. The action of typical doses used in humans lasts approximately 25 minutes, about one-half to one-third less than that of atracurium. Mivacurium also shows marked differences in potency among species, being much more potent in dogs than in people. In dogs, one-third of the human dose is associated with blockade that is five times longer. The differences in duration of action between species may in part reflect the reduced activity of pseudocholinesterase in dogs, because normal plasma cholinesterase concentrations for dogs are reportedly from 19% to 76% of human values. Also, canine pseudocholinesterase enzyme might have differing affinity for the three primary isomers of mivacurium. Clinical observations indicate that mivacurium has a much briefer action in cats than in dogs.

Precautions

Because the muscles of respiration are paralyzed, ventilation must be controlled, either by a mechanical ventilator or by a staff member who can manually ventilate the patient until muscle strength is restored. Muscle relaxants have no sedative, anesthetic, or analgesic properties, so it is critical that the animal be adequately anesthetized to render it completely unconscious. Assessing the level of anesthesia in a paralyzed patient is more difficult than in a nonparalyzed patient because the usual indicators of depth (e.g., purposeful movement in response to a noxious stimulus, palpebral response, and jaw tone) are abolished. When including an NMBA in an anesthetic protocol, anesthetists must be certain they can reliably maintain an adequate plane of surgical anesthesia and level of ventilation.

Reversal of neuromuscular blockade

As previously reviewed, acetylcholinesterase is present in high concentrations at the neuromuscular junction. It hydrolyzes ACh into choline and acetic acid, terminating the effects of ACh. The effects of nondepolarizing muscle relaxants are antagonized by administering an anticholinesterase (also known as an acetylcholinesterase inhibitor). This class of drugs inhibits the enzyme acetylcholinesterase, increasing the concentration of ACh molecules at the neuromuscular junction. Since nondepolarizing muscle relaxants and ACh compete for the same postsynaptic binding sites, the ACh increase can tip the balance of competition in favor of ACh, and neuromuscular transmission is restored.

The anticholinesterase drugs used to antagonize neuromuscular blockade include edrophonium, neostigmine, and pyridostigmine. They differ in how they inhibit acetylcholinesterase activity. Edrophonium produces a reversible inhibition by electrostatic attachment to the anionic site and by hydrogen bonding at the esteratic site on acetylcholinesterase. The action of edrophonium is relatively brief because a covalent bond is not formed and ACh can easily compete with edrophonium for access to the enzyme. Neostigmine and pyridostigmine inhibit acetylcholinesterase by forming a carbamylester complex at the esteratic site of acetylcholinesterase. This bond lasts longer when compared with the bond of the enzyme with ACh, thereby preventing acetylcholinesterase from accessing ACh.

The ACh accumulation following the administration of an anticholinesterase drug is not specific to the neuromuscular junction. While nicotinic effects occur at the neuromuscular junction and autonomic ganglia, muscarinic cholinergic effects occur because of inhibition of acetylcholinesterase at the sinus node, smooth muscle, and glands. Clinical effects of increased ACh concentrations at these sites include bradycardia, sinus arrest, bronchospasm, miosis, intestinal hyperperistalsis, and salivation. For this reason, it is advised that an anticholinergic drug, either atropine or glycopyrrolate, be administered immediately prior to reversal of neuromuscular blockade with an anticholinesterase.

Recovery from succinylcholine (phase I block) is rapid and spontaneous because of succinylcholine hydrolysis by plasma cholinesterases. Recovery may be delayed in patients with decreases in plasma cholinesterase levels or activity. The administration of an anticholinesterase would actually prolong the depolarizing block. On the other hand, a phase II block from succinylcholine can be antagonized similarly to the nondepolarizing muscle relaxants, emphasizing the need for determining the type (phase I or phase II) of block present when using succinylcholine.

Revised from "Cardiovascular System" by William W. Muir; "Respiratory System" by Wayne N. McDonell and Carolyn L. Kerr; "Nervous System" by Kurt A. Grimm and Anne E. Wagner; "Anticholinergics and Sedatives" by Kip A. Lemke; "Injectable and Alternative Anesthetic Techniques" by Keith R. Branson; "Dissociative Anesthetics" by Hui-Chu Lin; "Inhalation Anesthetics" by Eugene P. Steffey and Khursheed R. Mama; and "Muscle Relaxants and Neuromuscular Blockade" by Elizabeth A. Martinez and Robert D. Keegan in Lumb & Jones' Veterinary Anesthesia and Analgesia, Fourth Edition.

Chapter 3

Pain physiology, pharmacology, and management

Peter W. Hellyer, Sheilah A. Robertson,
Anna D. Fails, Leigh A. Lamont, Karol A. Mathews,
Roman T. Skarda, Maria Glowaski, Dianne Dunning,
and Duncan X. Lascelles

Introduction

The prevention and control of pain are central to the practice of veterinary medicine. It is essential that clinicians have an understanding of the physiological processes leading to the perception of pain and the responses of patients to this process. Ultimately, anesthetic patient management is the control of pain and maintenance of homeostasis in the face of noxious stimuli. The perioperative analgesic protocol has an impact on patient well-being that often extends far beyond the immediate anesthetic period. Appropriate pain management is not only integral to an anesthetic plan; it is a fundamental component of good medical practice.

Definition of pain

Pain is an unpleasant sensory and emotional experience (perception) associated with actual or potential tissue damage or is described in terms of such damage. The inability to communicate in no way negates the possibility that an individual is experiencing pain and is in need of appropriate pain-relieving treatment.

Nociceptive pain arises from the activation of a discrete set of receptors and neural pathways by noxious stimuli that are actually or potentially damaging to tissues. Pain is a conscious awareness of acute or chronic nociceptive stimulation occurring in varying degrees of severity resulting from injury and disease, or abnormal neural processing associated with emotional distress as evidenced by biologic or behavioral changes or both. Pain elicits protective motor actions, results in learned avoidance, and may modify

Essentials of Small Animal Anesthesia and Analgesia, Second Edition. Edited by Kurt A. Grimm, William J. Tranquilli, Leigh A. Lamont.

species-specific traits of behavior, including social behavior. Acute pain is the result of a traumatic, surgical, or infectious event that begins abruptly and is relatively brief. It is generally alleviated by analgesic drugs. Chronic pain is pain that persists beyond the usual course of an acute disease or beyond a reasonable time for an injury to heal, or that is associated with a chronic pathological process or neurological dysfunction that persists or recurs for months or years (e.g., osteoarthritis). Chronic pain is seldom permanently alleviated by analgesics, but may respond to a combination of analgesics, tranquilizers or psychotropic drugs, physical therapy, environmental manipulation, and behavioral conditioning. Acute pain is a symptom of disease, whereas chronic pain, in and of itself, is a disease of altered neuroprocessing. Acute pain has a biologic function in that it serves as a warning that something is wrong and leads to protective behavioral changes. Chronic pain does not serve a biologic function and imposes severe detrimental stresses. Because pain is a perception, it is always subjective.

In people, pain experience has three dimensions—sensory-discriminative, motivational-affective, and cognitive-evaluative—that are subserved by physiologically distinct systems. The sensory-discriminative dimension provides information on the onset, location, intensity, type, and duration of the pain-inducing stimulus. This aspect is subserved primarily by the lateral ascending nociceptive tracts, thalamus, and somatosensory cortex. The motivational-affective dimension disturbs the feeling of well-being of the individual, resulting in the unpleasant experience of pain and suffering, and triggers the organism into action. This dimension is closely linked to the autonomic nervous system, and cardiovascular, respiratory, and gastrointestinal responses are associated with it (although these can also occur reflexly). This dimension is subserved by the medial ascending nociceptive tracts and their input into the limbic system. The cognitive-evaluative dimension encompasses the effects of prior experience, social and cultural values, anxiety, attention, and conditioning. These activities are largely caused by cortical activity, although cortical activation is dependent on reticular activity. The cognitive-evaluative dimension of the pain experience in lower mammals may be the only one that differs significantly from that in people.

To discuss pain physiology and its management requires a review of the definitions commonly used to describe this perception.

Agology The science and study of pain phenomena.
Allodynia Pain caused by a stimulus that does not normally provoke pain.
Analgesia The absence of pain in the presence of stimuli that would normally be painful.
Analgesics Drugs that produce analgesia.
Anesthesia The absence of all sensory modalities.
Anesthetics Drugs that induce regional anesthesia (i.e., in one part of the body) or general anesthesia (i.e., unconsciousness).
Cancer pain Pain that is caused by primary tumor growth, metastatic disease, or the toxic effects of chemotherapy and radiation, such as neuropathies caused by neurotoxic antineoplastic drugs.
Causalgia A syndrome of prolonged burning pain, allodynia, and hyperpathia after a traumatic nerve lesion, often combined with vasomotor and sudomotor (sweating) dysfunction and later trophic changes.

Central pain Pain associated with a lesion or altered neurophysiology of the central nervous system (CNS).

Chronic pain Pain that persists for longer than the expected time frame for healing or pain associated with progressive nonmalignant disease (such as osteoarthritis).

Deafferentation pain Pain caused by loss of sensory input into the CNS, as occurs with avulsion of the brachial plexus or other types of peripheral nerve lesions, or caused by pathology of the CNS.

Dermatome The sensory segmental supply to skin and subcutaneous tissue.

Distress The external expression through emotion or behavior (i.e., fear, anxiety, hyperactivity, or aggression) of suffering.

Dysesthesia An unpleasant abnormal sensation, whether spontaneous or evoked.

Hyperalgesia An increased response to a stimulation that is normally painful.

Hyperesthesia An increased sensitivity to stimulation, excluding special senses.

Hypoalgesia A diminished sensitivity to noxious stimulation.

Hypoesthesia A diminished sensitivity to stimulation, excluding special senses.

Inflammatory pain Spontaneous pain and hypersensitivity to pain in response to tissue damage and inflammation.

Neuralgia Pain in the distribution pathway of a nerve or nerves.

Neuritis Inflammation of a nerve or nerves.

Neuropathic pain Spontaneous pain and hypersensitivity to pain in association with damage to or a lesion of the nervous system.

Neuropathy A disturbance of function or a pathological change in a nerve.

Nociception The reception, conduction, and central nervous processing of nerve signals generated by the stimulation of nociceptors. It is the physiological process that, when carried to completion, results in the conscious perception of pain.

Nociceptive pain Transient pain in response to noxious stimuli.

Nociceptor A receptor preferentially sensitive to a noxious stimulus or to a stimulus that would become noxious if prolonged.

Nociceptor threshold The minimum strength of stimulus that will cause a nociceptor to generate a nerve impulse.

Noxious stimulus One that is actually or potentially damaging to body tissue. It is one of intensity and quality that are adequate to trigger nociceptive reactions in an animal, including pain in people.

Pain (detection) threshold The least experience of pain that an individual can recognize. The point at which an individual just begins to feel pain when a noxious stimulus is being applied in an ascending trial or the point at which pain disappears in a descending trial. The pain-detection threshold is relatively constant among individuals and species. In most cases, it is higher than the nociceptor threshold.

Pain tolerance The greatest level of pain that an individual will tolerate. Pain tolerance varies considerably among individuals, both human and animal. It is influenced greatly by the individual's prior experience, environment, stress, and drugs.

Pain-tolerance range The arithmetic difference between the pain-detection threshold and the pain-tolerance threshold.

Paresthesia An abnormal sensation, whether spontaneous or evoked. Paresthesias are not painful (as opposed to dysesthesias).

Radiculalgia Pain along the distribution of one or more sensory nerve roots.

Radiculitis Inflammation of one or more nerve roots.

Radiculopathy A disturbance of function or pathological change in one or more nerve roots.

Reactions A combination of reflexes designed to produce widespread movement in relation to the application of a stimulus. Reactions are mass reflexes not under voluntary control and therefore do not involve the cerebral cortex.

Reflexes Involuntary, purposeful, and orderly responses to a stimulus. The anatomical basis for the reflex arc consists of a receptor, a primary afferent nerve fiber associated with the receptor, a region of integration in the spinal cord or brain stem (synapses), and a lower motor neuron leading to an effector organ such as skeletal muscles (somatic reflexes), smooth muscles, or glands (visceral reflexes).

Responses Willful movement of the body or parts of the body. A response cannot occur without involvement of the somatosensory cerebral cortex. A decerebrate animal can give a reaction but not a response. Reflexes and reactions may or may not be perception linked (i.e., the stimulus perceived as painful). Because responses require a functioning somatosensory cortex, the initiating stimulus must first be perceived.

Somatic Usually used to describe input from body tissues other than viscera.

Suffering An unpleasant emotional state that is internalized and not expressed outwardly. It is described as an undesirable mental state or as an unpleasant emotion that people or animals would normally prefer to avoid. Suffering can refer to a wide range of intense and unpleasant subjective states, such as fear and frustration. It can be of either physical or psychological origin. Suffering can be provoked by pain or by pain-free nontissue-damaging external stimuli such as denial of the fulfillment of an animal's natural instincts or needs, such as maternal deprivation, social contacts, and so on.

Neuroanatomy of nociceptive pathways

Nociceptors and stimuli

Nociception is the reception of signals from activation of nociceptors, which are receptors that detect tissue-damaging (noxious) stimuli. Pain implies that noxious stimuli have been perceived at the cortical level. Activating stimuli for nociceptors can include mechanical, thermal, or chemical stimuli. Some nociceptors respond only to one of these modalities, whereas others are sensitive to a variety of them (polymodal nociceptors). Nociceptors are naked (nonencapsulated) nerve endings, widely distributed in skin and deep tissues. These represent the peripheral termini of nociceptive primary afferent neurons that possess lightly or unmyelinated, small-diameter axons. Activation of fast-conducting (5–30 m/s), A-δ fibers are associated with sharp, pricking pain (as reported by humans). Slow-conducting (0.5–2.0 m/s), unmyelinated C fibers are associated with a slower, burning type of pain. Both types of nociceptive fibers innervate the skin (superficial pain) and deep somatic or visceral structures (deep pain). The distinction between superficial and deep pain is not just an arbitrary one based on "outside" and "inside." Each is associated with an anatomically and functionally segregated central pain pathway; they are differentially susceptible to injury, and they are examined separately in a neurological exam.

Pain research has revealed the presence of a particular functional type of nociceptor referred to as a silent nociceptor. The high threshold of this nerve ending ensures that under normal circumstances it is relatively insensitive to any stimuli. Following release of tissue-inflammatory mediators, however, the threshold is markedly reduced, and these previously silent nociceptors can be activated by a variety of thermal and mechanical stimuli. The presence of silent nociceptors is one mechanism by which inflammation produces primary hyperalgesia.

Divergence in nociceptive pathways

In addition to the connections of ascending nociceptive pathways with somatosensory cortex for conscious perception, nociceptive pathways exhibit variable degrees of connectivity with a number of subcortical regions of the brain, and through these connections elicit a variety of nonconscious responses.

A behaviorally important aspect of nociception (and other sensory modalities) is the degree to which it affects mental alertness. This relationship between sensation and consciousness is orchestrated in the reticular formation (RF), a loose aggregate of nuclei in the central core of the brain stem, extending from the diencephalon through the medulla oblongata. Functions of the RF include regulation of heart and respiratory rates, selective attention to stimuli, and maintenance of consciousness and cortical alertness. The RF is critical to the regulation of the level of consciousness through its rostral projections to the diencephalon, which, in turn, diffusely excites the cerebral cortex. The RF receives input from all afferent pathways, although the degree to which these connections are made is variable, depending on the pathway. Stimuli—but most especially noxious stimuli—increase alertness and autonomic functions, such as heart and respiratory rates.

Nociceptive information is simultaneously directed to the hypothalamus, which is the brain's coordinator of elaborate autonomic responses and the primary integrator of physiological and emotional responses. Input from nociceptive pathways to the hypothalamus produces activity in the sympathetic nervous system and the pituitary gland and thus increases circulating epinephrine/norepinephrine and glucocorticoids. The catabolic and other endocrinologic manifestations of this activation can have negative effects on health.

Both the hypothalamus and the RF have projections to other parts of the limbic system, a group of cortical and subcortical regions that produce the behavioral, cognitive, and physiological changes that people describe as emotions.

Nociceptive pathways send collateral projections to the mesencephalon (midbrain). One set of nuclear targets in the midbrain consist of motor neurons that coordinate orienting movements of the head and eyes toward the noxious stimulus (the visual grasp reflex). Other neurons that form the periaqueductal gray matter (PAG) of the midbrain activate important descending pain modulatory systems.

Ascending spinal pathways

Multiple nociceptive pathways that have been described in the spinal cord of domestic animals are present in all funiculi of the cord and with a confusing degree of overlap in their functions. None of these pathways are exclusive for transmission of nociception (all have fibers conducting tactile information). For clinical purposes, only two need be understood fully: the spinocervicothalamic and spinoreticular tracts.

The spinocervicothalamic tract is concerned with the transmission of superficial pain and tactile sensations and is regarded as the primary conscious pain pathway in carnivores. The primary afferents of this pathway synapse in the dorsal horn, from which secondary afferents then mediate local reflexes and project craniad in an ipsilateral tract in the dorsal part of the lateral funiculus. The axons in this tract ascend to spinal cord segments C1 and C2, where they synapse in the lateral cervical nucleus. The fibers arising from this nucleus will then decussate and project through the brain stem to the thalamus. Some collaterals of the ascending fibers will terminate in the RF. From the thalamus, fibers project to the somatosensory cortex.

The sensations transmitted by the spinocervicothalamic tract are touch and superficial pain. This pathway is discriminative in that the location of the painful stimulus can be precisely determined by the animal, which is a quality linked to the high degree of somatotopy exhibited by this pathway. Clinically, the function of the spinocervicothalamic tract is tested by lightly pinching the skin with fingers or a mosquito hemostat. This stimulus is applied lightly and briefly so as to activate the spinocervicothalamic pathway preferentially.

The spinoreticular tract is primarily concerned with transmission of deep-pain and visceral sensations. The primary afferents of this pathway enter the cord and immediately diverge to send collaterals several segments rostral and caudal to the segment of entry. This spreading of information across several spinal cord segments enables these afferents to participate in intersegmental reflexes (various manifestations of withdrawal and postural reflexes in response to painful stimuli). Second-order neurons are found in the dorsal horn. Axons of projection neurons in this system are present diffusely in the lateral and ventral funiculi. These projections are bilateral; decussation of axons in this system occurs diffusely throughout the long axis of the spinal cord.

Most ascending projections of the spinoreticular tract that reach the brain stem do not project directly to the thalamus; rather, they terminate in the RF. Therefore most deep pain that is consciously perceived arrives at the cortex via diffuse reticular projections to the thalamus. Activation of this pathway increases arousal and activates the limbic system, a connection that in humans is associated with emotional responses to pain.

Visceral pain is particularly poorly localized. Visceral afferent fibers travel in sympathetic nerves, have large overlapping receptor fields, and respond primarily to stretch, ischemia, dilation, or spasm (direct trauma to viscera—including surgical trauma—is a surprisingly ineffective stimulus for nociceptors). Pain of visceral origin tends to be dull, aching, or burning. Primary afferents from viscera follow autonomic nerves (e.g., the vagus and sympathetic nerves) to the CNS. The deep nociceptive pathway is tested in the neurological examination by application of a hemostat across the base of a toenail (taking care to exclude skin), a manipulation that stimulates nociceptors in the periosteum of the third phalanx.

Trigeminal system

For the head, nociception and tactile information are transmitted by the trigeminal system. Cell bodies of primary afferent fibers reside within the trigeminal (semilunar) ganglion. Their central processes enter the pons with the trigeminal nerve and course caudal along the lateral surface of the medulla. A nuclear column lies medial to the spinal tract throughout its length. At its rostral extent in the pons, this group of cell bodies comprises the pontine sensory nucleus. More caudally, the column is known as the spinal nucleus of V. The pontine and spinal nuclei of V contain somata of the second-order neurons in this system. There is a rostral-to-caudal segregation of function in these nuclei; the pontine nucleus is primarily concerned with discriminative tactile and proprioceptive stimuli, and the rostral part of the spinal nucleus of V sends somato-sensory information to the cerebellum. The majority of neurons in the spinal nucleus of V, however, are concerned with nociception. Many of these will project to motor nuclei of cranial nerves to participate in reflex arcs (e.g., corneal and palpebral reflexes), and many more will project to the RF to affect autonomic responses and increase arousal. Fibers for conscious perception, however, cross the midline of the medulla diffusely and join the contralateral quintothalamic tract, adjacent to the medial lemniscus. The quintothalamic (also known as the trigeminal lemniscus) tract projects to the thalamus, and, from there, nociceptive information reaches the somatosensory cortex via the internal capsule.

Pain modulation

There is a tendency to conceive of somatosensory pathways as electrical circuits that respond to stimuli in predictable ways and that consistently produce a sensory perception that is a faithful recording of the stimulus in the periphery. This is a useful model but it grossly oversimplifies the actual condition, wherein activity in the CNS can modulate somatosensory processing. This ability to alter activity in sensory systems is especially well developed in nociceptive pathways. The ability of a given stimulus to produce a perception of pain is a highly labile property and can be modified in the periphery, in the spinal cord, in the brain stem, and in higher centers.

Modulation in the periphery (nociceptors)

Nociceptor threshold is not a constant. As was described above, the presence of so-called silent nociceptors is one example of how conditions in the cellular environment of the naked nerve ending can change the sensitivity of the receptor to stimulus. The high threshold of silent nociceptors ensures that, under normal circumstances, they are relatively insensitive to any stimuli, but, upon exposure to inflammatory mediators, this threshold is markedly reduced, and previously silent nociceptors can be activated.

Similarly, many inflammatory mediators (e.g., prostaglandins [PGs] and leukotrienes), collectively referred to as nociceptor sensitizers, will lower the threshold of other populations of nociceptors. Thus, in damaged or inflamed tissue, stimuli that would normally be subthreshold may produce activity in nociceptive afferents. Likewise, certain inflammatory mediators (e.g., bradykinin and serotonin) or substances released by damaged cells (e.g., potassium ions and adenosine triphosphate) directly stimulate nociceptors and can thus be considered nociceptor activators. Interestingly, stimulated free-nerve endings can release substances directly into the surrounding tissues. Notable among these is substance P. Substance P (which is also an important neurotransmitter in central nociceptive pathways) dilates blood vessels and degranulates mast cells (neurogenic edema), both of which contribute to inflammation and increased sensitization of local nociceptors. All of these events contribute to the development of primary hyperalgesia (resulting from the increased responsiveness of nociceptors to noxious stimuli) and a related phenomenon, allodynia (wherein normally nonnoxious stimuli, such as those that elicit a touch sensation, become capable of activating nociceptors).

Modulation in the dorsal horn

Considerable processing of nociceptive information occurs in the dorsal horn, although precisely what happens there is debated. One of the fundamental concepts of dorsal horn processing is that one population of second-order neurons is dedicated to nociception (nociceptive-specific cells) and an additional, smaller group receives input from primary afferents conducting both noxious and nonnoxious tactile information. It is suspected that the nociceptive-specific neurons are primarily involved in discriminative nociception (i.e., localization). The second group, referred to as wide-dynamic-range or WDR neurons, responds both to noxious and nonnoxious stimuli, and is likely to be recruited in pathways that exhibit less somatotopy (i.e., are less discriminative). The WDR neurons appear to be relatively insensitive to tactile information, discharging at one rate in response to innocuous touch stimuli, while responding more vigorously (at a greater frequency) to noxious stimulation. These neurons also receive information from both somatic and visceral structures, which is a feature believed to underlie the phenomenon of referred pain. In referred pain, noxious stimuli originating in viscera are perceived as originating instead from a somatic region (body wall or skin). This perception is thought to result from the fact that information from that region of viscera converges on WDR neurons and pathways that also convey information from somatic structures.

The WDR neurons are probably the cells most important in the expression of spinal facilitation of pain, or windup (Figure 3.1). Windup occurs with rapid, continuous firing of primary nociceptive afferents, probably most especially small-diameter, unmyelinated fibers (C fibers). The high-frequency volley of action potentials (APs) in the primary afferent terminal stimulates the release of increased amounts of glutamate and is also associated with the release of substance P and brain-derived neurotrophic factor (BDNF). The increased exposure to glutamate in the synaptic cleft activates N-methyl-D-aspartate (NMDA) receptors (inactive except under conditions of persistent membrane depolarization) on the postsynaptic membrane. This particular variety of glutamate receptor is unique in that it exhibits a calcium conductance; its activation is therefore associated

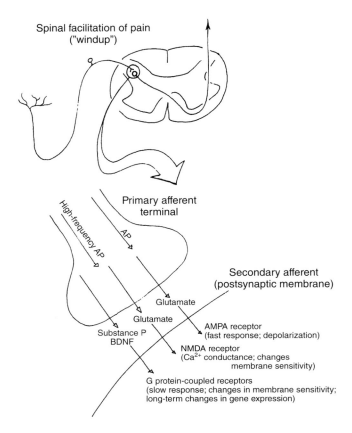

Figure 3.1. Processes involved in the spinal facilitation of pain or windup. AMPA, α-amino-3-hydroxy-5-methyl-4-isoxazolepropionic acid; AP, action potential; BDNF, brain-derived neurotrophic factor; NMDA, *N*-methyl-ᴅ-aspartate.
Source: Hellyer P.W., Robertson S.A., Fails A.D. 2007. Pain and its management. In: *Lumb and Jones' Veterinary Anesthesia and Analgesia*, 4th ed. W.J. Tranquilli, J.C. Thurmon, and K.A. Grimm, eds. Ames, IA: Blackwell Publishing, p. 37.

with the influx of calcium ions onto the postsynaptic neuron, leading to a series of intracellular cascades that ultimately results in the upregulation of receptors. Substance P and BDNF are neuromodulatory neurotransmitters that bind with G protein-coupled receptors. These, too, activate intracellular signaling cascades that increase the membrane's sensitivity to subsequent stimulation.

The net effect of these events is that high-frequency APs in the primary afferent neuron "train" the second-order neurons to respond more vigorously to subsequent stimulation. This change can last from hours to days (and longer) after the causative event ends. Effectively, then, prolonged noxious stimuli produce greater sensitivity to subsequent stimuli. What is especially significant about this phenomenon is that general anesthesia does not prevent windup, as it does not prevent generation of APs in the primary afferents. This observation has been used as a compelling argument for the use of analgesics preoperatively or intraoperatively as a preemptive strike against the development of windup during surgeries likely to activate C fibers.

Suprasegmental modulation

Activity in spinal nociceptive pathways is also strongly influenced by antinociceptive systems that originate in the brain stem. The midbrain (mesencephalon) and medulla both possess a series of midline nuclei that modulate the transmission of nociception. Input from higher cerebral centers and collaterals from ascending nociceptive pathways, particularly those conveying deep pain (spinoreticular tract), activate these nuclei. Among the nuclei that give rise to descending pain modulatory pathways, of particular note are the mesencephalic PAG and the nucleus raphe magnus of the rostroventral medulla.

The PAG receives input from ascending nociceptive tracts and higher centers (including limbic structures and cerebral cortex) and sends axons to the nucleus raphe magnus, to other medullary reticular nuclei, and, to a much lesser extent, to the dorsal horn of the spinal cord. These axons release multiple neurotransmitters, most notably endorphins, which are transmitters with powerful antinociceptive properties. The PAG input to the nucleus raphe magnus activates (through disinhibition) the monoaminergic pathways that arise here and descend the cord to modulate nociception at the level of the dorsal horn. The primary neurotransmitters of the nucleus raphe magnus and other medullary nuclei are serotonin and norepinephrine. Activity in these systems will recruit a pool of inter-neurons whose neurotransmitters (endorphin, enkephalin, and dynorphin) inhibit transmission in spinal cord pain pathways at the level of the dorsal horn.

Neuropathic pain

This is pain that is caused by injury to the nervous system. Damage leading to neuropathic pain can result from a variety of insults, including trauma (e.g., amputation and crushing injury), vascular injury (e.g., thromboembolic disease), endocrinopathy (e.g., diabetes mellitus), or infection (e.g., postherpetic neuralgia). Neuropathic pain resulting from these many different causes is probably not a single entity. Several mechanisms are thought likely to contribute to neuropathic pain; not all of these necessarily underlie any given case of neuropathic pain, although they are not mutually exclusive.

Hyperalgesia and allodynia are both commonly associated with neuropathic pain. Dysesthesias, which are unpleasant, abnormal sensations often characterized as tingling or "electric," are sometimes described by affected people, although neuropathic pain is most usually described as having a burning, lancinating quality. In the peripheral nervous system, injury to primary afferents (up to and including the dorsal root ganglia) can cause neuropathic pain. The mechanisms producing this pain are not clearly understood and, like all facets of neuropathic pain, are likely to be multiple. In at least some cases, the damaged primary afferent produces an increased frequency of spontaneous APs (most neurons do this to some extent, but normal nociceptive afferents typically do so at a very low rate), a phenomenon called ectopic discharge. Damaged primary afferents are also apt to develop collateral sprouting, perhaps in response to neurotrophic factors released by damaged tissues. Aberrant collaterals of nociceptive neurons may spread into adjacent skin or other tissues, where their activation can produce an abnormal perception of pain. One line of inquiry has revealed a phenomenon of electrical coupling between somatosensory and sympathetic fibers in the periphery (including the dorsal root ganglia). This coupling, called sympathetically maintained pain, activates nociceptive pathways (and pain perception) with activity in sympathetic neurons.

Centrally, the alterations described in the discussion of windup (spinal facilitation of pain) are likely to play a role in the development of sustained, neuropathic pain, inasmuch as the upregulation of receptors on postsynaptic membranes can persist for a prolonged time. Since activation of NMDA glutamate receptors is a key part of spinal facilitation of pain, use of NMDA antagonists shows potential as a therapy for neuropathic pain. Additionally, there is evidence that tactile (i.e., nonnociceptive) A-β afferent fibers sprout collateral connections in the dorsal horn (again, probably in response to neurotrophic factors released by injured nervous tissue), making aberrant connections with projection neurons that are normally associated with nociception. Activity in these fibers will therefore produce activity in nociceptive pathways, leading ultimately to the perception of increased pain.

There is also ample evidence that the repertoire of neurotransmitters and/or receptors within the dorsal horn undergoes changes in response to injury. Some researchers have documented a decrease in γ-aminobutyric acid (GABA, an inhibitory neurotransmitter) in animal models of neuropathic pain. Experimental techniques that increase levels of GABA in the spinal cord are associated with an attenuation of allodynia, which is characteristic of neuropathic pain.

A particularly frustrating aspect of neuropathic pain is the extent to which it is refractory to opioids. This is likely because of a loss of opioid receptors, which is a phenomenon that has been reported in the dorsal root ganglion and the dorsal horn. Simultaneously, cholecystokinin and its receptors appear to be upregulated by nervous tissue injury; cholecystokinin has documented opioid antagonist activity.

Measuring pain in veterinary patients

As previously mentioned, pain is an extremely complex multidimensional experience with both sensory and affective elements. Obviously, there are distinct populations, including human neonates, nonverbal adults, and animals, that cannot express their pain overtly. However, all mammals possess the neuroanatomical and neuropharmacological components necessary for transduction, transmission, and perception of noxious stimuli; therefore, it is commonly assumed that animals experience pain even if they cannot exactly perceive or communicate it in the same way people do.

There is presently no gold standard for assessing pain in animals. Many different scoring methods that include physiological variables (in an attempt to identify objective measures) and behavioral variables have been published, but few have been rigorously validated. The issue of pain assessment in animals is especially complex because consideration must include differences in gender, age, species, breed, strain, and environment. Assessment systems must also take into account the different types and sources of pain, such as acute versus chronic or neuropathic pain and visceral compared with somatic pain. For example, if a pain scale were developed to evaluate acute postoperative pain in dogs following routine abdominal surgery, such as ovariohysterectomy, then the scale might be inappropriate for assessing pain after orthopedic surgery or pain associated with chronic osteoarthritis in that species. There is no question that as more studies focus on species-specific pain behaviors and the different types of pain, the ability of the veterinary community to recognize and treat pain in animals will improve. Nevertheless, the assessment of pain in animals will remain a subjective and inaccurate undertaking for the foreseeable future.

Behavioral responses to pain vary greatly between species, and these differences may be linked to an animal's innate behaviors. For example, because rats and mice are prey animals, overt signs of pain or injury draw the attention of predators, so the rodents have evolved to where they instinctively disguise their pain. The subtle signs of pain exhibited by these species, such as abdominal pressing and back arching, can be easily missed by an inexperienced observer. Because of behavioral distinctions, pain assessment tools must be species specific.

Acute pain

Most studies in dogs and cats have focused on assessing acute postoperative pain. Not all of the systems used have been validated or rigorously tested, however; and the key question for a busy practitioner is "How well do these scoring systems perform in clinical practice?"

Objective measures

In both cats and dogs, the correlation between easily measured physiological variables (heart rate, respiratory rate, blood pressure, and pupil diameter) and pain scores have been evaluated. No study found a consistently reliable objective measure, which is not surprising as these parameters can be affected by many factors other than pain. For example, an opioid alone causes mydriasis in cats but miosis in dogs. Pupil size is also affected by fear and ambient light. In a tightly controlled research setting, blood pressure looked promising as an indirect indicator of pain in cats, but, in a clinical environment, this variable was an unreliable indicator of pain.

Changes in plasma cortisol and β-endorphins are components of the "stress response" to anesthesia and surgery, and much effort has been expended trying to correlate these hormones with pain in laboratory and clinical analgesia trials. Plasma cortisol was not a useful pain marker in dogs and is extremely unreliable in cats. Mechanical nociceptive threshold testing with various devices (palpometers and algometers) has proved to be useful for evaluating both primary (wound) and secondary (remote area) hyperalgesia in cats and dogs. Changes in wound sensitivity have correlated with visual analog scoring in cats, suggesting that assessing wound tenderness is a valuable tool and should be incorporated into an overall assessment protocol. Force plate gait analyses have been widely used to assess lameness in dogs objectively. This technique has also been used to evaluate response to different surgical procedures and to assess the efficacy of a variety of analgesics.

Subjective scoring systems

Because animals cannot self-report, all scoring systems that depend on a human observer must, by definition, be subjective to some degree and leave room for error, which could be either underassessment or overassessment of the animal's pain. Any system used should be valid, reliable, and sensitive. Without strictly defined criteria and the use of well-trained and experienced observers, many scoring systems are too variable, which is one of the main criticisms of multicenter clinical trials. One scoring system may show an analgesic agent to be effective, and another shows that same analgesic to be ineffective. If a system is insensitive, then these differences are inevitable and result in large interobserver variability.

Simple descriptive scales These are the most basic pain scales. These usually have four or five descriptors from which observers choose, such as no pain, mild pain, moderate pain, severe pain, or very severe pain. Although simple to use, these scales are extremely subjective and do not detect small changes in pain behavior.

Numerical rating scales These are essentially the same as simple descriptive scales, but assign numbers for ease of tabulation and analyses; for example, absence of pain is assigned the number 0 and very severe pain the number 5. This system implies equal difference or weighting between each category, which is not the case. These are discontinuous scales; therefore, a dog experiencing pain that is "just in" category 2 is in a quite different condition from a dog that is also in category 2 but almost in category 3. A further development of the simple descriptive and numerical rating systems is a categorized numerical rating system where certain behaviors are chosen and assigned a value. For example, vocalization can be divided into none (score = 0), crying but responsive (score = 1), and crying but nonresponsive (score = 2); other categories may include movement, agitation, and posture.

Visual analog scale In an attempt to improve on discontinuous scales, the visual analog scale (VAS) has been widely used in veterinary medicine (Figure 3.2). This tool consists of a continuous line (usually 100 mm long) anchored at either end with a description of the limits of the scale, for example no pain or no sedation at one end and severe pain or asleep at the other end. An observer places a mark on the line at the point that he/she thinks correlates with the degree of pain in the animal under observation, and this point is later translated into a number by measuring the distance to the mark from zero. Without training and experience, the VAS results in wide interobserver variation.

Dynamic and interactive visual analog scale (DIVAS) are an extension of the classic VAS system in dogs. With the DIVAS system, animals are first observed from a distance undisturbed and then approached, handled, and encouraged to walk. Finally, the surgical incision and surrounding area are palpated, and a final overall assessment of sedation and pain is made. This approach overcomes some of the deficiencies of purely observational systems; for example, a dog may lie very still and quiet because a wound is painful,

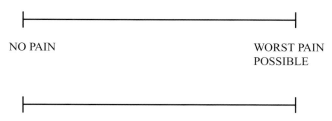

Figure 3.2.   The VAS used to assess pain in animals.
Source: Hellyer P.W., Robertson S.A., Fails A.D. 2007. Pain and its management. In: *Lumb and Jones' Veterinary Anesthesia and Analgesia*, 4th ed. W.J. Tranquilli, J.C. Thurmon, and K.A. Grimm, eds. Ames, IA: Blackwell Publishing, p. 43.

and this would go undetected unless the observer interacted with the animal. The DIVAS system has also been used to assess postoperative pain in cats and, when performed by one individual unaware of treatments, it detected differences between analgesics and between treated and untreated cats. So far, the scoring systems discussed in this section are regarded as one-dimensional in that they assess only intensity of pain.

Considering the complexity of pain, it is not surprising that simple, subjective, one-dimensional systems have not proven ideal. In humans, multidimensional systems—such as the McGill Pain Questionnaire—that account for not only intensity but also sensory and affective (emotional) qualities of pain have provided a more comprehensive assessment of a patient's pain. Multidimensional systems are particularly important when self-reporting is not possible, but reports must incorporate components that are proven to be sensitive and specific to pain (e.g., facial expressions in infants) in the species being studied.

The University of Melbourne Pain Scale (UMPS) has been developed to incorporate objective physiological data (heart rate, respiratory rate, pupil size, and rectal temperature) and behavioral responses (activity, response to palpation, posture, mental status, and vocalization). By assigning numbers to each factor, a score between 0 and 27 is derived. This scale has been tested on dogs following ovariohysterectomy and demonstrated good agreement between different assessors. It could differentiate between dogs that were anesthetized but not subjected to surgery and those undergoing surgery. With some refinement to detect smaller differences, the system shows promise for clinical use.

To date, the most vigorously validated scale for assessing acute postoperative pain in dogs is the Glasgow Composite Measures Pain Scale. The original 279 words or expressions that could describe pain in dogs have been reduced to 47 well-defined words placed in one physiological category and seven behavioral categories. The behavioral categories comprise evaluations of: posture, comfort, vocalization, attention to the wound, demeanor and response to humans, mobility, and response to touch. Each descriptor is well defined to avoid misinterpretation. Assessment involves both observation from a distance and interaction with the patient (e.g., palpation of the wound). Frequent assessments are necessary because pain is not a static process, and the benefits of intervention with analgesics must be evaluated. In a busy practice, time-consuming assessments are the biggest drawbacks to effective pain management. For this reason, a short form of the Glasgow composite pain scale, which takes only a few minutes to perform, has been developed (Figure 3.3).

How often should animals be assessed

The health status of the animal, extent of surgery/injuries, and anticipated duration of analgesic drugs determine the frequency and interval of evaluations. In general, evaluations should be made at least hourly for the first 4–6 hours after surgery, provided the animal has recovered from anesthesia, has stable vital signs, and is resting comfortably. Animals not recovering as anticipated from anesthesia/surgery and critically ill animals require much more frequent evaluations until they are stabilized. Patient response to analgesic therapy and expected duration of analgesic drug(s) administered help to determine frequency of evaluations. For example, if a dog is resting comfortably following the postoperative administration of morphine, it may not need to be reassessed for 2–4 hours. Animals should be allowed to sleep following analgesic therapy. Vital signs can often be checked without unduly disturbing a sleeping animal. In general, animals are not awakened to check their pain status; however, that does not mean they should not receive their scheduled analgesics.

Continuous, undisturbed observations, coupled with periodic interactive observations (open the cage, palpate the wound, etc.) are likely to provide more information than occasionally observing the animal through the cage door. It is regrettable that continuous observations are not practical for most clinical situations. In general, the more frequent the observations, the more likely that subtle signs of pain will be detected.

Chronic pain

Chronic pain can affect an animal's quality of life. Because of the nature of chronic pain, such as that associated with osteoarthritis in dogs and cats, the accompanying behavioral changes can be insidious and easily missed. Indeed, many owners assume these changes are inevitable with advancing age. Preliminary data based on owner interviews revealed changes in 32 types of behavior in dogs with chronic pain. This study also indicated that

Figure 3.3.   The short-form composite measure pain score (CMPS-SF) can be applied quickly and reliably in a clinical setting and has been designed as a clinical decision-making tool that was developed for dogs in acute pain. It includes 30 descriptor options within six behavioral categories, including mobility. Within each category, the descriptors are ranked numerically according to their associated pain severity and the person carrying out the assessment chooses the descriptor within each category that best fits the dog's behavior/ condition. It is important to carry out the assessment procedure as described on the questionnaire, following the protocol closely. The pain score is the sum of the rank scores. The maximum score for the six categories is 24, or 20 if mobility is impossible to assess. The total CMPS-SF score has been shown to be a useful indicator of analgesic requirement and the recommended analgesic intervention level is 6/24 or 5/20.
Source: Reproduced with the permission of Jacky Reid, Professor of Veterinary Anaesthesia, University of Glasgow.

SHORT FORM OF THE GLASGOW COMPOSITE PAIN SCALE

Dog's name _____

Hospital Number _____ **Date** / / **Time**

Surgery Yes/No (delete as appropriate)

Procedure or Condition_____

_____

In the sections below please circle the appropriate score in each list and sum these to give the total score.

A. Look at dog in Kennel

Is the dog?

(i)		(ii)	
Quiet	0	Ignoring any wound or painful area	0
Crying or whimpering	1	Looking at wound or painful area	1
Groaning	2	Licking wound or painful area	2
Screaming	3	Rubbing wound or painful area	3
		Chewing wound or painful area	4

> In the case of spinal, pelvic or multiple limb fractures, or where assistance is required to aid locomotion do not carry out section **B** and proceed to **C**
> *Please tick if this is the case* ☐ then proceed to C.

B. Put lead on dog and lead out of the kennel.

When the dog rises/walks is it?

(iii)	
Normal	0
Lame	1
Slow or reluctant	2
Stiff	3
It refuses to move	4

C. If it has a wound or painful area including abdomen, apply gentle pressure 2 inches round the site.

Does it?

(iv)	
Do nothing	0
Look round	1
Flinch	2
Growl or guard area	3
Snap	4
Cry	5

D. Overall

Is the dog?

(v)		(vi)	
Happy and content or happy and bouncy	0	Comfortable	0
Quiet	1	Unsettled	1
Indifferent or non-responsive to surroundings	2	Restless	2
Nervous or anxious or fearful	3	Hunched or tense	3
Depressed or non-responsive to stimulation	4	Rigid	4

Total Score (i+ii+iii+iv+v+vi) = _____

the owners are the best evaluators of their pet's pain. The Glasgow University Health-Related Dog Behavior Questionnaire has identified some key indicators of chronic pain, including, but not limited to, decreases in mobility, activity, sociability, and curiosity, and increases in aggression, anxiety, daytime sleeping, and vocalizing.

Chronic pain is undoubtedly a clinical problem in cats, but is not well documented. Compared with dogs, very little is known about degenerative joint disease in cats, but radiographic evidence in geriatric cats suggests the incidence may be as high as 90%. Because of a pet cat's lifestyle, lameness is not a common owner complaint; but changes in behavior, including decreased grooming, reluctance to jump up to favorite places, and soiling outside the litter box, should prompt veterinarians to look for sources of chronic pain. It is common for owners not to realize how debilitated their pet is until they see dramatic improvements following treatment.

Management of pain

Analgesia in the strictest sense is an absence of pain but clinically is the reduction in the intensity of pain perceived (hypoalgesia). The goal should not be to eliminate pain completely, but to make the pain as tolerable as possible without undue depression of patients. Analgesia in the clinical setting may be induced by obtunding or interrupting the nociceptive process at one or more points between the peripheral nociceptor and the cerebral cortex.

Nociception involves four physiological processes that are subject to pharmacological modulation. Transduction is the translation of physical energy (noxious stimuli) into electric activity at the peripheral nociceptor. Transmission is the propagation of nerve impulses through the nervous system. Modulation occurs through the endogenous descending analgesic systems, which modify nociceptive transmission. These endogenous systems (opioid, serotonergic, and noradrenergic) modulate nociception through inhibition of the spinal dorsal horn cells. Perception is the final process resulting from successful transduction, transmission and modulation, and integration of thalamocortical, reticular, and limbic function to produce the final conscious subjective and emotional experience of pain.

Transduction can be largely abolished by use of local anesthetics infiltrated at the site of injury or incision, or by intravenous, postthoracotomy intrapleural, or postlaparotomy intraperitoneal injection.

Nonsteroidal anti-inflammatory drugs (NSAIDs) will obtund transduction by decreasing production of endogenous algogenic substances such as PGs at the site of injury. Transmission can be abolished by local anesthetic blockade of peripheral nerves or nerve plexuses or by epidural or subarachnoid injection. Modulation can be augmented by subarachnoid or epidural injection of opioids, and/or alpha$_2$ adrenergic agonists. Perception can be obtunded with general anesthetics or by systemic administration of opioids and alpha$_2$ agonists, either alone or in combination with tranquilizer-sedatives.

Balanced or multimodal analgesia results from the administration of analgesic drugs in combination and at multiple sites to induce analgesia by altering more than one part of the nociceptive process. Multimodal analgesia relies on the additive or synergistic effects of two or more analgesic drugs working through different mechanisms of action. When multimodal analgesia is used, doses of individual drugs can usually be reduced, thereby theoretically decreasing the potential for any one drug to induce adverse side effects.

Preemptive analgesia refers to the application of balanced analgesic techniques prior to exposing patients to noxious stimuli (surgical trespass). By so doing, the spinal cord is not exposed to the barrage of afferent nociceptive impulses that induce the neuroplastic changes leading to central hypersensitivity. By consensus, this concept has gained acceptance as the most effective means of controlling postoperative pain.

There are three major classes of analgesic agents employed in veterinary medicine for the management of pain: opioids, NSAIDs, and local anesthetics. In addition to these three traditional drug classes, another diverse group of agents used to manage pain is known collectively as analgesic adjuvants.

Opioids

All opioid analgesics are chemically related to a group of compounds that have been purified from the juice of a particular species of poppy: *Papaverum somniferum*. The unrefined extract from the poppy is called opium and contains approximately 20 naturally occurring pharmacologically active compounds, including familiar ones like morphine and codeine. This group of purified natural agents is specifically referred to as opiates. In addition, numerous semisynthetic and synthetic analogs of the opiates have been developed for clinical use. The word opioid is used broadly to cover all drugs that are chemical derivatives of the compounds purified from opium and is the term that is used throughout this chapter.

The opioids continue to be the cornerstone of effective pain treatment in veterinary medicine. They are a versatile group of drugs with extensive applications in the management of pain in patients with acute trauma, in patients undergoing surgical procedures, in patients with painful medical conditions or disease processes, and in patients suffering from chronic pain that require long-term therapy.

It is well known that exogenously administered opioids such as morphine exert their effects by interacting with specific opioid receptors and mimicking naturally occurring molecules known as endogenous opioid peptides. There are three well-defined types of opioid receptors, most commonly known by their Greek letter designations as μ (mu), δ (delta), and κ (kappa). This classic system of nomenclature has been under reconsideration for a number of years and, during this time, several alternative naming systems have been proposed, leading to considerable confusion. In addition, a fourth type of opioid receptor, the nociceptin receptor (also known as the orphanin FQ receptor), has been characterized. According to the most recent recommendations of the International Union of Pharmacology Subcommittee on Nomenclature, variations based on the Greek letters remain acceptable. Thus, mu, μ, or MOP (for mu opioid peptide); delta, δ, or DOP (for delta opioid peptide); kappa, κ, or KOP (for kappa opioid peptide); and NOP (for nociceptin opioid peptide) are considered interchangeable abbreviations. Distinct complementary DNA (cDNA) sequences have been cloned for all four opioid receptor types, and each type appears to have a unique distribution in the brain, spinal cord, and periphery.

The diversity of opioid receptors is further extended by the existence of several subtypes of μ, δ, and κ receptors. Based on pharmacological studies, there are thought to be at least three μ-receptor subtypes, μ_1, μ_2, and μ_3; two δ-receptor subtypes, δ_1 and δ_2; and perhaps as many as four κ-receptor subtypes, κ_{1a}, κ_{1b}, κ_2, and κ_3. The discovery of opioid receptor subtypes generated great enthusiasm among researchers and introduced the possibility of developing subtype-specific therapeutic agents with favorable side-effect profiles. At this point, however, the functional significance of these receptor subtypes remains unclear, and distinct cDNA sequences corresponding to these subtypes have not yet been identified.

In general, it appears that the μ receptor mediates most of the clinically relevant analgesic effects, as well as most of the adverse effects associated with opioid administration. Drugs acting at the δ receptor tend to be poor analgesics, but may modify μ receptor-mediated antinociception under certain circumstances and mediate opioid receptor "cross-talk." The κ receptor mediates analgesia in several specific locations in the CNS and the periphery, but distinguishing μ- and κ-mediated analgesic effects has proven to be difficult.

In contrast to the classic opioid receptors, the nociceptin receptor does not mediate typical opioid analgesia, but instead produces antiopioid (pronociceptive) effects. Because of the considerable structural homology among the three classically described opioid receptors, it is likely that there are significant interactions among these receptors in different tissues, and the loosely defined physiological roles ascribed to each receptor type still require further clarification.

Endogenous receptor ligands

The aforementioned opioid receptors discussed are part of an extensive opioid system that includes a large number of endogenous opioid peptide ligands. Endogenous opioid peptides are small molecules that are naturally produced in the CNS and in various glands throughout the body, such as the pituitary and the adrenal. Three distinct families of endogenous opioid peptides have been identified: the enkephalins, the dynorphins, and β-endorphin. Each of these is derived from a distinct precursor polypeptide: proenkephalin, prodynorphin, and proopiomelanocortin, respectively. These endogenous opioid peptides are expressed throughout the CNS, and their presence has been confirmed in peripheral tissues, as well. There are considerable structural similarities among these three groups of peptides, and each family demonstrates variable affinities for μ, δ, and κ receptors. None of them bind exclusively to a single opioid receptor, and none of them have any significant affinity for the nociceptin receptor. The physiological roles of these peptides are not completely understood at this time. They appear to function as neurotransmitters, neuromodulators, and, in some cases, as neurohormones. They mediate some forms of stress-induced analgesia and also play a role in analgesia induced by electrical stimulation of discrete regions in the brain, such as the periaqueductal gray area of the mesencephalon.

Nociceptin (also known as orphanin FQ) is the endogenous ligand for the more recently discovered nociceptin receptor. Nociceptin is derived from pronociceptin, and its amino acid sequence is closely related to that of the aforementioned endogenous opioid peptides. Despite this homology, nociceptin binding is specific for the nociceptin receptor, and the peptide does not appear to interact with μ, δ, or κ receptors. Furthermore, the physiological effects of nociceptin are in direct contrast to the actions of the classical endogenous opioid peptides, with nociceptin producing a distinctly pronociceptive effect. The functional significance of nociceptin and its receptor remains to be elucidated, but additional insight into this novel opioid peptide may have substantial implications in future therapeutic drug development.

In addition to the enkephalins, dynorphins, β-endorphin, and nociceptin, there are now two other recently discovered endogenous opioid peptides called endomorphin 1 and endomorphin 2. These peptides are putative products of an as yet unidentified precursor and have been proposed to be the highly selective endogenous ligands for the μ receptor. The endomorphins are small tetrapeptides that are structurally unrelated to the endogenous opioid peptides. Their identification has heralded a new era in research of the μ opioid system, which may contribute to our understanding of the neurobiology of opioids and provide new avenues for therapeutic interventions.

Signaling and mechanisms of analgesia

Binding of an opioid agonist to a neuronal opioid receptor, regardless of whether the agonist is endogenous or exogenous, typically leads to several events that serve to inhibit the activation of the neuron. Opioid receptors are part of a large superfamily of membrane-bound receptors that are coupled to G proteins. As such, they are structurally and functionally related to receptors for many other neurotransmitters and neuropeptides that act to modulate the activity of nerve cells. Opioid receptor binding, via activation of various types of G proteins, may inhibit adenylyl cyclase (cyclic adenosine monophosphate) activity, activate receptor-operated potassium ion (K^+) currents, and suppress voltage-gated calcium ion (Ca^{2+}) currents.

At the presynaptic level, decreased Ca^{2+} influx will reduce release of transmitter substances, such as substance P, from primary afferent fibers in the spinal cord dorsal horn, thereby inhibiting synaptic transmission of nociceptive input. Postsynaptically, enhanced K^+ efflux causes neuronal hyperpolarization of spinal cord projection neurons and inhibits ascending nociceptive pathways. A third potential mode of opioid action involves upregulation of supraspinal descending antinociceptive pathways in the PAG. It is now known that this system is subject to tonic inhibition mediated by GABAergic neurons, and opioid receptor activation has been shown to suppress this inhibitory influence and augment descending antinociceptive transmission. The proposed cellular basis for this involves μ receptors that activate voltage-dependent K^+ ions present on presynaptic GABAergic nerve terminals that inhibit GABA release into the synaptic cleft. It is important to note that although our collective understanding of opioid receptor-mediated signaling has increased dramatically in recent years, the relationship of such subcellular events to clinical analgesia at the level of the organism continues to require further clarification.

Distribution and therapeutic implications

Although cellular and molecular studies of opioid receptors and ligands are invaluable in understanding their function, it is critical to place opioid receptors in their anatomical and physiological context to fully appreciate the opioid system and its relevance to pain management. It has long been a principle tenet of opioid analgesia that these agents are centrally acting, and this understanding has shaped the way we use opioid analgesics clinically. It has been well established that the analgesic effects of opioids arise from their ability to directly inhibit the ascending transmission of nociceptive information from the spinal cord dorsal horn, and to activate inhibitory pathways that descend from the midbrain via the rostral ventromedial medulla to the spinal cord. Within the CNS, evidence of μ, δ, and κ opioid receptor messenger RNA and/or opioid peptide binding has been demonstrated in supraspinal sites, including the mesencephalic PAG, the mesencephalic RF, various nuclei of the rostral ventromedial medulla, and forebrain regions including the nucleus accumbens, as well as spinally within the dorsal horn. The interactions between groups of opioid receptors at various spinal and supraspinal locations, as well as interactions among different receptor types within a given location are complex and incompletely understood at this time.

Systemic administration of opioid analgesics via intravenous, intramuscular, or subcutaneous injection will induce a relatively rapid onset of action via interaction with these CNS receptors. Oral, transdermal, rectal, or buccal mucosal administration of opioids will result in variable systemic absorption, depending on the characteristics of the particular agent, with analgesic effects being mediated largely by the same receptors within the CNS. In addition, neuraxial administration, either into the subarachnoid or epidural space, is an efficacious route of administration. Small doses of opioids introduced via these routes readily penetrate the spinal cord and interact with spinal and/or supraspinal opioid receptors to produce profound and potentially long-lasting analgesia, the characteristics of which will depend on the particular drug used.

Even though opioids have long been considered the prototype of centrally acting analgesics, a body of evidence has emerged that clearly indicates that opioids can produce potent and clinically measurable analgesia by activation of opioid receptors in the peripheral nervous system. Opioid receptors of all three major types have been identified on the processes of sensory neurons, and these receptors respond to peripherally applied opioids and locally released endogenous opioid peptides when upregulated during inflammatory pain states. Furthermore, although sympathetic neurons and immune cells have also been shown to express opioid receptors, their functional role remains unclear. Although the binding characteristics of peripheral and central opioid receptors are similar, the molecular mass of peripheral and central μ opioid receptors appears to be different, suggesting that selective ligands for these peripheral receptors could be developed that would produce opioid analgesia without the potential to induce centrally mediated adverse side effects.

Adverse effects

Although opioids are used clinically primarily for their pain-relieving properties, they also produce a host of other effects on a variety of body systems. This is not surprising in light of the wide distribution of endogenous opioid peptides and their receptors in supraspinal, spinal, and peripheral locations. Some of these adverse effects, such as sedation, may be classified as either desirable or undesirable depending on the clinical circumstances. The following is a brief summary of these major side effects as they relate to opioids as a class of drugs.

CNS   There are considerable species differences in the CNS response to opioid analgesics that cannot be attributed to pharmacokinetic variations alone. CNS depression (i.e., sedation) is typically seen in dogs, monkeys, and people, whereas CNS stimulation (i.e., excitement and/or spontaneous locomotor activity) may be elicited in cats, horses, goats, sheep, pigs, and cows after systemic administration of various opioids, most notably morphine. Reasons for these different responses are not entirely clear at this time, but are presumably related to differing concentrations and distributions of μ, δ, and κ receptors in various regions of the brain in these species. Despite these fundamental differences, it must be remembered that there are numerous factors that may affect the CNS response to opioids within a given species, including the temperament or condition of the patient; the presence or absence of pain; the dose, route, and timing of drug administration; and the specific opioid administered.

The hypothalamic thermoregulatory system is also affected by opioid administration. Hypothermia tends to be the most common response, particularly when opioids are used during the perioperative period in the presence of other CNS-depressant drugs. Under some clinical circumstances, however, opioid administration causes hyperthermia in cats. Part of this increase in body temperature may be attributed to an increase in muscle activity associated with CNS excitation in this species; however, a specific central hypothalamic mechanism has also been implicated, but remains poorly understood. Panting is seen commonly after opioid administration, most often in dogs, but this effect tends to decrease with the onset of hypothermia.

Nausea and vomiting associated with opioid administration are caused by direct stimulation of the chemoreceptor trigger zone for emesis located in the area postrema of the medulla. As with the other centrally mediated side effects, species plays a role in determining an individual's tendency to vomit after an opioid is administered. Cats may vomit, but usually at doses that are greater than those which stimulate vomiting in dogs. Dogs will commonly vomit after opioid administration, especially with morphine. Emesis is rarely seen when opioids are administered in the immediate postoperative period or in any patient that may be experiencing some degree of pain.

Opioids have variable efficacy in depressing the cough reflex, at least in part by a direct effect on a cough center located in the medulla. Certain opioids are more effective antitussives than others, and drugs like codeine, hydrocodone, and butorphanol are occasionally prescribed specifically for this indication.

As a general rule, opioids tend to produce mydriasis in those species that exhibit CNS excitation, and miosis in those that become sedated after opioid administration. Miosis is produced by an excitatory action of opioids on neuronal firing in the oculomotor nucleus. In cats, and presumably in other species that exhibit mydriasis, this increase in activity in the oculomotor nuclear complex still occurs, but the miotic effect is masked by increased release of catecholamines, which produces mydriasis.

Respiratory system   Opioids produce dose-dependent depression of ventilation, primarily mediated by $μ_2$ receptors, leading to a direct depressant effect on brain stem respiratory centers. This effect is characterized by decreased responsiveness of these centers to carbon dioxide and is reflected in an increased resting arterial carbon dioxide partial pressure and displacement of the carbon dioxide response curve to the right. This effect is compounded by the coadministration of sedative and/or anesthetic agents, meaning that significant respiratory depression and hypercapnia are much more likely to occur in anesthetized patients that receive opioids compared with those that are conscious. It should be noted that, in general, humans tend to be more sensitive to the respiratory depressant effects of opioids when compared with most veterinary species, and the risk of hypoventilation would rarely constitute a legitimate reason for withholding opioid treatment in clinical practice; however, careful patient monitoring is prudent.

Cardiovascular system   Most opioids have minimal effects on cardiac output, cardiac rhythm, and arterial blood pressure when clinically relevant analgesic doses are administered. Bradycardia may be caused by opioid-induced medullary vagal stimulation and will respond readily to anticholinergic treatment. Particular opioids (morphine and meperidine) can cause histamine release, especially after rapid intravenous administration, which may lead to vasodilation and hypotension. Because of their relatively benign effects on cardiovascular function, opioids commonly form the basis of anesthetic protocols for patients with preexisting cardiovascular disease.

Gastrointestinal system   The gastrointestinal effects of the opioids are mediated by μ and δ receptors located in the myenteric plexus of the gastrointestinal tract. Opioid administration will often stimulate dogs and, less frequently, cats to defecate. After this initial response, spasm of gastrointestinal smooth muscle predisposes patients to ileus and constipation. These side effects tend to be most significant with prolonged administration of opioids in dogs and cats experiencing chronic pain, and such patients may require dietary modifications and stool-softening medications to manage these adverse effects.

In human patients, opioids (most notably fentanyl and morphine) have been shown to increase bile duct pressure through constriction of the sphincter of Oddi. The incidence of this side effect in people is, however, quite low. Despite anatomical differences, this observation has led to concerns about opioid administration to dogs and cats with pancreatitis and/or cholangitis. A study reviewing the body of human literature found that, despite widespread clinical practice, there was no evidence to indicate that morphine is contraindicated for use in acute pancreatitis. As there are no studies that specifically evaluate the effects of opioids in dogs and cats with pancreatitis, it does not at this time seem appropriate to withhold this class of drugs from this subset of severely painful patients.

Genitourinary system   Opioids, particularly when administered neuraxially, may cause urinary retention through dose-dependent suppression of detrusor contractility and decreased sensation of urge. Manual expression of the urinary bladder or catheterization may be required in certain individuals until urodynamic function returns to normal. Urine volume may also be affected by opioids, and the mechanism of this effect appears to be multifactorial. μ-Agonists tend to produce oliguria in the clinical setting, and this is in part due to increased antidiuretic hormone release leading to altered renal tubular function. Elevations in circulating plasma atrial natriuretic peptide may also play a role in morphine-induced antidiuresis. Conversely, κ-agonists tend to produce a diuretic effect, possibly through inhibition of antidiuretic hormone secretion. Other peripheral mechanisms involving stimulation of renal alpha$_2$ adrenergic receptors may also contribute to this κ-agonist effect.

Agonists

Almost all clinically useful opioids exert their analgesic effects by acting as agonists at μ receptors. Although a few opioids act as κ-agonists, these drugs also tend to have antagonist or partial agonist effects at μ and/or δ receptors and are thus not classified as pure agonists. Pure or full opioid agonists can elicit maximal activation of the receptor when they bind it, and the subsequent downstream processes produce a maximal analgesic effect (Figure 3.4). Clinically, the full μ-agonists are superior analgesics and are the drugs of choice for pain of moderate to severe intensity in many veterinary species (see Table 3.1 for recommended dosages).

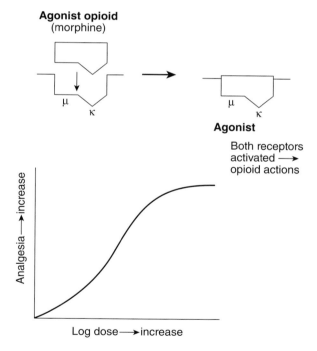

Figure 3.4.   A lock-and-key analogy is used to illustrate full agonist drug interactions at opioid receptors, with a relative dose–response curve for analgesic effectiveness shown. A full opioid agonist (in this example morphine) stimulates both μ- and κ-receptor types, which produces increased analgesic effect with increased dose.
Source: Modified from Nicholson A., Christie M. 2002. Opioid analgesics. In: *Small Animal Clinical Pharmacology*. J. Maddison, S. Page, and D.B. Church, eds. Philadelphia, PA: WB Saunders, pp. 271–292.

Table 3.1. Dosage ranges (milligram per kilogram) for opioid agonists in several domestic species

Opioid	Dogs	Cats	Horses	Cattle	Swine
Morphine	0.3–2.0 IM, SC 0.1–0.5 IV 0.1–0.3/h IV CRI 0.1–0.2 epidural[a] 1.5–3 PO[b]	0.05–0.2 IM, SC 0.1–0.2 epidural[a]	0.1–0.3 IM, SC 0.1–0.2 epidural[a]	?	0.5–2.0? IM, SC
Oxymorphone	0.05–0.2 IV, IM, SC	0.05–0.1 IV, IM, SC	0.01–0.03 IV, IM, SC	NR	0.05–0.2? IM, SC
Hydromorphone	0.05–0.2 IV, IM, SC	0.05–0.1 IV, IM, SC	0.01–0.03 IV, IM, SC	NR	0.05–0.2? IM, SC
Meperidine	3–5 IM, SC	3–5 IM, SC	1–3 IM, SC 0.2–1.0 IV	3–4? IM, SC	1–2? IM, SC
Fentanyl	0.002–0.01 IV 0.002–0.03c/h IV CRI 0.001–0.005/h epidural[a] CRI 0.002–0.005/h transdermal[d]	0.001–0.005 IV 0.002–0.03[c]/h IV CRI 0.001–0.005/h epidural[a] CRI 0.002–0.005/h transdermal[d]	0.001–0.002/h transdermal[d]	0.001–0.002/h transdermal[d]	NR
Alfentanil	?	?	NR	NR	?
Sufentanil	0.001–0.005 IV loading dose 0.001–0.01[c]/h IV CRI	?	NR	NR	?
Remifentanil	0.004–0.01 IV loading dose 0.004–0.06[c]/h IV CRI	?	NR	NR	?
Methadone	0.05–0.2 PO, IM, SC	0.05–0.2 PO, IM, SC	NR	NR	NR
Codeine	1–2 PO	0.1–1.0 PO	NR	NR	NR
Oxycodone	0.1–0.3? PO	?	NR	NR	NR
Hydrocodone	0.5 mg/kg PO q 8–12 h	?	NR	NR	NR

[a] Preservative-free formulations are recommended for epidural administration.

[b] Doses are for sustained-release product (MS Contin, Purdue Pharma L.P., Stamford, CT), which should be dosed every 12 hours.

[c] Lower IV infusion rates are suitable for management of most types of pain, whereas higher rates will produce profound analgesia suitable for surgery.

[d] Fentanyl transdermal patches are available in 0.025-, 0.05-, 0.075-, or 0.1-mg/h sizes.

CRI, continuous rate infusion; IM, intramuscular; IV, intravenous(ly); NR, not recommended for administration in this species; PO, per os (orally); SC, subcutaneous(ly); ?, reliable doses have not been established for this species.

Source: Lamont L.A., Mathews K.A. 2007. Opioids, nonsteroidal anti-inflammatories, and analgesic adjuvants. In: *Lumb and Jones' Veterinary Anesthesia and Analgesia,* 4th ed. W.J. Tranquilli, J.C. Thurmon, and K.A. Grimm, eds. Ames, IA: Blackwell Publishing, p. 245.

Morphine   Morphine is the prototypical opioid analgesic and acts as a full agonist not only at μ receptors, but also at δ and κ receptors. Despite the development of numerous synthetic opioids, many of which are more potent than morphine and may have other characteristics that make them desirable alternatives to morphine in certain circumstances, no other drug has been shown to be more efficacious than morphine at relieving pain. Compared with the synthetic opioid agonists, morphine is relatively hydrophilic and crosses the blood–brain barrier more slowly than fentanyl or oxymorphone, thereby delaying the peak effect somewhat even after intravenous administration. Clinically, this lag is not likely to be significant under most circumstances, with the onset of analgesia occurring reasonably promptly after a single dose of morphine and typically lasting 3–4 hours. Morphine's poor lipid solubility means that it can produce long-lasting analgesia when administered into the epidural or subarachnoid space, with effects persisting for 12–24 hours. The first-pass effect is significant after oral administration, and the bioavailability of oral morphine preparations is only in the range of 25%. If dose adjustments are made, adequate pain relief can be achieved with oral morphine administration, and the duration of action tends to be somewhat longer with this route.

In most species, the primary metabolic pathway for morphine involves conjugation with glucuronic acid, leading to the formation of two major metabolites: morphine 6-glucuronide and morphine 3-glucuronide. Despite the low levels of glucuronyl transferase in cats, the pharmacokinetics of morphine in this species seem to be broadly comparable to those in dogs and people, though clearance rates may be marginally slower. This suggests that morphine must undergo a different type of conjugation reaction in this species. Morphine 6-glucuronide has pharmacological activities that are indistinguishable from those of morphine in animal models and in people, whereas morphine 3-glucuronide appears to have little affinity for opioid receptors, but may contribute to the excitatory effects of morphine in some situations. With chronic morphine administration, it is likely that the active metabolite, morphine 6-glucuronide, contributes significantly to clinical analgesia.

The adverse effects associated with morphine administration are typical of most opioid agonists and have been discussed previously in this chapter. In particular, the increased incidence of vomiting after morphine administration, as well as its potential to cause histamine release after intravenous administration, helps to distinguish morphine from other full opioid agonists.

Clinically, morphine is a useful analgesic in dogs and cats. It is often administered at fixed dosing intervals via the intramuscular, subcutaneous, or, less commonly, intravenous routes to manage pain associated with a variety of traumatic injuries and disease processes. Morphine has also been used extensively throughout the perioperative period in these species to manage pain associated with surgical procedures. In dogs and cats, the sparing effect of morphine on both injectable and inhalant anesthetic requirements can be significant. Morphine is particularly effective in dogs when administered intravenously as a continuous infusion, which facilitates more precise dose titration to achieve optimal analgesic effects. Subcutaneous infusions of morphine and other opioids are being employed in human patients experiencing cancer pain, and, as subcutaneous infusion devices are developed that are applicable to dogs and cats, this route of administration may be accessed by veterinarians in the future. Administration of the drug into the epidural or, less commonly, subarachnoid space is a common analgesic technique employed in both dogs and cats in a variety of clinical situations. More recently, the discovery of peripheral μ opioid receptors has led to the clinical practice of instilling morphine locally into inflamed joints and even topically onto damaged corneas to supplement analgesia in canine patients.

Oxymorphone   Oxymorphone is a synthetic opioid that acts as a full agonist at μ receptors and is comparable with morphine in its analgesic efficacy and duration of action. It is a more lipid-soluble drug than morphine and is readily absorbed after intramuscular or subcutaneous administration. Oxymorphone is not available as an oral formulation.

When compared with morphine, oxymorphone is less likely to cause dogs and cats to vomit, and tends to produce more sedation when administered to these species. Its respiratory depressant effects are similar to those induced by morphine, but oxymorphone seems more likely to cause dogs to pant. It does not produce histamine release, even when administered intravenously. Oxymorphone's other side effects are typical of other full μ-agonist opioids and have been discussed previously.

Oxymorphone has been used extensively in dogs and cats, and is most often administered at fixed dosing intervals, either intramuscularly, subcutaneously, or intravenously, to manage pain in a variety of clinical settings. It is also commonly used in the preanesthetic, intraoperative, and postoperative periods in surgical patients. Oxymorphone has been administered epidurally in dogs, but its relative lipid solubility means that its analgesic action is briefer when administered by this route compared with the action of morphine.

Hydromorphone   Hydromorphone is a synthetic opioid that acts as a full agonist at μ receptors and is used in both human and veterinary medicine. Clinically, hydromorphone and oxymorphone have similar efficacy, potency, duration of analgesic action, and side-effect profiles, but hydromorphone remains significantly less expensive. Like oxymorphone, hydromorphone is not associated with histamine release, so bolus intravenous administration is considered safe, although it can lead to brief excitation and vocalization.

In dogs and cats, hydromorphone can be used in any clinical situation where oxymorphone is used. Evidence from the human literature suggests that hydromorphone may be suitable for administration via a continuous infusion, either intravenously, subcutaneously, or epidurally, and these routes of administration may further expand the use of hydromorphone in veterinary patients in the future.

Meperidine   Meperidine is a synthetic opioid that exerts its analgesic effects through agonism at μ receptors. Interestingly, it also appears able to bind other types of receptors, which may contribute to some of its clinical effects other than analgesia. Meperidine can block sodium channels and inhibit activity in dorsal horn neurons in a manner analogous to local anesthetics. Meperidine also exerts agonist activity at alpha$_2$ receptors, specifically the alpha$_{2B}$ subtype, suggesting that it may possess some alpha$_2$ agonist-like properties.

Meperidine has a shorter analgesic action compared with morphine, oxymorphone, or hydromorphone, typically not extending beyond 1 hour. Metabolic pathways vary among different species, but, in general, most of the drug is demethylated to normeperidine in the liver and then undergoes further hydrolysis and ultimately renal excretion. Normeperidine is an active metabolite and has approximately one-half the analgesic efficacy of meperidine. Normeperidine has produced toxic neurological side effects in human patients receiving meperidine for prolonged periods, especially in the presence of impaired renal function.

Unlike most of the other opioids in clinical use, meperidine has been shown to produce significant negative inotropic effects when administered alone to conscious dogs. Because of its modest atropine-like effects, meperidine tends to increase heart rate rather than predispose patients to bradycardia, as is often seen with other opioids. The clinical significance of these cardiovascular effects in the perianesthetic period has never been clearly ascertained. Like morphine, meperidine also causes histamine release when administered intravenously.

A rare, but life-threatening, drug interaction that may have relevance in veterinary medicine has been reported in human patients receiving meperidine. The combination of meperidine (and perhaps other opioids) with a monoamine oxidase inhibitor may lead to serotonin syndrome, which is characterized by a constellation of symptoms, including confusion, fever, shivering, diaphoresis, ataxia, hyperreflexia, myoclonus, and diarrhea. A monoamine oxidase inhibitor, selegiline (or deprenyl), has been used in canine patients to treat pituitary-dependent hyperadrenocorticism or to modify behavior in patients with canine cognitive dysfunction. Though there have not, to date, been any scientific studies of adverse meperidine–selegiline interactions in dogs, veterinarians must be aware of the potential for complications if analgesia is required in patients receiving monoamine oxidase inhibitors. A recent study that evaluated the effects of other opioids (oxymorphone and butorphanol) in selegiline-treated dogs did not identify any specific adverse drug interactions in these animals.

Clinically, meperidine has been used primarily in dogs and cats during the preanesthetic period, often in combination with sedatives or tranquilizers. In patients undergoing surgery, administration of another full μ-agonist opioid with a longer duration of action is recommended for use postoperatively. Meperidine appears to offer few, if any, advantages over other opioids, such as oxymorphone or hydromorphone, in these species during the perioperative period.

Fentanyl   Fentanyl is a highly lipid soluble, short-acting synthetic μ opioid agonist. A single dose of fentanyl administered intravenously has a more rapid onset and a much briefer action than morphine. Peak analgesic effects occur in about 5 minutes and last approximately 30 minutes. Rapid redistribution of the drug to inactive tissue sites, such as fat and skeletal muscle, leads to a decrease in plasma concentration and is responsible for the prompt termination of clinical effects. In most veterinary species, the elimination half-life after a single bolus or a brief infusion is in the range of 2–3 hours. Administration of very large doses or prolonged infusions may cause saturation of inactive tissues, with termination of clinical effects becoming dependent on hepatic metabolism and renal excretion. Thus, the context-sensitive half-life of fentanyl increases significantly with the duration of the infusion, and clinical effects may persist for an extended period following termination of a long-term intravenous infusion.

Adverse effects associated with fentanyl administration are similar to those of the other full μ-agonist opioids. In general, cardiovascular stability is excellent with fentanyl, and intravenous administration is not associated with histamine release. Bradycardia may be significant with bolus doses, but readily responds to anticholinergics if treatment is warranted. In human patients, muscle rigidity, especially of the chest wall, has been noted after administration of fentanyl or one of its congeners. The potential significance of this adverse effect in animal patients is not clear at this time, and the risk is considered minimal if large, rapid bolus administrations are avoided.

Clinically, fentanyl is used most frequently in dogs and cats, but is also a potentially useful analgesic in other species. Because of its shorter action, fentanyl is typically administered as a continuous infusion to provide analgesia. Intravenous fentanyl can be infused at relatively low doses to supplement analgesia intraoperatively and/or postoperatively in dogs and cats. It is also useful for management of nonsurgical pain, such as that associated with pancreatitis. Alternatively, larger doses can be administered, often in combination with a benzodiazepine like midazolam, to induce general anesthesia in canine patients with cardiovascular or hemodynamic instability. Similarly, higher infusion rates of fentanyl can be used as the primary anesthetic agent for surgical maintenance in patients who will not tolerate significant concentrations of volatile inhalant anesthetics.

In addition to intravenous administration, fentanyl may be deposited into the epidural space to produce analgesia. Because of its high lipid solubility, epidural fentanyl, unlike morphine, is rapidly absorbed into the systemic circulation. Consequently, the clinical effects associated with a single bolus of epidural fentanyl resemble those of an intravenous injection. However, the benefits of neuraxial administration can be achieved by administering epidural fentanyl as a continuous infusion through an indwelling epidural catheter, often in combination with other analgesic agents. This technique is typically used in canine patients for management of severe acute pain, but it may have additional applications for the management of chronic pain as well.

The development of novel, less invasive, routes of opioid administration for use in human patients led to the marketing of transdermal fentanyl patches. The patches are designed to release a constant amount of fentanyl per hour that is then absorbed across the skin and taken up systemically. Fentanyl patches are designed for human skin and human body temperature, but their use has been evaluated in a number of veterinary species. Though transdermal fentanyl appears to be an effective means of providing analgesia in a number of clinical settings, substantial variations in plasma drug concentrations have been documented, and significant lag times after patch placement are common prior to onset of analgesia. Furthermore, changes in body temperature have been shown to affect fentanyl absorption significantly in anesthetized cats, and it is likely that other factors associated with skin preparation and patch placement have the potential to alter plasma fentanyl levels and analgesic efficacy substantially. Two recent studies evaluating the efficacy of pluronic lecithin organogel (PLO gel) delivery of fentanyl through skin in dogs and cats concluded that this method of administration did not result in measurable plasma concentrations and thus could not be justified as an effective means of systemic administration.

Alfentanil, sufentanil, and remifentanil   Alfentanil, sufentanil, and remifentanil are all structural analogs of fentanyl that were developed for use in human patients in an effort to create analgesics with a more rapid onset of action and predictable termination of opioid effects. All three are similar with regard to onset, and all have context-sensitive half-lives that are shorter than that of fentanyl after prolonged infusions. Remifentanil is unique among opioids because it is metabolized by nonspecific plasma esterases to inactive metabolites. Thus, hepatic or renal dysfunction will have little impact on drug clearance, and this, in combination with the robust nature of the esterase metabolic system, contributes to the predictability associated with remifentanil infusion.

All three of these drugs are used during general anesthesia for procedures requiring intense analgesia and/or blunting of the sympathetic nervous system response to noxious stimulation. As yet, they have limited applications for postoperative or chronic pain management. Like fentanyl, they can be administered at relatively low infusion rates as adjuncts to general anesthetic protocols based on volatile inhalant or other injectable agents, or they can be administered at higher rates as primary agents for total intravenous anesthesia. The minimum alveolar-sparing properties of these agents have been demonstrated in both dogs and cats. There is little evidence to suggest that any of the fentanyl analogs offer advantages over morphine when administered into the epidural space for analgesia.

Methadone   Methadone is a synthetic μ opioid agonist with pharmacological properties qualitatively similar to those of morphine, but possessing additional affinity for NMDA receptors. Methadone's unique clinical characteristics include excellent absorption after oral administration, no known active metabolites, high potency, and an extended duration of action. In human patients, the drug has been used primarily in the treatment of opioid-abstinence syndromes, but is being used increasingly for the management of chronic and acute pain. Although methadone undergoes CYP 450 metabolism in dogs and the potential for drug interactions exist, at this time only chloramphenicol has been shown to significantly delay methadone biotransformation in dogs. Additional studies may identify a role for oral methadone in the management of acute and chronic pain syndromes in veterinary patients.

Codeine   Codeine is the result of the substitution of a methyl group onto morphine, which acts to limit first-pass hepatic metabolism and accounts for codeine's higher oral bioavailability. Codeine is well known for its excellent antitussive properties and is often combined in an oral formulation with a nonopioid analgesic, such as acetaminophen, for the management of mild to moderate pain in human patients. Codeine, alone or in combination with acetaminophen (Tylenol 3, Ortho-McNeil Pharmaceuticals, Titusville, NJ), has been used in dogs for the management of mild pain on an outpatient basis. Acetaminophen combinations should not be prescribed for cats due to the potential for acetaminophen toxicity.

Oxycodone and hydrocodone   Oxycodone and hydrocodone are opioids that are typically administered orally for the treatment of pain in human patients. Though oxycodone is available as a single-drug continuous-release formulation (Oxycontin, Purdue Pharma L.P., Stamford, CT), these drugs are most often prepared in combination with nonopioid analgesics, such as aspirin and acetaminophen (e.g., Percocet, Endo Pharmaceuticals, Chadds Ford, PA; Percodan, Endo Pharmaceuticals; and Vicodin, Abbott Laboratories, Abbott Park, IL). Little has been published regarding the use of these opioids in veterinary patients.

Agonist-antagonists and partial agonists

This group includes drugs that have varying opioid receptor-binding profiles, but that have one thing in common: They all occupy μ opioid receptors, but do not initiate a maximal clinical response. Drugs such as butorphanol and nalbuphine are classified as agonist-antagonists. They are competitive μ-receptor antagonists, but exert their analgesic actions by acting as agonists at κ receptors (Figure 3.5). Buprenorphine, on the other hand, is classified as a partial agonist and binds μ receptors, but produces only a limited clinical effect (Figure 3.6). These mixed agonist-antagonist drugs were developed for the human market in an attempt to create analgesics with less respiratory depression and

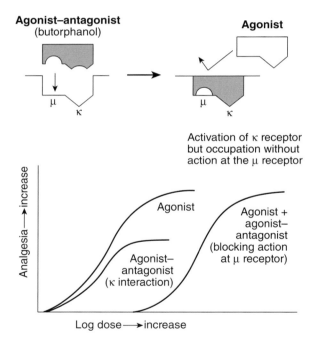

Figure 3.5.   A lock-and-key analogy is used to illustrate agonist–antagonist drug interactions at opioid receptors, with a relative dose–response curve for analgesic effectiveness shown. An agonist–antagonist opioid (in this case, butorphanol) has agonist activity at κ receptors and antagonist activity at μ receptors. In the presence of a full μ agonist, these opioids tend to have antagonistic effects and will increase the dose of full agonist required to achieve maximal analgesic effect.
Source: Modified from Nicholson A., Christie M. 2002. Opioid analgesics. In: *Small Animal Clinical Pharmacology*. J. Maddison, S. Page, and D.B. Church, eds. Philadelphia, PA: WB Saunders, pp. 271–292.

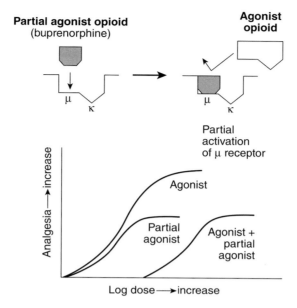

Figure 3.6. A lock-and-key analogy is used to illustrate partial agonist drug interactions at opioid receptors, with a relative dose–response curve for analgesic effectiveness shown. A partial opioid agonist (in this case buprenorphine) weakly stimulates μ receptors, which produces a reduced maximal analgesic effect compared with a full agonist. A large dose of partial agonist will interfere with the receptor actions of a full agonist, moving its dose–response curve to the right and depressing its maximal analgesic effect.
Source: Modified from Nicholson A., Christie M. 2002. Opioid analgesics. In: *Small Animal Clinical Pharmacology*. J. Maddison, S. Page, and D.B. Church, eds. Philadelphia, PA: WB Saunders, pp. 271–292.

addictive potential. Because of their opioid receptor-binding affinities, the adverse effects associated with these drugs demonstrate a so-called ceiling effect, whereby increasing doses do not produce additional adverse responses. Unfortunately, the benefits of this ceiling effect on ventilatory depression come at the expense of limited analgesic efficacy and only a modest ability to decrease anesthetic requirements.

The coadministration of opioids with differing receptor-binding profiles is currently an active area of research that deserves further attention. The interactions in this setting are complex, and opioid coadministration appears to have the potential to produce additive, synergistic, or antagonistic analgesic effects, depending on the particular species, dosage, drugs, and pain model being evaluated. The following section contains brief descriptions of opioid agonist-antagonists and partial agonists that are currently in clinical use.

Butorphanol Butorphanol is a synthetic agonist-antagonist opioid and has been used extensively in a wide variety of veterinary species. The drug was originally labeled as an antitussive agent in dogs and, even now, is approved as an analgesic in cats and horses only. Butorphanol exerts its relevant clinical effects through its interactions at κ receptors and acts as an antagonist at μ receptors. The duration of butorphanol's analgesic effects remains somewhat debatable and likely varies with species, type and intensity of pain, dosage, and route of administration. In general, its effects are shorter-lived than those of morphine and are probably in the range of 1–3 hours. Butorphanol is typically administered via the intramuscular, subcutaneous, or intravenous route, though an oral formulation is available and is occasionally prescribed for outpatient analgesia in dogs.

Butorphanol does not induce histamine release when administered intravenously and has minimal effects on cardiopulmonary function. There is conflicting evidence regarding the effects of butorphanol on inhalant anesthetic requirements in the dogs and cats. Earlier studies failed to demonstrate a significant sparing effect on MAC when butorphanol was coadministered with halothane in dogs. More recently, isoflurane MAC reductions have been documented after administration of clinically relevant doses of butorphanol in both dogs and cats. Reasons for these discrepancies are probably related to differences in study techniques, and, in dogs and cats specifically, it seems that butorphanol can induce at least modest reductions in inhalant anesthetic requirements.

When administered alone to healthy dogs and cats, butorphanol produces minimal sedation only. However, the drug is commonly used in combination with a variety of sedatives and tranquilizers, such as acepromazine, dexmedetomidine, or midazolam, to produce sedation and analgesia for minimally invasive procedures. It is also used during the preanesthetic and postoperative periods to provide analgesia for surgical procedures associated with mild to moderate pain. Butorphanol does not appear to be an effective monoanalgesic for moderate to severe pain in these species, especially when pain is orthopedic in origin.

Traditionally, it was thought that the simultaneous or sequential administration of butorphanol with a pure μ opioid agonist such as morphine or hydromorphone would be counterproductive from an analgesic standpoint because butorphanol's ability to antagonize μ receptors could inhibit or even reverse the effects of the agonist drug. Certainly, it has been clearly demonstrated that excessive sedation associated with a pure μ-agonist can be partially reversed by the administration of low doses of butorphanol, and it was presumed that butorphanol would similarly reverse the μ-mediated analgesic effects as well. It would now appear that the potential interactions between butorphanol and full μ opioid agonists are more complex than originally believed. The clinical effects produced by such coadministration likely depend on many factors, including species, type of pain, dose, and the specific drugs involved.

Nalbuphine and pentazocine Nalbuphine and pentazocine are classified as agonist-antagonist opioids and are clinically similar to butorphanol. They induce mild analgesia accompanied by minimal sedation, respiratory depression, or adverse cardiovascular effects. In human patients, nalbuphine is used more commonly than butorphanol, whereas in veterinary medicine, butorphanol is used far more frequently. Like butorphanol, nalbuphine is occasionally used to partially reverse the effects of a full μ-agonist opioid while maintaining some residual analgesia.

Buprenorphine Buprenorphine is a semisynthetic, highly lipophilic opioid derived from thebaine. Unlike other opioids in this category, buprenorphine is considered to be a partial agonist at μ opioid receptors. The drug binds avidly to, and dissociates slowly from, μ receptors, but cannot elicit a maximal clinical response. Because of its receptor-binding characteristics, buprenorphine has a delayed onset of action and takes at least 1 hour to attain peak effect after intramuscular administration. It also has a relatively long action, with clinical analgesic effects persisting for 6–12 hours in most species. Also, its high affinity for the μ receptor means that it may be difficult to antagonize its effects with a drug such as naloxone. Buprenorphine has most often been administered intravenously or intramuscularly; however, because of the long lag time before clinical effects are achieved after intramuscular administration, the intravenous route is preferred. A recent study has documented comparable plasma drug levels and analgesic efficacy with oral transmucosal administration in cats. This route seems to be well tolerated by feline patients and is becoming increasingly popular in clinical practice. A transdermal buprenorphine patch is now commercially available and currently being evaluated.

In dogs and cats, buprenorphine is used most often in the postoperative period to manage pain of mild to moderate intensity. As with the other opioids in this category, buprenorphine may not be adequate for management of severe pain such as that associated with thoracotomies or invasive orthopedic procedures. The drug is a popular analgesic in laboratory animal species because it can be formulated with a variety of foodstuffs and given orally to rodents.

Antagonists

These drugs have high affinities for the opioid receptors and can displace opioid agonists from μ and κ receptors. After this displacement, the pure antagonists bind to and occupy opioid receptors, but do not activate them. Under ordinary circumstances, in patients that have not received exogenous agonist opioids, the opioid antagonists have few clinical effects when administered at clinically relevant dosages. It is important to recognize that these drugs will rapidly reverse all opioid-induced clinical effects, including analgesia. Therefore, use of pure opioid antagonists should be reserved for emergency situations such as opioid overdose or profound respiratory depression. Their routine use for reversal of excessive sedation in patients experiencing prolonged anesthetic recoveries or in patients that develop bradycardia secondary to opioid administration may cause the development of intense acute pain and activation of the sympathetic nervous system.

Naloxone The use of this pure opioid antagonist can reverse all opioid agonist effects, producing increased alertness, responsiveness, coordination and, potentially, increased perception of pain. Naloxone's effects are shorter than that of many of the opioid agonists, with recommended intravenous doses lasting between 30 and 60 minutes. Consequently, animals need to be closely monitored for renarcotization after a dose of naloxone. Occasionally, excitement or anxiety may be seen after naloxone reversal of an opioid agonist. Premature ventricular contractions have also been documented after reversal, but are not common and seem to be more likely if there are high levels of circulating catecholamines. This drug is sometimes administered sublingually to neonatal patients exhibiting respiratory depression that have been delivered by cesarean section after maternal administration of an opioid agonist.

Naloxone has also been shown in animal models and human patients to produce a dose-related improvement in myocardial contractility and mean arterial blood pressure during shock. Further studies are needed to clarify the role of the endogenous opioid system in the pathophysiology of various forms of shock.

Nalmefene and naltrexone   Both of these drugs are pure opioid antagonists with clinical effects that last approximately twice as long as those of naloxone. Though little is published about the use of these drugs in veterinary patients, they may be advantageous in preventing renarcotization when used to antagonize the effects of a long-acting opioid.

Nonsteroidal anti-inflammatories

The NSAIDs relieve mild to moderately severe pain, with efficacy dependent on the particular NSAID administered. The NSAIDs appear to confer synergism when used in combination with opioids and may demonstrate an opioid-sparing effect should lower dosages of opioid be required. Their extended duration of action, in addition to their analgesic efficacy and lack of CNS alterations (sedation or dysphoria), make the NSAIDs ideal for treating acute and chronic pain in veterinary patients. Careful patient and drug selection is critical, however, because of their potential for harmful adverse effects.

Cyclooxygenases and PG synthesis

In 1971, Vane discovered the mechanism by which aspirin exerts its anti-inflammatory, analgesic, and antipyretic actions. He proved that aspirin and other NSAIDs inhibited the activity of a cyclooxygenase (COX) enzyme that produced PGs involved in the pathogenesis of inflammation, swelling, pain, and fever. Twenty years later, a second COX enzyme was discovered and, more recently, a newly identified COX-3 has been identified. COX (previously termed PG synthase) oxidizes arachidonic acid (previously termed eicosatetraenoic acid) to various eicosanoids (including PGs and other related compounds) (Figure 3.7). Oxidation of arachidonic acid by 5-lipoxygenase (5-LOX), the most biologically important of the mammalian oxygenases, produces the series of eicosanoids termed leukotrienes. The release of arachidonic acid from membrane phospholipid is catalyzed by the enzyme phospholipase A_2 and is the rate-limiting step in PG and leukotriene synthesis. PGG_2 is the initial prostenoid formed, followed by PGH_2, which serves as a substrate for PGE synthetase, PGD isomerase, PGF reductase, prostacyclin synthetase, and thromboxane synthetase for conversion to a variety of other prostenoids ubiquitous throughout cells and tissues in the body. These include the PGs PGE_2, PGD_2, PGF_2, and PGI_2 (prostacyclin), and the thromboxanes TXA_2 and TXB_2, all with diverse functions. The PGs are not stored, but are synthesized at a constant rate. They have short half-lives of 4–6 minutes at 37°C and act locally at the site of production.

The PGs produced by both COX-1 and COX-2 are ubiquitous throughout the body and serve to facilitate many physiological functions during both health and illness. Consequently, the clinical use of NSAIDs has the potential to disrupt these functions, with the possibility of significant organ dysfunction. Thus, in addition to their role as analgesics, the effects of NSAIDs on the constitutive functions of the PGs must always be

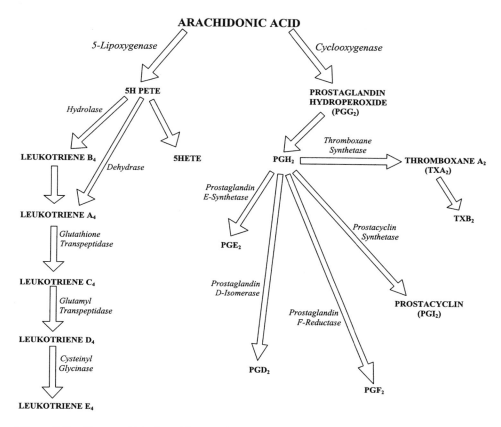

Figure 3.7. The arachidonic acid cascade and eicosanoid synthesis. 5-HETE, 5-hydroxy-6,8,11,14-eicosatetraenoic acid; and 5-HPETE, 5-hydroperoxy-6,8,11,14-eicosatetraenoic acid.
Source: Lamont L.A., Mathews K.A. 2007. Opioids, nonsteroidal anti-inflammatories, and analgesic adjuvants. In: *Lumb and Jones' Veterinary Anesthesia and Analgesia*, 4th ed. W.J. Tranquilli, J.C. Thurmon, and K.A. Grimm, eds. Ames, IA: Blackwell Publishing, p. 253.

considered. There are several key points to note: (1) COX-1 generates PGs that are responsible for mucosal defense (i.e., secretion of bicarbonate and mucus, mucosal blood vessel attenuation of constriction, and mucosal epithelial regeneration), as well as TXA_2, which is necessary for platelet function; (2) COX-2 produces PGs that function in the prevention and promotion of healing of mucosal erosions, and exert anti-inflammatory effects by inhibiting leukocyte adherence, as well as play a role in renal protection and maturation; and (3) COX-3 produces PGs that exert a protective function by initiating fever. Thus, depending on the NSAID selected, primary plug formation of platelets, modulation of vascular tone in the kidney and gastric mucosa, cytoprotective functions within the gastric mucosa, smooth muscle contraction, and regulation of body temperature will all be affected. In this regard, however, not all NSAIDs are created equal. As already noted, the COX-1, COX-2, and COX-3 enzymes make variable contributions to these functions, and individual NSAIDs inhibit each of these enzymes differently. Some

NSAIDs inhibit both COX-1 and COX-2 (i.e., aspirin, phenylbutazone, ketoprofen, ketorolac, and flunixin meglumine); other NSAIDs preferentially inhibit COX-2 with only weak inhibition of COX-1 (i.e., meloxicam, carprofen, etodolac, vedaprofen, and tolfenamic acid); and others inhibit COX-2 exclusively (i.e., deracoxib, firocoxib, and rofecoxib); whereas still another drug, acetaminophen, only weakly inhibits both COX-1 and COX-2 while inhibiting COX-3 activity preferentially.

Several *in vitro* studies investigating NSAID-selective inhibition of the COX-1 and COX-2 isoenzymes have been published, but their findings are very difficult to interpret because of inconsistencies in the assays used. Clinically, this information is confusing because it does not consider the pharmacokinetics of particular drugs and their concentrations in various tissues. Most NSAIDs that inhibit COX have been shown to result in diversion of arachidonate to the 5-LOX pathway. The 5-LOX is principally found in polymorphonuclear cells, mast cells, monocytes, basophils, and B lymphocytes that are recruited during inflammatory and immune reactions. This enzyme catalyzes the initial step in leukotriene biosynthesis, which subsequently produces various eicosanoids, with leukotriene B_4 (LTB_4) being the most notable potent mediator of inflammation. The excessive production of leukotrienes has been implicated in the creation of NSAID-induced ulcers. As always, however, the biologic system is not clear-cut. Although the LOX pathway is proinflammatory, there is also an anti-inflammatory pathway, which is discussed in more detail later.

The contribution of the leukotrienes to the inflammatory process would seem to suggest that inhibition of both the COX and 5-LOX pathways by a therapeutic agent would enhance the safety profile and may confer even greater analgesic efficacy because of broader anti-inflammatory and antinociceptive effects. Data available show that dual-acting compounds are effective in arthritic models, where they also retain antithrombotic activity, produce little or no gastrointestinal damage, and do not adversely affect the asthmatic state. A dual COX–5-LOX inhibitor (tepoxalin) has undergone clinical trials and is now approved for veterinary use. Tepoxalin has demonstrated gastrointestinal anti-inflammatory activity in mice, which supports the theory that 5-LOX inhibition can play a vital role in preventing NSAID-induced gastric inflammation.

Mechanisms of analgesia

PGs, notably PGE_2 and prostacyclin, are potent mediators of inflammation and pain. These molecules exert hyperalgesic effects and enhance nociception produced by other mediators, such as bradykinin. The NSAIDs' analgesic mechanism of action is through inhibition of COX-1, COX-2, and COX-3 activity, with subsequent prevention of PG synthesis.

The antinociceptive effects of the NSAIDs are exerted both peripherally and centrally. The NSAIDs penetrate inflamed tissues, where they have a local effect, which makes them excellent analgesic choices for treatment of injuries with associated inflammation, as well as conditions such as synovitis, arthritis, cystitis, and dermatitis. The central action is at both the spinal and the supraspinal levels, with contributions from both COX-1 and COX-2. This central effect may account for the overall well-being and improved appetite that are often observed in patients receiving parenterally administered NSAIDs for relief of acute pain.

The rational use of NSAIDs as analgesics should be based on an understanding of physiology and pathophysiology. Nociceptive pathways may involve either the COX-1 or COX-2 gene, and these genes are expressed in different locations and under different circumstances. The COX-2 isoenzyme, which is known as the inducible isoform because it is upregulated in inflammatory states, is known to play a key role in nociception. Although the COX-1 gene has traditionally been thought of as being expressed constitutively, this isoenzyme also plays an integral role in the pain experience.

The COX-2 or inducible isoenzyme can increase by 20-fold over baseline in the presence of tissue injury and inflammation. Proinflammatory cytokines and mitogens, such as interleukin-1b (IL-1b), interferon γ, and tumor necrosis factor-α (TNF-α), induce COX-2 expression in macrophages, as can platelet-activating factor and PGE_2. These events may also occur in chondrocytes, osteoblasts, and synovial microvessel endothelial cells. Higher COX levels increase prostenoid production where these compounds serve as amplifiers of nociceptive input and transmission in both the peripheral and central nervous systems. The COX-2-selective NSAIDs have been shown to be clinically useful in managing inflammatory pain in human and animal patients. This has been a focus of the pharmaceutical industry, as a more selective COX-2 inhibitor might show efficacy in alleviating pain and hyperalgesia while sparing COX-1-constitutive activity and potential adverse effects traditionally associated with NSAID administration. Unfortunately, this biologic system is not as simple as first envisioned. Although COX-2 is induced during inflammation, it has also been shown to be induced during resolution of the inflammatory response where the anti-inflammatory PGs (PGD_2 and PGF_2), but not proinflammatory PGE_2, are produced. Potentially, inhibition of COX-2 during this phase may actually prolong inflammation. As is the case for COX-1, it now appears that the COX-2 isoenzyme also has important constitutive functions. Studies indicate there may be a protective role for COX-2 in the maintenance of gastrointestinal integrity, in ulcer healing, and in experimental colitis in rats. In addition, the COX-2 isoenzyme appears to have constitutive functions associated with nerve, brain, ovarian and uterine function, and bone metabolism. Therefore, the potential for NSAID-associated side effects with these systems is of concern. Of major importance are the COX-2-constitutive functions within the kidney, which differ from those of COX-1 in hypotensive and hypovolemic states. Also, COX-2 appears to be important in nephron maturation. The canine kidney is not fully mature until 3 weeks after birth, and administration of a NSAID during this time, or to the bitch prior to birth, may cause a permanent nephropathy. In fact, in COX-2 null mice, which lack the gene for COX-2, all animals die of renal failure before 8 weeks of age. Renal failure does not occur in COX-1-null-developing mice, and they do not develop gastric pathology.

Dissecting out the details of the derivation and specific actions of COX-1 and COX-2 continues to provide important insight into the management of pain with NSAIDs. The picture, however, remains incomplete because some NSAIDs do not significantly inhibit these enzymes. This finding stimulated the search for a potential COX-3 isoenzyme. Based on studies using canine cortex, a COX-3 isoenzyme was discovered that was derived from the same gene as COX-1. The COX-3 isoenzyme is also present in human brain and heart tissues. It is distinct from COX-1 and COX-2 as demonstrated in studies using common analgesic–antipyretic NSAIDs in suppressing COX production.

Acetaminophen inhibited COX-3 activity, but not COX-1 and COX-2, as does dipyrone. Both of these agents are frequently used to reduce fever in animals. Other analgesic–antipyretic NSAIDs found to be effective COX-3 inhibitors are diclofenac (the most potent) and aspirin and ibuprofen (which preferentially inhibit COX-3 over COX-1 and COX-2). The overall conclusion of this particular study was that COX-3 possesses COX activity that differs pharmacologically from both COX-1 and COX-2, but is more similar to COX-1. These findings indicate that the COX-3 isoenzyme is more susceptible to inhibition by drugs that are analgesic and antipyretic, but that lack anti-inflammatory activity.

Fever inhibition

Just as the relationship between pain and the various activities of the COX system is complex, so too is the association between fever and the COX isoenzymes. The mechanisms leading to the generation of fever vary depending on the inciting factor, which may be peripheral (i.e., endotoxin) or central (i.e., endogenous pyrogens, such as IL-1). Interspecies variation is also substantial, and the definitive role of the COXs in pyresis remains to be clearly elucidated. Evidence suggests that COX-2 plays a role in endotoxin pyrexia, whereas based on the antipyretic effects of acetaminophen and aspirin, COX-1 and COX-3 appear to function in endogenous pyrexia. Both of these drugs are effective in reducing fever in dogs. As an alternative in feline patients, ketoprofen and meloxicam have been shown to be effective antipyretic agents. Ketoprofen appears to be a good antipyretic in both cats and dogs, and this action can often be achieved at a relatively low dose.

Endogenous anti-inflammatory mechanisms

Endogenously generated small chemical mediators, or autacoids, play a key role in controlling inflammation by inhibiting polymorphonuclear cell recruitment and enhancing monocyte activity in a nonphlogistic manner. Arachidonic acid-derived lipoxins, particularly lipoxin A_4, have been identified as anti-inflammatory mediators, indicating that the LOX pathway has a dual proinflammatory and anti-inflammatory function.

The NSAIDs may amplify or decrease this endogenous anti-inflammatory system. Aspirin is more COX-1 selective and can impair many components of mucosal defense and enhance leukocyte adherence within the gastric and mesenteric microcirculation. However, with chronic use of aspirin, an adaptation of the gastric mucosa is associated with a marked upregulation of COX-2 expression and lipoxin production. This lipoxin is specifically termed aspirin-triggered lipoxin (ATL). Aspirin is unique among current therapies because it acetylates COX-2, thereby enabling the biosynthesis of 15(R)-hydroxyeicosatetraenoic acid from arachidonic acid, which is subsequently converted to ATL by 5-LOX. Inhibition of either the COX-2 or 5-LOX enzymes causes blockade of ATL synthesis. Lipoxin A_4 and ATL (a carbon-15 epimer of lipoxin) attenuate aspirin-induced leukocyte adherence, whereas administration of selective COX-2 inhibitors blocks ATL synthesis and has been shown to augment aspirin-induced damage and leukocyte adherence to the endothelium of mesenteric venules in rats.

In addition to the lipoxins, aspirin-induced COX-2 acetylation generates numerous other endogenous autacoids derived from dietary omega-3 fatty acids. Some of these local autacoids are potent inhibitors of neutrophil recruitment, thereby limiting the role of these cells during the resolution phase of inflammation, and thus are referred to as resolvins. The identification of both the lipoxins and the resolvins has introduced new potential therapeutic avenues for the treatment of inflammation, cardiovascular disease, and cancer.

Pharmacological considerations

The NSAIDs are effective analgesics as indicated by the human consumption of 120 billion aspirin tablets per year in addition to the many other NSAIDs currently on the market. Despite this, the safety profile of these analgesics remains a concern. A search for the NSAID without adverse gastrointestinal effects is still ongoing. Incorporation of a nitric oxide-generating moiety into the molecule of several NSAIDs has shown attenuation of the ulcerogenic effects of these drugs. However, nitric oxide has also been implicated in the pathogenesis of arthritis and subsequent tissue destruction.

Because of their high protein binding, NSAIDs can displace other drugs from their plasma protein-binding sites and potentially increase their plasma concentration. This is rarely a concern unless NSAIDs are administered to patients with organ dysfunction or in those receiving other highly protein-bound medications with a narrow therapeutic index. Interference with the metabolism and excretion of certain coadministered drugs may occur; therefore, verifying the safety of combination therapy is always mandatory.

NSAID-induced renal insufficiency is usually temporary and reversible with drug withdrawal and administration of intravenous fluids. Accidental ingestion of NSAIDs should be managed with gastric lavage (if within 1 hour) followed by administration of activated charcoal and gastric protectants. If evidence of gastric ulcers exist, aggressive sucralfate therapy is necessary. Intravenous fluid therapy should continue for at least 1 day. Therapy beyond this period will depend on the renal and gastric status of the individual patient.

Patient selection and therapeutic considerations

The general health of a patient greatly influences the decision to use NSAIDs. Cats and dogs are more susceptible than people to the adverse effects of this class of drugs. Thus, the reported safety of any one NSAID in human patients should not be assumed to be so in veterinary patients. Most NSAIDs have a narrow safety margin, so accurate dosing is necessary.

The administration of NSAIDs for perioperative pain management should be restricted to animals older than 6 weeks that are well hydrated and normotensive. Patients should have normal hemostatic function, no evidence or concern for gastric ulceration, and normal renal and hepatic function. Although these are general guidelines, future studies may indicate that short-term management of acute pain by using COX-1-sparing and, to some degree, COX-2-sparing NSAIDs may prove safe in animals with minimally compromised liver or renal function. Patients should not receive corticosteroids and NSAIDs concurrently, nor should different NSAIDs be administered concurrently.

The preemptive use of NSAIDs is controversial because of their potential for harm. An earlier study assessing the effects on the kidney of preoperative administration of ketorolac, ketoprofen, or carprofen resulted in variable alterations in parameters measured. The conclusions of the study were that, in clinically normal dogs undergoing elective surgery, the use of these NSAIDs was not contraindicated, although renal function was not measured and two dogs in each of the ketoprofen and ketorolac groups were azotemic. Another study assessing effects of preoperative administration of ketoprofen on whole blood platelet aggregation, buccal mucosal bleeding time, and hematologic indices in dogs undergoing elective ovariohysterectomy showed a decrease in platelet aggregation for at least 1 day after surgery.

The benefit of preoperative administration of NSAIDs is the potential for a preemptive effect and the presence of analgesia upon recovery. When NSAIDs are administered postoperatively, opioids are often given concurrently, as 45 minutes is required to obtain a therapeutic effect with an NSAID, regardless of route. Another potential approach could be to administer the NSAID parenterally prior to completing the surgical procedure at least 45 minutes prior to extubation. Often it is difficult to distinguish the difference in the analgesic effects produced by preoperative versus intraoperative NSAID administration. For prolonged operative procedures, the benefit of a longer postoperative effect may be seen with administration of the NSAID upon completion, rather than at the start, of the procedure.

Postoperative pain

The NSAIDs are extremely valuable in selected orthopedic and soft tissue surgical procedures, especially where extensive inflammation or soft tissue trauma is present. Opioid administration is preferred immediately after any surgical procedure, because the sedative–analgesic effects of this class of drugs help to ensure a smooth recovery. Injectable NSAIDs (carprofen, ketoprofen, meloxicam, or tolfenamic acid) can be coadministered initially with an opioid and subsequently used alone following orthopedic and selected soft tissue surgery; however, this depends on the degree of pain an animal is experiencing. Oral NSAIDs may be administered when an animal is able to eat. The initial dose of NSAID depends on the expected severity of pain.

Inflammatory conditions

For relief of pain caused by meningitis, bone tumors (especially after biopsy), soft tissue swelling (mastitis), polyarthritis, cystitis, otitis, or severe inflammatory dermatologic diseases or injury (e.g., degloving and animal bites), the NSAIDs may be more efficacious than opioids. However, as many of these patients may be more prone to NSAID toxicity, careful patient selection and management are advised. The combination of an opioid with a low dose of NSAID is also effective in these conditions. An exception is necrotizing fasciitis, where NSAIDs may actually increase morbidity and mortality.

Osteoarthritis

The major adverse effects associated with long-term use of NSAIDs for osteoarthritis in dogs are predominantly associated with the gastrointestinal tract. Gastroduodenal pathology associated with buffered aspirin, carprofen, etodolac, and placebo has been evaluated in healthy dogs after a 4-week course of administration. Two independent studies concluded that the administration of carprofen, etodolac, or placebo produced significantly fewer gastroduodenal lesions in dogs than did buffered aspirin. Similar studies comparing ketoprofen with aspirin and placebo, and comparing carprofen, meloxicam, and ketoprofen to aspirin and placebo, noted that these NSAIDs produced mild to moderate gastrointestinal lesions that were similar to placebo, but significantly less severe than those produced by aspirin.

As many patients with osteoarthritis are geriatric, a rapid reduction of the dose to affect a comfortable state is advised to reduce potential toxicity. For example, alternating every-third-day therapy of meloxicam with half the recommended label dose proved efficacious in some dogs during a 1-year period. If an individual patient requires persistent high doses of a particular NSAID to manage pain, prescribing a different NSAID may be more effective because of individual variation in response and effect, as previously discussed. When the adverse effects of an NSAID are a concern, reducing the dose and adding an analgesic of a different class (e.g., tramadol) may be equally effective for the treatment of chronic severe pain. However, for many geriatric animals with renal insufficiency, NSAIDs may be the only effective class of analgesic. For these animals, quality of life is a major issue. Informed consent of the owner is imperative in these situations because of the prescribing of the drug in contradiction to the approved label information.

During NSAID therapy, all patients should be monitored for hematochezia or melena, vomiting, increased water consumption, and nonspecific changes in demeanor. If any of these occur, the owner should be instructed to stop the medication and consult a veterinarian. Intermittent monitoring of creatinine and alanine aminotransferase (ALT) is recommended when the use of NSAIDs is prescribed on a chronic basis.

Another important consideration for chronic use is the potential effect of NSAID therapy on joint and cartilage metabolism. Studies investigating the effects of carprofen and meloxicam at therapeutic doses found no toxicological or pharmacological actions on cartilage proteoglycan metabolism. In addition, meloxicam may have the potential for controlling cellular inflammatory reactions at inflamed sites in the joints of patients with osteoarthritis.

Miscellaneous conditions

Other indications for the use of NSAIDs are panosteitis, hypertrophic osteodystrophy (HOD), cancer pain (especially of bone), and dental pain. The NSAIDs with selective COX-1 inhibition should be used with caution after dental extractions where bleeding is, or may be, of concern. Meloxicam, carprofen, and the coxibs have minimal, if any, antithromboxane activity and should, therefore, not interfere with platelet adhesion. For severe panosteitis and HOD, the full loading dose of an NSAID is required to obtain a suitable effect. The HOD of Weimaraners is poorly responsive to NSAID therapy and is better treated with high-dose, short-term corticosteroids, provided infectious disease has been ruled out and clinical signs are consistent with HOD alone.

Contraindications

NSAIDs should not be administered to patients with acute renal insufficiency, hepatic insufficiency, dehydration, hypotension, or conditions associated with low effective circulating volume (e.g., congestive heart failure or ascites), coagulopathies (e.g., factor deficiencies, thrombocytopenia, or von Willebrand's disease), or evidence of gastric ulceration (i.e., vomiting with or without the presence of "coffee ground material" or melena). Administration of NSAIDs following gastrointestinal surgery must be determined by the overall health of the gut at the time of surgery. As the COX-2 isoenzyme is important for healing, intuitively NSAIDs producing potent COX-2 enzyme inhibition would be contraindicated where compromised bowel is noted. Concurrent use of other NSAIDs (e.g., aspirin) or corticosteroids is not recommended. The use of COX-1 preferential NSAIDs is contraindicated in patients with spinal injury (including herniated intervertebral disc) because of the potential for hemorrhage and neurological deterioration, and because of excessive bleeding at the surgical site should surgical treatment be pursued. The NSAIDs should never be administered to patients in shock, trauma patients upon presentation, or patients with evidence of hemorrhage (e.g., epistaxis, hemangiosarcoma, or head trauma) until the patient can be stabilized and organ function assessed. The condition of patients with severe or poorly controlled asthma, such as feline asthma, or other types of moderate to severe pulmonary disease, may deteriorate with NSAID administration. Aspirin administration has been documented to exacerbate asthma in human patients, but the administration of COX-2-specific NSAIDs did not worsen clinical signs. It is unknown whether animals may be affected in this way.

Because of inhibition of PG activity, the NSAIDs may be detrimental to reproductive function. Indomethacin may block PG activity in pregnant women, causing cessation of labor, premature closure of the ductus arteriosus in the fetus, and disruption of fetal circulation. These effects may also occur in animals, so NSAIDs should not be administered during pregnancy. As COX-2 induction is necessary for ovulation and subsequent implantation of the embryo, the use of NSAIDs should also be avoided in breeding females during this stage of the reproductive cycle. As previously mentioned, the COX-2 isoenzyme is required for maturation of the embryological kidney, so COX-2 administration to lactating mothers should be avoided.

Specific NSAIDs

Recommended dosages are listed in Table 3.2.

Meloxicam   Meloxicam is a COX-2 preferential NSAID approved for oral use in dogs in Australasia, Europe, and North America. The parenteral formulation is approved for cats in Australasia and the United States. Studies indicate no permanent renal or hepatic

Table 3.2. Dosage ranges (milligram per kilogram unless otherwise indicated) for NSAIDs in dogs and cats

NSAID[a]	Indication	Species, dose, route	Frequency
Ketoprofen	Surgical pain	Dogs, ≤2.0 IV, SC, IM, PO	Once
		Cats, ≤2.0 SC	Once
		then dogs and cats, ≤1.0 IV, SC, IM, PO	q 24 hours
		Dogs and cats, ≤2.0 PO	
	Chronic pain	then ≤1.0	Once
Meloxicam	Surgical pain	Dogs, ≤0.2 IV, SC	Once
		then ≤0.1 IV, SC, PO	q 24 hours
	Chronic pain	Dogs, ≤0.2 PO	Once
		then ≤0.1 PO	q 24 hours
	Surgical pain	Cats, ≤0.2 SC, PO	Once
		then ≤0.1 SC, PO lean weight	q 24 hours for 2–3 days
	Chronic pain[b]	Cats, ≤0.2 SC, PO	Once
		then ≤0.1 PO lean weight	q 24 hours for 2–3 days
		then 0.025 PO or (0.1 mg/ CAT max) lean weight	3–5 × weekly
Carprofen	Surgical pain	Dogs, ≤4.0 IV, SC, IM	Once at induction
		then ≤2.2 PO	Repeat q 12–24 hours
		Cats, ≤1.0 SC lean weight	Once at induction only
	Chronic pain	Dogs, ≤2.2 PO	q 12–24 hours
Robenacoxib	Surgical and chronic pain	Dogs, ≤1 PO, SC	q 24 hours
		Cats, 1 PO up to 3 days	
Tolfenamic acid	Acute, chronic pain	Dogs and cats, ≤4 SC, PO	q 24 hours for 3 days, 4 days off, then repeat cycle
Firocoxib	Chronic pain	Dogs, 5.0 PO	q 24 hours
Flunixin meglumine	Surgical pain	Dogs, ≤1.0 IV, SC, IM	Once
		Cats, 0.25 SC	q 12–24 hours PRN × 1 or 2 doses
	Pyrexia	Dogs and cats, 0.25 SC	q 12–24 hours PRN × 1 or 2 doses
	Ophthalmologic procedures	Dogs, 0.25–1.0 SC, IM	q 12–24 hours PRN × 1 or 2 doses
Ketorolac	Surgical pain	Dogs, 0.3–0.5 IV, IM	q 8–12 hours × 1 or 2 doses
		Cats, 0.25 IM	q 12 hours × 1 or 2 doses
	Panosteitis	Dogs, 10-mg total dose in dogs ≥30 kg PO, 5-mg total dose in dogs >20 kg <30 kg PO	q 24 hours for 2–3 days
Deracoxib	Surgical pain	Dogs, ≤3–4 PO	q 24 hours for 3–7 days
	Chronic pain	Dogs, ≤1–2 PO	q 24 hours
Tepoxalin	Chronic pain	Dogs, 10 PO	q 24 hours
Piroxicam	Inflammation of the lower urinary tract	Dogs, 0.3 PO	q 24 hours × 2 doses then q 48 hours
Acetaminophen	Acute, chronic pain	Dogs, 15 PO (contraindicated in cats)	q 8 hours
Aspirin	Acute, chronic pain	Dogs, 10 PO	q 12 hours

[a] See the text for details on contraindications for use.
[b] Repeated dosing of meloxicam to cats is specifically not recommended by the manufacturer.
CAT max, maximal dose in cats; IM, intramuscular; IV, intravenously; NSAID, nonsteroidal anti-inflammatory drug; PO, per os (orally); PRN, as necessary; SC, subcutaneously.

Source: Lamont L.A., Mathews K.A. 2007. Opioids, nonsteroidal anti-inflammatories, and analgesic adjuvants. In: *Lumb and Jones' Veterinary Anesthesia and Analgesia*, 4th ed. W.J. Tranquilli, J.C. Thurmon, and K.A. Grimm, eds. Ames, IA: Blackwell Publishing, p. 259.

abnormalities with acute administration; however, concern exists (as with all NSAIDs) that cats may develop acute renal damage with one or more doses).

Carprofen   Although classified as an NSAID, carprofen administration to beagles did not inhibit PGE_2, 12-hydroxyeicosatetraenoic acid, or TXB_2 synthesis in an experimental study using subcutaneous tissue cage fluids. It was concluded that the principle mode of action of carprofen must be by mechanisms other than COX or 12-LOX inhibition. However, more recent studies indicate that it is a COX-2 preferential NSAID. Carprofen is approved for perioperative and chronic pain management in dogs in Australasia, Europe, and North America. Carprofen is approved for single-dose, perioperative use in cats in Europe. Antithromboxane activity is minimal, suggesting that induced coagulopathy may not be a problem in patients with intact hemostatic mechanisms.

Acute hepatotoxicity and death after carprofen administration have been reported among dogs with previously reported normal liver function (with Labrador retrievers highly represented). The potential for hepatotoxicity appears to be a general characteristic of NSAIDs and not specific to any one product. Carprofen provides good analgesia from 12 to 18 hours after a variety of orthopedic procedures. In cats undergoing ovariohysterectomy, carprofen administration provided profound analgesia between 4 and 20 hours postoperatively.

Ketoprofen   Ketoprofen is approved for treatment of postoperative and chronic pain in both dogs and cats in Europe and Canada. As ketoprofen is an inhibitor of both COX-1 and COX-2, adverse effects are a potential problem requiring careful patient selection. Although several studies using ketoprofen preoperatively indicate its effectiveness in controlling postoperative pain, a general consensus among practitioners has restricted its use primarily to the postoperative period to reduce the potential for hemorrhage. Ketoprofen should not be administered to patients with risk factors for hemorrhage. It is often administered to animals immediately after orthopedic procedures (e.g., fracture repair, cruciate repair, or onychectomy); however, it is advised to restrict administration after laparotomy or thoracotomy until such time that hemorrhage is not a concern and when intracavitary drainage tubes have been removed.

In a study investigating the efficacy of NSAIDs in controlling postoperative pain, ketoprofen conferred a very good to excellent analgesic state for up to 24 hours when compared with butorphanol. Ketoprofen administration has also been suggested for management of pain associated with HOD and panosteitis in dogs. Gastroprotectants should be coadministered. Occasional vomiting may be seen when ketoprofen is administered chronically.

Etodolac   Etodolac is a COX-2-preferential NSAID approved in the United States for oral use in dogs for the management of pain and inflammation associated with osteoarthritis. Most adverse effects appear to be primarily restricted to the gastrointestinal tract. However, keratoconjunctivitis sicca (KCS) has been reported following etodolac administration to dogs; and its use has been limited.

Robenacoxib, deracoxib, and firocoxib   The coxib-class COX-2-specific inhibitors are approved in the United States and Canada for control of postoperative pain and inflammation associated with orthopedic surgery and chronic osteoarthritic pain in dogs.

Robenacoxib is approved for use in dogs in Europe, but it is currently the only coxib-class NSAID approved for use in the cat. Robenacoxib is approved for up to 3 days of oral administration to cats in the United States and up to 6 days in Europe. It has a relatively short half-life which should limit drug accumulation with repeated dosing. The coxib class of NSAIDs was originally marketed as being more gastroprotective in human patients when compared with the less COX-1-sparing NSAIDs such as aspirin. However, more recent findings and large-scale usage in human patients have indicated that the coxib class of NSAIDs does not guarantee gastroprotection. In a more recent canine study comparing the gastrointestinal safety profile of licofelone (a dual COX–LOX inhibitor) with rofecoxib (a similar coxib-type COX-2 inhibitor to deracoxib and firocoxib), rofecoxib was found to induce significant gastric and gastroduodenal lesions.

Tepoxalin   Tepoxalin is a COX-1, COX-2, and LOX inhibitor of varying degrees with efficacy comparable to meloxicam or carprofen and safety comparable to placebo. Tepoxalin has been approved for management of osteoarthritic pain in dogs. The safety profile of tepoxalin showed no difference from that of placebo when administered prior to a 30-minute anesthesia period and a minor surgical procedure in dogs.

Tolfenamic acid   Tolfenamic acid is approved for use in cats and dogs in Europe and Canada for controlling acute postoperative and chronic pain. The dosing schedule is 3 days on and 4 days off, which must be strictly adhered to. Reported adverse effects are diarrhea and occasional vomiting. Tolfenamic acid has significant anti-inflammatory and antithromboxane activity, so posttraumatic and surgical hemostasis may be compromised during active bleeding after administration of this NSAID.

Vedaprofen   The oral form is approved for use in dogs in Europe and Canada. The parenteral form is approved for use in horses in Europe and North America and has very similar pharmacokinetic and pharmacodynamic properties to those of ketoprofen.

Ketorolac   Ketorolac, which is a COX-1 and COX-2 inhibitor, is not approved for use in veterinary patients, but is included for the benefit of those working in the research setting where the availability of ketorolac is more likely than other NSAIDs. Ketorolac is comparable to oxymorphone in efficacy and to ketoprofen in duration and efficacy in managing postlaparotomy and orthopedic pain in dogs. Only one to two doses should be administered to dogs or cats. Ketorolac has been used successfully for treatment of severe panosteitis in dogs where all other therapies had failed. It is recommended that ketorolac be administered with food or gastroprotectants to decrease the incidence of gastric irritation (which is relatively common).

Piroxicam   Piroxicam is not approved for use in veterinary patients, but has proven valuable for its anti-inflammatory effects on the lower urinary tract in dogs with transitional cell carcinoma or cystitis and urethritis. The administration of gastroprotectants is often recommended.

Acetaminophen   Acetaminophen is a COX-3 inhibitor with minimal COX-1 and COX-2 effects. It is not approved for use in veterinary patients. It should not be administered to cats because of deficient glucuronidation of acetaminophen in this species. It may be administered to dogs as an antipyretic and analgesic for mild pain and can be used in combination with opioids for a synergistic analgesic effect or opioid-sparing effect. When prescribed as an individual drug it can be coadministered with an opioid (this approach allows more flexibility in dosing of the opioid), or it can be dosed in a proprietary combined formulation with an opioid (e.g., codeine plus acetaminophen, or oxycodone plus acetaminophen).

Aspirin Aspirin, which is primarily a COX-1 inhibitor, is most commonly used as an analgesic for osteoarthritic pain in dogs. It is also available in proprietary combinations with various opioids (aspirin plus codeine, or aspirin plus oxycodone) to achieve a synergistic effect for the treatment of moderate pain. It is also used as an antipyretic and anticoagulant in dogs and cats.

Dipyrone Dipyrone, which is a COX-3 inhibitor, is approved for use in cats and dogs in Europe and Canada. It should be given intravenously to avoid the irritation experienced when given intramuscularly. The analgesia produced is not usually adequate for moderate to severe postoperative pain, and dipyrone is reserved for use as an antipyretic in cases where other NSAIDs are contraindicated. Nephrotoxicity or gastric ulceration is not a major concern in the short term even in critically ill patients. Dipyrone administration induces blood dyscrasias in human patients, but this has not been reported in animals.

Analgesic adjuvants

Analgesic adjuvants are defined as drugs that have primary indications other than pain, but that possess analgesic actions in certain painful conditions. This definition encompasses a very diverse group of drugs and distinguishes the analgesic adjuvants from the so-called traditional analgesics, which include the opioids, the NSAIDs, and the local anesthetics. It is only recently that analgesic adjuvants have begun to be used in veterinary medicine, and most therapeutic recommendations have been extrapolated from experience with human patients and subsequently applied to companion animals.

As the name implies, these agents are typically coadministered with the traditional analgesics. They have been used most often in the management of chronic pain states; however, their use in acute pain settings is increasing, and certain adjuvant agents have become common analgesic supplements during the perioperative period. In the chronic pain setting, the adjuvant analgesics are administered (1) to manage pain that is refractory to traditional analgesics, (2) to enable the dose of traditional analgesics to be reduced in order to lessen side effects, and (3) to concurrently treat a symptom other than pain. In some clinical settings, such as chronic neuropathic pain syndromes, adjuvant analgesics have become so well accepted that they are administered as the first-line therapy in human patients.

When contemplating administration of an adjuvant analgesic, veterinarians must be aware of the drug's clinical pharmacology and its particular use in patients with pain. The following information about the drug is necessary: (1) approved indications, (2) unapproved indications (e.g., for analgesia) that are widely accepted in veterinary medical

Table 3.3. Dosage ranges (milligram per kilogram) for analgesic adjuvants in selected domestic species

Analgesic adjuvant	Dogs	Cats
Ketamine	0.5 IV loading dose 0.1–0.5/h IV CRI	0.5 IV loading dose 0.1–0.5/h IV CRI
Dexmedetomidine	0.001–0.015 IV, IM	0.0025–0.02 IV, IM
Gabapentin	2–10 PO q 8–12 hours	2–10 PO q 8–12 hours
Amantadine	3–5 PO q 24 hours	3–5 PO q 24 hours
Tramadol	2–10 PO q 12–24 hours	?

CRI, continuous rate infusion; IM, intramuscular(ly); IV, intravenous(ly); PO, per os (orally); ?, reliable doses have not been established for this species.
Source: Lamont L.A., Matthews K.A. 2007. Opioids, nonsteroidal anti-inflammatories, and analgesic adjuvants. In: *Lumb and Jones' Veterinary Anesthesia and Analgesia*, 4th ed. W.J. Tranquilli, J.C. Thurmon, and K.A. Grimm, eds. Ames, IA: Blackwell Publishing, p. 263.

practice, (3) common side effects and uncommon but potentially severe adverse effects, (4) important pharmacokinetic features, and (5) specific dosing guidelines for pain.

Numerous drugs may be considered as analgesic adjuvants in veterinary medicine today. Some of these, such as ketamine and the alpha$_2$ agonists, are familiar to practitioners, whereas others have not been used historically in veterinary medicine. Much of the evidence substantiating the use of these agents comes from laboratory animal research, clinical trials in humans, or anecdotal reports in human or animal patients. The following section briefly reviews the current state of knowledge regarding selected analgesic adjuvants in veterinary medicine (see Table 3.3 for recommended dosages).

Ketamine

Ketamine is a dissociative anesthetic used for decades in veterinary medicine. More recently, it has been recognized as an NMDA receptor antagonist and, at very low doses, can contribute substantially to analgesia by minimizing CNS sensitization.

Alpha$_2$ adrenergic agonists

Xylazine and, more recently, medetomidine, dexmedetomdine, and romifidine, have been used extensively to provide sedation in a variety of veterinary species. Medetomidine and dexmedetomidine in particular have considerable analgesic potential, even in microdoses, and can be administered via a number of novel routes and techniques to supplement analgesia and enhance the analgesic actions of other agents.

Gabapentin

Gabapentin is a human antiepileptic drug that has been approved by the U.S. Food and Drug Administration since 1993. Several years later, reports of its antihyperalgesic effects in rodent experimental pain models, as well as case reports and uncontrolled clinical trials involving human patients suffering from neuropathic pain, began to appear in the literature. Gabapentin's mechanism of analgesic action is unknown, but there is evidence suggesting it is a voltage-dependent Ca^{2+} channel blocker and may increase central inhibition or reduce the synthesis of glutamate, even though it does not appear to interact directly with NMDA receptors.

Despite the lack of controlled data available at this time, gabapentin administration has been advocated for the management of a variety of human neuropathic pain syndromes and more recently for management of incisional pain and arthritis. In human clinical trials, side effects occur in approximately 25% of patients, are usually mild and self-limiting, and include drowsiness, fatigue, and weight gain with chronic administration. Dosing guidelines in dogs and cats have been extrapolated from human dosing recommendations and some preliminary pharmacokinetic data. Dosage modifications are often based on the clinical efficacy achieved in individual veterinary patients.

Amantadine

Amantadine is an antiviral agent developed to inhibit the replication of influenza A in human patients. It has efficacy in the treatment of drug-induced extrapyramidal effects and in the treatment of Parkinson's disease. More recently, amantadine has been advocated for the treatment of various types of pain. It exerts its analgesic effects through antagonism of NMDA receptors in a manner analogous to ketamine. Though controlled clinical human trials are lacking, amantadine seems most efficacious in the management of chronic neuropathic types of pain characterized by hyperalgesia and allodynia. Patients suffering from opioid tolerance may also respond favorably to amantadine therapy. Dosing recommendations are based largely on anecdotal reports; however, a 2008 study by Lascelles et al. demonstrated improved activity in dogs with NSAID-refractory osteoarthritis when added to meloxicam. As the management of chronic pain in companion animals continues to receive much attention, amantadine and other drugs with a similar mechanism of action are likely to become more prevalent.

Tramadol

Tramadol is a synthetic codeine analog that is a weak μ-receptor agonist. In addition to its opioid activity, tramadol also inhibits neuronal reuptake of norepinephrine and 5-hydroxytryptamine (serotonin), and may actually facilitate 5-hydroxytryptamine release. It is thought that these effects on central catecholaminergic pathways contribute significantly to the drug's analgesic efficacy. Tramadol is recommended for the management of acute and chronic pain of moderate to moderately severe intensity associated with a variety of conditions, including osteoarthritis, fibromyalgia, diabetic neuropathy, neuropathic pain, and even perioperative pain in human patients.

A study published in 2003 compared the effects of intravenous tramadol and morphine administered prior to ovariohysterectomy in dogs. Tramadol was comparable to morphine in its analgesic efficacy for this type of surgical pain. Clearly, additional studies are necessary before definitive therapeutic recommendations can be made for the management of perioperative pain in a variety of species. Anecdotal reports of managing chronic pain in dogs and cats with tramadol when NSAID usage is contraindicated are widespread. Because of its inhibitory effect on 5-hydroxytryptamine uptake, tramadol should not be used in patients that may have received monoamineoxidase inhibitors (MAOIs) such as selegiline (see also the section on meperidine), patients on selective serotonin reuptake inhibitor (SSRI), or in those patients with a recent history of seizure activity.

Tapentadol

Tapentadol is a multimodal analgesic approved for use in human patients experiencing pain. It has significant noradrenergic effects as well as opioid actions. Its use in veterinary medicine has not been reported to date, but it holds promise as an alternative to tramadol in animals that are intolerant. The disadvantages to its use at this time are considerable expense and its status as a controlled substance.

Acupuncture and traditional Chinese medicine

A veterinarian's training often leads to skepticism of Eastern traditional medical practices because of the apparent conflicts with Western scientific methodology and the feeling that Eastern medical practice is somewhat faith based. It is important that novices to traditional Chinese medicine (TCM) understand that much of the theory and vocabulary, although similar to Western terminology, have little direct correlation. Much of the practice of TCM developed before the advent of Western medical science and publication of medical textbooks, so a simplified method had to be devised for the practice of TCM based on diagnostic and treatment strategies observable on the external surfaces of the body. Consequently, it is best to think of the description of acupuncture points and TCM diagnostics as metaphors or teaching aids rather than as anatomical or pathophysiological correlates to Western medicine.

Treatment strategies have evolved over millennia of trial and error in many species and represent a consensus among TCM practitioners as to what is effective. Current Western medical teaching is that TCM is complementary to Western medicine rather than an alternative to it. Acupuncture is traditionally viewed as one treatment modality among several used by TCM practitioners.

Most Western acupuncture charts show transpositional acupuncture points and meridians on animals, meaning the points are adapted from anatomical correlates on the human body. This creates some interesting adaptations, since animal anatomy varies from humans. Some acupuncturists prefer to use the points described for animals in the early Chinese veterinary texts. These may or may not be aligned with modern points. They are difficult for many Westerners to learn because the names are in Chinese and often describe the anatomy in terms of natural objects (rivers, branches, etc.). Some acupuncturists only use points located on the distal limbs. These are often referred to as Ting points and are the ends of the meridians and are usually extremely painful when needled (like sticking needles under fingernails), so they would be expected to produce a pronounced response.

Any patient being treated with acupuncture should be evaluated using the standards of care established for Western-based veterinary medicine. This includes a thorough physical examination, chest auscultation, blood work if necessary, and any other diagnostics that are required. Failure to maintain this standard of care could lead to malpractice. Acupuncture is often used in conjunction with Western treatments such as surgery or pharmacological therapy. It is recommended that written refusal of a Western-based standard of care be obtained from clients who seek to use acupuncture exclusively. Such clients have caused much concern and ethical debate among veterinarians.

History

Interest in acupuncture surged in the United States in the early 1970s, in part because James Reston, a *New York Times* reporter covering President Richard Nixon's trip to China, developed acute appendicitis. After his postoperative pain was treated with acupuncture, he described his experience on the front page of the newspaper, igniting an interest in acupuncture in the Western medical community. Subsequently, American and European physicians visiting China witnessed surgeries in which the only anesthetic used was acupuncture. A number of articles in newspapers and magazines about the use of acupuncture instead of general anesthesia followed. Basic research on acupuncture's mechanisms in Western societies started in 1976 after the endorphin hypothesis of acupuncture's mechanism of action was introduced. Further advancement of acupuncture research was prompted by the introduction of functional magnetic resonance imaging (fMRI) and positron emission tomographic scanning, which revealed the relation between acupuncture stimulation and activation of certain brain structures. Interest in the United States led the National Institutes of Health to create the National Center for Complementary and Alternative Medicine (NCCAM), which has funded basic and clinical acupuncture studies.

In 1997, the World Health Organization issued a list of human medical conditions that may benefit from treatment with acupuncture. Applications include prevention and treatment of postoperative and chemotherapy-associated nausea and vomiting, treatment of pain, therapy for alcohol and other drug addiction, treatment of asthma and bronchitis, and rehabilitation from neurological damage such as that caused by stroke. Scientific information on the effectiveness of acupuncture for veterinary disorders is limited. The effectiveness of treatment is based on a consensus among veterinarians commonly performing acupuncture in specific species.

Skepticism about the effectiveness of acupuncture therapy in humans and animals remains among some Western medical practitioners. Some factors contributing to this skepticism are: (1) the scientific basis of acupuncture remains unclear, (2) the philosophical basis of acupuncture is difficult for a modern industrial society to accept, (3) the operational language is unusual, and (4) the traditional system of acupuncture points does not correspond to Western concepts of anatomy or neurology. Moreover, traditional Chinese acupuncture remains a mix of philosophy and science and teaches that many factors can profoundly influence the outcome of the treatment. In addition to the signs related to the disease, a practitioner might consider a patient's gender and psychological profile, the season, the time of the day, and even the environment in which the treatment is administered. Because of these differences, it is believed that the efficacy of interventions may differ substantially among patients with similar symptoms, and thus it is difficult to standardize procedures. Scientific exploration of these factors remains limited.

Another problem associated with acupuncture studies is defining an adequate placebo as a control intervention for them. Some trials compare acupuncture with drugs, and others use sham acupuncture (acupuncture at random spots on the body surface that are thought to be inactive). There is substantial controversy, however, about the use of sham acupuncture as a control treatment because the procedure itself can provide neurohormonal and clinical effects, though usually of lower effectiveness compared with treatment at defined acupuncture points.

Basic concepts

The theory of TCM, of which acupuncture is one part, is complex and beyond the scope of this review. Unlike Western biomedical science, TCM does not make a distinction between physical, mental, and emotional components of life. Moreover, it considers a being as an integral part of the universe. It is believed that everything within the universe, including animals, obeys the same laws. Therefore, health and disease result from balance or imbalance.

Organs and meridians

Most modern acupuncture schools teach meridian theory. However, early practitioners (and some modern practitioners) do not recognize meridians or do not agree on their path. Meridians are most useful in remembering locations of points, although they are used in developing treatment protocols. Meridians were identified based on observations in a small percentage of people who are extremely sensitive to acupuncture. A meridian can describe the course of a tingling or burning sensation along a path that roughly corresponds to the meridian. Most of the meridians are not obviously associated anatomically with nerve pathways, although many of the relationships observed seem to be explained by the way peripheral nerves enter the spinal cord and neural pathways converge in the brain. For example, many people that have heart attacks describe a pain across the chest and down the arm. The heart meridian courses down the chest and arm. The pain (origin in the heart muscle) is felt in the arm because some of the afferent fibers enter the spinal cord near the location of afferents from the thoracic limb. Other observations indicate that distant areas of the body have complementary effects because many areas in the somatosensory cortex of the brain colocalize. Associations between internal organs and meridians (and superficial points) are very common and make sense if the concept of referred pain is understood.

The theory of traditional Chinese acupuncture recognizes 12 main meridians with corresponding organs in the human body. In addition, eight so-called curious meridians can be distinguished. Most acupuncture "organs" have names similar to organs of Western medicine but only an approximate correlation with physiological functions and anatomical structures. Organs, as seen in ancient Chinese traditions, are functional systems rather than anatomical structures, with broader and sometimes peculiar physiological functions and anatomical representations. For example, two traditional acupuncture organs, namely "triple warmer" and "pericardium" ("heart governor"), do not have a distinct anatomical representation at all. All meridians and organs are connected and related to one another directly or indirectly according to various rules and principles:

- Each organ has a corresponding meridian with acupuncture points located along it.
- Meridians travel inside the body and on the body's surface and are connected to one another and organs by a complex network of accessory collateral connections.
- The function of the meridians is to regulate and modify the corresponding organ or group of related organs. It is believed that meridians can control pain along the areas they traverse.

Points

In Chinese acupuncture, points are called *xue*, which means "cave" or "hole." In Chinese acupuncture tradition and language, the names of points are important and informative. Western acupuncture practitioners rarely use Chinese names because of unfamiliarity with the Chinese languages. Instead, the points are identified by number and capital letter abbreviation of the meridian to which they belong: 365 classic points are located along the meridians and at least the same number of extrameridian points. The exact location of the points is important, because according to classic theory, even small deviations from the intended location can nullify the response. The distance of acupoints to anatomical landmarks is usually described as *cun*.

Investigation into the anatomy and physiology of acupuncture points has resulted in a hypothesis that most recognized acupuncture points coincide with tissues that are capable of eliciting a strong neurohumoral response when irritated. These include nerves, neurovascular complexes, Golgi tendon apparatuses, and other sensitive tissues. Stimulation of these tissues might cause acute and intense irritation that triggers endogenous analgesic, immune, and behavior-adapting systems to be activated, resulting in the clinical effectiveness of acupuncture.

Several factors have been associated with precise location of acupuncture points:

- Points are located in a small hollow or depression on the skin surface.
- Acupuncture points are usually tender compared with the surrounding area, and a response (probably associated with discomfort) can often be elicited with deep palpation. Human patients describe a feeling of slight pain or numbness radiating circumferentially for at least a centimeter when the point is pressed.
- A subjective roughness or stickiness can be appreciated when an acupuncture point is brushed slightly with the finger.
- A specific feeling called the *De-Qi* sensation is usually felt by human patients, and the acupuncturist feels a change in the resistance to needle movement, when a needle stimulates an acupuncture point.

In humans, the *De-Qi* sensation may be described as soreness, numbness, warmth, heaviness, or distension around the area where a needle is inserted. Sometimes this sensation radiates along the pathway of the meridian to which the stimulated point belongs. An experienced practitioner also feels tightness and some heaviness in the fingers when the needle hits the point. This change in needle resistance coupled with the animal's reaction to needle placement is what most veterinary acupuncturists rely on to assess the attainment of *De-Qi* sensation. Most human and veterinary acupuncturists consider *De-Qi* sensation to be crucial in achieving the effect of acupuncture.

The descriptions of the diameter and depth of acupuncture points vary among various species. Traditionally, the size depends on the individual point, the patient's condition, the time of day, and possibly the season. The depth depends on the amount of hair on the patient, skin thickness (e.g., the thin skin of cats vs. the rather thick skin of stallions), location of the point, and duration of the disease. In veterinary acupuncture, most clinically used points in most species are believed to be 3–15 mm below the skin surface.

Point stimulation

Traditional Chinese acupuncture teaches that each point has specific functions and indications for use. For example, stimulation of certain acupuncture points distant from the source of pain can provide analgesia, whereas stimulation of inappropriately selected points in close proximity to the source of pain might be ineffective or even aggravate the symptoms. Stimulation of site-specific acupoints usually induces spatially restricted analgesia. Although this aspect of acupuncture has yet to be studied in detail, Benedetti et al. demonstrated that in people, placebo or treatment expectation provides an analgesic response with a highly spatial presentation, which is completely abolished by systemic naloxone administration. These data indicate that this type of analgesic response is mediated by endogenous opioid release but that the effect is regional rather than systemic. Acupuncture might manifest a similar mechanism of action. Point specificity was also questioned in an fMRI study by Cho et al., where meridian and sham acupuncture were both involved in the transmission and perception of pain. Meridian acupuncture demonstrated more profound pain control than did sham-point stimulation, but the effect may not have been entirely point specific. Point specificity, as stated in traditional acupuncture literature and demonstrated by clinical practice and some experimental studies, is not fully supported by other studies and therefore remains a controversial issue. For any species being treated with acupuncture therapy, only careful systematic research using site-, organ-, and function-specific acupuncture points with carefully selected sham control points can resolve this issue.

Mechanisms of analgesic action

Starting in the 1960s, Western-trained Chinese physicians began to study acupuncture analgesia, particularly acupuncture-induced physiological changes in the CNS. This, and subsequent research in Western countries, resulted in the discovery of several plausible mechanisms of acupuncture analgesia, receptors, and several endogenous opioids involved in the process; hence, a comprehensive hypothesis of acupuncture analgesia was formed. Experimental studies on animals and clinical studies on humans have since identified numerous clinical and physiological responses to acupuncture stimulation.

Types of acupuncture

Invasive methods include skin penetration with an acupuncture needle with subsequent manual stimulation of needles, electroacupuncture, or chronic intradermal needle insertion. These methods are considered dry needle techniques. Drugs can be injected into acupoints, a technique considered as wet needle acupuncture or aquapuncture. Noninvasive methods include acupressure, transcutaneous electrical stimulation, moxibustion, and application of various stimulating patches and pellets.

Because the traditional theory of acupuncture is based on the concept that diseases are caused by an imbalance of *Qi*, the goal of needle insertion is, in the context of TCM, to disperse excessive *Qi* or to replenish it. These two goals can be achieved by several means: applying needles of different sizes or lengths, using needles made of different material, changing the direction of needle insertion, selecting different points for stimulation, and so forth. For strong stimulation, a bigger needle, more intense needle manipulation, or directing the needle tip against the hypothetical energy flow along the meridian is believed to disperse the excessive energy, whereas for mild stimulation, a smaller needle, gentle and more superficial needle insertion, or directing the needle toward the energy flow is used to replenish it. Manual stimulation techniques can be altered to provide the desired effect by using strong vertical up-and-down movements, rotational movements, or mild vibrating movements, for example. Some practitioners believe that selecting the proper acupuncture maneuvers and appropriate points is key to producing a satisfactory therapeutic effect.

Electrical stimulation

Electrical stimulation of acupuncture points (electroacupuncture) was developed as an alternative to manual stimulation of acupuncture points. Electrical stimulation has several advantages in that it (1) is less painful than manual stimulation, (2) requires less practitioner time directly spent with the patient, (3) provides better analgesia, and (4) facilitates standardization. Transcutaneous and percutaneous electrostimulation are now the most common types of acupuncture analgesia performed in people.

In humans, the *De-Qi* sensation depends on the type of acupuncture stimulation. Manual stimulation produces mainly soreness, fullness, and distension, whereas electroacupuncture generally produces tingling and numbness. How various stimulation modalities influence brain networks in companion animal species such as dogs and cats has not been evaluated.

Electroacupuncture with high-frequency stimulation (100–200 Hz) provides rapid-onset analgesia that is not cumulative and cannot be blocked by naloxone. This type of analgesia is probably mediated by norepinephrine, serotonin, and dynorphins. In contrast, low-frequency stimulation (2–4 Hz) and medium-frequency stimulation (15–30 Hz) produce an analgesic effect that is reversed by naloxone (and therefore presumably mediated by enkephalin and endorphins), have a tendency to accumulate, and last at least 1 hour after treatment ceases. Reportedly, antinociception induced by low-frequency stimulation is mediated by both μ opioid and δ opioid receptors; high-frequency electroacupuncture stimulation induces antinociception mediated by κ opioid receptors; and medium-frequency stimulation (e.g., 30 Hz) induces antinociception mediated by all three opioid receptor types.

Needles

Most modern acupuncture needles are made of stainless steel, although needles made of gold or silver are also available. Most acupuncture needles are between 1.3 and 12.7 cm long and range from 26 to 36 gauge in diameter. The tips of the needles are rounded and thus separate fibers rather than cutting tissues. For this reason, even capillary bleeding from an acupuncture site is rare unless a needle accidentally penetrates a vessel. In the treatment of human patients, special needles have been developed for intradermal use, auricular acupuncture, and hand and foot acupuncture.

Veterinary acupuncture

Probably the most commonly treated species is the dog, although historically, equine acupuncture was more widely used because horses were important for the daily survival of people (similar to the history for Western veterinary medicine). Dogs tend to be cooperative, and most relax during the treatment. If an animal becomes severely distressed, it is unlikely that the treatment will have the desired effect. The most commonly treated problems are related to the musculoskeletal system. It is important for beginners to recognize that pain and disuse in many musculoskeletal diseases— especially chronic degenerative diseases, including low-grade intervertebral disk disease—often wax and wane. This, coupled with the placebo effect, would suggest that some of the patients treated (whether with acupuncture or NSAIDs) should improve, at least for a while. One should be careful to not interpret a positive response as possession of superior TCM skills. However, some scientific evidence supports the use of acupuncture alone or in conjunction with other Western treatments such as NSAIDs. Other common uses for acupuncture in canine patients include treatment of signs associated with chronic diseases such as cancer, nervous system degeneration, and organ failure, such as chronic renal disease. Unless functional tissue is present, reversal of the course of disease is unlikely. Acupuncture cannot miraculously regenerate tissue. Owners should be educated on what the treatment capabilities are of any form of therapy before administering it.

Owners should be informed about the complications and contraindications to treatment. Complications are rare, but include infection, tissue or organ trauma, and needle breakage. Acupuncture needles are extremely flexible and strong, so breakage is rare. It is more common for hypodermic needles to break. An animal's behavior can change after treatments, so owners should be educated on what to expect. Some practitioners have suggested that acupuncture treatment can be problematic in cancer patients. Increased blood flow and needle trauma might spread cancer. However, many people find acupuncture useful for symptomatic treatment of paraneoplastic conditions. Acupuncture-associated stress and physiological responses can cause extremely ill animals to decompensate. It is suggested that very ill animals be treated very conservatively at first until they can tolerate more aggressive treatment. Implants for chronic acupoint stimulation (e.g., gold beads) should not be used when animals are subject to prepurchase examinations (mostly horses). The beads will show up on radiographs and are usually diagnostic for preexisting lameness. Pregnancy can be a contraindication to acupuncture, because it is believed that stimulating points distal to the elbow and knee may induce labor.

Application in a perioperative setting

Perioperative acupuncture and related techniques have been advocated for preoperative sedation, to reduce intraoperative opioid use, and to decrease postoperative pain. There is compelling evidence that acupuncture reduces postoperative nausea and vomiting in human patients, and it has been used to decrease vomiting associated with opioid administration to dogs. It may also stabilize cardiac function and ameliorate some consequences of anesthesia and surgery.

Perioperative acupuncture can be divided into three components: preoperative preparation, intraoperative acupuncture-assisted anesthesia, and postoperative care.

Preoperative preparation

The goals of preoperative preparation with acupuncture are to optimize the conditions for patients, reduce preoperative anxiety, and trigger release of endogenous opioids to enhance analgesia. One way that acupuncture might help preoperative preparation is by producing relaxation and sedation. For example, Ekblom et al. demonstrated that although acupuncture did not produce intraoperative and postoperative analgesia for dental surgery in humans, it caused significant relaxation and drowsiness. Ulett et al. reported that electroacupuncture to classic acupoints is associated with a deep calming effect. In people, postoperative pain intensity and consumption of postoperative analgesics both correlate with the amount of anxiety that patients experience.

Intraoperative assisted anesthesia

Reduction in volatile anesthetic or opioid requirement is a clinically important outcome because it can reduce anesthetic toxicity and duration of recovery. Evidence suggests that inadequately treated pain, even during general anesthesia, activates nociceptive pathways. Subsequent release of local mediators then primes the nociceptive system and aggravates postoperative pain. To the extent that intraoperative acupuncture inhibits activation of nociceptive pathways and provides analgesia, it may similarly reduce postoperative pain and the requirement for postoperative opioids.

It is important to emphasize that acupuncture does not provide true anesthesia or unconsciousness, because it preserves all normal sensory, motor, and proprioception sensations. It does not provide adequate muscle relaxation or suppress autonomic reflexes caused by intra-abdominal visceral pain. Instead, acupuncture produces analgesia and sedation as long as patients are cooperative. For these reasons, acupuncture cannot be recommended for use as a sole anesthetic technique in veterinary patients.

Postoperative pain control

Acupuncture and related techniques can potentially serve as important adjuvants for pain control and for relieving opioid-related adverse effects during the postoperative period. However, controversial results, dissimilar study designs, and diverse modes of acupuncture-point stimulation make it difficult to evaluate the clinical importance of perioperative acupuncture analgesia across a wide array of species. The results of few randomized, controlled clinical trials on acupuncture-related postoperative pain relief have been published in English. Interpretation of these available studies is complicated by the fact that acupuncture success depends on numerous factors, including adequate patient selection and the acupuncturist's knowledge and skill level.

As previously mentioned, in human patients, point selection and mode of stimulation perform important roles in the outcome of acupuncture for postoperative pain relief. It seems that different components of postoperative pain respond to different combinations of acupuncture points. *Shu* points of the internal organs are located bilaterally 3 cm lateral to the posterior midline. *Shu* points are associated with the viscera and traditionally have been used for treatment of internal organ diseases. Stimulation of these points may alleviate pain associated with visceral organ dysfunction.

Transcutaneous electrical nerve stimulation (TENS) near the incision site significantly reduces postoperative pain. However, this treatment seems to be most effective for the superficial cutaneous component of postoperative pain, leaving the deep visceral pain component largely intact. It seems likely that high-frequency TENS near the incision site mainly stimulates specific afferent nerve fibers instead of triggering endogenous opioid-release mechanisms. Combining TENS and stimulation of viscera-associated *Shu* points in the treatment plan is therefore promising for reducing postoperative superficial and deep visceral pain, respectively.

Both high-frequency and low-frequency electroacupuncture at the Zusanli (ST 36) point performed 20 minutes immediately before induction of anesthesia reduces morphine consumption after abdominal surgery in human patients. This point is traditionally considered effective for the treatment of abdominal disorders. The high-frequency acupuncture group had a 61% reduction in 24-hour patient-controlled analgesia morphine consumption. Pain scores postoperatively did not significantly differ between groups, but cumulative morphine consumption for the first 24 hours, number of patient-controlled analgesia demands, and intervals for the first request for analgesic were significantly less in both the high-frequency and low-frequency electroacupuncture groups. The aforementioned parameters were also reduced in the sham acupuncture group compared with the control group, although they were greater than in the acupuncture groups. This is not surprising because sham acupuncture seems to have an analgesic effect in 40–50% of patients compared with 60–70% for real acupuncture and 30–35% for placebo (control). The extrapolation or translation of human clinical trial findings to veterinary patients is controversial, although similar responses and mechanisms of action are plausible.

Acupuncture for the treatment of postoperative nausea and vomiting is one of its most common and investigated uses in human patients. This application has not been adequately assessed for use in animals during the perioperative period to date. Acupuncture may reduce nausea and vomiting through endogenous β-endorphin release into the cerebral spinal fluid or through a change in serotonin transmission via activation of seritonergic and noradrenergic fibers. The exact mechanisms have yet to be established.

Miscellaneous perioperative uses

Cardiopulmonary resuscitation

In a study using 35 dogs anesthetized with halothane, acupuncture reversed cardiovascular depression induced by morphine and halothane. Acupuncture at point Jen Chung (GV 26) significantly increased cardiac output, stroke volume, heart rate, mean arterial pressure, and pulse pressure while simultaneously significantly decreasing total peripheral resistance and central venous pressure. The authors concluded that stimulation of the GV 26 acupoint could be helpful in resuscitating patients whose cardiovascular system is depressed by opioids and volatile anesthetics.

GV 26 (also called Renzhong) is in the midline of the nasal philtrum, one-third of the way from the nose to the edge of the upper lip. The point is in the center of the horizontal line joining the lower edge of the nostrils. GV 26 has many clinical uses, the best known being its use in emergencies (coma, shock, apnea, anesthetic emergencies, drowning, etc.).

In human patients, the Neiguan (P 6) point has long been considered a primary point for treatment of various cardiovascular diseases. It has been shown to be effective as an adjunct therapeutic modality in conservative treatment of severe angina pectoris. Electroacupuncture at Neiguan (P 6) was effective in maintaining the hemodynamics and cardiac contractility in anesthetized open-chest dogs. Stroke volume and cardiac output were slightly increased compared with the control group. The end-systolic pressure and end-systolic elastance increased markedly in the Neiguan (P 6) acupuncture group. No analogous data support acupuncture-induced cardiovascular benefits in human patients.

Impaired intestinal function

A major side effect of general anesthesia and opioid administration for postoperative pain control is the impairment of intestinal function. To the extent that intraoperative and postoperative acupuncture for pain relief decreases perioperative opioid consumption, it may be beneficial for speeding postoperative recovery of intestinal function. Acupuncture treatment has also been shown to promote postoperative recovery of impaired intestinal function after abdominal surgery in people.

Rehabilitation therapy

Companion animal rehabilitation is a rapidly growing area aimed at improving supportive care in veterinary patients. In the veterinary setting, rehabilitation is essentially akin to the human-oriented profession of physical therapy. Similar to physical therapy, rehabilitation uses physical and mechanical methods such as light, heat, cold, water, electricity, massage, and exercise to improve function and reduce pain and morbidity in a variety of conditions, including orthopedic and neurological disease. Other terms commonly used to describe rehabilitation are physical rehabilitation, physical therapy, and physiotherapy. Because pain and discomfort may be elicited by some techniques on occasion, therapists should be prepared to administer an appropriate analgesic, if necessary. Advanced training and certification in rehabilitation are available for certified veterinary technicians, physical therapists, and veterinarians. Practice acts vary from state to state, with most requiring that animal rehabilitation be supervised and in some cases implemented by a veterinarian.

Until recently, rehabilitation has not played an important role in the management of pain in veterinary medicine. Standard postoperative care has focused on basic nursing and support care, confinement, and pharmaceutical intervention. With the incorporation of rehabilitation into overall supportive care and pain management, many patients are recovering sooner and more completely from medical, surgical, and traumatic events. To date, however, the benefits of nondrug therapies in the management of pain, including those of rehabilitation, have been relatively undocumented in the veterinary literature. Similarly, the analgesic effects and overall benefits of therapies such as acupuncture and electroacupuncture, acupressure, and TENS are relatively undefined. Despite this lack of experimental scientific evidence for their efficacy, clinical experience in veterinary patients suggests that the use of such therapeutic modalities in conjunction with drug therapy can be beneficial. The desired clinical outcome is better control of discomfort and reduction in the overall pharmacological requirement of patients.

Therapeutic modalities

Seven therapeutic modalities are used to decrease pain, reduce inflammation, and stimulate normal healing responses in veterinary patients: (1) local hypothermia and hyperthermia, (2) passive range-of-motion activity, (3) massage, (4) therapeutic exercise, (5) hydrotherapy, (6) ultrasound, and (7) electrical stimulation.

Local hypothermia

Local hypothermia therapy, or cryotherapy, entails the application of therapeutic cold to a musculoskeletal tissue. Common forms of therapeutic cold include commercially available reusable ice and gel packs, continuously circulating cold-water blankets, homemade ice packs and towels, ice massage, and cold-water hydrotherapy. The application of local hypothermia is indicated in the acute (<72 hours) postinjury period to ameliorate inflammation, irritation, pain, swelling, and edema. The primary purported method of action of cryotherapy is via vasoconstriction, which reduces arterial and capillary blood flow, thereby minimizing fluid leakage and edema. Because cryotherapy also decreases enzyme activity and metabolism in tissues, it is effective against local inflammation in periarticular and articular tissues. Analgesia is provided by alteration of sensory nerve conduction and skeletal muscle relaxation.

The cooling effects of local hypothermia on deeper tissues are less profound and unpredictable, depending on the application method, the initial temperature of the treated area, and the duration of treatment. Regardless, application of local hypothermia should be limited to multiple short sessions (5–15 minutes up to four times daily) to prevent reflex vasodilation and edema. Overzealous cryotherapy causing a 10.0°C (18.0°F) or more decrease in tissue temperature may cause protein degradation, local hyperemia, epithelial and nerve damage, and muscle atrophy and contracture. The use of local hypothermia should be avoided in hypothermic animals. If body core temperature is further dropped, peripheral vasoconstriction and increased blood pressure may ensue. Furthermore, cryotherapy is contraindicated in people and presumably animals that have diabetes mellitus, ischemic injuries, vasculitis, or indolent wounds.

Local hyperthermia

This technique uses heat to promote capillary dilation and increase capillary hydrostatic pressure, permeability, and filtration. The cellular and vascular changes produced by heat also stimulate inflammation and invigorate wound healing. Tissues treated with local hyperthermia increase in temperature, which causes a local histamine release while simultaneously enhancing cellular metabolism. Heat therapy provides pain relief by increasing blood flow and capillary permeability, decreasing edema, increasing local metabolic rate, increasing extensibility of collagen in articular and ligamentous tissues, and decreasing muscle tension and spasm, as well as providing general relaxation.

Common forms of therapeutic heat used in veterinary medicine include the application of hot packs, heat lamps, warm towels, warm-water blankets, therapeutic ultrasound, laser therapy, circulating warm-water baths, and hydrotherapy units. The therapeutic protocol for heat is similar to that for cryotherapy, with application durations varying from 15 to 20 minutes, two to four times a day. Other types of less frequently used heat therapy include incandescent, infrared, ultraviolet, and microwave radiation, all of which require special equipment and training. As the primary method of action of heat therapy is inflammatory, local hyperthermia should be used only once acute inflammation has subsided, typically 24–72 hours after injury or surgery. Heat therapy is indicated to remove the inflammatory mediators and edema present in the peri-injury site tissues. It is important to note that local hyperthermia has a narrow therapeutic temperature window (40–45°C [104–113°F]) and warrants careful monitoring. Care should be taken not to prematurely apply heat too soon after a traumatic injury, because that can induce vascular leakage, exacerbate the inflammatory response, augment edema and seroma formation, and potentiate hemorrhage and pain. Local hyperthermia has few indications in the immediate postoperative period and should be combined with other forms of physical therapy (massage or exercise) in the later stages of convalescence (>72 hours after surgery). Therapeutic heat is also contraindicated in neurological or vascularly impaired patients. Direct nerve injury from local hyperthermia and burns is possible, especially with prolonged application or the use of electric heating pads.

Passive range of motion

Passive range of motion (PROM) exercise refers to the controlled movement of the limbs and joints in flexion, extension, adduction, and abduction by the therapist with no effort being exerted by the animal. The goals of PROM are to stretch and manipulate the periarticular structures of the appendicular skeleton to maintain normal joint range of motion (ROM) while preventing soft tissue and muscle contracture. Experimental evidence evaluating the effects of prolonged immobilization and restricted weight bearing on canine cartilage reveals chondrocyte atrophy and deterioration of the supportive matrix, which in many cases is irreversible. In addition to direct benefits to cartilage, PROM improves blood flow and sensory awareness of the affected joints and limbs. However, PROM is not a replacement for normal weight bearing and the superior affects of voluntary active movement. In comparison to PROM, active exercise produces superior cartilage, better prevents muscle atrophy, and improves muscle strength and endurance.

PROM should be instituted immediately after surgery and continued until the patient begins to ambulate within normal limits. If the animal has decreased ROM, as documented by goniometry, the PROM exercises can be prolonged to improve the function of the limb. Typically, PROM is performed with the animal in relaxed lateral recumbency. The joint or joints are flexed or extended to their nonpainful end point and held for 10–30 seconds and returned to a normal or functional standing position. These cycles are repeated for 10–15 complete cycles of flexion and extension. Caution should be taken not to overstretch the periarticular tissues, because overzealous PROM may tear the joint capsule and surrounding tissues and result in pain and unintentional fibrous scar formation. Contraindications to the use of PROM include unstable fractures, luxations, hypermotile joints, or skin grafts.

Therapeutic massage

This involves the manual or mechanical manipulation of soft tissues and muscle by rubbing, kneading, or tapping. Benefits of massage include increased local circulation, reduced muscle spasm, attenuation of edema, and breakdown of irregular scar tissue formation. The method of action of this therapeutic technique is based on both reflexive and mechanical effects. The reflexive effects are due to stimulation of peripheral receptors, which produces the central effects of relaxation while simultaneously producing muscular relaxation and arteriolar dilation. The mechanical effects are due to increased lymphatic and venous drainage removing edema and metabolic waste, increased arterial circulation enhancing tissue oxygenation and wound healing, and manipulation of restrictive connective tissue enhancing ROM and mobility.

The most common techniques of massage used in veterinary medicine are effleurage, pétrissage, cross fiber, and tapotement. Effleurage (Latin, *effluere*, "to flow out") is a form of superficial or light stroking massage and is generally used in the beginning of all massage sessions to relax and acclimatize the animal. Pétrissage is characterized by deep kneading and squeezing of muscle and surrounding soft tissues. Cross fiber is also a deep massage that is concentrated along lines of restrictive scar tissue and designed to promote normal ROM. This type of massage has limited use in veterinary medicine because it requires sedation of the animal during therapy and most often temporarily exacerbates lameness because of an inflammatory response to the tissue manipulation. Tapotement involves the percussive manipulation of soft tissues with a cupped hand or massage equipment and is most commonly used to relax spastic muscle contraction or enhance postural drainage for respiratory conditions. Contraindications to massage therapy include unstable or infected fractures or tissue and the direct manipulation of a malignancy. In most instances, massage is an indispensable therapy when animals are in intensive care and have restricted mobility.

Therapeutic exercise

The potential for catastrophic failure associated with uncontrolled activity has previously limited the role of therapeutic exercise in the recovery of veterinary patients, particularly in postoperative orthopedic animals. Controlled active therapeutic exercise, however, may be safely performed in most cases, even orthopedic, when closely assisted and attended to by the therapist or the attentive owner. The benefits of therapeutic exercise are abundant. Exercise helps build strength, muscle mass, agility, coordination, and cardiovascular health. In addition, therapeutic exercise may be used as a preventive measure to improve general health, reduce obesity, and increase performance in all veterinary patients. Prior to initiating therapy, all animals must be fully evaluated and assessed, because it is imperative to match the intensity of the activities to the animal's level of function and ability. Included in the repertoire of controlled active exercise are assisted standing; facilitated walking; prolonged, momentary, and repeated sits and downs; stair walking; walking on inclines and hills; and weight shifting. When performed appropriately and in consultation with the primary care clinician or surgeon, these activities can be performed early in the postoperative recovery period and modified and intensified to promote cardiovascular and musculoskeletal fitness.

Aquatic-based rehabilitation

Aquatic-based therapeutic techniques for veterinary patients include local therapeutic massage with warm or cold water, underwater treadmill exercise, and swimming. Massage in water is particularly beneficial for postoperative animals because it is an efficacious method for removing lymphedema from extremities. Water-based massage is also relaxing and effective for cleansing surgical incisions. Cold-water hydrotherapy may be employed as soon as a surgical incision has established a fibrin seal, which is generally within 24 hours of surgery. This form of hydrotherapy is a relatively low-tech, high-yield form of rehabilitation in that it requires little equipment, other than a washtub and a hose.

Increasing the water depth and the temperature to 30–32°C (86–90°F) provides a nongravitation environment that is ideal for performing nonconcussive active-assisted exercise such as underwater treadmill and swimming activity. The natural properties of water provide both buoyancy and resistance, which can be manipulated to improve limb mobility, joint ROM, gait, and cadence. Caution should be used with any water exercise in order to minimize the risk of aspiration or drowning. It is wise to acclimatize animals to water before initiating any therapy regimen.

Therapeutic ultrasound

The method of action of therapeutic ultrasound is based on the delivery of energy to tissue in the form of acoustic vibrations. Sound waves can produce both physiological heat and cellular inflammation. The net physiological effects of ultrasound may be divided into two categories: thermal and nonthermal. The thermal effects of ultrasound increase connective tissue extensibility and vascularity and provide a form of temporary nerve blockage, thus promoting muscular relaxation and pain relief. The nonthermal effects of ultrasound include the acceleration and compressing of the inflammatory phase of healing; an increase in local circulation; a decrease in edema; an increase in endorphins, enkephalins, and serotonin; and the stimulation of collagen synthesis and bone growth. Therapeutic ultrasound is primarily indicated in the treatment of chronic scar tissue and indolent decubital ulcers. It may also be effective for palliation of muscle spasms and for enhanced tendon healing. Contraindications for the use of therapeutic ultrasound include tissue infection or inflammation. Prior to its application, therapeutic ultrasound should be thoroughly investigated because there are a wide variety of continuous-wave or pulsed-wave delivery modes, wave intensities, and therapy regimens to choose from. Complications are associated with operator inexperience and error that can produce excessive heat, free radicals, and subsequent tissue destruction.

Electrical stimulation

This entails the delivery of electrical current to a selected treatment area. Common uses for electrical stimulation include muscle reeducation, pain palliation, and edema reduction. There are a variety of waveforms and devices available, varying in cost and versatility. The nomenclature is quite confusing and does little to improve one's understanding of the fundamentals of electrical stimulation. Essentially, however, there are two forms: neuromuscular electrical stimulation (NMES) and TENS.

NMES is indicated in animals that are neurological, debilitated, recumbent, or immobile or need prolonged joint immobility. It prevents disuse atrophy and improves limb performance by recruiting contracting fibers and increasing maximum contractible force of affected muscles. The electrical stimulation device consists of a simple pulse generator and electrodes, which are placed over selected weakened or paralyzed muscle groups to create an artificial contraction. Pulse amplitude, rate, and cycle length may be varied to suit the comfort of the patient. Muscular pain and edema may also be reduced because of improved blood flow. Combining neuromuscular stimulation with PROM exercises improves joint ROM and prevents muscle contracture, and is particularly indicated in fractures of the distal femur of young dogs. This technique has proven effective in promoting muscle reeducation after prolonged disuse.

TENS has been used widely to identify neural stimulators that modify pain. Electrical stimulation to alter pain sensation involves the application of an electrical current to a sensory nerve. There are various suggestions as to the mechanism(s) responsible for altered pain sensation: the gate control theory, which involves the increased activity of the sensory afferents causing presynaptic inhibition of pain transmission; an endogenous opiate release; the counterirritant theory; and the placebo effect. In most patients, altered pain sensation via TENS is probably due, in part, to all of the aforementioned mechanisms. TENS should be considered an adjunctive pain management modality, to be combined with other pain-management techniques rather than as a sole therapy to control pain.

Revised from "Pain and Its Management" by Peter W. Hellyer, Sheilah A. Robertson, and Anna D. Fails; "Opioids, Nonsteroidal Anti-inflammatories, and Analgesic Adjuvants" by Leigh A. Lamont and Karol A. Mathews; "Acupuncture" by Roman T. Skarda and Maria Glowaski; and "Rehabilitation and Palliative Analgesia" by Dianne Dunning and Duncan X. Lascelles in Lumb and Jones' Veterinary Anesthesia and Analgesia, Fourth Edition.

Chapter 4

Chronic pain management

Duncan X. Lascelles and James S. Gaynor

General considerations

While the importance of acute perioperative pain management for dogs and cats has been embraced by veterinarians in recent years, chronic pain management has lagged behind. Barriers to effective chronic pain control in animals include the following:

- lack of appreciation that many chronic disease processes and cancers are associated with significant pain (Table 4.1);
- inability to assess chronic pain in dogs and cats;
- lack of knowledge of drugs, drug therapy, and other pain-relieving techniques;
- lack of communication with clients and lack of involvement of clients in the assessment and treatment phases;
- underuse of nursing staff for assessment and re-evaluation of pain in hospitalized patients.

There are four main steps in overcoming these barriers and assuring that chronic pain management is optimized in veterinary patients:

(1) Assure that veterinarians have the appropriate education and training about the importance of alleviating pain, assessment of pain, available drugs and potential complications, and interventional techniques.
(2) Educate the client about realistic expectations surrounding pain control and quality of life and convey the idea that most patients' pain can be managed. This involves letting the client know that owner involvement in evaluating the pet and providing feedback on therapy is crucial to success. The veterinarian and owner should both participate in developing effective strategies to alleviate pain. The clients' involvement also helps decrease their feelings of helplessness.
(3) Thoroughly assess the pet's pain at the start and throughout the course of therapy, not just when it becomes severe.
(4) Have good support from the veterinary practice or institution for the use of opioids and other controlled substances.

Essentials of Small Animal Anesthesia and Analgesia, Second Edition. Edited by Kurt A. Grimm, William J. Tranquilli, Leigh A. Lamont.

Table 4.1. Common conditions that may be associated with chronic pain in dogs and cats

Condition	Examples
Cancer	• Osteosarcoma • Chondrosarcoma • Nerve sheath tumor • Spinal cord tumor • Transitional cell carcinoma
Soft tissue inflammation/injury	• Otitis media and interna • Traumatic degloving injury • Radiation therapy induced
Musculoskeletal inflammation/injury	• Coxofemoral, stifle, elbow, shoulder osteoarthritis • Spinal osteoarthritis (spondylosis) • Cruciate ligament rupture • Luxating patella(s)
Nervous tissue inflammation/injury	• Cervical, thoracic, lumbar intervertebral disk disease • Postamputation (phantom limb) • Postthoracotomy
Visceral inflammation/injury	• Pancreatitis • Cystitis
Dental disease	• Feline odontoclastic resorptive lesions • Stomatitis • Gingivitis
Ocular disease	• Glaucoma

Although pharmacological treatment is a mainstay of chronic pain treatment, adjunctive nondrug therapies such as acupuncture may play an important role in patient management. It must also be remembered that surgery is an important treatment modality for many types of chronic pain and radiation therapy may be useful for treatment or palliation of neoplastic disease.

A basic approach to chronic pain management can be summarized as follows:

(1) Assess the pain. Ask for the owner's perceptions of the pet's pain or of any compromise in its quality of life.
(2) Believe the owner. The owner sees the pet every day in its own environment and knows when alterations in behavior occur. Owners can rarely suggest diagnoses but do know when something is wrong. The veterinarian should become familiar with the owner's terminology when explaining the pet's abnormal behaviors to establish a baseline of communication for further assessment in the home environment once therapy has been initiated.
(3) Choose appropriate therapy depending on the stage of the disease. Anything other than mild pain should be treated with more than one class of analgesic or with an analgesic drug combined with nondrug adjunctive therapy. Also consider concurrent problems and drug therapy; be aware of potential drug interactions and toxicity.
(4) Deliver the therapy in a logical, coordinated manner and explain carefully to the owner about any possible side effects.

(5) Empower the clients to participate actively in their pet's treatment; ask for feedback and updates on how the therapy is working.

The importance of alleviating pain

The alleviation of pain is important from physiological and biologic standpoints as well as from an ethical perspective. Pain can induce a stress response in patients that is associated with elevations in adrenocorticotropic hormone, cortisol, antidiuretic hormone, catecholamines, aldosterone, renin, angiotensin II, and glucose, along with decreases in insulin and testosterone. A prolonged stress response can decrease the rate of healing. In addition, the stress response can adversely affect the cardiovascular and pulmonary systems, fluid homeostasis, and gastrointestinal (GI) tract function.

Veterinarians have an ethical obligation to treat animal pain. Most undertreatment of chronic pain is probably a result of lack of adequate knowledge and resources rather than a lack of concern. Outward show of concern for the pet and family is important for demonstrating a bond-centered approach to chronic therapy and pain management. It is important for the veterinarian to foster good communication surrounding primary therapy and pain treatment and at the same time demonstrate empathy for the owner. In cancer patients especially, pain prevention and treatment are not the only aspects that impact animal welfare, and veterinarians must evaluate all aspects of welfare when making treatment decisions. The five freedoms have been suggested as a rubric for the evaluation of an animal's welfare (Table 4.2).

The approach to the treatment of chronic pain in dogs and cats should be one that considers *all* aspects of welfare. For each freedom, the severity, incidence, and duration of perturbation should be considered. In the case of pain, the longer the pain lasts, such as in long-standing painful cancers, the more welfare is compromised.

It is of significant interest that the provision of analgesics significantly reduces the tumor-promoting effects of undergoing and recovering from surgery. Surgery is well known to suppress several immune functions, including natural killer (NK) cell activity in animals and people, probably as a result of substances released such as catecholamines and prostaglandins. This suppression of NK cell activity can enhance metastasis. The reduction of the tumor-promoting effects of surgery by analgesics seems to be due to the alleviation of pain-induced reductions in NK cell function, but unrecognized factors other than immune cells probably also play a role. Thus, the provision of adequate perioperative pain management in oncological surgery may protect clinical patients against

Table 4.2.   Five freedoms for evaluation of animal welfare

Freedom from hunger and thirst
Freedom from physical and thermal discomfort
Freedom from pain, injury, and disease
Freedom to express normal behavior
Freedom from fear and distress

metastatic sequelae. Pain therapy itself may protect against metastasis and possibly the local extension of cancer.

Assessment of chronic pain

Assessment of pain in animals can be difficult and frustrating. The tolerance of pain in a veterinary patient probably varies greatly from individual to individual as it does in humans. Coupled with the innate ability of dogs and particularly cats to mask significant disease and pain, the task becomes even more challenging. Often veterinarians need to rely on pet owner experience to help define pain in animals. The mainstay of chronic pain assessment in cats and dogs involves recognizing changes in behavior. Table 4.3 outlines behaviors that are indicative of pain. The main point to remember is that *any* change in behavior can be associated with pain. Veterinarians should also allow technicians and other staff members to be involved in the assessment. Technicians and other staff members are usually better able to evaluate pain and quality of life in animals

Table 4.3.   Behaviors that may be associated with chronic pain in dogs and cats

Behavior	Comments
Activity	• Less activity than normal • Very specific activities may be changed: decreased jumping, less playing, less venturing outside, less willingness to go on walks (dogs) • Stiff gait, altered gait, or lameness can be associated with general pain but more often are associated with appendicular or axial musculoskeletal system • Slow to rise and get moving after rest
Appetite	• Often decreased
Attitude	• Aggression, dullness, shyness, "clinginess," increased dependence, and so on
Facial expression	• Head hung low, squinted eyes (cats) • Head carried low, sad expression (dogs)
Grooming	• Failure to groom may be caused by generalized pain
Response to palpation	• Palpation or manipulation of affected area temporarily exacerbates low grade pain and elicits an aversion response (such as attempts to escape, yowls, cries, hisses, bites)
Respiration	• Respiratory rate may be elevated with severe pain
Self-traumatization	• Licking an affected area (such as a joint, bone, or abdomen) • Scratching an affected cutaneous lesion or biting at the flank with prostatic or colonic pain • May also be observed with neuropathic or referred pain
Urinary and fecal elimination	• Failure to use litter box (cats) • Urinating and defecating inside (dogs)
Vocalization	• Whining, grunting, groaning (dogs) • Hissing, spontaneous meowing, growling (cats)

because they spend more time with the patients in the hospital. Thus, they are more likely to be able to converse in a relaxed and informal way with pet owners.

The best and most important people to assess their animal's behavior are the owners. Often owners need education as to what signs to look for or be informed that certain behaviors may be indicative of pain. Once very specific changes in behavior can be identified and recorded, these can be used to monitor the effectiveness of analgesic therapy. This approach has proved very sensitive in the evaluation of chronic pain caused by osteoarthritis. In cases where pain does not cause a specific behavioral change and only vague signs are observed, the owner is still the best person to assess the pet's pain or quality of life. Owner feedback can also be used as an indicator of the effectiveness and appropriateness of therapy. Physiological variables such as heart rate, respiratory rate, temperature, and pupil size have been shown to be unreliable measures of acute perioperative pain in dogs and are therefore unlikely to be useful in chronic pain patients.

Principles of alleviation of chronic pain

Drugs are the mainstay of chronic pain management although nondrug adjunctive therapies are becoming recognized as increasingly important. The World Health Organization (WHO) has outlined a general approach to the management of chronic cancer pain based on the use of the following groups of analgesics: (1) nonopioids (such as nonsteroidal anti-inflammatory drugs [NSAIDs] and acetaminophen), (2) weak opioids (such as codeine), (3) strong opioids (such as morphine); and (4) adjuvant drugs (such as corticosteroids, tricyclic antidepressants, anticonvulsants, and *N*-methyl-D-aspartate antagonists [NMDA]).

The general approach of the WHO ladder is a three-step hierarchy (see Figure 4.1). Within the same category of drugs there can be different side effects for individuals. Therefore, if possible, it may be best to substitute drugs within a category before switching therapies. It is always best to try to keep dosage scheduling as simple as possible.

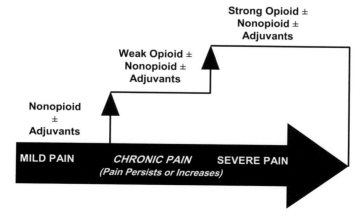

Figure 4.1. WHO "analgesic ladder" for treatment of cancer pain in humans.

The more complicated the regimen, the more likely owner noncompliance. Drugs should be dosed on a regular basis, not just as needed as pain becomes moderate to severe. Continuous analgesia will facilitate maintaining patient comfort. Additional doses of analgesics can then be administered as pain is intermittently more severe. Adjuvant drugs can be administered to help with specific pathophysiologies of pain and anxiety.

There are two potential problems with the use of the WHO analgesic ladder in veterinary medicine. First, there is very little information from human medicine and virtually none from veterinary medicine on which drugs are most effective for a particular type of chronic pain. It may well be that third-tier drugs are the most effective for a particular chronic pain state.

Many veterinary patients present at an advanced stage of disease and thus are already in severe pain. Once pain has been present for an extended period, changes may have occurred in the central nervous system (CNS) that alter the way pain signals are processed. This alteration in processing (called central sensitization) makes traditional analgesics less effective and requires that multiple classes of drugs be used concurrently to minimize pain. This is known as multimodal pain therapy. Once pain is minimized and central changes are addressed, some drugs may be discontinued. This approach has been termed the "analgesic reverse pyramid approach." It is currently unknown which of these two approaches (the WHO ladder or the reverse pyramid) is most appropriate and, indeed, one approach may be best at one disease stage and the other later on. The most important aspect in the treatment of chronic pain is that, in the majority of situations, multimodal therapy (the concurrent use of more than one class of drug or physical modality) is required for successful alleviation of the pain.

NSAIDs

NSAIDs have been the mainstay of therapy for chronic pain in veterinary medicine, especially osteoarthritis, for many years. For chronic pain, the choice among available NSAIDs can be bewildering, but a few key points should be remembered. On a population basis, all NSAIDs appear equally effective in relieving pain associated with osteoarthritis, but for a given patient one drug may be more effective than another. This is probably especially relevant for cancer pain where the mechanisms of pain may be very different from one patient to another.

In human patients GI side effects associated with NSAID use appear to be more common with drugs that preferentially block cyclooxygenase-1 (COX-1) over cyclooxygenase-2 (COX-2), although COX-2-inhibiting drugs have the potential to exacerbate GI injury when there is preexisting pathology. This results from inhibition of a beneficial role that the COX-2 enzyme likely plays in GI healing. The significance of COX selectivity and its association with GI adverse events is still debated in veterinary pharmacology.

There may be no difference in renal toxicity between COX-1 selective drugs and COX-2 selective drugs. Both COX-1 and COX-2 are constitutively expressed in the kidney. Liver toxicity with NSAIDs is an idiosyncratic event that can happen with *any* NSAID.

Monitoring NSAID therapy

If the NSAID chosen is effective and does not cause significant adverse effects it should be continued. If not, therapy may be changed to another NSAID provided the animal did not experience a serious side effect (such as GI bleeding, azotemia, or hepatopathy). If any toxicity occurs the patient should be carefully evaluated and the benefits of continued NSAID therapy weighed against the potential for further adverse events. Changing therapy to another class of drugs (such as opioids) may be the safest strategy if the patient's tolerance for NSAIDs is low. If another NSAID is chosen the patient should be monitored closely for toxicity. This involves informing the owner of the potential for further toxicity and signs to watch for (e.g., lethargy, anorexia, depression, vomiting, melena, and increased water ingestion). Periodic blood work (and urinalysis) to evaluate renal status (urea, creatinine, and urine specific gravity) and liver status (alkaline phosphatase and alanine aminotransferase and, if these enzymes are raised, bile acids) should also be performed. A baseline should be obtained when NSAID therapy is initiated and parameters monitored regularly thereafter. Reevaluation is done more frequently if multiple drugs are being used. Little information is available on the potential of clinical toxicity when combinations of analgesics are administered chronically.

NSAIDs in cats

Cats have longer but more variable and inconsistent rates of NSAID biotransformation and excretion when compared with other species. Most of the kinetic studies performed in cats have involved single doses. Given that most of the NSAIDs have a relatively long half-life in cats, chronic dosing at the dosing level and frequency described for dogs is likely to be more dangerous for cats than for dogs.

Meloxicam is the only NSAID labeled for chronic use in cats (and only in the European Union) at a dose of 0.05 mg/kg per os (PO) every 24 hours. Lower doses may result in clinical improvements in many cats. It should be noted that in the United States there is a specific bold type label advisory warning against more than one injection of meloxicam to cats. One strategy to minimize risk associated with chronic NSAID administration in cats is to individualize the dose by using the smallest effective dose or extend the dosing interval relative to other species. Some cats may metabolize drug at a rapid rate, requiring more frequent dosing, whereas other cats may accumulate drug to toxic levels unless the dosing interval is increased or the dose is reduced. This seems especially true with carprofen. Cats are more prone to toxicity associated with NSAIDs than are dogs; therefore, blood and urine should probably be analyzed even more frequently than recommended for dogs.

Other analgesics

If pain relief with NSAIDs is inadequate, oral opioid medications such as morphine or tramadol can be administered. Transdermal fentanyl or buprenorphine patches can also be used. Fentanyl, morphine, or tramadol can be used for dogs that cannot be given

NSAIDs although adverse effects may be more common. Acetaminophen has been used in conjunction with NSAIDs (except in cats) although safety data on combined use are lacking. Other agents to treat chronic pain include amantadine (an NMDA antagonist); anticonvulsants, such as gabapentin; and tricyclic antidepressants, such as amitriptyline. Each of these have been combined with NSAIDs.

Acetaminophen

Acetaminophen is a nonacid NSAID though many pharmacologists do not consider it an anti-inflammatory because it acts by different mechanisms than do most currently marketed NSAIDs. Although its mechanism of action is poorly understood it likely acts on a variant of the cyclooxygenase enzyme (cyclooxygenase-3 [COX-3]), which is present in CNS tissues of dogs. With any type of chronic pain there is always potential for CNS changes, so centrally acting analgesics can be very effective for what might seem like a peripheral problem. Although highly toxic in cats, even in small quantities, acetaminophen can be effectively used to control pain in dogs. No studies of toxicity in dogs have been done but if toxicity is seen it will probably affect the liver. Consequently, the drug should be used cautiously in dogs with liver dysfunction. It can be used on its own or in combination with codeine and is initially dosed at 10 to 15 mg/kg PO every 12 hours. The authors often use it as the first line of analgesic therapy in dogs with renal compromise where NSAIDs cannot be used, or in dogs that appear susceptible to the GI-associated side effects of NSAIDs.

Opioids

Many veterinarians may be unfamiliar with the use of opioids outside the perioperative period but they can be a very effective part of a multimodal approach. Adverse effects of opioids can include behavior changes, diarrhea, vomiting, occasionally sedation, urine retention, and constipation with long-term use. It is very often the urine retention, constipation, and occasionally the sedation, which owners seem to object to most. This is especially problematic with the administration of oral morphine. Opioids most often used clinically to alleviate chronic cancer pain are oral morphine, transdermal fentanyl, oral butorphanol, transmucosal buprenorphine, and oral codeine. Oral oxycodone has been used recently to control severe cancer pain in dogs. None of these drugs has been fully evaluated for clinical toxicity or for efficacy of chronic pain alleviation. It is important to realize that dosing must be done on an individual basis and adjustment of the dose to produce analgesia without undesirable side effects requires excellent communication with clients. Recent studies have indicated that certain preparations of prolonged-release oral morphine and oral methadone may not reach effective plasma concentrations in dogs when dosed at the currently recommended levels. Much work has to be done to better evaluate the efficacy and safety of long-term oral opioids in dogs.

Opioid use in cats

Currently no information on the long-term use of oral opioids for chronic pain in cats is available. Interestingly, there seems to be significant individual variation in the level of analgesia obtained with certain opioids, especially morphine and butorphanol, in the acute setting. Buprenorphine appears to produce predictable analgesia when given sublingually in cats. The sublingual route appears to result in near 100% bioavailability in cats, which may be a result of differences in ionization in the alkaline environment (pH 8–9) of the cat mouth compared to that of humans (pH 6.5–7.0). Sublingual administration of buprenorphine is well accepted by cats with no resentment or salivation, so there is no need to compound the injectable solution. The small volume required makes administration simple. Based on clinical feedback from owners, this is a very acceptable technique for them to perform at home. However, inappetence may occur after several days of treatment. Slightly lower doses can usually overcome this problem. When administered concurrently with other drugs longer dosing intervals appear to be all that is required to minimize the potential for adverse effects.

NMDA antagonists

Since the NMDA receptor appears to be important for the induction and maintenance of central sensitization, the use of NMDA receptor antagonists may offer benefits where central sensitization has become established.

Ketamine, tiletamine, dextromethorphan, amantadine, and methadone possess NMDA-antagonist properties among their other actions. Ketamine is not useful for the management of chronic pain in the injectable formulation that is currently available. However, intraoperative microdose ketamine appears to provide beneficial effects for a variety of surgical procedures, including limb amputations, and may decrease the incidence of chronic pain following surgery. Other recent publications suggest a benefit of using ketamine perioperatively (an intravenous bolus of 0.5 mg/kg followed by a continuous intravenous infusion of 0.01 mg/kg/min prior to and during surgery), particularly in patients that have pain associated with neoplasia. A lower continuous intravenous infusion rate (0.002 mg/kg/min) may be beneficial for the first 24 hours postoperatively and an even lower rate (0.001 mg/kg/min) for the next 24 hours. In the absence of an infusion pump, ketamine can be mixed in a bag of crystalloid fluids for administration during anesthesia.

Dextromethorphan has received attention as an orally administered NMDA receptor antagonist for use in human patients suffering from chronic pain. Although it appears effective in some people, dogs do not make the active metabolite after oral administration, negating its use as an analgesic in this species.

Amantadine has been used for the treatment of neuropathic pain in humans. It does not appear to have the undesirable CNS adverse effects associated with ketamine administration. Amantadine has been used in dogs as an adjunctive drug for the alleviation of chronic pain, particularly in osteoarthritis and cancer. As an adjunct to NSAIDs it appears to augment pain relief with a low incidence of adverse effects (mainly agitation and diarrhea over the first few days of administration). It may take 5–7 days to be effective. Amantadine should probably not be used in patients with congestive heart failure, or in patients on selegiline, sertraline, or tricyclic antidepressants.

Combination analgesics

Tramadol is a synthetic derivative of codeine and is classified as an opioidergic–monoaminergic drug. It has been found to be effective in the alleviation of pain associated with osteoarthritis in humans as part of a multimodal approach. Studies establishing dosing regimens and effectiveness in veterinary species are limited. Tramadol and its metabolite have agonist action at the mu opioid receptor and also facilitate the descending serotonergic system, which is part of the body's endogenous analgesic system. Tramadol has been used in many parts of the world to treat perioperative pain in animals and is occasionally used to treat chronic pain. Recent pharmacokinetic studies suggest that only low levels of the active *O*-desmethyl-tramadol metabolite are present in dogs after oral administration. While cats appear to make the active metabolite, drug clearance is lower in this species. The immediate release formulation is recommended for dogs, as the pharmacokinetics of the oral sustained-release formulation do not appear to be favorable for once-daily dosing. Toxicity has not been thoroughly evaluated in dogs or cats but clinical experience suggests that the adverse effects usually resemble those of other opioids.

Anticonvulsants

Gabapentin is a structural analogue of gamma-aminobutyric acid (GABA) and was introduced as an antiepileptic drug, although its GABAergic actions appear minimal. It is thought to act by modulating the alpha$_2$-delta subunit of calcium channels, thereby decreasing calcium influx and neurotransmitter release. It appears to be useful for treating neuropathic pain and central sensitization in some patients, although effectiveness in humans (and probably veterinary patients) is unpredictable. It is metabolized rapidly in dogs and is most often used for its anticonvulsive properties. It appears to have some analgesic properties at low doses administered two or three times daily.

A similar drug, pregabalin, has been approved by the U.S Food and Drug Administration (FDA) for treatment of neuropathic pain in human patients. It has the benefit of more predictable absorption following oral administration. Its clinical evaluation in dogs and cats has not been published to date.

Tricyclic antidepressants

The tricyclic antidepressant amitriptyline appears to be effective in cats for pain alleviation in interstitial cystitis, and many practitioners have anecdotally reported efficacy in other chronically painful conditions in cats and dogs. Amitriptyline has been used daily for periods of up to 1 year for interstitial cystitis and few side effects have been reported. There are no other studies of its possible analgesic effects in dogs or cats. Tricyclics should probably not be used concurrently with tramadol until more is known about drug interactions.

Steroids

These have a mild analgesic action, are anti-inflammatory, and can produce a state of euphoria. Steroids are often used to palliate cancer and cancer pain in cats and dogs.

They should not be used concurrently with NSAIDs because of the increased risk of serious adverse effects.

Bisphosphonates

Bone and periosteal pain induced by primary or metastatic bone tumors is thought to be caused mainly by osteoclast activity; therefore, drugs that block osteoclast activity should markedly reduce bone pain. Bisphosphonates inhibit osteoclast activity and can thus produce analgesia. There is very little information on their use in dogs for palliation of bone pain but drugs such as pamidronate are being used, and early anecdotal reports suggest effectiveness in approximately 40% of cases.

Other chronic pain-relieving modalities

Local or whole body radiation can enhance analgesic drug effectiveness by reducing metastatic or primary-tumor bulk in cancer patients. Radiation dose should be balanced between the amount necessary to kill tumor cells and that which would affect normal cells. Mucositis of the oral cavity and pharynx can develop after radiation to the neck, head, or oral cavities, resulting in impaired ability to eat and drink. Therapies to treat mucositis include analgesics, sucralfate, 2% viscous lidocaine, and green tea rinses. Intravenous administration of strontium 89 has also been shown to provide analgesia related to bony metastases in approximately 50% of humans but its use is uncommon in veterinary patients.

Acupuncture can be used as a pain-relieving modality when conventional therapy does not work. While some practitioners have difficulty accepting acupuncture because of traditional Chinese medical explanations that may be scientifically untenable, it is important to remember that there are documented physiological theories and evidence for its clinical effects in animals.

In general, acupuncture analgesia is extremely useful for treatment of pelvic, radius/ulna, and femoral bone pain, as well as cutaneous discomfort secondary to radiation therapy. Acupuncture may help to alleviate nausea associated with chemotherapy and some analgesics while promoting general well-being. Acupuncture analgesia can be provided through simple needle placement. Needle placement efficacy can be enhanced with electrical stimulation of high or low frequency (most types of pain respond to low frequency stimulation).

Nutraceutical products may contain a variety of compounds but the main ones are glucosamine and chondroitin sulfate. There is some evidence that they provide mild anti-inflammatory and analgesic effects. Interestingly, based on the authors' experience, the analgesic effect appears to be more predictable in cats than in dogs.

Revised from "Cancer Patients" by Duncan X. Lascelles and James S. Gaynor in Lumb and Jones' Veterinary Anesthesia and Analgesia, Fourth Edition.

Chapter 5

Anesthesia equipment

Craig Mosley

Introduction

Inhalant anesthesia forms the basis of most modern anesthetic protocols in veterinary medicine. The administration of potent inhaled anesthetics requires specific delivery techniques. The anesthetic machine enables the delivery of a precise yet variable combination of inhalant anesthetic and oxygen. The basic components and functions of all anesthetic machines are similar but significant design differences exist among them. Machines can be very simple, for example, those used for mobile applications to very complex anesthetic workstations with built-in ventilators, monitors, and safety systems (see Figure 5.1). Regardless of the complexity of the design, all anesthetic machines share common components: a source of oxygen, a regulator for oxygen (this may be part of the gas supply system), flow meter for oxygen, and a vaporizer. If additional gases are used (i.e., nitrous oxide) there will also be a source, regulator, and flow meter for each gas that generally parallels the path of oxygen with some exceptions (i.e., oxygen flush valve). The basic anesthetic machine is then used in conjunction with a breathing circuit and anesthetic waste gas scavenging system for anesthetic delivery to the patient.

Safety and design

Since 2000, human anesthetic machines sold in North America must meet minimum design and safety standards established by organizations such as the American Society for Testing and Materials (ASTM) and the Canadian Standards Association (CSA). Anesthetic machines designed for veterinary use are not required to meet any specific design or safety standards beyond those associated with basic hazards to the operator (i.e., electrical safety requirements). Safety features are often added on an ad hoc basis and there are no requirements for demonstrating equipment efficacy. Ideally, safety features, such as airway pressure alarms, should be designed into the anesthetic machine itself. The inclusion of some of these safety systems on anesthetic machines may help

Essentials of Small Animal Anesthesia and Analgesia, Second Edition. Edited by Kurt A. Grimm, William J. Tranquilli, Leigh A. Lamont.

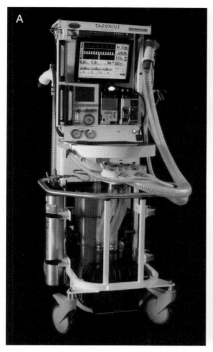
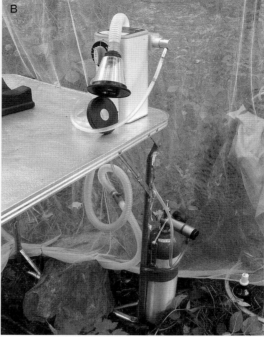

Figure 5.1. Anesthetic machines for veterinary use can vary considerably in their complexity and sophistication. (A) A complete veterinary anesthetic workstation for large animal use. (B) A portable anesthetic system for field use. Both systems provide all the components necessary for the controlled delivery of inhalant anesthetics. Photo A courtesy of Hallowell EMC, Pittsfield, MA.

eliminate preventable anesthetic accidents. However, until safety and design standards are adopted by the manufacturers of veterinary anesthetic equipment, there will remain numerous equipment options of varying quality, efficacy, and safety available for delivering inhalant anesthetics to veterinary patients. Regardless of the presence of standards, it will always be incumbent upon the veterinary anesthetist to thoroughly understand the function of each component of the anesthesia machine and to ensure that the machine is designed suitably well to accomplish these tasks safely.

It is beyond the scope of this chapter to describe in detail all the anesthesia machines and equipment currently available and used in veterinary medicine. There are many excellent textbooks devoted to describing in great detail the anesthetic equipment available for use in human anesthesia.[1,2] This chapter aims to provide the reader with a general working overview of the anesthetic machine, vaporizers, breathing circuits, and ventilators. In addition, there are products that have been designed specifically for veterinary use that are not described elsewhere, and some of these will be described here.

Endotracheal tubes and laryngoscopes

Endotracheal tubes

Endotracheal tubes are commonly used to maintain an airway in patients anesthetized with inhalant anesthetics. However, laryngeal masks have been evaluated in a number of domestic species and may be suitable alternatives in some instances.[3–6] A properly placed endotracheal tube or laryngeal mask with a properly inflated cuff provides a patent airway, facilitates positive pressure ventilation, protects the airway from aspiration of fluids, and prevents contamination of the work environment with waste anesthetic gases.

There are many styles and types of endotracheal tubes available that can be used in veterinary medicine (Figure 5.2A). Most are manufactured for humans but can be used in most small animal patients. For patients requiring tube sizes larger and smaller than those available for human use, there are some veterinary-specific products available. Endotracheal tubes manufactured for use in humans must have various markings and abbreviations directly on the tube that fully describes each tube. The markings may include the manufacturer, internal (ID) and outer (OD) tube diameter, length, and codes indicating tissue toxicity or implantation testing (e.g., F29) (Figure 5.2B). There is no requirement for similar markings on tubes manufactured solely for veterinary use but it is common for them to minimally list tube diameters and length. Endotracheal tubes are normally sized according to their IDs. For example, a size 6.0 endotracheal tube refers to a tube with an ID of 6.0 mm. The OD for any given tube size may vary depending upon the construction of the tube. Endotracheal tubes having thicker walls will have greater differences between the IDs and ODs. This can become important when selecting tubes for very small patients. Very thick-walled tubes will effectively reduce the internal airway diameter compared with a thin-walled tube, as ultimately the size of the endotracheal tube that can be placed in a patient is limited by the OD of the tube and not the ID. However, very thin-walled soft tubes are susceptible to obstruction by external compression (i.e., tube tie) or kinking (Figure 5.3).

Common endotracheal tubes materials include polyvinyl chloride, silicone, or red rubber. Clear endotracheal tubes are generally preferred so that they can be visually inspected for the presence of mucous or blood intraoperatively, or debris within the tube lumen after cleaning. Generally, the largest size endotracheal tube that will fit in the patient's trachea should be used. Although various "rules of thumb" for selecting tube size exist, it is probably easiest to estimate the most appropriate tube size by palpating the individual patient's trachea. The tube should not extend distally beyond the thoracic inlet and ideally should not extend rostrally significantly beyond the patients incisors, as this will increase mechanical dead space. If the endotracheal tube is too long and further insertion would lead to the possibility of endobronchial intubation, it can be cut and the endotracheal tube connector replaced.

The most commonly used type of endotracheal tube in both large and small animals is the cuffed Murphy-type tube shown in Figure 5.2B. Cole-type and guarded (spiral embedded, armored) tubes are also occasionally used in veterinary medicine. Cole tubes are an uncuffed tube that has a smaller diameter at the patient (distal) end relative to the machine (proximal) end. The distal smaller diameter portion of the tube is inserted into

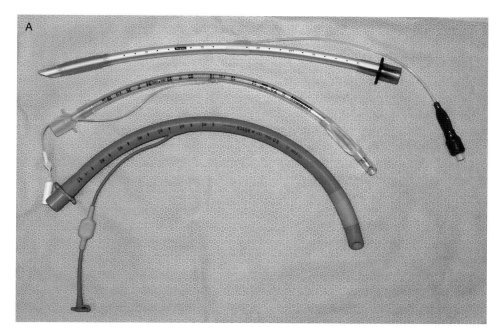

A

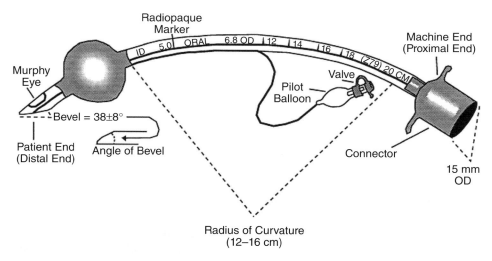

B

Characteristics of Common Endotracheal Tubes

Radiopaque Marker

ID 5.0 ORAL 6.8 OD 12 14 16 18 (279) 20 CM

Machine End (Proximal End)

Murphy Eye

Valve

Pilot Balloon

Bevel = 38±8°

Angle of Bevel

Patient End (Distal End)

Connector

15 mm OD

Radius of Curvature (12–16 cm)

Figure 5.2. (A) The tubes include tubes made of silicone, polyvinyl chloride, and red rubber (top to bottom). (B) Diagram illustrating the parts and desirable characteristics (e.g., radius of curvature and angle of the bevel) of a Murphy endotracheal tube. OD, outer diameter. From Dorsch J.A., Dorsch S.E. Tracheal tubes. 1994. In: *Understanding Anesthesia Equipment*, 3rd ed. J.A. Dorsch and S.E. Dorsch, eds. Baltimore, MD: Williams and Wilkins, p. 439.

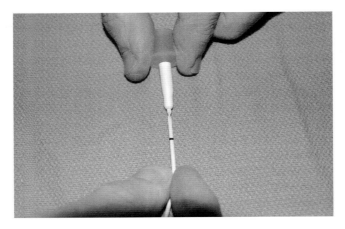

Figure 5.3.   Very thin-walled endotracheal tubes are prone to occlusion from external compression or twisting. Continual evaluation of the endotracheal tube for patency is required when thin pliable walled endotracheal tubes are used.

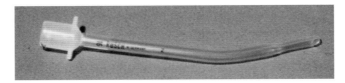

Figure 5.4.   A 10-French Cole endotracheal tube appropriate for small veterinary patients. Note the smaller diameter of the laryngotracheal portion of the tube (distal end of the tube, right side of the figure).

the trachea to a point where the shoulder contacts the larynx, forming a seal. However, Cole tubes will not produce the same degree of airway security compared with a standard cuffed tube and are normally only used in very small patients for short-term intubation (see Figure 5.4). Guarded tubes incorporate a metal or nylon spiral reinforcing wire into the endotracheal tube wall that helps prevent tube collapse and occlusion. Guarded tubes are useful in situations where the tube is likely to be compressed or kinked, such as procedures requiring extreme flexing of the head and neck (i.e., cerebrospinal fluid [CSF] taps) or those that involve compression of the trachea (i.e., tracheal retraction during ventral approach to the cervical spinal cord).

The machine end contains the endotracheal tube connector. The most proximal portion of the connector is a uniform size (15 mm OD) facilitating universal connection to all standard anesthetic circuits. The distal end of the connector varies in size according to the diameter of the endotracheal tube.

The patient (distal) end of the endotracheal tube is normally beveled. Murphy-type tubes have a hole in the endotracheal tube wall opposite the bevel, referred to as a Murphy eye or hole. The purpose of the hole is to provide an alternate route for gas flow should the beveled opening become occluded. Endotracheal tubes without a Murphy eye are referred to as Magill-type tubes. The cuff is located rostral to the Murphy eye for cuffed tubes, and can be a low-volume, high-pressure or high-volume, low-pressure design. In general, high-volume, low-pressure cuffs are preferred to minimize the risk of ischemic tracheal injury that may result from excessive pressure against the tracheal wall. When a properly fitting endotracheal tube with a high-volume, low-pressure cuff is used, the pressure exerted by the cuff on the tracheal wall is similar to the intracuff pressure. This allows for better estimation of the anticipated pressure on the tracheal wall exerted by the cuff. When using a high-pressure, low-volume cuffed endotracheal tube, the intracuff pressure does not reflect the pressure on the tracheal wall but rather the pressure created by the elastic recoil of the cuff, making estimates of pressure exerted by the cuff on the tracheal wall difficult. Tracheal wall pressures exceeding 48 cm H_2O may impede capillary blood flow, potentially causing tracheal damage, and pressure below 18 mm Hg may increase the risk of aspiration.[7] The best method for ensuring cuff pressures are within the recommended range is to use a cuff monitor to inflate the cuff. A cuff monitor is essentially a low-pressure manometer similar to those used for Doppler blood pressure measurement that are attached to the pilot balloon of the cuff and provide a measure of intracuff pressure. Other commercially available cuff inflation guides are available for the human market and have been adapted to veterinary use (Figure 5.5). Alternatively, it is common to use a leak test, performed by inflating the cuff until a leak is no longer audible at airway pressures of 20–30 cm H_2O. The pilot balloon used for inflating the endotracheal tube cuff is connected to the cuff via a channel incorporated into the endotracheal tube and normally includes a syringe-activated self-sealing valve system. However, there are also pilot balloons that do not self-seal and require some sort of manual occlusion using either a clamp or plug.

Laryngoscopes

Laryngoscopes consist of a handle and lighted blade; and are used to aid tracheal intubation and oropharyngeal evaluation during intubation. Unfortunately, laryngoscopes are often considered an optional piece of anesthetic-related equipment but their proper use can be vital for successful intubation in some patients (i.e., brachycephalics, patients with laryngeal/oral trauma). Regardless of the absolute need for laryngoscope-assisted intubation, its use is recommended for all intubations to ensure the anesthetist maintains the motor skills and coordination to properly use a laryngoscope and that a cursory oropharyngeal evaluation can be performed.

There are several styles and types of laryngoscopes and blades available. Some disposable laryngoscopes have a fixed blade (i.e., one blade type and size) and may be made of plastic while others are designed for use with multiple blade types and styles of blades and made of stainless steel. Because there is such a range of patient sizes, with different oral cavity configurations found in veterinary medicine, the option to use multiple blades is a significant advantage when selecting a laryngoscope. The handle may also vary in size and although this rarely impacts the functional use of the laryngoscope, a smaller handle may be more comfortable and easier to manipulate for some anesthetists, particularly when used for intubating very small patients. The handles are usually specific for either fiber-optic or bulb-in-blade illumination, although there are some handles that can

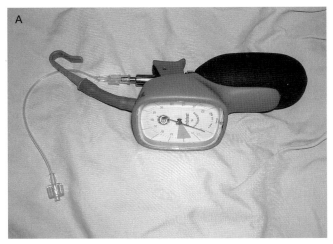

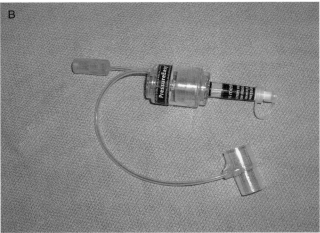

Figure 5.5.   An endotracheal tube inflation guide or monitor can be used to evaluate the intracuff pressures of the endotracheal tube and may help avoid tracheal injury secondary to excessive tracheal wall pressures. Several styles are available, including (A) an incorporated manometer and (B) a visual indicator.

accept either type of blade illumination system. There is no clear advantage of one lighting system over the other.

There are two main types of blades that are used in veterinary medicine, the MacIntosh and the Miller blade. Both come in a wide range of sizes (000–5). The MacIntosh is a curved blade with a prominent vertical flange, whereas the Miller is a straight blade with a less prominent vertical flange; both are suitable for intubation of most patients and the decision to use one over the other is often determined by personal preference. However, the prominent flange of the MacIntosh blade can potentially interfere with laryngeal visualization when used for intubating veterinary patients. In addition to the standard-sized blades available in human medicine, extremely long (~300 mm)

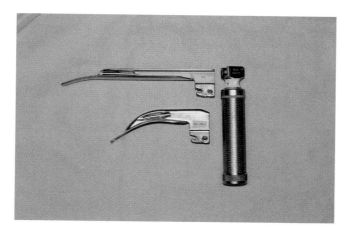

Figure 5.6.   Laryngoscope handle with Miller (upper) and MacIntosh (lower) blades. Note the more prominent vertical flange on the MacIntosh blade. This flange may impair visualization of the larynx when intubating a patient in sternal recumbency using the right hand.

Miller-style blades (useful for intubating swine, camelids, sheep, and goats) are also available (Figure 5.6).

Interestingly the majority of human-designed laryngoscope blades and endotracheal tubes are designed for anesthetists using their right hand to pass the endotracheal tube while their left hand holds the laryngoscope. The endotracheal tube bevel faces the left when viewing the tube from the concave aspect and the laryngoscope blade flange is normally on the right side of the blade when viewing the blade from the top. This configuration provides optimal visualization of the larynx when intubating a patient in the supine position (dorsal recumbency), where the laryngoscope is held with the blade in a downward position (inverted) and the endotracheal tube is held with the concave surface directed upwards. However, most veterinary patients are intubated in sternal recumbency, where the flange of the laryngoscope when held in the left hand can obscure visualization and the bevel of the endotracheal tube will do little to improve visualization when held in the right hand. There are left-handed MacIntosh blades available that may be more appropriate for intubation in veterinary species, as these blades place the flange on the left side of the blade, improving visualization of the laryngeal area when the laryngoscope is held in the left hand in an upright position. Since the Miller blade's flange is far less prominent, there is no real need for a left-handed design.

Medical gas supply

Anesthetic machines normally have two gas supplies, one from small high-pressure tanks attached directly to the machine and a second source often originating from a hospital's central pipeline supply. The small tanks mounted directly to the anesthesia machine are normally intended to be used as back up or reserve gas sources should the pipeline malfunction or for working in an area without access to the pipeline. Oxygen is by far the most commonly used medical gas during anesthesia, with nitrous oxide being used in conjunction with oxygen as an adjunct carrier gas for the inhalants much less frequently. Most medical gases are normally stored under high pressure in gas cylinders of various sizes or in low-pressure insulated cryogenic liquid bulk tanks. The characteristics (i.e., working pressure) and capacity of the gas cylinders varies with the type of gas they contain (see Table 5.1). Alternatively, oxygen concentrators can be used to supply a hospital with its oxygen requirements in circumstances where obtaining and storage of tanks is inconvenient, impossible, or prohibitively expensive (i.e., remote communities). Most oxygen concentrators use a system of absorbing nitrogen from air to produce gas with an oxygen concentration between 90% and 96%.

Most modern veterinary facilities will have some form of central gas supply and pipeline distribution system delivering medical gases to various work sites. The complexity of these systems can vary significantly; from a small bank of large (G or H) cylinders and a regulator to more complex systems consisting of multiple large liquid oxygen tanks, automatic manifolds, regulators, alarms, and banks of large high-pressure cylinders for back up. The size and complexity of the gas distribution system will depend upon the gas needs, area of required gas distribution, and the number of work sites required. Proper installation of large gas distribution systems is essential for safety and efficacy. All gas installations should be properly evaluated by those with expertise in this area prior to using them to deliver gas to patients.

Medical gas safety

There are several international (ASTM), national, and local documents related to the safe use, transport, and storage of pressurized gases. There are also standards surrounding the installation of medical gas piping systems and some of these provisions have been incorporated into hospital accreditation requirements in veterinary medicine. However, the specific guidelines can vary significantly among jurisdictions and regions. There have

Table 5.1. Characteristics of medical gas cylinders

Size	Gas	Gas symbol	Color code (U.S.)	Capacity and pressure (at 70°F)	Empty cylinder weight (lb.)
E	Oxygen	O_2	Green	660 L 1900 psi	14
E	Nitrous oxide	N_2O	Blue	1590 L 745 psi	14
G	Nitrous oxide	N_2O	Blue	13,800 L 745 psi	97
H	Oxygen	O_2	Green	6900 L 2200 psi	119
H	Nitrous oxide	N_2O	Blue	15,800 L 745 psi	119

been several well-documented medical accidents related to the inappropriate use of medical gases. Consequently, there are several safety systems that have been developed to help reduce and eliminate these problems. For example, all anesthetic equipment has a gas-specific noninterchangeable connector that is part of the base unit (anesthetic machine, ventilator). These connectors—diameter index safety system (DISS), pin index safety system (PISS), and quick connector—are described below.

Color coding

Gas cylinders and gas lines are commonly colored coded to avoid improper use, but color coding systems can vary among countries. For example, oxygen is colored white in Canada and green in the United States. In addition to color coding, all tanks have a labeling scheme consisting of various shaped labels, key words, and colors that are all used to identify hazards associated with the gas they contain. Most tanks originating from gas supply facilities normally have perforated tags (full, in use, empty) to track the cylinder's use status.

DISS

The DISS is a noninterchangeable, gas-specific threaded connection system. DISS is the gas connection used almost universally by all equipment and cylinder manufactures for the connection of medical gases.

Quick connectors

There are many proprietary (manufacturer specific) quick-connect systems that have been developed. These are standardized within a manufacturer but are not generally compatible with the quick-connect systems of another manufacturer. These systems facilitate rapid connecting and disconnecting of gas hoses and may be useful in situations where frequent connects and disconnects are required.

PISS

The PISS uses gas-specific pin patterns that only allow connections between the appropriate cylinder yokes and small gas cylinders (E size). The PISS is commonly found on the yokes mounted on anesthesia machines and some cylinder-specific regulator/flow meters.

Pressure reducing valve (regulator)

The pressure reducing valve (regulator) is a key component required to bring the high pressures of gas cylinders down to a more reasonable and safe working pressure (i.e., 35–50 psi). Regulators also reduce or prevent fluctuations in pressure as the tank empties. Regulators are normally found wherever a high-pressure gas cylinder is in use (i.e., gas pipelines, cylinder connected directly to machine). The regulators used for pipelines are normally adjustable, whereas those on most anesthesia machines are set by the manufacturer. The ASTM standard requires that regulators on anesthesia machines be set to preferentially use pipeline gases before using gas from the backup cylinder on the anesthesia machine. However, since neither pipeline systems nor veterinary anesthesia machines are required to meet ASTM standards, it is not uncommon for machines to draw from the reserve or backup tank preferentially rather than the pipeline. This problem can be avoided by ensuring that the pipeline pressure is set approximately 5 psi higher than the anesthesia machines regulator for the reserve oxygen cylinder.

Pressure gauges

Pressure gauges are commonly used to measure cylinder pressures, pipeline pressures, anesthetic machine working pressures and pressures within the breathing system. Cylinder, pipeline and anesthetic machine working pressures are normally expressed in pounds per square inch (psi) or kiloPascals (kPa), whereas the pressures within the breathing system of the anesthetic machine are normally expressed in centimeters of water (cm H$_2$O). The gauge measuring the pressure of the breathing system is often also referred to as a pressure manometer. The information provided by these gauges is vital for the safe operation of anesthesia equipment.

The modern anesthetic machine

Gas flow within the anesthetic machine

The basic anesthesia machine is made up of a series of parts that work collectively to safely deliver inhalant anesthetics and support breathing. These components include: the basic anesthetic machine (gas delivery system), the vaporizer, the breathing circuit, and the waste gas scavenge system. Perhaps the simplest way to describe an anesthetic machine is to describe the components in order of the flow of gas through the machine, from source to patient. However, prior to describing these components, it is important recognize that the pressures of gas vary at different locations in an anesthesia machine and knowledge of these pressures facilitates the evaluation and safe operation of these machines. There are high-, intermediate-, and low-pressure areas. The high-pressure area accepts gases at cylinder pressure and reduces and regulates the pressure; this area includes gas cylinders, hanger yokes, yoke blocks, high-pressure hoses, pressure gauges, and regulators, and the pressure may be as high as 2200 psi. The intermediate-pressure area accepts gases from the central pipeline or from the regulators on the anesthesia machine and conducts them to the flush valve and flow meters; this area includes pipeline inlets, power outlets for ventilators, conduits from pipeline inlets to flow meters, and conduits from regulators to flow meters, the flow meter assembly, and the oxygen-flush apparatus. The pressure usually ranges from 40 to 55 psi. The low-pressure area consists of the conduits and components between the flow meter and the common gas outlet; this area includes vaporizers, piping from the flow meters to the vaporizer, conduit from the vaporizer to the common gas outlet, and the breathing system. The pressure in the low-pressure area is essentially equivalent to ambient pressure and the pressures being experienced by the patient. Pressures within the low-pressure area can vary depending upon how the system is being used (i.e., positive pressure ventilation) but should generally never exceed 30 cmH$_2$O, as these pressures are transmitted directly to the patient's lungs (Figure 5.7).

Occasionally in veterinary medicine, multiple sources of medical gases (i.e., oxygen, air, nitrous oxide) are used with the anesthetic machine. However, 100% oxygen is normally the only gas used to deliver anesthesia and power anesthetic equipment (i.e., ventilators) in veterinary medicine. If the reader plans to use multiple gases for delivering anesthesia, it is the responsibility of the user to fully understand the implications of their use (indications and contraindications) and to ensure that the anesthetic equipment is properly designed and monitored to prevent the possibility of delivering a hypoxic gas mixture to the patient.

The flow of gas within an anesthetic machine may take multiple routes once it enters the intermediate-pressure areas of the anesthetic machine. Minimal gas must be delivered to the flow meter, where it is then directed to the vaporizer and subsequently to the patient. However, in addition to this route of movement, there may be several more routes available for gas distribution in the anesthesia machine. Normally on most anesthesia machines intermediate-pressure gas is also diverted to a fresh gas flush valve that bypasses the flow meter and vaporizer and delivers fresh gas directly to the breathing circuit. There are circumstances where flush valves may not be present or unavailable on veterinary anesthesia machines. Also, where present, gas from the intermediate pressure area may be diverted to one or more auxiliary oxygen outlets that may be used as the driving gas for a built-in or external ventilator or an oxygen flow meter.

Flow meter

Flow meters control the rate of gas delivery to the low-pressure area of the anesthetic machine and determine the fresh gas flow (FGF) to the anesthetic circuit. There must be a separate flow meter for each gas type used with the anesthetic machine. The type of breathing system used, the volume of the breathing circuit, and the size of the patient are all factors that influence the rate of FGF. There are several flow meter designs available but most are based on a tapered gas tube with a moveable float. The gas normally flows in the bottom of the tube and out the top. The tube is narrower at the bottom and wider at the top so as the float moves up the tube more gas can flow around the float, producing higher flow rates. The gas flow rates are normally expressed in liters per minute. The spatial distance between vertical markings on the flow meter does not necessarily correspond to equal changes in flow rate. In other words, the distance between 0 and 1000 mL as measured vertically on the flow meter may not be the same as the vertical distance between 1000 and 2000 mL. This is similar to the spatial separation of the percentages found on many vaporizers, where there is a greater spatial allocation on the dial for normal working percentages than for those rarely used. Some anesthetic machines may also have two flow meters for the same gas placed in series for allowing even greater precision at lower gas flow rates.

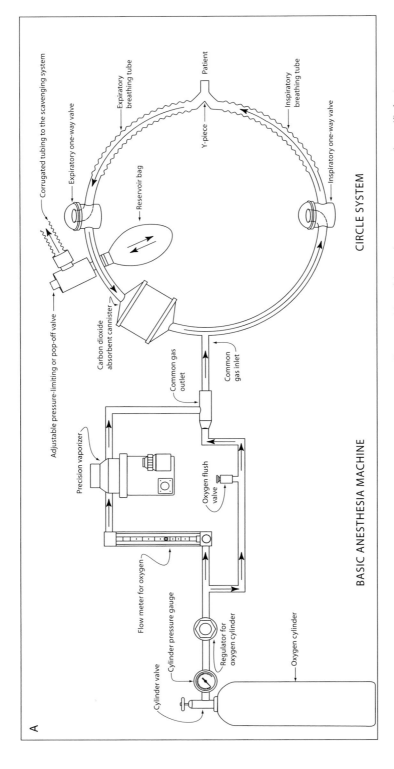

Figure 5.7(A). Diagram of the basic anesthetic machine: the circle system. Exact position of the various components and specific features can vary markedly among manufacturers. Illustration by Kath Klassen, BSc (Agr), DVM.

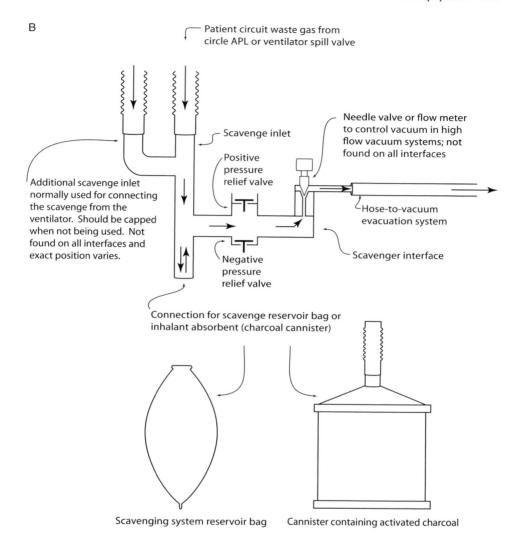

SCAVENGING SYSTEM

Figure 5.7(B). Diagram of the basic anesthetic machine: the scavenge interface. Exact position of the various components and specific features can vary markedly among manufacturers. Illustration by Kath Klassen, BSc (Agr), DVM.

Vaporizer

Vaporizers change liquid anesthetic into vapor and control the amount of vapor leaving the vaporizer. Most modern vaporizers are agent specific, concentration-calibrated, variable-bypass, flow-over the wick, out of the circuit vaporizers that are compensated for temperature, flow, and back pressure. Nonprecision, low-resistance, in the circle vaporizers continue to be found in veterinary medicine, but without proper inspired inhalant gas monitoring these vaporizers would seem to pose unnecessary risks during anesthesia and their use should probably be discouraged. Vaporizers essentially work by splitting the carrier gas to flow into either the vaporizing chamber where it picks up anesthetic vapor or to the bypass channel where it does not. The ratio of the amount of gas that picks up inhalant to the gas that does not pick up inhalant, along with the vapor pressure of the volatile anesthetic, will determine the final concentration of the gas leaving the vaporizer. The output from the vaporizer is expressed as a concentration (e.g., volume percent) of vapor in the gas leaving the vaporizer.

Temperature, flow, and pressure are all factors that can potentially alter vaporizer output. The mechanisms for temperature, flow, and pressure compensation vary among vaporizer manufacturer and model. In general, most precision-compensated vaporizers will maintain consistent output at flows between 0.5 and 10 L/min, temperatures between 15 and 35°C, and pressure changes associated with positive pressure ventilation and the use of the flush valve.

Temperature compensation

Temperature compensation is achieved through using materials for vaporizer construction that supply and conduct heat, efficiently promoting greater thermostability. In addition, most vaporizers have mechanical thermocompensation systems. These vaporizers compensate for temperature changes by altering the splitting ratio so that a greater or lesser amount of gas is conducted through the vaporizing chamber as the temperature changes during use. As the vaporizer cools, the thermal element restricts gas flow to the bypass chamber, causing more carrier gas to enter the vaporizing chamber. The opposite will occur if the vaporizer becomes too warm. The exact thermocompensation systems vary among manufacturers but the thermal element is normally a heat-sensitive metal that will reliably expand and contract when subjected to temperature changes.

Flow rate

Changes in gas flow rate through the vaporizer could potentially lead to changes in output. For example, if the flow was excessively high, complete saturation of the gas moving through the vaporizing chamber may not occur, leading to a reduction in output. Flow rate compensation is achieved by ensuring reliable and consistent saturation of all gas flowing through the vaporization chamber by using a series of wicks, baffles, and spiral tracks to facilitate liquid gas vaporization. These techniques are used to increase the surface area of the carrier gas–liquid interface, ensuring that all the gas exiting the vaporization chamber is fully saturated. All properly functioning modern vaporizers have very predictable outputs within a clinically useful range of gas flow rates.[2]

Back pressure

Back pressure on the vaporizer can occur during intermittent positive pressure ventilation or with the use of the flush valve, and this effect can increase vaporizer output if compensation mechanisms were not in place. There are a number of ways that the effects of back pressure are minimized in modern vaporizer. One is to reduce the size of the vaporizing chamber relative to the bypass chamber. Another option is to use a long, spiral or large-diameter tube leading to the vaporizing chamber; both will reduce the amount of pressurized gas reaching the vaporizing chamber. The use of one-way check valves immediately upstream from the vaporizer can also prevent the effects of back pressure and are incorporated into some machines. One-way check valves are also sometimes used downstream of the flush valve (upstream of the vaporizer) to prevent back pressure.

There are many vaporizers available for use in veterinary anesthesia but most are based on three main styles of vaporizers: the Ohmeda Tec (GE Healthcare, Fairfield, CT), Drager Vapor (Dräger Medical, Inc., Telford, PA), and Penlon Sigma (Penlon, Inc., Minnetonka, MN) series of vaporizers. The primary differences among vaporizer series include capacity of the vaporization chamber (larger chambers allow greater time between fillings, particularly useful for large animal applications), susceptibility to alterations in output due to tipping (rarely a consideration under normal circumstances), and mounting options.

Most vaporizers are mechanical devices requiring no external power to function normally. However, as a result of the unique vapor properties of desflurane, specially designed heated vaporizers are required to ensure consistent output. Additionally, there are electronic vaporizers available for use in both human and veterinary anesthesia. These vaporizers function as variable bypass vaporizers, but the splitting ratio of the carrier gas is determined electronically rather than mechanically. Since the system is electronic, various manufacturer and user alarm settings can be incorporated. For example, the vaporizer may alert the user if unusually high concentrations of anesthetic are being delivered from the vaporizer or that the vaporizer setting has not been altered within a specified time period, potentially avoiding inadvertent anesthetic overdoses (i.e., vaporizer output is momentarily increased and the user forgets to reduce the setting). Although electronic systems arguably provide additional information that may be valuable to the anesthetist, they may also be more prone to problems and damage related to the fact that they rely on properly operating electronics to function.

Vaporizers can be filled using a standard screw capped filler port or an agent-specific keyed filler port. Keyed filler ports are intended to prevent inadvertently filling a vaporizer with the wrong anesthetic agent. Most modern vaporizers are extremely dependable and durable, requiring very little routine maintenance and care. However, maintenance and care should be done according to the manufacturers' recommendations and only performed by a certified technician.

Oxygen flush

Oxygen flush valves are found on most but not all veterinary anesthetic machines. Flush valves are designed to rapidly deliver large volumes of nonanesthetic-containing gas to the patient circuit in emergency situations. The flow originates downstream of the regulator within the intermediate pressure area of the anesthetic machine ($\sim$50 psi) and bypasses the flow meter and vaporizer, delivering gas at rates ranging between 35 and 75 L/min to the patient circuit. To avoid overpressuring the patient circuit, the flush valve should not be used, or should be used very cautiously in nonrebreathing circuits, circuits attached to mechanical ventilators, and circuits with very low volumes (i.e., pediatric circle systems), as pressures within the breathing circuit may temporarily rise, creating dangerously high pressures to the patients lungs. The adjustable pressure-limiting (APL) valves should be fully open at all times to help prevent overpressurizing the breathing circuit.

Common gas outlet

The common gas outlet leads from the anesthetic machine to the breathing circuit. Gas reaching the common gas outlet has traveled from the gas supply (cylinder or pipeline), through the regulator, flow meter, and vaporizer. The gas flowing from the common gas outlet normally delivers the anesthetic to the patient circuit at the concentration and flow rate determined by the vaporizer setting and flow meter flow rate. However, the concentration of inhalant gas from the common gas outlet is not usually equivalent to the gas concentration inhaled by the patient when using rebreathing circuits, particularly when using low FGF rates, due to dilution of incoming gases with those already in the patient circuit. When depressed, the flush valve also delivers gas to the common gas outlet, bypassing the flow meter and vaporizer.

Breathing systems

Although some breathing systems are often built-in to anesthesia machines (i.e., the circle system), they are frequently considered separately from the actual anesthesia machine (i.e., gas regulating and inhalant deliver components). This is a particularly convenient way to discuss breathing systems in veterinary medicine, as on any single anesthetic machine, the breathing system may be frequently changed depending upon the needs of the patient or the circumstances in which anesthetic is delivered. The primary purposes of the breathing circuit are to: direct oxygen to the patient, deliver anesthetic gas to the patient, remove carbon dioxide from inhaled breaths (or prevent significant rebreathing of carbon dioxide), and to provide a means of controlling ventilation.

Breathing systems have been classified using numerous schemes. However, for clarity, it is suggested that the breathing circuit be classified into one of two groups: those designed for rebreathing of exhaled gases (rebreathing or partial rebreathing system) and those designed to be used under circumstances of minimal to no rebreathing (nonrebreathing systems). Some have argued that this classification is a bit of a misnomer, since depending upon the specific system used and the FGF rates used, a rebreathing system may have minimal rebreathing occurring (i.e., excessively high FGFs) or a nonrebreathing system may not completely prevent rebreathing (i.e., inadequate/low FGF). To help circumvent this debate it has been suggested that in addition to describing the design of the breathing circuit, the FGF rate should be provided to fully describe how the system is being used.[8] The FGF rate should be expressed in milliliters per kilogram per minute in veterinary medicine, owing to the vast range of patient sizes encountered. Additionally, the degree of rebreathing with breathing circuits can be affected by other factors such as the equipment dead space and the patient's respiratory pattern. Suffice it to say that breathing systems have been designed to function as rebreathing or nonrebreathing systems and should be used in the manner they were originally intended.

Rebreathing (circle system)

The circle system is the most commonly used rebreathing system and will be the only one described here, although other types of rebreathing systems have been used (i.e., to-and-fro). The circle system is designed to produce a unidirectional flow of gas through the system and has a means of absorbing carbon dioxide. The components of the circle system include: fresh gas inlet, inspiratory one-way valve, breathing tubes, expiratory one-way valve, APL valve, reservoir bag, and carbon dioxide absorber.

   The FGFs used with a circle system determine the amount of rebreathing; full rebreathing (closed), partial rebreathing (semiclosed, low flow), and minimal rebreathing. Historically, many terms have been applied to describe the amount of rebreathing, but there is no universally accepted standard or description of these terms. However, it has been suggested by several authors that the use of the terms open, semiopen, and semiclosed be dropped to avoid confusion.[9]

Full (complete) rebreathing

This describes a circle system using flow rates equal to the metabolic consumption of the patient between 3 and 14 mL/kg/min.[10] This is sometimes also described as a closed system; however, it may be best to avoid using such terms to avoid confusion.

Partial rebreathing

This describes a circle system using a flow rate greater than metabolic oxygen consumption (~20 mL/kg/min) but less than that required to prevent rebreathing (~200–300 mL/kg/min). Since this is a very large range it is often divided arbitrarily into low flow (20–50 mL/kg/min), mid-flow (50–100 mL/kg/min), and high flow (100–200 mL/kg/min) although this is not a universally accepted description.

Non (minimal)-rebreathing circle system

This would describe a circle system using flow rates greater than 200 mL/kg/min. Flow rates that would not normally be used in most circumstances. However, this flow rate may result when circle systems are used for maintenance of anesthesia in very small patients (<5 kg) with flow rates of 1000 mL/min or greater. Frequently in veterinary medicine it is suggested that flow rates below 1000 mL/min should not be used and although this recommendation may be clinically useful for preventing anesthetic-related errors by increasing the margin of anesthetic safety, most modern anesthetic systems (i.e., vaporizers) continue to function optimally down to flow rates of 500 mL/min. With the availability of low volume, low dead-space pediatric and neonatal circle systems, it is becoming increasingly common to use circle systems with partial rebreathing flow rates (i.e., <1000 mL/min) in small patients (<5 kg).

Obviously it is most economical in terms of both oxygen and gas anesthetic use to employ low flow rates when possible. Lower flow rates are also associated with less environmental contamination by halogenated hydrocarbons (all commonly available inhaled anesthetics) and the better maintenance of body temperature. However, lower flow rates are also associated with lower volumes of anesthetic delivery to the circuit, leading to slower changes of the inspired gas concentrations by the patient. Low FGF rates can be offset by using higher vaporizer settings.

Most anesthetics are delivered initially by relatively high gas flow rates to ensure rapid attainment of sufficient anesthetic concentration within the circle to maintain anesthesia in the patient following intravenous anesthetic induction. The flow rates are normally decreased after the first 10–20 minutes to economize on gas use and waste. The use of high FGFs enables the anesthetist to deliver large volumes of anesthetic vapor during the initial period of uptake by the patient and allows rapid changes in anesthetic depth. This ensures the patient's inspired gas concentration is more reflective of the concentration of anesthetic gas delivered from the vaporizer. This is in contrast to using low FGF, where the inspired patient anesthetic concentration will not necessarily reflect the vaporizer concentration of gas until nearing equilibration (i.e., anesthetic uptake, distribution, and metabolism are nearly equal to anesthetic delivery). The interaction between the vaporizer output, circuit volume, patient size, and flow rate is often an unfamiliar and difficult concept to grasp. Equating anesthetic delivery to a constant rate infusion of an intravenous drug is perhaps a more familiar comparison for understanding inhalant anesthetic delivery.

The actual configuration and features of each circle system vary somewhat depending upon the manufacturer, but in general a common pattern of gas flow is followed through the fresh gas inlet, the inspiratory one-way valve, the inspiratory and expiratory breathing tubes, the expiratory one-way valve, the APL valve, the reservoir bag, and the carbon dioxide absorbing canister back to the fresh gas inlet.

Fresh gas inlet

The fresh gas inlet is the site of gas delivery to the circle system from the common gas outlet of the anesthetic machine. The fresh gas inlet is normally found after the carbon dioxide absorber and before the inspiratory one-way valve.

Inspiratory one-way valve

During inspiration, the inspiratory one-way valve opens, allowing gas to move from the fresh gas inlet and reservoir bag to move through the valve into the inspiratory limb of the breathing circuit. During expiration, the inspiratory valve is forced closed, preventing exhaled gas from entering the inspiratory limb of the breathing circuit, forcing it into the expiratory limb of the breathing circuit.

Breathing circuit/tubing

The most basic breathing circuit is made up of a corrugated plastic or rubber inspiratory and expiratory limbs. The corrugated tubing helps prevent kinking and allows for some expansion if the breathing circuit is subjected to any compression or traction. The two breathing limbs are connected via a Y-piece and the Y-piece connects to endotracheal tubes and facemasks. There are also various coaxial designs that place the inspiratory limb within the expiratory limb of the breathing circuit. Coaxial systems reduce the bulk associated with the breathing system and at least theoretically the design facilitates warming the cold inspired gases by the warm expired gases. The Universal F-circuit (a coaxial breathing system) is designed to function with standard circle systems (i.e., 22 mm OD connectors of the circle system). Most breathing circuits can be adapted for use with all circle systems as the fitting diameters are standardized. However, there is a proprietary coaxial circuit available that utilizes nonstandard-sized circle system connectors requiring the use of a proprietary circle system. There are also several sizes of breathing circuits available that vary in length, volume, and the amount of dead space to meet various anesthetic requirements. Pediatric and neonatal rebreathing circuits are normally low volume and low dead space systems, allowing them to function optimally in small patients (i.e., those with small tidal volumes).

Expiratory one-way valve

The expiratory one-way valve functions together with the inspiratory one-way valve, closing upon inspiration and opening during expiration. This valve helps direct gas into the expiratory limb of the breathing system, through the expiratory valve, and into the reservoir bag. At least one system also incorporates a negative pressure relief valve, providing an alternative path of gas flow (room air) to the patient should the inspiratory valve become stuck in the closed position.

Reservoir bag

The reservoir bag is also referred to as a breathing or rebreathing bag. The purpose of the reservoir bag is to provide a compliant reservoir of gas that will expand and collapse with the patient's expiration and inspiration. It is commonly recommended that the reservoir bag be a volume equal to or greater than six times the patient's normal tidal volume (10–20 mL/kg). Ultimately the reservoir bag should be large enough to provide a reasonable-sized reservoir of gas, but not so large that it becomes difficult to quantify the size of the breath by observing movements of the bag. In addition, a very large reservoir bag will contribute to the overall functional volume of the rebreathing system (i.e., circle system), contributing to slower rates of change in anesthetic concentration within the breathing system when the vaporizer output is altered. This would not be the case when using a nonrebreathing system.

APL valve

The APL valve is also commonly referred to as the overflow, pop-off, or pressure relief valve. The APL is a safety valve allowing excess gas to escape from the patient circuit. If the valve is functioning properly gas should escape if pressures exceed 1–3 cm H_2O and it should be left fully open at all times. It may be closed slightly if the rebreathing

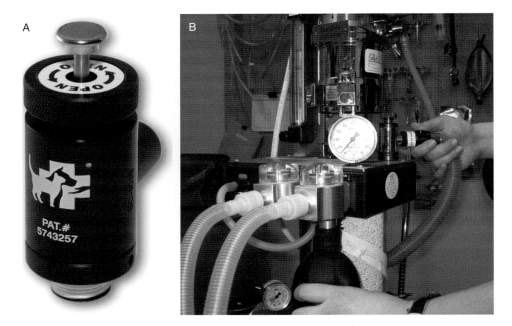

Figure 5.8. (A) An example of a momentary closure valve built into the adjustable pressure-limiting (APL) valve and (B) a momentary closure valve that can be added to any standard APL valve demonstrating its use to deliver a breath.

bag collapses completely but gas should still escape if pressures exceed $1–3\,cm\,H_2O$. The APL valve may be closed temporarily to deliver positive pressure ventilation but should be immediately reopened to prevent excessive pressure from building in the patient circuit.

Recently several manufacturers have designed products that allow momentary closure of the APL system. These products allow temporary closure of the system when a button is depressed, but the system automatically becomes fully open again once the button is released. These momentary closure systems are built directly into some APL valves or can be added to currently used APL valves. These are invaluable additions to the APL valve system and help to prevent inadvertent APL valve closure, potentially causing excessive pressure to build in the patient circuit that can lead to patient barotrauma or death (Figure 5.8).

Carbon dioxide absorber

The carbon dioxide absorber contains the chemical absorbent for removing carbon dioxide from exhaled gases. There are many types (dual canister, disposable, etc.) and sizes of carbon dioxide absorbers available. All contain some type of screen to prevent absorbent granules from entering the breathing circuit and most contain a baffling system to prevent channeling of gases within the absorber canister. However despite the screens, absorbent granules and/or dust will occasionally enter the breathing circuit; this is probably most commonly encountered in large animal systems where relatively high peak flows of gas (associated with inspiration and expiration) are more common. It is commonly suggested in veterinary medicine that the absorber canister must be twice the patient's tidal volume to ensure complete absorption of carbon dioxide, but there seems to be little evidence to support this statement. In fact, most large animal canisters rarely have a volume equal to twice the patient's tidal volume and may in fact have a volume equivalent or less than the patient's tidal volume. Moreover, many carbon dioxide absorbers used in human anesthetic machines normally have volumes less than the patient's tidal volume. However, the relative efficiency of absorption (i.e., the carbon dioxide load absorbed when an absorbent appears exhausted) may improve with larger carbon dioxide absorbers.[11] Smaller carbon dioxide absorbers will reduce the internal volume of the breathing circuit, leading to vaporizer concentration changes being reflected more rapidly in the inspired gas concentration but will require more frequent absorbent changes.

Carbon dioxide absorbents

The general principle of carbon dioxide absorption involves a base (absorbent) neutralizing an acid (CO_2). The end products of the reaction are water, carbonate, and heat production. The principle component of most commonly used absorbents is calcium hydroxide. The two most common absorbent materials used are soda lime and barium lime (baralyme) with absorptive capacities of 25 and 27 L of carbon dioxide per 100 g, respectively. However, when in continuous use the absorbents appear exhausted (i.e., indicator color change) before the absorbing capacity of the granules is exceeded. Granules normally turn from white to purple or pink as they become exhausted depending upon the indicator used. Ethyl violet (purple) or phenolphthalein (red) are pH-sensitive indicators commonly added to the granules to help identify absorbent exhaustion. The color change should not be used as the only indicator of absorbent exhaustion. It is common for the absorbent that has changed color to turn back to white if allowed to stand unused for several hours. Fresh absorbent is normally easily crumbled under pressure, whereas used absorbent becomes hard (carbonate). Additionally, since the reaction of carbon dioxide absorption produces heat and moisture, activity of the absorbent may be evaluated by looking for evidence of both heat and moisture development within the canister. Also, where available, capnography can be used to detect absorbent exhaustion. The rate of absorbent exhaustion will be determined by the size of the patient (CO_2 production) and the rate of FGF (mL/kg/min). Absorbent exhaustion will occur faster in larger patients and when low FGFs are used. Under most circumstances, various criteria (i.e., hours of use) for routinely changing the absorbent are adopted. The absorbent canister should be filled carefully to avoid overfilling, packing granules in the canister and spilling granules into the breathing system.

Some degradation of inhalant anesthetics occurs with their exposure to carbon dioxide absorbents. Normally this degradation is insignificant. However, sevoflurane can decompose to a potentially nephrotoxic compound, Compound A. Factors associated with increasing production of Compound A include high concentration of sevoflurane, low FGFs, dry absorbent, high temperature, and use of barium lime. The significance of

Compound A production for human and other animal health effects has been widely debated, but its clinical significance appears to be of little concern in dogs and cats. Carbon monoxide can also be produced when desflurane, enflurane, or isoflurane are passed through dry absorbents containing a strong alkali (potassium or sodium hydroxide). Most human cases of carbon monoxide poisoning have been reported to occur during the first general anesthetic administered from a little-used anesthetic machine. In human anesthesia, it is recommended to use only nondesiccated absorbents containing no potassium hydroxide and little or no sodium hydroxide. Although carbon monoxide poisoning associated with anesthetic use in veterinary medicine seems to be a very rare occurrence (or it is simply not recognized), similar recommendations are probably applicable.

Nonrebreathing systems

Nonrebreathing systems are characterized by the absence of unidirectional valves and a carbon dioxide absorber. Rather than relying on carbon dioxide absorption for removal of CO_2, these systems depend on high FGFs to eliminate CO_2 from the circuit. Nonrebreathing systems are normally not used for patients exceeding 10 kg as they become far less economical to use owing to the high FGF rates required to prevent rebreathing of CO_2 compared to the circle system. Recommended flow rates required to prevent the rebreathing of expired CO_2 range from 130 to 300 mL/kg/min, although values as high as 600 mL/kg/min have been recommended. The wide range of recommended flow rates likely has something to do with fact that in addition to the FGF rate, the patient's intrinsic respiratory pattern will influence whether rebreathing occurs (discussed later). Nonrebreathing systems have historically been recommended, somewhat arbitrarily, for use in all patients less than 5 kg, citing lower resistance during breathing, less equipment dead space, and less total circuit volume. However, by using newer pediatric, neonatal, and small-patient-specific rebreathing circuits, many of the advantages normally associated with nonrebreathing systems are eliminated and it is possible to safely maintain patients less than 5 kg using rebreathing systems as long as the patient's tidal volume is adequate to actuate the unidirectional valves. Small patient-specific circuits generally have no more—and in some case less—dead space and total volume than standard nonrebreathing systems (see Figure 5.9).

There is no generally accepted minimum patient size for using a rebreathing system accepted among anesthesiologists. The minimum patient size generally ranges between 3 and 7 kg, although an individual anesthetist may choose values outside this range depending upon monitoring available (i.e., capnography for evaluation of rebreathing) and intended ventilation mode (spontaneous, controlled).

Although there are often three or more nonrebreathing systems commonly described for use in veterinary medicine in North America, all are functionally nearly identical and based on two of the six historically described Mapleson systems: D and F (see Figure 5.10).

Parts of the nonrebreathing system include fresh gas conducting tubing, patient connection, exhalation conducting tubing (normally corrugated), excess gas venting system, and reservoir bag. All commonly used systems have the FGF entering near the patient's

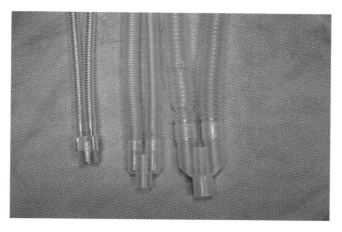

Figure 5.9. The Y-piece of three different-sized circle system circuits demonstrating the difference in dead space. Circle system circuits are commonly available in neonatal/pediatric and adult configurations, middle and right, respectively. The circle system on the left is a veterinary specific circuit designed specifically for very small patients and has minimal dead space associated with its use.

mouth and rely on the fresh gas inflow to push the CO_2-containing expired breath down a variable length of conducting tubing toward the reservoir bag and ultimately into the scavenge system. The FGF is delivered by the fresh gas conducting tube and the exhaled and excess FGF are conducted down the exhalation conducting tube toward the reservoir bag. The high FGFs are necessary to help minimize the rebreathing of expired gases (i.e., CO_2). During the expiratory pause the high FGF from the fresh gas conducting tube pushes the exhaled gas from the previous expiration down the exhalation conducting tube away from the patient toward the reservoir bag. When the patient inspires, they inspire gas coming from both the fresh gas conducting tube and the exhalation conducting tube. Under normal circumstances (i.e., patient with a normal respiratory pattern), the majority of the inspired breath actually comes from the exhalation conducting tube. In some circumstance (i.e., patients with unusual respiratory patterns), a patient may rebreathe exhaled gases despite seemingly sufficient FGFs. For example, a patient with rapid deep breathing may not have an expiratory pause of sufficient duration for CO_2 to be washed distal enough from the patient end of the tube to prevent rebreathing, particularly if a sufficiently large breath is taken, creating a high peak inspiratory flow rate.

The Bain system and the Modified Jackson–Rees are probably the names most commonly applied to nonrebreathing systems but they do not adequately describe the systems as they are frequently used in veterinary medicine. Neither system is a specifically defined system in that they are not always reliably configured in the same manner. Based on the historical descriptions of these circuits the Bain circuit (based on a Mapleson D system) would have an APL valve proximal to the rebreathing bag, whereas the Modified Jackson–Rees (based on a Mapleson F system) would have a pinch or stopcock valve located distal to the rebreathing bag. However, both breathing systems can be adapted for use with a mounting block and various reservoir bag and venting system

a. Bain with Bain mount and APL
   (Mapleson D-type configuration — coaxial)

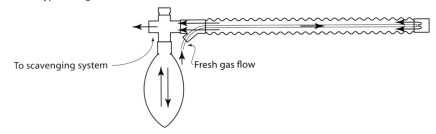

To scavenging system

Fresh gas flow

b. Bain with pinch valve distal to bag
   (Mapleson F-type configuration — coaxial)

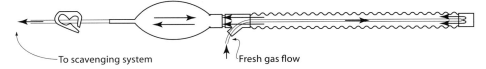

To scavenging system

Fresh gas flow

c. Modified Jackson–Ree's with relief valve proximal to bag
   (Mapleson D-type configuration — non coaxial)

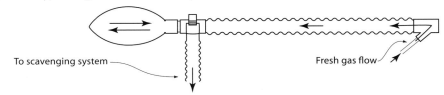

To scavenging system

Fresh gas flow

d. Modified Jackson–Ree's with pinch valve distal to bag
   (Mapleson F-type configuration — non coaxial)

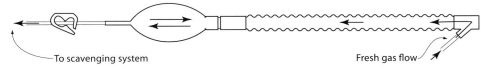

To scavenging system

Fresh gas flow

COMMONLY USED NONREBREATHING SYSTEM CONFIGURATIONS

Figure 5.10. Diagrams of the Mapleson systems (D and F) used most commonly as the foundation for modern nonrebreathing systems. Most modern nonrebreathing systems are modifications of the Mapleson classification and can no longer be strictly classified as one type or the other. For example, a Bain system is a coaxial system like the Mapleson D system but can be configured with (a) the exhaust gas exiting prior to the rebreathing bag—Mapleson D or (b) after the rebreathing bag—Mapleson F. The Jackson–Rees system, a noncoaxial system, can be configured similarly with the exhaust gas exiting either (c) before—Mapleson D or (d) after the rebreathing bag—Mapleson F. Illustration by Kath Klassen, BSc (Agr), DVM.

combinations, making strict classification nearly impossible. Essentially, the main difference between how the two systems can be used functionally is that one is a coaxial design (Bain) and the other is not (Modified Jackson–Rees). Perhaps a less confusing way to classify the commonly used nonrebreathing circuits in veterinary medicine would be based on the configuration of the conducting tubing (i.e., coaxial or noncoaxial), location of scavenging system (i.e., proximal or distal to the reservoir bag), and method of scavenging (APL valve, pinch valve or stopcock type valve).

The coaxial design of the Bain system reduces the overall bulk and provides a method for potentially warming the cold inspired gases. Mounting blocks are convenient methods for arranging nonrebreathing systems by providing fixed connections points for the breathing circuit, reservoir bag, and scavenge tubing. The use of a mounting block minimizes the potential for misconnections, disconnections, or kinked hoses. The fixed positioning relative to the anesthetic machine also allows the anesthetist to readily assess the integrity of all connections. Nonrebreathing systems used without a mounting block can be placed anywhere in the anesthetic work area and run the risk of being covered by drapes, hanging off surgical tables, or being pulled or caught by moving legs or equipment in the operating room, all increasing the possibility for anesthetic complications. Most mounting blocks also have a pressure manometer built into the system; this is an invaluable addition enabling the user to monitor and assess changes in airway pressure. Most nonrebreathing systems sold to veterinarians are not configured with a pressure manometer as part of the standard system, which, along with high FGFs and relatively small circuit volumes, exposes patients to the potential for accidental barotrauma. One solution to overcome this problem if a mounting block with manometer is not available is to purchase disposable pressure manometers designed for use with a resuscitation bag. These can be easily placed within all nonrebreathing systems, used many times over and are an inexpensive method of evaluating airway pressures (Figure 5.11).

Waste gas scavenge system

The scavenging system includes the APL valve, an interface, and a waste gas elimination system. The waste gas elimination system may be either an active or passive system. A passive system does not use negative pressure, whereas an active system uses either high or low negative pressure. The type of waste gas elimination system will determine the need and type of waste gas interface required. Passive waste gas systems may use an activated charcoal canister to inactivate halogenated anesthetics or they may divert the waste anesthetic gases through a short conduit outside the work environment directly to the atmosphere.

Negative pressure scavenge (vacuum) systems are increasingly being used in veterinary medicine. All negative pressure scavenge systems require some type of scavenge interface to operate properly. Ideally, waste gas scavenge interfaces should have the means of managing both excessive positive and negative pressure, a reservoir system to accommodate changes in waste gas delivery to the scavenge system, and a means of inactivating any halogenated gas that escapes the scavenging system. Most scavenge interfaces fail to meet all these specifications under extreme circumstances of use (i.e.,

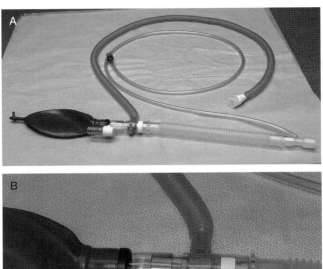

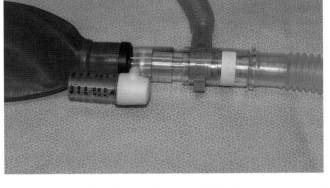

Figure 5.11. (A) An example of a disposable resuscitation bag manometer that can be adapted for use with most nonrebreathing systems. (B) A closer view of the markings on the manometer. The presence of the manometer will allow the anesthetist to better evaluate airway pressures within the breathing system.

high negative pressure scavenge systems, pressure alterations within the vacuum system, marked alterations in the rate of waste gases exhausted to the scavenge system) but most perform adequately under normal operating conditions.

Low negative pressure (vacuum) scavenging systems work well with most scavenge interfaces. These systems are often dedicated for waste gas scavenge only and may be centrally located or located at the machine itself. High negative pressure scavenge systems are most commonly found in larger facilities with centrally located medical vacuum systems and the active scavenge system works off the same high negative pressure system used for medical suction. Although it is often seen as more convenient and cost-effective to use the same vacuum system for all functions in the hospital, there are some unique challenges associated with this type of installation. Since these systems are under a tremendous amount of negative pressure relative to that needed for scavenging, these systems require adjustable scavenge interfaces to regulate the level of suction at the scavenge interface and frequent minor adjustments to prevent collapsing of the reservoir bag (compliant component) of the breathing system, making it difficult or impossible for the patient to fully inspire. Regardless of the type of scavenging system used, canisters of activated charcoal should be available for situations where other modes of waste anesthetic gas scavenge are not available (i.e., when moving patients attached to the anesthetic machine or when working in areas without scavenging facilities).

Routine anesthesia machine checkout procedure

Routine evaluation of the anesthetic machine and associated systems prior to and throughout the anesthetic period should be part of every anesthetist's standard operating procedures (SOP). Equipment failures appear to be a relatively common cause of anesthetic-related morbidity and mortality.[12] Standards of safety and the development of preanesthetic equipment checkout recommendations for human anesthetic equipment have been developed in conjunction with regulatory, industry, and anesthesia personnel and published in many countries. Unfortunately, there is no generally recognized standard for preanesthetic checkout recommendations in veterinary medicine. However, there is an excellent checklist proposed for veterinary anesthetists developed by Hartsfield that is based on the U.S. Food and Drug Administration's Center for Devices and Radiological Health "Anesthesia Apparatus Checkout Recommendations".[10,13] Table 5.2 presents a modified summary of the checklist proposed by Hartsfield.

Table 5.2. Veterinary anesthesia apparatus checkout recommendations[a]

High-pressure system
  Central gas supplies (oxygen, nitrous oxide, air) should be adequate in quantity and pressure. The central pipeline pressure should not fluctuate and should remain at its preset level (normally about 50 psi) when flow meters on the anesthesia machine are adjusted to a 3–5 L/min flow rate.
  Portable gas supplies (oxygen cylinders on the anesthesia machine) should be adequate in quantity and pressure. These cylinders should be evaluated for leaks. With the flow meter off and the cylinder valve open, there should be no audible leaks or decrease in cylinder pressure over time (i.e., 10 minutes).

Low-pressure system
  Test the flow meters of each gas. With the flow control off, the float should rest on the bottom of the glass tube. Adjust the flow meter throughout its full range; the float should move smoothly with no sticking or erratic movements.
  Vaporizers should be filled, filler caps tightened, and the control dial in the off position. The inlet and outlet connections should be in place and secure.
  Leak test the low pressure system.
  (1) Attach a "suction bulb" to the common gas outlet.
  (2) Squeeze the bulb until fully collapsed.
  (3) Verify the bulb stays fully collapsed for at least 10 seconds.
  (4) Open each vaporizer one at a time, if more than two vaporizers, and repeat steps 2 and 3 with each vaporizer.

Scavenging system
  Ensure proper connection between the scavenging system and the APL valve.
  Adjust the waste gas vacuum flow, if possible, to meet the needs of the individual case.
  (Continued)

Table 5.2. (*Continued*)

With the APL fully open and the Y-piece occluded.
(1) Allow the scavenge reservoir back to fully collapse and verify that the circuit pressure gauge reads about zero.
(2) With the oxygen flush valve activated, allow the scavenge reservoir bag to distend fully and then verify that the circuit pressure gauge reads less than $10\,cm\,H_2O$.
If the scavenging system involves a charcoal canister, the quality of the charcoal absorbent should be ensured.

Breathing system
  Rebreathing (circle) system
    Ensure the selected circuit and reservoir bag size are appropriate for the patient.
    Check the breathing system is complete, undamaged, and unobstructed.
    Verify that the carbon dioxide absorbent is adequate.
    Perform a leak test of the breathing system.
    (1) Set all gas flows to zero (or minimum).
    (2) Close the APL valve and occlude the Y-piece.
    (3) Pressurize the breathing system using the flush valve to a pressure of about $30\,cm\,H_2O$.
    (4) Ensure the pressure remains fixed for at least 10 seconds. Alternatively, the leak rate required to maintain at $30\,cm\,H_2O$ should be less than $300\,mL/min$.
    (5) Open the APL and ensure the pressure decreases appropriately.
  Nonrebreathing system
    Ensure the selected circuit and reservoir bag size are appropriate for the patient.
    Check the breathing system is complete, undamaged, and unobstructed.
    Perform a leak test of the breathing system.
    (1) Set all gas flows to zero (or minimum).
    (2) Close the APL valve and occlude the patient port.
    (3) Pressurize the breathing system using the flush valve to a pressure of about $30\,cm\,H_2O$. If there is no pressure gauge associated with the breathing system, the reservoir bag should remain fully distended with no loss of pressure.
    (4) For Bain systems (coaxial Mapleson D), the integrity of the inner tube should be evaluated. With the flow meter set to $1\,L/min$, the inner tube should be briefly occluded and the float of the flow meter should fall to near zero.
    (5) Open the APL and ensure the pressure decreases appropriately.

Ventilator
  Place a second reservoir bag on the patient circuit, appropriate for the size of the patient.
  Set the appropriate ventilator parameters for the patient.
  Connect the ventilator as directed by the manufacturer and fill the bellows and reservoir bag using the flush valve.
  Turn the ventilator on and ensure adequate tidal volumes are delivered and that during expiration the bellows fill completely.
  Check for the proper action of the unidirectional valves of the circle, if applicable.
  Manipulate ventilation parameters to ensure all are functioning normally.
  Turn off the ventilator and disconnect as directed by the manufacturer.

Monitors
  Ensure all cables and connectors are present.
  Ensure all alarms are appropriately set.

This anesthesia checkout list does not replace the experience of a knowledgeable operator continuously monitoring the anesthetic equipment. All parts of the anesthesia machine and breathing system should be present, properly functioning, free of defects, and correctly connected. This checklist includes the assessment of automated ventilators and patient monitors if they are present.
[a] Owing to the significant variability and lack of standards among veterinary anesthesia equipment, not all checkout procedures will apply to all anesthetic machines.

Anesthesia ventilators

The anesthesia ventilator is an automated device designed to provide patient ventilation in the perianesthetic period. Most of these ventilators lack the sophistication of control and function found in intensive care unit (ICU) ventilators and work best when used to ventilate patients with relatively normal lung function and simple ventilation needs. However, some human- and veterinary-specific anesthesia ventilators now offer features and performance rivaling that of a basic ICU ventilator. In North America, anesthesia ventilators designed for use in humans are subject to a series of international and national standards, whereas ventilators designed for the veterinary market are under no obligations to meet any similar design standards. Once again this makes it imperative that the veterinary anesthetist not only fully understand the physiological and practical implications of ventilator use but that they are also intimately familiar with the design, function, and troubleshooting of any ventilator used. There are two primary types of ventilators used in veterinary anesthesia, the dual-circuit ventilator that uses gas to compress the bellows (i.e., the second gas circuit) and the piston-driven ventilators that lack a second gas circuit. An anesthesia ventilator replaces the reservoir bag and APL valve with a bellow (or piston) and spill valve, respectively.

Piston-driven ventilators use electronically controlled pistons to compress gas in the breathing circuit. The use of an electronically controlled piston eliminates the need for a second circuit (i.e., the driving gas) and this typically enables the ventilator to more precisely deliver tidal volumes since it will not be influenced by the presence of a compressible driving gas. Electrical power is used to raise and lower the piston using a servomotor and ball screw assembly (linear actuator). Piston-driven ventilators can offer the user a very wide range of sophisticated ventilation options typically unavailable using common dual-circuit ventilators.

Each piston-driven ventilator is unique in its specific design but many will share some of the following features: cylinder, piston, linear actuator, rolling diaphragms, and positive/negative pressure relief valves. The exact configuration of each component and mechanism for facilitating expiration and spontaneous breathing will vary among manufacturers. The Tafonius large animal anesthestic workstation ventilator (Hallowell EMC, Pittsfield, MA) is a veterinary-specific, piston-driven ventilator and will be used as an example for describing the operation of a piston-driven anesthetic ventilator. Descriptions of other piston-driven ventilators designed for human use such as the Drager Apollo, Divan, or Fabius GS ventilators (Dräger Medical, Inc.) are available elsewhere.[14] There are two rolling diaphragms that seal the piston of the Tafonius ventilator to prevent mixing of ambient and patient circuit gas. The lower diaphragm seals the breathing gas below the piston in the breathing system. The upper diaphragm seals the upper side of the lower diaphragm from ambient air, creating a space between the two diaphragms. A vacuum is applied to this space that holds the two diaphragms tightly against the piston and cylinder walls. As the piston moves downward the space below the lower diaphragm decreases, forcing gas into the patient's lungs, and as the patient exhales, the piston rises. During controlled ventilation the piston drives the inspiration as per the ventilator settings. When the patient expires, the piston moves in response to the measured airway pressure, measured at the patient Y-piece. When the airway pressure increases by

0.5 cm H₂O, the piston is moved up enough to bring the airway pressure back to zero. This correction is made every 5 ms (200 times per second). This ensures that unless desired there is no resistance to exhalation (i.e., positive end-expiratory pressure [PEEP]). Most standard standing bellows will have a mandatory PEEP (2–4 cm H₂O) due to the design of the ventilator spill valve that is required to compensate for the weight of the bellows. During spontaneous breathing, the piston moves both upward (expiration) and downward (inspiration) in response to changes in measured airway pressure, ensuring that airway pressure is maintained at zero. Expiration will occur as noted above while conversely, during inspiration when the airway pressure decreases by 0.5 cm H₂O, the piston will move down enough to bring the airway pressure back to zero. Electronic positive and negative relief valves are located at the scavenging manifold to protect against excessive positive or negative pressure within the patient circuit (Figure 5.12).

Dual-circuit ventilators

Dual-circuit ventilators are basically comprised of the bellows assembly and the control mechanism for the driving gas. The control mechanism is normally an electronic microprocessor for most modern ventilators but some earlier ventilators used pneumatics and mechanics to control the driving gas. The bellows assembly replaces the reservoir bag

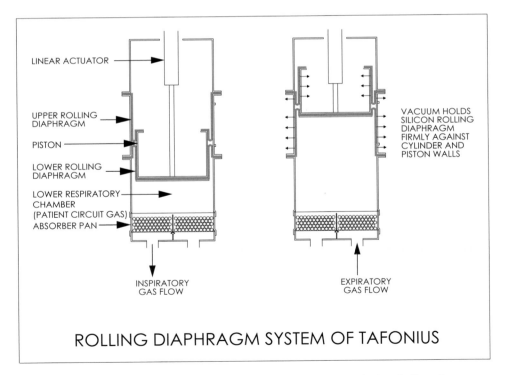

Figure 5.12.   Configuration of a piston-driven ventilator during inspiration (left) and expiration (right). Modified from a diagram courtesy of Hallowell EMC, Pittsfield, MA.

and APL valve and is comprised of the following components: bellows, housing, exhaust valve, spill valve, and ventilator hose connection. The primary circuit is continuous with the patient circuit and consists of the bellows and the spill valve. The second circuit contains the driving gas used to compress the bellows. The breathing circuit and the driving gas circuit are not connected; the bellows acts as a compliant interface between these two circuits. Driving gas is allowed into the bellows housing for a specific period of time and delivered at a specific rate compressing the bellow and closing the spill valve; this forces gas from the bellow to move toward the patient's lungs, expanding the chest. During expiration the driving gas is discontinued (housing pressure and consequently patient circuit pressure drops) and the gas in the bellows housing is allowed to escape from an exhaust valve, allowing the patient to exhale passively into the bellows. The spill valve reopens, allowing excess FGF into the patient circuit to escape, preventing pressure from building within the patient circuit. Although there are specific design differences in the way these functions are accomplished among dual-circuit ventilators, the general principles are similar (see Figure 5.13).

Bellows (configuration)

The bellows is an accordion-like device attached to either the top or bottom of the bellows assembly. Anesthesia ventilators can be configured with ascending (standing) or descending (hanging) bellows. The terms ascending and descending refer to the direction the bellows moves during exhalation and have been used historically to describe the orientation of the bellows. However, it is becoming increasingly common to replace these terms with standing (ascending) or hanging (descending) to describe the position of the bellows during the expiratory pause; this is often considered a more intuitive description of the configuration of the bellows. The majority of modern ventilators use a standing (ascending) bellows configuration where the bellows moves toward the base of the ventilator during inspiration, and upon exhalation they expand upwards. The tidal volume may be set by adjusting the inspiratory time and/or flow rate, or by a plate or other limiting device that limits the upward excursion of the bellows (see Figure 5.13B).

The spill valves on these ventilators normally pose slight resistance (2–4 cm H_2O) to opening, creating a slight PEEP in the system. This is to counteract the tendency of the bellows to collapse due to their weight and their elastic nature. In the case of very large and heavy bellows this may have the effect of producing a clinically relevant amount of PEEP. In some cases this may be considered desirable (i.e., horses), but at least one manufacturer has developed a method to overcome this PEEP effect by providing the option of applying a slight vacuum to the interior of the bellows housing to offset this effect. A desirable feature of the standing bellows configuration is that should a leak occur in the system, the bellows will fail to fully expand and progressively collapse toward the bottom. A leak is readily detected by an observant anesthetist. In addition, the patient's tidal volume can be estimated quite easily, in most cases by reading from the calibrated markings on the bellows housing.

The hanging (descending) bellows is attached to the top of the ventilator assembly and is compressed upwards during inspiration. During exhalation the bellows falls passively downward; this is usually facilitated by a weight placed in the dependent portion

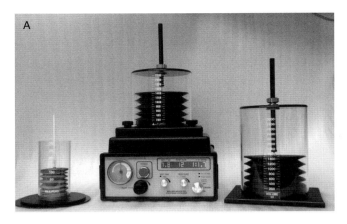

A

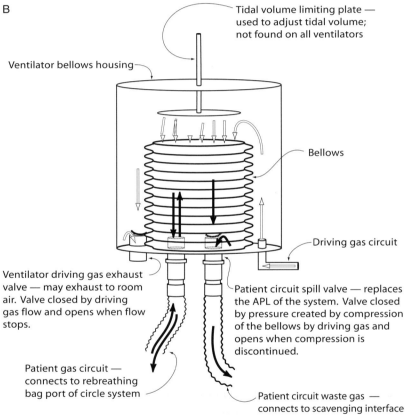

B

Tidal volume limiting plate — used to adjust tidal volume; not found on all ventilators

Ventilator bellows housing

Bellows

Driving gas circuit

Ventilator driving gas exhaust valve — may exhaust to room air. Valve closed by driving gas flow and opens when flow stops.

Patient circuit spill valve — replaces the APL of the system. Valve closed by pressure created by compression of the bellows by driving gas and opens when compression is discontinued.

Patient gas circuit — connects to rebreathing bag port of circle system

Patient circuit waste gas — connects to scavenging interface

DUAL-CIRCUIT ANESTHESIA VENTILATOR

Figure 5.13. (A) Example of a standing (ascending) bellows configured ventilator with a plate system that can be used to limit the tidal volume. Alternatively, the tidal volume can be limited by adjusting the inspiratory gas flow and/or inspiratory time. Courtesy of Mallard Medical, Redding, CA. (B) Schematic of generic dual circuit ventilator demonstrating the gas flows within the ventilator during inspiration and expiration. Note that the exact position and design of various components varies among manufacturers. Illustration by Kath Klassen, BSc (Agr), DVM.

of the bellows. As the bellows descends, it can cause a slight negative pressure in the bellows and breathing system. If a leak or disconnection develops in the breathing system, the weight of the bellows will cause it to expand normally, drawing room air into the breathing system through a negative pressure relief valve. During the subsequent inspiration, not only will the gas in the breathing circuit be diluted by the room air, but all or some of the inspiration will be lost to the room. Leaks (particularly large leaks) in the breathing system are not as readily identified by visually assessing the bellows using this type of ventilator configuration compared with the standing configuration. However, it is possible to detect small leaks that are made more significant by high pressure. For example, a small leak between the ETT cuff and the trachea of the patient will become much more significant as the airway pressures associated with intermittent positive pressure ventilation (IPPV) rise; this will direct some of the tidal volume intended for the patient into the room. Upon exhalation, a volume of gas inadequate to replace the volume lost from the bellows during inspiration will be expelled from the animal's lungs. The bellows will then attempt to fall but will do so more slowly if the rate of aspiration of room air through a small leak (and volume contributed to the system via the FGF) is less than that required for the bellows to fall normally. The result will be a bellows that falls very slowly or does not fall completely before the next inspiration occurs. This effect is most commonly recognized during ventilation of large animal patients where the leak is often relatively small (and is increased with positive pressure), the tidal volume is relatively large, and the FGFs are low relative to the patient's tidal volume.

There is at least one unique dual-circuit ventilator designed specifically for patients requiring tidal volumes of less than 100 mL that replaces the bellows with a floating disc. The floating disc separates the two circuits, patient breathing circuit and driving gas circuit. In this configuration, the driving gas and patient circuit do not come into contact with one another but they do move back and forth across the same surface of the ventilation tube. This configuration requires very precise machining of both the ventilation tube and the floating disc to ensure that gas remains separated within their respective circuits and that the disc moves freely without resistance.

Housing

A housing made of clear plastic that surrounds the bellows and allows observation of its movement by the anesthetist. The housing is a sealed container around the bellows that can be pressurized, causing compression of the bellows. A scale is normally found on the side of the bellows indicating the approximate tidal volume delivered. However, this volume is not always equivalent to the actual tidal volume received by the patients (see factors affecting tidal volume below).

Exhaust valve

The exhaust valve communicates with the inside of the housing and the room on dual circuit ventilators. During inspiration the exhaust valve is closed, allowing pressure from the driving gas to build within the housing. During exhalation the exhaust valve opens (and driving gas delivery stops), allowing the pressurized driving gas to escape and the bellows to re-expand. Piston-driven ventilators have no need for an exhaust valve.

Spill valve

The spill valve replaces the APL valve and is sometimes also referred to as a vent valve, dump valve, overflow valve, expired gas outlet, pop-off valve, relief valve, or pressure relief valve. The valve is used to direct excess fresh gas from the breathing circuit into the scavenge system. During the ventilator's inspiratory cycle, the spill valve is closed to prevent the escape of gas into the scavenge system. This is similar to closing the APL valve in order to deliver a manual breath using the reservoir bag. During exhalation, and once the bellows have fully expanded to their original preinspiratory volume, the spill valve reopens. With a standing bellows configuration, the spill valve normally has a minimal opening pressure of between 2 and 4 cm H_2O to offset the downward force created by the weight of the bellows. This allows the bellows to fill fully during exhalation. The spill valve is normally controlled pneumatically in ventilators using gas to compress the bellows, but in the case of piston-driven ventilators it may be opened and closed electronically.

Ventilator hose connection

The ventilator hose connection is a standard size outlet (22 mm male conical fitting) normally found on the back of the ventilator bellows assembly. A length of standard-sized tubing is used between the ventilator hose connection and the fitting that normally holds the reservoir bag on the anesthesia machine to attach the ventilator to the breathing system. In anesthetic machines with built-in ventilators, this connection is often accomplished through the use of a switch or dial, minimizing the potential for misconnections, disconnections, or kinked hoses (Figure 5.14).

Control of ventilator driving gas

The driving gas supplied to the ventilator is normally under intermediate pressure (i.e., 35–55 psi) and is delivered at a specific flow rate for a specific period of time to produce a volume of gas sufficient to compress the bellows and ventilate the patient's lungs. The driving gas is normally 100% oxygen and is used to minimize the potential for reducing the oxygen concentration of the breathing circuit should a leak develop between the two ventilator circuits (breathing and driving gas circuit).

   The driving gas flow to the ventilator is normally controlled electronically with dials variably labeled to adjust three essential variables: duration of time driving gas is allowed into the bellows housing (inspiratory time), rate that the driving gas flows into the bellows housing (inspiratory flow rate), and the pause between inhalations (expiratory time). By manipulating these three variables, the more commonly described variables respiratory frequency (f), tidal volume (Vt), and the inspiratory/expiratory ratio (I/E) can be controlled.

   Pneumatically controlled ventilators are slightly less intuitive to operate but essentially through manipulations related to pressure thresholds, flow rates, and time, the same

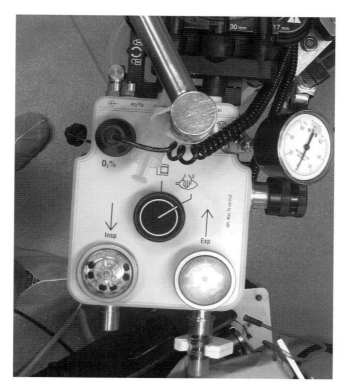

Figure 5.14. In anesthetic machines with built-in ventilators, a simple switch is often used to engage the ventilator. This minimizes the potential for misconnections, disconnections, or kinked hoses.

variables list above can be controlled. Pneumatically controlled ventilators are sometimes also referred to as pressure-limited ventilators as the tidal volume is determined by reaching a pressure limit rather than a volume limit.

Factors that affect delivered tidal volume

Unless mechanisms for compensation are built into the anesthesia ventilator, various factors can affect the actual tidal volume delivered to the patient. Under most circumstances and by using proper ventilation, monitoring, and set-up procedures, these factors are insignificant.

FGF

Although many modern human anesthesia ventilators compensate for changes in FGF, most veterinary ventilators do not. The electronics of most veterinary anesthesia ventilators are designed to deliver a set amount of driving gas regardless of the actual compression of the bellows. During inspiration the FGF will continue in to the patient circuit, contributing to the patient's actual tidal volume. Increasing the FGF or prolonging the inspiratory time will lead to larger tidal volumes, and although this effect may be insignificant in most patients, it can become significant in very small patients where an FGF of 1000 mL/min will contribute roughly 17 mL/s of gas to the patient's tidal volume during inspiration.

Compliance and compression volumes

Changes in compliance of the breathing system can be accompanied by changes in the tidal volume of gas delivered to the patient. Increases in the compliance of a breathing system can be accompanied by decreases in tidal volume as more of the gas volume is expended, expanding the breathing components. In addition, changes in airway pressures associated with ventilation may alter the actual tidal volume of gas the patient receives as gas volume is compressible when subjected to increasing pressures.

Leaks

Leaks within the system (i.e., around the endotracheal tube) will impact the delivered tidal volume as some volume will escape through these leaks, leading to a reduction in the delivered tidal volume. Although side-stream airway gas monitors are not considered leaks, they do aspirate a small volume of gas from the breathing system that may marginally reduce tidal volume. This effect is normally negligible but may be significant in patients requiring extremely small tidal volumes (i.e., <50 mL).

Alarms

There are no standard alarm configurations for veterinary anesthesia ventilators. Some of the more commonly found alarms are described below.

Low driving gas pressure alarm

This alarm is sometimes also referred to as the low-pressure alarm and will detect when the driving gas pressure falls below a preset value (i.e., 35 psi). A drop in driving gas pressure below a certain level may lead to a decrease in delivered tidal volume.

Airway pressure alarms

Both high and low airway pressure alarms are available on some ventilators. These are important variables that can help protect a patient from barotrauma (high airway pressure) and help detect leaks or disconnects. These alarm settings can be either preset by the manufacturer or can be adjusted by the user. Occasionally, preset alarms are not compatible with the ventilation requirements in some patients. For example, a minimum airway pressure alarm set at 6 cm H$_2$O may exceed the maximum airway pressures obtained when ventilating very small patients with extremely compliant chests (i.e., kittens, puppies, reptiles, and birds).

Proper ventilator setup and monitoring

Prior to using an anesthesia ventilator, it is important for the anesthetist to clearly determine desired ventilator settings. The anesthetist should have a solid understanding of the indications, contraindications, and physiology of IPPV prior to initiating ventilation. In addition, the anesthetist should ensure that they are familiar with all the features and proper operation of the ventilator they are using by reviewing the manufacturer's instructions. Improper use of positive pressure ventilation equipment can lead to unnecessary morbidity and mortality. The following steps are intended as a general overview to ventilator setup and may not be applicable for all ventilators, patients, and circumstances.

- Ensure power is available to the ventilator. Most ventilators will require a source of compressed gas and an electrical supply.
- Connect the scavenge hose from the ventilator to a scavenge system. Many scavenge interfaces have two scavenging ports, one for the anesthetic machine and the other for a ventilator.
- Empty the reservoir bag into the scavenge system, remove the reservoir bag, and connect the ventilator breathing hose to the reservoir bag mount. Close the APL valve. Some machines with built-in ventilators do not require removal of the reservoir bag and closure of the APL; instead, a switch or dial are used to isolate the reservoir bag and APL from the ventilator.
- Allow the bellows to fill. This can be facilitated by momentarily increasing the FGF rate. The flush valve should not normally be used for this purpose unless the FGF cannot be suitably increased to fill the bellows in a relatively rapid fashion (i.e., large animal ventilator).
- Initiate ventilation based on the predetermined ventilation parameters. It is generally best to start with tidal volumes in the lower end of the range to avoid barotrauma or volutrauma. Under all circumstances, it is vital to immediately and then routinely evaluate the peak airway pressures generated during inspiration to assess changes in respiratory compliance and avoid barotrauma.
- Further adjustments in ventilation should be made based on the assessment of peak airway pressures, end tidal CO_2, pulse oximetry, and/or blood gas analysis.

References

1. Davey A.J., Diba A., eds. 2005a. *Ward's Anaesthetic Equipment*. Philadelphia, PA: Elsevier Ltd.
2. Dorsch J.A., Dorsch S.E., eds. 2008d. *Understanding Anesthesia Equipment*. New York: Lippincott Williams & Wilkins.
3. Cassu R.N., Luna S.P., Teixeira Neto F.J., Braz J.R., Gasparini S.S., Crocci A.J. 2004. Evaluation of laryngeal mask as an alternative to endotracheal intubation in cats anesthetized under spontaneous or controlled ventilation. *Vet Anaesth Analg* **31**: 213–221.
4. Fulkerson P.J., Gustafson S.B. 2007. Use of laryngeal mask airway compared to endotracheal tube with positive-pressure ventilation in anesthetized swine. *Vet Anaesth Analg* **34**: 284–288.

5. Kazakos G.M., Anagnostou T., Savvas I., Raptopoulos D., Psalla D., Kazakou I.M. 2007. Use of the laryngeal mask airway in rabbits: placement and efficacy. *Lab Anim (NY)* **36**: 29–34.
6. Wiederstein I., Moens Y.P. 2008. Guidelines and criteria for the placement of laryngeal mask airways in dogs. *Vet Anaesth Analg* **35**: 374–382.
7. Stewart S.L., Secrest J.A., Norwood B.R., Zachary R. 2003. A comparison of endotracheal tube cuff pressures using estimation techniques and direct intracuff measurement. *AANA J* **71**: 443–447.
8. Hamilton W.K. 1964. Nomenclature of inhalation anesthetic systems. *Anesthesiology* **25**: 3–5.
9. Dorsch J.A., Dorsch S.E. 2008c. The breathing system: general principles, common components, and classifications. In: *Understanding Anesthesia Equipment*. J.A. Dorsch and S.E. Dorsch, eds. New York: Lippincott Williams & Wilkins.
10. Hartsfield S.M. 2007. Anesthetic machines and breathing systems. In: *Lumb and Jones' Veterinary Anesthesia and Analgesia*, 4th ed. W.J. Tranquilli, J.C. Thurmon, and K.A. Grimm, eds. Ames, IA: Blackwell Publishing.
11. Davey A.J., Diba A. 2005b. Working principles of breathing systems. In: *Ward's Anaesthetic Equipment*. A.J. Davey and A. Diba, eds. Philadelphia, PA: Elsevier.
12. Dorsch J.A., Dorsch S.E. 2008b. Equipment checkout and maintenance. In: *Understanding Anesthetic Equipment*, 5th ed. J.A. Dorsch and S.E. Dorsch, eds. New York: Lippincott Williams & Wilkins.
13. Hartsfield S.M. 2008. Anesthesia equipment. In: *Small Animal Anesthesia and Analgesia*. G.L. Carroll, ed. Ames, IA: Blackwell Publishing.
14. Dorsch J.A., Dorsch S.E. 2008a. Anesthesia ventilators. In: *Understanding Anesthetic Equipment*, 5th ed. J.A. Dorsch and S.E. Dorsch, eds. New York: Lippincott Williams & Wilkins.

Chapter 6

Patient monitoring

Steve C. Haskins

Introduction

The purpose of anesthesia is to provide a reversible alteration in central nervous system (CNS) function characterized by unconsciousness, amnesia, analgesia, and immobility suitable for completion of a wide variety of procedures including invasive surgery. Unfortunately, the drugs needed to produce these changes in CNS function also compromise patient homeostasis. Thus, anesthetic management can be considered a balancing act whereby adequate anesthetic depth is weighed against depression of other key organ systems. The ability to monitor the function of both the CNS and these other organs, notably the cardiovascular and pulmonary systems, is crucial in maintaining this balance.

Statistics regarding anesthetic risk, morbidity, and mortality in dogs and cats are presented in Chapter 1. The traditional method for measuring anesthetic outcomes in veterinary medicine has been anesthetic mortality. While mortality clearly fits the definition of an adverse anesthetic outcome, lack of mortality is, at best, a very crude benchmark for defining a successful outcome. Instead, as the standard of veterinary care continues to advance, there is an increasing movement to focus on more suitable measures of anesthetic morbidity. By striving to minimize morbidity in the perianesthetic period, the quality of care can be substantially improved and mortality rates will inevitably fall.

This approach is predicated on the ability to define and identify key pathophysiological abnormalities that contribute to anesthetic morbidity, such as hypotension, hypoxemia, hypercapnia, and hypothermia, and to institute corrective measures and/or supportive care. In order to do this effectively, personnel specifically trained in anesthetic monitoring and appropriate monitoring equipment are required. For more information on the American College of Veterinary Anesthesiologists Recommendations for Monitoring Anesthetized Patients, please visit www.acva.org.

Essentials of Small Animal Anesthesia and Analgesia, Second Edition. Edited by Kurt A. Grimm, William J. Tranquilli, Leigh A. Lamont.
© 2011 John Wiley & Sons, Inc. Published 2011 by John Wiley & Sons, Inc.

Monitoring CNS function

In general, the transition from a light to a deep plane of anesthesia is associated with the following: loss of recall, loss of awareness, lack of movement in response to a noxious stimulus, and finally lack of a hemodynamic or electroencephalographic (EEG) response to a noxious stimulus. Anesthetic depth represents the balance between the administered doses of anesthetic and adjuvant drugs, the intensity of surgical stimulation (which tends to awaken patients), and the severity of illness (which tends to augment anesthesia). For longer procedures, anesthetic requirements tend to decrease over time within a single anesthetic episode. In these situations, it is appropriate to make repeated attempts to incrementally decrease the amount of anesthetic administered and observe the patient's response.

Subjective methods

The physical signs of anesthetic depth depend largely on evaluation of muscular tone and reflex activity. In dogs and cats, these will vary from moment to moment, from individual to individual, and between anesthetic drugs. Since no one sign alone defines anesthetic depth, it is important to assess as many signs as possible and integrate the information they provide.

The following are key points for evaluation of the physical signs of anesthetic depth:

(1) Careful selection of administered doses of injectable and inhalant anesthetic drugs is mandatory, but in no way guarantees an appropriate depth of anesthesia will be achieved. Measurement of end-tidal inhalant anesthetic concentration (ET_{agent}) is a relatively new monitoring modality in veterinary clinical anesthesia that measures the amount of anesthetic in the patient. It is analogous to measuring plasma concentrations of injectable drugs but is clinically applicable as it provides continuous, real-time data to the anesthetist. While ET_{agent} is not a measure of anesthetic depth, it does provide more insight than vaporizer setting, which simply estimates the amount of drug delivered to the breathing circuit.

(2) Spontaneous movement is a reliable sign of a light level of anesthesia with most anesthetics, though there are several exceptions to this rule. Focal myoclonus (muscle twitching) has been associated with etomidate and propofol administration and should not be interpreted as a light level of anesthesia. Spontaneous muscular movement is common with opioid-based anesthetic protocols and should also not be interpreted to indicate a light level. Muscle hypertonus can be a feature of ketamine-based protocols and should not be interpreted as a light level of anesthesia.

(3) Reflex movement in response to surgical stimulation is a reliable sign of a light level of anesthesia. It does not, however, mean that an animal is experiencing pain from a noxious stimulus.

(4) An abrupt increase in heart rate (HR), arterial blood pressure (ABP), respiratory rate (RR), or tidal volume (TV), specifically in response to surgical stimulation, is generally considered to be a reliable sign of a light level of anesthesia. In general,

these physiological parameters tend to trend upward as an animal becomes more lightly anesthetized and downward with deeper anesthesia. These are not, however, reliable premonitory indicators of anesthetic depth. In some situations, physiological parameters may remain relatively stable until after an animal abruptly awakens or suffers cardiovascular collapse. There are also numerous confounding factors that will impact these parameters, in either direction, that have nothing to do with anesthetic depth. Inappropriate anesthetic depth is only one differential to consider when an animal exhibits increases or decreases in HR, ABP, RR, and/or TV.

(5) Mandibular muscle tone ("jaw tone") should be substantial, moderate, and none at light, medium, and deep levels of anesthesia, respectively. The definitions of substantial, moderate, and none are relative and will vary in dogs versus cats, and in small versus large breed dogs. Mandibular muscle tone is assessed by the resistance encountered when trying to open the mandible. In neonatal puppies and kittens, mandibular muscle tone is usually minimal and this parameter is less useful in these patients.

(6) A change to an abdominal (diaphragmatic) breathing pattern usually signals a deeper level of anesthesia. This will be accompanied by changes in physiological parameters including decreased RR and TV.

(7) The presence of a palpebral reflex is a reliable indicator of a light level of anesthesia in most patients. The absence of it suggests a medium or deep level. Some individuals, however, fail to exhibit a palpebral reflex even though their anesthesia level is light. With ketamine use, the palpebral reflex is always present so this parameter is not a reliable indicator of anesthetic level in this situation.

(8) The presence of a pupillary light reflex (pupillary constriction in response to a bright light directed onto the retina) and the presence of a dazzle reflex (a blink in response to a bright light) are reliable indicators of a light to light-medium level of anesthesia. The pupillary light reflex may be minimized or eliminated by administration of anticholinergics (atropine or glycopyrrolate) so this parameter is not a reliable indicator of anesthetic level in this situation.

(9) The eyeball position is central (and the pupil size is medium) when the animal's anesthesia level is light, is rotated ventromedially when the level is medium, and is central again (and the pupil is dilated) when the level is deep. The eyeball does not rotate when ketamine is used so this parameter is not a reliable indicator of anesthetic level in this situation. Nystagmus does not normally occur in anesthetized dogs and cats at any depth.

(10) The gag and swallow reflexes are reliable indicators of a light level of anesthesia in virtually all circumstances in anesthetized dogs and cats.

Objective methods

Neurophysiological monitoring as a tool to quantify anesthetic depth is not a new field of study. One type of neurophysiological monitoring, EEG analysis, involves interpretation of brain waves recorded from the scalp during anesthetic delivery, which exhibit characteristic changes during the transition from light to medium to deep levels of anesthesia. In some cases, the raw EEG is studied directly or alternatively, EEG derivatives such as frequency or power distribution, amplitude, or correlations between recorded signals are analyzed. Unfortunately, EEG signal and pattern analysis have proved to be complex and difficult to accomplish in real time, making this approach impractical in a clinical setting.

Another approach to neurophysiological monitoring involves evoked potential (EP) studies. Both auditory (brain stem recordings in response to an auditory stimulus) and somatosensory (brain stem and cortical recordings in response to electrical stimulation of a peripheral nerve) EPs show progressive changes with alterations in anesthetic depth. This approach suffers from many of the same disadvantages as analysis of spontaneous EEG potentials and is not useful as a real-time monitor of anesthetic depth clinically.

The Bispectral Index™ (BIS) Monitoring System (Covidien-Nellcor, Boulder, CO) was introduced in 1994 as a novel measure of the level of consciousness and is based on an algorithmic analysis of a patient's EEG during anesthesia. BIS is a statistically based, empirically derived parameter based on the weighted sum of selected EEG sub-parameters. It includes a time domain, a frequency domain, and other high-order spectral variables. Essentially, the BIS monitor takes a complex signal (the EEG), analyzes it, and processes the result into a single dimensionless number between 0 (equivalent to EEG silence) and 100 (equivalent to awake and alert). The proprietary calculation algorithm used was based on the evaluation of numerous EEG recordings taken from healthy human volunteers at specific clinically important end points and plasma anesthetic drug concentrations. While the calculation is extremely complex, the more recent availability of cost-effective, rapid, powerful computer processors has facilitated clinical introduction of this technology and others like it.

Clinically, the BIS monitor displays a value that changes, with a minimal lag time, along with changes in anesthetic depth. In general, BIS values above 90 are compatible with an awake and alert state, 80–90 with anxiolysis, 60–80 with hypnotic or moderate obtundation, below 60 with loss of recall, below 50 with unresponsiveness to verbal stimuli, below 20 with burst suppression, and 0 with cortical silence (isoelectric EEG). Not all anesthetics affect BIS in the same way. Propofol, midazolam, and thiopental strongly depress it, inhalational anesthetics have an intermediate effect, opioids have little effect, and nitrous oxide and ketamine tend to increase the BIS value. BIS does not monitor analgesia and may not predict reflex movement or hemodynamic activity in response to noxious stimulation. The recent introduction of other systems also based on calculated EEG indices, such as the Narcotrend™ Monitor (Arbeitsgruppe Informatik/ Biometrie der Anästhesie, Hannover, Germany) and the Cerebral State™ Monitor (danmeter, DK-5000 Odense C, Denmark), appear to perform similarly to the BIS monitor.

While the use of BIS and other similar monitors continues to increase in human operating rooms worldwide, it is important to note that they have not replaced physical evaluation of patients and it is not likely that they ever will. The benefits of quantitative monitoring of anesthetic depth include minimizing the risk of patient awareness, reduction of anesthetic drug dosages, and shortened recovery times. While these tools are currently being used by veterinary anesthesia specialists in academic and private practice settings, their potential place in general practice remains to be determined.

Physiological consequences of the anesthesia

Although the specific pharmacodynamic effects of the various anesthetic drugs vary, the mechanisms by which they contribute to morbidity and mortality are similar. Excessive bradycardia, dysrhythmias, myocardial depression, vasodilation, hypotension, hypoventilation, hypoxemia, and hypothermia are among the most common examples. Since all of these (except hypothermia) can be classified as derangements in cardiopulmonary function and all may negatively impact other organ systems, perianesthetic monitoring tends to prioritize cardiovascular and pulmonary stability.

These two systems function, in a very broad sense, to deliver oxygen (O_2) and remove carbon dioxide (CO_2) from tissues. Oxygen delivery (DO_2) involves the pulmonary system, which is responsible for loading arterial blood with O_2 (i.e., oxygenation), and the cardiovascular system, which pumps oxygenated blood to tissues (i.e., circulation). Carbon dioxide removal is also accomplished by the lungs through atmospheric gas exchange (i.e., ventilation). It is useful to consider this big picture when monitoring individual patient parameters and always strive to put a particular measurement or trend into context. Figure 6.1 is a simplified illustration of the key factors determining circulation and oxygenation, including their relationships to each other and to O_2 delivery. Figure 6.2 illustrates the key factors determining ventilation and how they relate to CO_2 removal.

Monitoring DO_2

DO_2 is the product of cardiac output (CO) and arterial oxygen content (CaO_2) as shown below. Reported DO_2 values are indexed to body surface area (i.e., milliliter of O_2 per minute per square meter) to facilitate comparisons as CO will vary depending on patient size. Estimates for normal dogs are approximately $800\,mL/min/m^2$ (or about 25–35 mL/min/kg).

$$DO_2 \text{ (mL } O_2/\text{min)} = CO \text{ (dL / min)} \times CaO_2 \text{ (mL } O_2/\text{dL)}$$

Note that CaO_2 represents the total amount of oxygen present in blood and is a function of arterial O_2 saturation (defined as the percent of O_2-bound hemoglobin binding sites to total hemoglobin binding sites; SaO_2), the concentration of hemoglobin and, to a minor extent, the amount of oxygen dissolved in blood (defined as the arterial partial pressure of oxygen; PaO_2). Normal CaO_2 values are approximately 20 mL of O_2 per deciliter of blood based on the following formula:

$$CaO_2 \text{ (mL } O_2/\text{dL)} = [SaO_2 \text{ (decimal)} \times Hb \text{ (g / dL)} \times 1.34 \text{ mL / } O_2/\text{g}]$$
$$+ [PaO_2 \text{ (mm Hg)} \times 0.003 \text{ mL } O_2/\text{dL / mm Hg}]$$

Based on these equations, a decrease in CaO_2 does not necessarily result in a decrease in DO_2 if CO is augmented. In human critical care, there has been a movement toward perioperative "targeted oxygen delivery" or "oxygen delivery optimization" in high-risk patients as a means of improving outcomes. Whether such strategies are actually effective

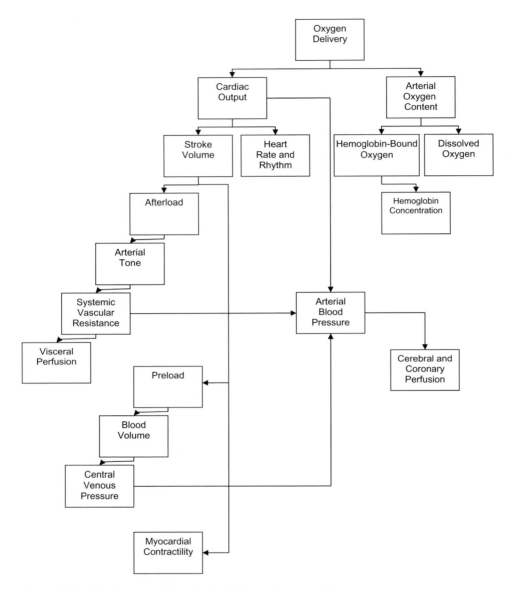

Figure 6.1. Key factors relating to circulation and oxygenation.

on a population basis remains controversial and further work is needed to determine the appropriate end points and timing of interventions. Because calculation of DO_2 requires measurement of CO, SaO_2, hemoglobin, and PaO_2, it is infrequently used during veterinary clinical anesthesia monitoring.

Oxygen consumption (VO_2) is the amount of oxygen consumed by tissues each minute and can be calculated by multiplying the difference between CaO_2 and mixed venous

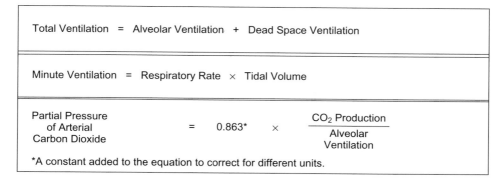

Figure 6.2. Key factors relating to ventilation.

oxygen content (CvO_2) by CO as shown below. Estimates of VO_2 in normal dogs are approximately 150 mL/min/m² (or about 4–10 mL/min/kg).

$$VO_2 \text{ (mL } O_2/\text{min)} = [CaO_2 - CvO_2 \text{ (mL } O_2/\text{dL)}] \times CO \text{ (dL/min)}$$

VO_2 is not normally limited by DO_2 as tissues can extract a greater proportion of oxygen from arterial blood (i.e., the $CaO_2 - CvO_2$ difference increases) in the face of lowered CO. As CO decreases to critically low values, however, VO_2 becomes DO_2 (or flow) dependent.

The oxygen extraction ratio (OER) is the proportion of O_2 consumed to O_2 delivered as shown below:

$$OER = \frac{VO_2}{DO_2} = \frac{[CaO_2 - CvO_2] \times CO}{CaO_2 \times CO}$$

Because CO appears in both the numerator and denominator and because hemoglobin is assumed to be the same in both arterial and venous blood, the above equation can be simplified to include only saturation instead of oxygen content. The simplified equation is shown below:

$$OER = \frac{SaO_2 - SvO_2}{SaO_2}$$

For optimal accuracy, this equation requires measurement of SaO_2 and SvO_2 using co-oximetry to analyze arterial and mixed venous blood samples drawn from the patient. While an estimate of SaO_2 is routinely calculated and reported by commercial blood gas analyzers using the measured parameters (pH, PO_2, and PCO_2), an arbitrary default hemoglobin concentration, and an algorithm based on the oxyhemoglobin dissociation curve, this method is less accurate than co-oximetry. Since SvO_2 values fall on the steep part of the dissociation curve, estimation of SvO_2 using the blood gas analyzer method is associated with an even greater margin or error. The fact that the oxyhemo-globin dissociation curve used by commercial blood gas analyzers is based on data from normal human adults introduces further potential error when extrapolating to dogs and cats.

The OER is a clinically useful method for assessing the adequacy of CO without actually measuring it (though it does require mixed venous sampling). Its primary utility is in critical care settings as opposed to clinical anesthesia monitoring. Under normal resting physiological conditions OER is approximately 0.25 and ratios >0.4 suggest serious impairment of CO.

Monitoring circulation, oxygenation, and ventilation

While measurement (or at least estimation) of DO_2 and OER may be indicated in critically ill veterinary patients requiring intensive care, they are not practical in the context of routine veterinary anesthesia monitoring. Consequently, measurement of other parameters is necessary to ensure and maintain cardiovascular and pulmonary stability. These parameters can be broadly classified into one of three categories: monitors of circulation, monitors of oxygenation, and monitors of ventilation. Regardless of the techniques used, patient monitoring must involve regular repeated assessments and documentation of trends in order to make appropriate interpretations and management decisions. Provision of a suitably trained individual dedicated to anesthetic monitoring and case management is recommended for all patients, wherever possible.

Monitoring circulation

Circulatory efficiency would ideally be monitored using CO as a global indicator of blood flow in combination with measurement of organ-specific blood flow to ensure adequate perfusion to individual tissue beds. Unfortunately, this is not currently feasible in a clinical setting. There are, however, numerous parameters, both subjective and objective, that when used collectively constitute a reasonable approximation of circulatory efficiency in most patients.

Subjective methods

The assessment of mucous membrane color and capillary refill time (CRT) provides subjective information about peripheral vascular tone and perfusion. Pale mucous membranes (in the absence of anemia) suggest vasoconstriction and impaired perfusion while dark pink or red mucous membranes suggest vasodilation and increased perfusion. Similarly, prolonged CRT suggests vasoconstriction and impaired perfusion while rapid CRT suggests vasodilation. While subjective and qualitative in nature, these assessments should be part of the preanesthetic patient evaluation and should be performed in all patients at regular intervals (usually every 5 minutes) during anesthesia and the immediate recovery period.

Palpation of a peripheral arterial pulse provides subjective, qualitative information about the pulse pressure. Pulse pressure or "strength" is a function of the difference between systolic (SAP) and diastolic arterial pressures (DAP). Animals with large gradients between their systolic and diastolic pressures will have large pulse pressures and their peripheral pulses will feel "strong." Patients with narrow gradients will have reduced pulse pressures and their peripheral pulses will feel "weak." Note that this does not guarantee that patients with a strong peripheral pulse have adequate mean arterial pressure and peripheral perfusion. Thus, pulse palpation is not a substitute for quantitative ABP measurement.

Palpation of peripheral pulses for the purpose of assessing pulse rate (PR) and rhythm is, however, a clinically valuable skill and should be performed at frequent regular intervals in anesthetized animals for this purpose. Common sites for peripheral pulse palpation include the dorsal pedal, digital, and lingual arteries. In anesthetized cats, appreciation of peripheral pulses at these sites may be challenging and requires practice.

Objective methods

There are a number of different parameters that can be used to monitor circulatory status objectively. Some provide continuous data while others are performed intermittently and most require some sort of specialized equipment.

HR or PR

HR is one of the principle determinants of CO and maintenance of HR within a range appropriate for the individual patient and clinical scenario is necessary to ensure adequate circulatory stability. Normal resting HR in conscious dogs will vary among breeds but usually ranges from 70 to 120 beats per minute. In conscious cats, a true resting HR may be difficult to obtain in many clinical settings, but a range of 120–180 beats per minute is reasonable. Both bradycardia and tachycardia can have significant detrimental effects on CO and should be prevented and/or treated when they occur. Maintenance of HR within a "normal" range, however, in no way guarantees an adequate CO and other monitors are required to provide a more complete picture of circulatory status.

There are numerous techniques available for measurement of HR or PR. Some require the anesthetist to interact directly with the patient while some employ automated monitoring devices. Some techniques facilitate intermittent evaluations only while others provide continuous visual data and/or auditory signals. Regardless of the technique chosen, HR or PR should be monitored at least every 5 minutes in all anesthetized patients.

Thoracic auscultation of the heartbeat using a stethoscope is performed as part of the routine preanesthetic patient evaluation and may be used to document HR during anesthesia as well. This technique is simple and involves direct interaction with the patient on an intermittent basis. It is often a challenge for the anesthetist to access the patient's thorax during various procedures, surgical and otherwise, so other alternatives must also be available.

Arterial pulse palpation is another technique that is useful in anesthetized patients. In dogs, common locations for pulse palpation include the femoral, dorsal pedal, digital, and lingual arteries. In cats, peripheral pulses are often more difficult to appreciate but can be located. As for auscultation, this technique involves direct patient interaction at frequent intervals and does not require any equipment. As there are a variety of arteries to choose from, at least one option is usually available in patients that are draped in for surgery. This technique is recommended for all anesthetized patients, even when other supplemental methods for HR assessment are used simultaneously.

The use of an esophageal stethoscope constitutes another low-cost method to evaluate HR. This technique involves esophageal placement of a probe that is attached to an earpiece and allows the anesthetist to appreciate heart sounds on an intermittent or semi-continuous basis. Alternatively, the probe may be attached to an electronic amplifier that projects a continuous audible signal. This method overcomes the inaccessibility issue for most patients and procedures and is recommended for routine use to supplement other automated monitoring techniques.

The Doppler system, though primarily utilized as a monitor of ABP, also provides an audible PR signal. This technique involves placement of a piezoelectric crystal over a peripheral artery (such as the palmar, dorsal pedal, or coccygeal) connected to an ultra-sonic Doppler flow detector, which translates and amplifies the sound of peripheral blood flow. If the Doppler system is also to be used for blood pressure measurement, an occlu-sive cuff and sphygmomanometer must also be applied (see below). The flow detector can be left on for continuous audio signaling or turned on and off for intermittent evalu-ations. PR is not digitally displayed so the anesthetist must count the rate based on the audible signal.

The electrocardiogram (ECG), though primarily utilized as a monitor of cardiac rhythm, also provides a continuous digital display of HR. Many ECG monitors can be programmed to emit an audible beep with each beat. The accuracy of the HR displayed by the ECG monitor depends on the unit itself and patient factors such as size, lead placement, and ECG waveform morphology. With low amplitude QRS complexes and/or high rates (both of which are often seen in cats), some monitors may count inaccurately low rates or may not display an HR at all. Similarly, with large T wave amplitudes rela-tive to the QRS complex, some monitors may double count and display an inaccurately high HR. Adjusting the settings on the ECG unit can often rectify these problems and produce a more reliable HR display. For these reasons; however, it is important to use supplemental techniques such as auscultation or pulse palpation to corroborate the HR displayed by an ECG unit.

The pulse oximeter, though primarily utilized as a monitor of oxygenation to measure percent hemoglobin saturation, also continuously displays a digital PR. Most pulse oximeters have an audible beep option corresponding to each detected pulse. The tongue is the most commonly used site for probe placement in anesthetized dogs and cats though other locations are possible. Some units also provide a plethysmographic waveform display, which, if consistently present, usually suggests that the displayed HR is reason-ably accurate. Despite this, the use of other supplemental techniques such as auscultation or pulse palpation is recommended to corroborate the displayed PR on a pulse oximeter. It is important to remember that pulse oximetry is designed to noninvasively monitor oxygenation and is not suitable for assessing circulatory adequacy (beyond simply docu-menting the presence of a pulse and counting the rate).

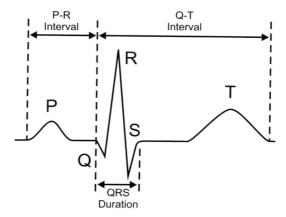

Figure 6.3. Components of the normal ECG waveform.

Cardiac rhythm

Abnormalities of cardiac rhythm have the potential to significantly impact stroke volume (SV) and CO and, therefore, DO_2. In some circumstances, documentation of a particular rhythm may signal an impending transition to a more serious, even life-threatening dysrhythmia. The challenge lies in not only recognizing that an abnormality is present but determining its potential significance. The only technique for quantitative evaluation of cardiac rhythm involves observation of cardiac electrical activity using the ECG. Figure 6.3 illustrates normal ECG waveform morphology. It is important to remember that cardiac electrical activity does not necessarily correlate with mechanical cardiac function. Documentation of normal cardiac rhythm in no way guarantees adequate CO and other methods of evaluating circulatory efficiency are required.

The most common approach to ECG monitoring in anesthetized dogs and cats involves placement of three surface electrodes, usually at the right forelimb (RA), left forelimb (LA), and left hind limb (LL) of the patient. This generates three bipolar limb leads for evaluation. Lead I is the voltage difference between the RA and LA electrodes, lead II the RA and LL electrodes, and lead III the LA and LL electrodes. Alternatively, a fourth electrode can also be placed on the right hind limb (RL) and this will generate three more leads referred to as augmented or unipolar limb leads (aVR, aVL, and aVF). Veterinary cardiologists may also place additional thoracic electrodes (rV2, V2, V4, and v10) to generate precordial leads that provide even more detailed diagnostic information regarding a particular dysrhythmia.

In most anesthetized patients, alligator clips with blunted teeth and relaxed spring mechanisms are used as electrodes. Alternatively, cutaneous adhesive pads may be placed after shaving an appropriate area of hair or by placing them on the foot pads. Depending on the procedure to be performed and patient positioning, electrode location may need to be adjusted. Application of conducting gel or 70% isopropyl alcohol where the electrodes contact the skin will improve signal transduction and may need to be repeated during long procedures.

Esophageal ECG electrodes are an alternative to standard surface electrodes in situations where skin placement may not be feasible (such as surgical procedures involving one or both proximal forelimbs) or where electrodes are likely to be disrupted during surgery. The electrode itself is placed in the esophagus and attached to a standard ECG cable.

With either surface or esophageal placement, the electrodes attach to a main cable that interfaces with a monitor. It may be a dedicated ECG monitor or, more likely, a multi-parameter patient monitor capable of evaluating other parameters such as ABP, pulse oximetry, capnometry, temperature, and so on. The monitor will display a real-time tracing of cardiac electrical activity and the operator can select which of the three (or more) leads is displayed. The most commonly used lead for rhythm analysis in an anesthesia setting is lead II, but any lead demonstrating distinct P waves, QRS complexes, and T waves may be utilized. The speed of the tracing can be adjusted by the operator and is usually set at 25 or 50 mm/s. Other parameters such as the size of the complexes displayed can also be controlled. Some monitors have the capability to print ECG tracings out on paper and many newer models can interface with other types of monitoring equipment and have advanced data storage capabilities.

Several small handheld ECG units are also available that are completely electrode and cable free (such as the Vet Biolog™ II, VetLogix, LLC, Plymouth, MN). These are particularly useful for routine preanesthetic screening, for rapid diagnosis in emergency situations, or for anesthetic monitoring in any situation where use of a standard ECG monitor with electrodes and cables is cumbersome and/or not feasible.

ABP

ABP refers to the force exerted by circulating blood against arterial walls and is measured in millimeters of mercury (mm Hg). During each cardiac cycle, ABP varies between a maximum (SAP) and a minimum (DAP). Mean arterial blood pressure (MAP) is the average pressure over the entire cardiac cycle and, at resting HRs, can be estimated from SAP and DAP values as follows:

$$MAP = DAP + 1/3(SAP - DAP)$$

At high HRs, MAP more closely approximates the arithmetic mean of SAP and DAP as the shape of the pulse pressure narrows. Reported normal values for SAP and DAP in dogs and cats vary from publication to publication but tend to be in the range of 120–140 and 60–80 mm Hg, respectively. Reported values for MAP in conscious dogs and cats are more consistent, usually in the range of 90–100 mm Hg. The MAP is physiologically the most important of the pressures as it is considered to be the driving pressure for organ perfusion. Inadequate MAP over a sustained period of time may result in end-organ ischemia and must be avoided. Hemodynamically, MAP is determined by three factors: CO, systemic vascular resistance (SVR), and central venous pressure (CVP) as illustrated in Figure 6.1 and shown below:

$$MAP = (CO \times SVR) + CVP$$

CO is a primary determinant of DO_2 while SVR is the resistance to blood flow within the systemic vasculature. It is primarily a function of vasomotor tone in small arterioles. CVP is the average pressure in the venous compartment and is a major determinant of right ventricular filling pressure and preload and therefore SV. Because CVP is usually at or near zero, the above relationship is often simplified as follows:

$$MAP = CO \times SVR$$

An appreciation of this relationship is crucial in understanding how ABP measurement fits into the larger circulatory picture. When monitoring ABP in anesthetized patients in the absence of CO data, as is usually the case, consideration must be given to the patient's vasomotor status. Inadequate MAP is referred to as hypotension and may be the result of inadequate HR or SV causing reduced CO, vasodilation, or a combination of both. High MAP is referred to as hypertension and may be the result of increased blood volume and CO according to the Frank–Starling relationship, or vasoconstriction. It is important to recognize that observation of a normal MAP does not imply that CO is adequate. Based on the above relationship, a patient may have very poor CO, but be normotensive if concurrently vasoconstricted. Thus, the clinician must make a judgment regarding the patient's myocardial function and vasomotor status in order to fully interpret the significance of a particular ABP measurement.

Clinical measurement of ABP may involve noninvasive approaches such as the oscillometric or Doppler techniques, or the invasive technique involving placement of an arterial catheter. All noninvasive techniques provide estimates of ABP and may not be absolutely accurate in all situations. In most cases, however, noninvasive methods effectively reflect trends in ABP and are recommended for routine use during anesthetic monitoring in all dogs and cats. Invasive ABP measurement is the most accurate approach but is not without limitations or complications. Each of these options is discussed below.

The oscillometric method for ABP determination is an automated, noninvasive (indirect) system that involves placement of a pneumatic occlusion cuff around a peripheral limb or the base of the tail. The cuff is automatically inflated to a suprasystolic pressure and then air is gradually released until characteristic arterial oscillations are detected by an electronic sensor. The computer interprets these oscillations and displays measured values for SAP, MAP, and DAP. Oscillometric monitors also display a PR as well. They can be programmed to automatically cycle at regular intervals, which is convenient when monitoring anesthetized patients. The width of the occlusion cuff is critical for accurate measurements and should be approximately 40% the circumference of the extremity around which it is placed. Cuffs that are too small will overestimate ABP while cuffs that are too large will underestimate it.

Traditionally, oscillometric ABP monitors available to veterinarians were designed for use in adult human patients, and the algorithms where not always able to detect oscillations in the arteries of very small canine and feline patients. In addition, the HR range was not appropriate for many small veterinary patients. Consequently, many such monitors were inaccurate or simply not able to provide measurements in small patients. As ABP monitoring has become increasingly common in veterinary medicine, a number of veterinary-specific oscillometric monitors have been marketed (such as the Cardell®

[MidmarkAnimal Health, Versailles, OH], PetMAP™ [Ramsey Medical, Inc. Tampa, FL], and BP-AccuGard™ [Vmed Technology, Mill Creek, WA] monitors). These monitors appear to function more reliably in a wider range of veterinary patients, though inaccuracy at extremes of ABP remains an issue. Oscillometric ABP monitors are available as stand-alone units or, as veterinary anesthetic monitoring becomes increasingly sophisticated, as part of multiparameter units that also have ECG, pulse oximetry, capnography, and temperature capabilities.

The Doppler system for ABP measurement is a noninvasive (indirect) system that involves placement of a piezoelectric crystal over a peripheral artery such as the digital, dorsal pedal, or coccygeal. Blood flow to and from the crystal reflects sound waves causing a change in frequency that is detected, translated, and amplified to a speaker. In order to use the Doppler system to determine ABP, an appropriately sized occlusive cuff (40% the circumference of the extremity) is then placed proximal to the probe location and connected to a sphygmomanometer. The cuff is inflated until the audible blood flow signal is lost and then incrementally deflated until the return of flow is recognized. The pressure displayed on the sphygmomanometer at the point when this occurs corresponds to the SAP.

Doppler systems (such as the Parks Medical Model 811 [Parks Medical Electronics, Las Vegas, NV] and VMed *Vet*-Dop™ [Vmed Technology] monitors) are not automated, so manual SAP determination by the anesthetist is required at intervals. It is not possible to determine MAP or DAP values with this system and its accuracy for determination of SAP is influenced by a number of factors. In anesthetized small patients (cats and small dogs), Doppler pressure readings tend to underestimate SAP. Some studies involving cats have suggested that SAP values are undervalued by approximately 15 mm Hg and that the Doppler measurement may actually be a more accurate reflection of MAP in these patients. Consequently, like any noninvasive ABP monitor, the Doppler system is best used as an indicator of trends when used for anesthetic monitoring.

Invasive or direct ABP measurement provides an accurate, quantitative, continuous assessment of SAP, MAP, and DAP, and also provides a graphical representation of the arterial pulse waveform as illustrated in Figure 6.4. This technique requires placement of an arterial catheter, usually in a peripheral artery such as the dorsal pedal, carpal or coccygeal, and thus is more technically challenging than noninvasive approaches. The catheter is then connected to saline-filled, semirigid arterial pressure tubing, which is in turn connected to an electronic resistance-type pressure transducer. The transducer should be placed at the level of the patient's right atrium to obtain accurate ABP measurements. Modern monitors typically have an offset pressure that allows the transducer to be moved to any convenient level and the monitor can compensate for any vertical difference between transducer and patient. The transducer connects to a cable that interfaces with a multiparameter patient monitor that displays the arterial pressure waveform in real time along with digital values for SAP, MAP, DAP, and PR. Recently, a number of veterinary-specific multiparameter patient monitors have been marketed with direct pressure capabilities.

While direct ABP measurement is considered the gold standard, it is not without potential sources for error and complications. The waveform can become dampened if

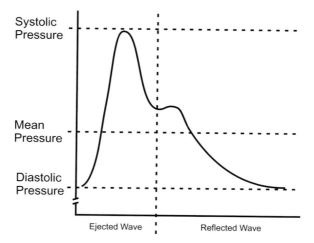

Figure 6.4. Components of the normal arterial pressure waveform.

the catheter tip is up against the arterial wall, if a clot forms at the catheter tip, if air bubbles are present within the catheter or tubing, or if the catheter or tubing becomes kinked. This will result in a flattened arterial waveform, lowered reported values for SAP, and higher reported values for DAP. The use of compliant tubing instead of semirigid arterial monitoring tubing will also negatively impact the fidelity of the system. Also, because this technique requires arterial catheterization, potential complications such as hematoma formation, infection, thrombosis, or necrosis of tissues distal to the catheter site are possible (though not common). Heparinization of the line to maintain its patency is required in most situations and this may be a concern in very small patients. Direct ABP measurement is also associated with an increased cost compared to noninvasive methods as it requires a number of consumable products (catheter, tubing, and transducer) in addition to the upfront cost associated with purchase of the monitor. In patients with preexisting or potential circulatory instability, however, this method is superior for monitoring during anesthesia and in critical care settings.

CVP

CVP is an estimate of mean right atrial pressure and reflects the balance between CO and venous return. Primary factors influencing CVP include blood volume, venous tone, cardiac contractility, HR, changes in intrathoracic or intrapericardial pressures, and body position. In dogs and cats, normal CVP ranges from 0 to 10 cm H_2O. Decreases in CVP generally indicate absolute or relative hypovolemia, while increases indicate hypervolemia or myocardial depression and/or heart failure.

CVP measurement requires placement of a catheter into the jugular vein extending to the level of the thoracic vena cava or, preferably, the right atrium. In cats, caudal vena cava pressures are a reasonable surrogate for CVP when a jugular catheter cannot be placed. The catheter is flushed with saline and connected to a commercially available manometer using saline-filled tubing attached to a three-way stopcock. A saline-filled fluid administration line is connected to the stopcock port immediately across from the catheter, and the manometer is attached to the remaining port. With the stopcock closed to the patient the graduated cylinder is filled with saline solution. To obtain an accurate measurement the three-way stopcock is positioned just below the base of the heart. In laterally recumbent animals this corresponds to the sternum, and in dorsally recumbent animals to the point of the shoulder. The stopcock is then closed to the fluid administration set and the resulting CVP measurement is read off of the gradations on the manometer in $cm\,H_2O$.

Alternatively, the catheter can be connected to a pressure transducer and interfaced with a multiparameter patient monitor similar to direct ABP measurement. Values for CVP and the characteristic CVP waveform will be digitally displayed. If using a standard pressure channel, most monitors will report CVP in millimeters of mercury, which must be converted to centimeters of water for interpretation ($1\,mm\,Hg = 1.36\,cm\,H_2O$). While CVP measurement is not indicated for routine anesthetic monitoring in healthy dogs and cats it does provide useful information in patients requiring aggressive volume resuscitation, especially in the face of concurrent myocardial dysfunction.

Cardiac output

CO is a principle determinant of DO_2 and an important indicator of global circulatory adequacy. Unfortunately, truly definitive conclusions about CO cannot be made on the basis of ABP and/or CVP measurements. Because CO is a flow parameter as opposed to a pressure parameter it is logistically more challenging to measure and, traditionally, has required invasive techniques such as cardiac catheterization. Consequently, normal values for CO in conscious dogs and cats based on large numbers of animals and indexed to body surface area are not well established but are probably in the range of $4.0\,L/min/m^2$ (or approximately 140–160 mL/min/kg).

Though measurement of CO has been impractical in most clinical veterinary settings, including anesthetic monitoring, this may change in the future. As the biomedical industry strives to find new noninvasive or minimally invasive methods of CO measurement for use in humans, veterinary patients may indirectly benefit. Note that the following discussion covers a few selected techniques only and is in no way meant to be an exhaustive review on the subject of CO measurement.

The traditional approach to clinical CO measurement is called the thermodilution technique. It is considered invasive as it involves placement of a balloon-tipped pulmonary arterial (Swan–Ganz) catheter. A small, known volume of fluid at a known temperature is injected into the catheter's proximal pulmonary arterial port and the blood temperature is subsequently measured at a thermistor located a known distance away along the catheter. A computer generates and interprets a temperature-time (thermodilution) curve and calculates CO as being inversely proportional to the area under this curve. Use of this method in human patients is in decline as more user-friendly, less invasive options with fewer potential complications are developed.

A newer system, also based on indicator dilution, avoids the need for cardiac catheterization. It requires peripheral venous and arterial catheterization only and incorporates the lithium dilution technique (LiDCO™, LidCO Ltd., Sawston, Cambridge UK). A small dose of lithium chloride is injected into the venous line and the resulting arterial lithium concentration-time curve is recorded by withdrawing blood past a lithium sensor attached to the arterial line. The computer than calculates and reports a value for CO.

A more recent technology has combined the LiDCO system with a variation on pulse contour analysis. Traditional pulse contour analysis systems attempted to measure SV on a beat-to-beat basis by analyzing the arterial pulse pressure waveform. There were a number of drawbacks associated with this approach but a new system, called arterial pulse power analysis (PulseCO™, LidCO Ltd.), uses an algorithm that overcomes many of these obstacles. The combination of these two technologies (LiDCO and PulseCO) into the LiDCOplus Hemodynamic Monitor (LidCO Ltd.) provides real-time, continuous assessment of CO for use in patients and requires peripheral venous and arterial access only.

An alternative technique is based on the Fick principle using partial rebreathing of CO_2. This monitor (NICO®, Philips Respironics, Murrysville, PA) estimates CO based on changes in end-tidal CO_2 ($ETCO_2$) concentration caused by brief intermittent periods of rebreathing through a specific disposable loop. The monitor consists of a carbon dioxide sensor (infrared light absorption), an airflow sensor (differential pressure pneumotachometer), and a pulse oximeter. The partial rebreathing reduces CO_2 elimination and increases $ETCO_2$. Patients must be mechanically ventilated and arterial blood sampling is required so that arterial oxygen tension (PaO_2) can be entered into the monitor for shunt estimation, which may otherwise skew CO results.

Transesophageal echocardiography (TEE) uses Doppler ultrasonography to measure blood velocity in the descending aorta using a transducer located at the tip of a flexible esophageal probe. The resultant velocity-time integral is multiplied by the measured aortic cross-sectional area to get blood flow, which is then multiplied by HR. Estimation of CO by this method assumes a fixed ratio of blood flow between the descending aorta and the left ventricular outflow tract since only descending aortic flow is actually measured. This technique requires training in obtaining appropriate echocardiographic images and making accurate aortic measurements.

More recently, a completely noninvasive continuous-wave Doppler ultrasound technology specifically designed to assess CO has been introduced (USCOM, USCOM Pty Ltd, Coffs Harbour, NSW, Australia). The USCOM monitor transcutaneously measures the Doppler flow profile velocity time integral but uses anthropometry to calculate aortic and pulmonary valve diameters so both right- and left-sided flows can be measured. This technique is technically simple to perform and does not require advanced training in ultrasonography. While it is unlikely that the anthropometric scaling used by the USCOM for human patients will translate well across all breeds of canine patients, which vary widely in stature, it is likely that some form of noninvasive CO assessment will be possible in veterinary medicine in the near future.

Monitoring oxygenation

Oxygenating efficiency would ideally be monitored by measurement of total CaO_2 as it incorporates the fraction of oxygen bound to hemoglobin as well as the fraction dissolved

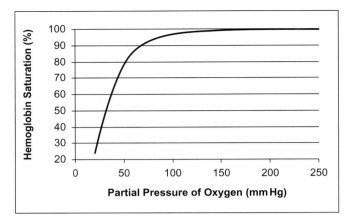

Figure 6.5.   Canine oxyhemoglobin dissociation curve under normal conditions (P_{50} approximately 28–30 mm Hg).

in plasma. Though the key contributors to CaO_2 (i.e., SaO_2, [Hb], and PaO_2) can be accurately measured, practically, it is not always necessary to evaluate all of them in the context of anesthetic monitoring. Because PaO_2 and SaO_2 are related to each other according to the oxyhemoglobin dissociation curve, measurement or estimation of one parameter offers insight into the other. Note that the position of the dissociation curve is, however, affected by a number of other factors. Increases in hydrogen ion concentration (i.e., decreased pH), pCO2, temperature, and 2,3-diphosphosglycerate (2,3-DPG) levels all shift the curve to the right. Figure 6.5 illustrates the canine oxyhemoglobin dissociation curve under normal conditions (i.e., with a P_{50} value of approximately 28–30 mm Hg). The feline curve under normal conditions appears similar but has a P_{50} value of approximately 32–37 mm Hg and thus is shifted rightward compared to dogs and humans.

Terminology describing inadequate oxygenation can be confusing. Hypoxemia is usually defined specifically as decreased PaO_2 which is invariability associated with decreased SaO_2. Note that this definition excludes a decrease in CaO_2 caused by anemia because PaO_2 is not decreased by anemia per se. The term hypoxia is more general, and refers to decreased oxygen availability and, as such, includes anemia as a potential cause.

In the context of clinical anesthesia monitoring, both subjective and objective assessments of oxygenating efficiency are recommended. The [Hb] (or some related surrogate measure such as packed cell volume or hematocrit) should be measured as part of the routine preanesthetic patient evaluation. From there, the decision to measure PaO_2 or SaO_2 directly, or to use a noninvasive estimate of oxygenation, depends on a number of factors that will be discussed in more detail below.

Subjective methods

Assessment of mucous membrane color is a simple, qualitative technique for evaluating oxygenation. Pink mucous membranes suggest adequate SaO_2. Cyanosis refers to the bluish discoloration caused by the presence of deoxygenated hemoglobin and is most frequently the result of hypoxemia. Note that because an absolute amount of deoxygenated hemoglobin (usually cited as 5 g/dL) is required for the patient to exhibit cyanosis, anemic patients can have profound hypoxemia but may not appear cyanotic. In general, the ability to detect cyanosis varies with the ambient light conditions and among observers and it is considered a very late, potentially life-threatening sign of oxygenating and/ or circulatory insufficiency. Consequently, mucous membrane color should only be used in combination with other more objective measures of oxygenation for anesthetic monitoring.

Objective methods

As mentioned above, objective measurement of oxygenating efficiency during anesthesia usually involves direct measurement of PaO_2 or SaO_2 or indirect estimation of the latter. Measurement of RR at regular 5-minute intervals is mandatory in all anesthetized patients and is discussed further under the section on monitoring ventilation. While bradypnea or apnea can lead to hypoxemia (depending on the inspired concentration of oxygen), it is also important to remember that a normal RR in no way guarantees adequate oxygenation.

Oxygen dissolved in arterial blood

At any given time, the PaO_2 constitutes only 1–2% of total CaO_2 (refer to the equation for calculating CaO_2 provided in the section on monitoring DO_2). However, because of its well-defined relationship to SaO_2, and the fact that it is easily and accurately measured using arterial blood gas analysis, PaO_2 is the most frequently cited parameter for evaluation of oxygenation. In order to interpret the significance of a particular PaO_2, value a number of factors must be considered concurrently.

First, the inspired concentration of oxygen (FiO_2) will affect PaO_2. Patients breathing enriched oxygen mixtures (as is the case for all patients that are intubated and anesthetized with an inhalant anesthetic using an anesthetic machine and breathing system) should be expected to have higher PaO_2 values than patients breathing room air (which is 21% oxygen). Second, the atmospheric pressure (P_{atmos}) also has an impact. Patients at sea level (760 mm Hg) are expected to have higher PaO_2 values than patients at altitude. Finally, the efficiency of ventilation also plays a role. Patients that are hypoventilating will have higher $PaCO_2$ values and consequently lower PaO_2 values compared with patients that are ventilating normally or hyperventilating. The impact of these factors on the partial pressure of alveolar oxygen (PAO_2), and consequently on PaO_2, is illustrated by the alveolar gas equation:

$$PAO_2 = FiO_2 \ (P_{atmos} - P_{H2O}) - PaCO_2/R$$

Note that P_{H2O} refers to the partial pressure of water, which is approximately 47 mm Hg at 37°C, and R refers to the respiratory quotient, which is assumed to be 0.8–0.9. This equation essentially determines the benchmark against which a particular PaO_2 value is compared depending on FiO_2, P_{atmos}, and $PaCO_2$.

Under normal circumstances, calculated values for PAO_2 are approximately 90–110 mm Hg. Normal measured PaO_2 values for patients under similar circumstances are approximately 80–100 mm Hg. The alveolar–arterial PO_2 gradient (A-a gradient) is defined as the difference between PAO_2 and PaO_2 and is a useful index of oxygenating efficiency. For patients breathing room air (i.e., $FiO_2 = 0.21$), the A-a gradient should be less than 10 mm Hg.

The situation is somewhat different when patients are inspiring enriched oxygen mixtures. In this situation PAO_2 will exceed 600 mm Hg so the expected PaO_2 will also be much higher and the criteria for evaluating the A-a gradient will differ. When FiO_2 approaches 1.0, the A-a gradient is considered to be normal if it is less than 100 mm Hg.

In clinical anesthesia monitoring, it may not be necessary to actually go through the calculations for the alveolar gas equation and the A-a gradient when assessing a given PaO_2 value. However, the clinician must always take into account the FiO_2 when interpreting PaO_2 values. It is impossible to make an accurate assessment of oxygenation based on PaO_2 if FiO_2 is not known.

Measurement of PaO_2 is considered a minimally invasive technique because it requires arterial sampling. Arteries commonly sampled in dogs and cats include the femoral and dorsal pedal. Samples should be collected into a heparinized syringe, sealed, and analyzed immediately using a blood gas machine. Blood gas analysis capabilities are becoming increasingly common in clinical veterinary practice and a number of portable, patient-side monitors are available. Such units use single-use cartridges that measure pH, PO_2, and PCO_2, as well as various other calculated parameters.

Though assessment of PaO_2 provides accurate quantitative information, the need for repeated arterial sampling and the associated cost make it impractical for routine anesthetic monitoring in healthy dogs and cats. In patients with preexisting pulmonary disease or injury or in any patient where impaired oxygenation is suspected, however, PaO_2 measurement is recommended.

Oxygen bound to hemoglobin

At any given time, the amount of oxygen bound to hemoglobin constitutes 98–99% of total CaO_2 (refer to the equation for calculating CaO_2 provided in the section on monitoring DO_2). This fraction is a function of the SaO_2 and the [Hb].

Hemoglobin measurement (or packed cell volume or hematocrit) is a required component of the preanesthetic patient evaluation in all patients to rule out anemia. Anemia can have a profound detrimental effect on CaO_2 and DO_2 in the absence of abnormalities in PaO_2 or SaO_2. This effect is illustrated in Table 6.1. Providing supplemental oxygen to increase PaO_2 as a strategy to improve CaO_2 in an anemic patient will be ineffective and efforts should focus on increasing [Hb] and oxygen-carrying capacity instead. In patients experiencing perioperative blood loss, serial evaluations of [Hb] or packed cell volume are indicated to track hemorrhage and the response to therapeutic interventions.

The SaO_2, like the PaO_2, is another way to look at the efficiency of oxygenation. In dogs, normal PaO_2 values of 80–100 mm Hg are associated with SaO_2 values of

Table 6.1. Impact of anemia of arterial oxygen content

PaO$_2$ (mm Hg)	SaO$_2$ (mm Hg)	[Hb] (g/dL)	CaO$_2$ (mL of O$_2$/dL)
100	98	15	20
100	98	12	16.1
100	98	10	13.4
100	98	8	10.8
100	98	6	8.1
100	98	4	5.6

approximately 95–98%. Unlike PaO$_2$, which changes dramatically, increasing FiO$_2$ has minimal impact on SaO$_2$ because the oxyhemoglobin dissociation curve has already flattened out at this point (see Figure 6.5). Assuming normal oxygenation, increasing FiO$_2$ from 0.21 to 1.0 causes PaO$_2$ to change from 100 mm Hg to >500 mm Hg, while SaO$_2$ changes from 97% to 99.9% only. Consequently, SaO$_2$ is a less discriminating index of oxygenation compared to PaO$_2$ in patients inspiring enriched oxygen mixtures.

The most accurate method for measurement of SaO$_2$ involves analysis of an arterial blood sample to directly quantify the concentrations of each hemoglobin species using co-oximetry. This parameter is sometimes referred to as fractional hemoglobin saturation. Alternatively, an estimate of functional SaO$_2$ is provided by most blood gas analyzers using measurements of pH, PaO$_2$, and PaCO$_2$ and an algorithm based on the human oxyhemoglobin dissociation curve. This calculated estimate is sometimes notated as ScO$_2$ to differentiate it from the fractional SaO$_2$. Because SaO$_2$ measurement requires arterial blood sampling and access to a co-oximeter, it is not used routinely for assessment of oxygenation in healthy anesthetized dogs and cats. The recent availability of portable, whole blood co-oximeters that require very small volumes of blood, however, has meant that this technology is being used increasingly in critically ill animals to more thoroughly evaluate oxygenation.

Pulse oximetry is an alternative approach to monitoring oxygenation that is completely noninvasive and offers a continuous, real-time estimation of SaO$_2$. A spectrophotoelectric device is applied directly to nonhaired skin over a peripheral arterial vascular bed (such as the tongue, esophagus, rectum, vulva, pinna, or digit). The light source emits both red and infrared wavelengths that pass through the tissue bed. Because oxygenated hemoglobin absorbs more light in the infrared band while deoxygenated hemoglobin absorbs more light in the red band, the two species can be differentiated. The monitor also separates the pulsatile components of each signal and uses the constant (nonpulsatile) components to normalize them. This ensures that only arterial hemoglobin is evaluated. The ratio between these two normalized signals is computed and an empirical algorithm is used to estimate SaO$_2$. Pulse oximetry-derived estimates of SaO$_2$ are notated as SpO$_2$ to differentiate them from saturations measured using co-oximetry. SpO$_2$ values consistent with normal oxygenation are the same as values for SaO$_2$ and range from 95% to 98% for animals inspiring room air.

It should be noted that because pulse oximetry estimates the ratio of oxyhemoglobin to the sum of functional hemoglobin, SpO$_2$ is sometimes referred to as functional hemoglobin saturation. This is in contrast to SaO_2, as measured by co-oximetry, which reports the ratio of oxyhemoglobin to the sum of all hemoglobin species present (including carboxyhemoglobin and methemoglobin), and is thus referred to as fractional hemoglobin saturation. In patients without dsyhemoglobinemias, the difference between functional and fractional hemoglobin saturations should be very small, but in patients with carboxy- or methemoglobinemia, SpO_2 readings will be inaccurate.

Any factor that decreases the strength of the pulsatile signal (such as hypotension, hypothermia, and altered SVR) may limit the ability of the monitor to estimate SpO_2. As mentioned previously, a normal SpO_2 value in an anemic patient does not guarantee adequate oxygenation as [Hb] has a major impact on CaO_2. Other limitations include motion artifact in conscious patients and signal loss after the probe is left in place for extended periods, leading to erroneously low readings. The latter can usually be rectified by moving the probe to an adjacent location.

Pulse oximeters are among the most commonly used anesthetic monitors in veterinary medicine. They are technically easy to operate and, in addition to continuous display of SpO_2, also measure PR. Pulse oximeters are available as small portable stand-alone units or, alternatively, are commonly incorporated into larger multiparameter patient monitors. While most units are accurate for their intended purpose, it is important to remember that the pulse oximeter does not assess circulatory adequacy and other monitoring modalities are required for this purpose (see the section on monitoring circulation). Though the use of pulse oximetry is strongly advocated for all anesthetized canine and feline patients, it should be considered mandatory for patients inspiring room air as these animals are at the greatest risk of desaturation. In this situation, early recognition of hypoxemia and institution of supportive interventions may be life saving.

Monitoring ventilation

Total ventilation (V_T) refers to the volume of gas flowing in and out of the lungs, which is related to CO_2 removal. Not all of this gas, however, actually participates in gas exchange so ventilation can be further broken down into alveolar ventilation (V_A; the portion participating in gas exchange and sometimes referred to as effective ventilation) and dead space ventilation (V_D; the portion not participating in gas exchange and sometimes referred to as wasted ventilation). Dead space ventilation includes the relatively constant volume of gas normally present in the upper conducting airways (i.e., anatomic dead space), and the more variable volume in alveoli, which are ventilated but not receiving pulmonary blood flow (i.e., alveolar dead space). In addition to this physiological dead space, airway instrumentation related to anesthesia can also contribute to wasted ventilation and this is referred to as equipment dead space.

Minute ventilation (MV) refers to the total volume of gas flowing in and out of the lungs in 1 minute including dead space. Normal values for MV in conscious dogs and cats are approximately 200 mL/kg/min. The two principle determinants of MV are RR and TV.

The effectiveness of ventilation is ultimately defined in terms of CO_2 removal by the lungs. The $PaCO_2$ has two principle determinants: CO_2 production and V_A. Because CO_2

production remains relatively stable in most clinical situations, $PaCO_2$ will vary inversely with changes in V_A. Thus, $PaCO_2$ can be considered the net result of the process of ventilation. Please refer to Figure 6.2 for a summary of important factors as they relate to ventilation.

While the consequences of inadequate ventilation (i.e., hypoventilation) to patient homeostasis may not be as obvious as those associated with impaired circulation or oxygenation, they can be just as significant. Hypercapnia induces acid–base derangements (i.e., respiratory acidosis), activation of the sympathetic nervous system, and cerebral vasodilation resulting in increased cerebral blood flow. Importantly, in patients inspiring room air (i.e., $FiO_2 = 0.21$), hypoventilation can also cause desaturation and hypoxemia. For this reason, pulse oximetry may be considered an indirect monitor of ventilation in that a normal SpO_2 value, in a patient breathing room air only, suggests that ventilation is reasonably normal. In patients inspiring greater than 30% oxygen (i.e., $FiO_2 > 0.3$), however, hypoventilation does not result in hypoxemia as illustrated by the alveolar gas equation.

Approaches to evaluation of ventilatory efficiency in anesthetized dogs and cats should include both subjective and objective assessments.

Subjective methods

Qualitative assessment of TV by observing thoracic wall movements or excursions of the breathing bag is routinely performed in anesthetized dogs and cats at frequent, regular intervals. In addition, the breathing pattern should also be evaluated. In conscious patients with restrictive types of lung disease (such as pulmonary edema, interstitial pneumonia, or pleural effusion), a rapid shallow breathing pattern is often observed. Conversely, in patients with airway obstruction (such as laryngeal paralysis or bronchoconstriction), a slow deep pattern of breathing may be seen. Note that anesthesia will usually depress ventilation and these patterns may be less distinct, especially at deeper levels of anesthesia. Because of the subjective nature of these methods and their lack of sensitivity, other objective methods of ventilation are required.

Objective methods

Objective methods for ventilatory monitoring may evaluate the components of MV (RR and TV) to infer conclusions regarding $PaCO_2$, or may directly measure or estimate $PaCO_2$ itself.

Respiratory rate

RR is a primary determinant of MV and therefore will impact $PaCO_2$. Normal RR values in conscious dogs and cats are approximately 10–20 and 20–30 breaths per minute, respectively. While extremes of RR (bradypnea or tachypnea) may precipitate decreases in MV and V_A, leading to hypercapnea, maintenance of RR within a so-called normal range in no way guarantees adequate ventilatory function. Evaluation of both RR and TV (see below) is necessary to estimate MV and make reasonable inferences regarding ventilation.

There are several techniques available for measurement of RR. Some require simple observation of the patient or breathing system while others employ automated monitoring devices. Regardless of the technique chosen, RR should be monitored at least every 5 minutes in all anesthetized patients.

The easiest way to assess RR is to observe thoracic wall excursions and/or breathing bag movements. Alternatively, auscultation of breath sounds using a standard or esophageal stethoscope can be performed.

Continuous assessment of RR is also possible using a respiratory monitoring device. This involves placement of a sensor between the endotracheal tube adaptor and the breathing system to detect changes in airway temperature or gas flow. Units digitally display RR on a continuous basis and can be programmed to emit an audible beep with each breath. Most monitors also have alarms that can be set to alert the anesthetist if RR decreases below a preset point.

Tidal volume

TV can be quantitatively assessed using a device known as a ventilometer (also variably known as respirometers or spirometers). By evaluating both TV and RR, MV can be determined and ventilatory efficiency can be estimated. In normal conscious dogs and cats, values for TV are approximately 15–20 and 10–15 mL/kg, respectively. Ventilometers can be very simplistic mechanical devices (such as the Wright's Respirometer) or computer-driven monitors where flow is converted into an electronic signal that is processed and digitally displayed.

In the case of the Wright's Respirometer, the device is inserted into the breathing system on the expiratory side where it attaches to the anesthetic machine. TV is read off a gauge and RR must be counted manually. More sophisticated ventilometers are available as components of multiparameter patient monitors. These units utilize side-stream spirometry to continuously measure pulmonary pressures, volumes, flows, compliance, and resistance. While advanced ventilometry is not indicated for routine anesthetic monitoring in healthy dogs and cats, it may provide useful insight into lung mechanics in patients with particular pulmonary abnormalities.

Arterial partial pressure of CO_2

Ultimately, it is the $PaCO_2$ that represents the net result of effective ventilation (i.e., V_A) so measurement of $PaCO_2$ directly provides the most accurate assessment of this process. According to the relationship illustrated in Figure 6.2, elevations in $PaCO_2$ imply hypoventilation while decreases in $PaCO_2$ imply hyperventilation. Compared to humans, normal ranges for $PaCO_2$ are marginally lower in dogs and significantly lower in cats (32–42 and 26–36 mm Hg, respectively).

Like PaO_2, measurement of $PaCO_2$ is considered minimally invasive as it involves arterial sampling from arteries such as the femoral or dorsal pedal. Samples should be collected into a heparinized syringe, sealed, and analyzed immediately using a blood gas machine. Blood gas analysis capabilities are becoming increasingly common in clinical veterinary practice, and a number of portable, patient-side monitors are available (such

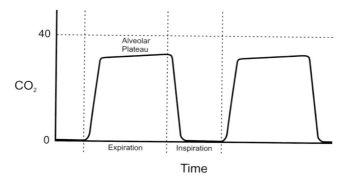

Figure 6.6.   Components of the normal capnograph waveform.

as IRMA TruPoint and i-Stat). Such units use single-use cartridges that measure pH, PO_2 and PCO_2 as well as various other calculated parameters.

While measurement of $PaCO_2$ provides accurate quantitative information, the need for repeated arterial sampling and the associated cost make it impractical for routine anesthetic monitoring in healthy dogs and cats. In patients where accurate determination of ventilatory status is critical and/or where other less invasive monitors such as end-tidal CO_2 (see below) are likely to be inaccurate, measurement of $PaCO_2$ is indicated.

End-tidal CO₂

Because diffusion of CO_2 in the lung is highly efficient, the $PaCO_2$ and the alveolar partial pressure of CO_2 (P_ACO_2) will be essentially equal. Furthermore, the partial pressure of CO_2 in the upper airway at the end of expiration closely approximates the $PACO_2$ and is called the end-tidal CO_2 tension ($ETCO_2$). Therefore, $ETCO_2$ constitutes a reasonable surrogate for $PaCO_2$ and can be measured continuously and noninvasively (though it does require endotracheal intubation in dogs and cats).

Capnometery refers to the measurement and numerical display of CO_2 concentrations during the respiratory cycle, and a capnometer is the device that performs the measurement and displays CO_2 readings. Capnography is the graphical record of CO_2 concentration on a screen or paper, and a capnograph is the device that generates the actual waveform. Please refer to Figure 6.6 for a schematic representation of a normal capnograph. Most monitoring devices specifically report the value for $ETCO_2$ (i.e., the concentration at the end of the expiratory plateau) and express it as a partial pressure (i.e., mm Hg). Contemporary units typically provide both capnometry and capnography capabilities.

Capnometers utilize infrared technology to measure $ETCO_2$ concentrations. Diverting or side-stream capnometers require a sampling line attached to an adaptor that fits onto the patient end of the endotracheal tube. Gas is continuously sampled and transferred to the monitor for analysis and display. Alternatively, nondiverting or mainstream capnometers use a small analyzer that similarly attaches to the end of the endotracheal tube but analyzes the gas locally and then transmits the information back to the monitor for display.

While both types of capnometers are used frequently in dogs and cats, there are some limitations to consider when they are used in very small patients. Conventional sidestream monitors with high sampling rates (150–200 mL/min) tend to underestimate $PaCO_2$ due to the relatively low TV in these patients, resulting in falsely low $ETCO_2$ readings. By using a capnometer with a lower sampling rate (50 mL/min) in these patients, this problem can be minimized. Conversely, mainstream capnography often competes for TV in very small patients due to increased dead space created by the airway adapter. The use of low-volume neonatal airway adaptors in small patients will minimize this problem.

Under normal circumstances, $ETCO_2$ is a reasonable noninvasive estimate of $PaCO_2$. Normal $ETCO_2$ values are expected to be 4–6 mm Hg lower than $PaCO_2$ (i.e., 27–37 and 22–32 mm Hg in dogs and cats, respectively) due to normal physiological dead space ventilation. In most anesthetized patients, increases in $ETCO_2$ accompanied by a normal capnographic waveform are a result of hypoventilation (see Figure 6.7A).

In some patients, however, it is not appropriate to infer adequate ventilation on the basis of a normal $ETCO_2$ value alone. Any factor that increases in the proportion of dead space (alveolar, anatomic, or equipment) will increase the $PaCO_2$–$ETCO_2$ gradient and make $ETCO_2$ less useful as an index of ventilation. Interestingly, conditions that increase shunt fraction (i.e., perfusion of alveoli in the absence of ventilation) tend to have minimal impact on the gradient. Table 6.2 summarizes key factors that may contribute to this phenomenon that must be considered when interpreting $ETCO_2$ in the absence of concurrently measured $PaCO_2$ values.

In addition to their primary use as a monitor of ventilation, capnometry and capnography also provide additional useful information about other aspects of pulmonary, circulatory, and anesthetic equipment function, making them a very versatile monitor.

A lack of $ETCO_2$ and the absence of a normal capnographic waveform reliably indicate esophageal intubation in a patient with reasonable pulmonary blood flow. Similarly, the presence of $ETCO_2$ and a normal capnographic waveform are usually interpreted as signs of correct tube placement.

Partial airway obstruction will result in an abnormal capnogram with potentially decreased $ETCO_2$ and an increased $PaCO_2$–$ETCO_2$ gradient (see Figure 6.7B). A progressively prolonged inspiratory upstroke is noted with inspiration beginning before expiration is complete, which lowers the $ETCO_2$ reading.

As stated above, impaired circulation for a wide variety of reasons will also impact $ETCO_2$. In the absence of increased ventilation, an exponential decline in $ETCO_2$ with a normal capnographic waveform may be seen with decreased CO and, if not addressed, may signal impending cardiovascular collapse (see Figure 6.7C). A return of $ETCO_2$ concentrations during cerebral cardiopulmonary resuscitation may be observed with return of spontaneous circulation.

The capnographic waveform can also provide valuable information about the function of the breathing system during anesthesia. Under normal circumstances, whether using a rebreathing or nonrebreathing system, the concentration of CO_2 in inspired gas should be at or near zero. With a circle (rebreathing) system, an incompetent one-way valve or

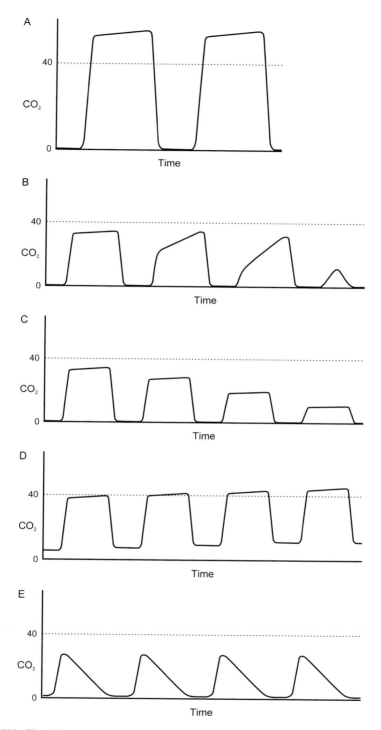

Figure 6.7(A–E). Variations in the normal capnograph. (A) Anesthetic-induced hypoventilation: elevated $ETCO_2$ with a normal waveform. (B) Partial airway obstruction: progressive prolongation of inspiratory upstroke and possibly decreased $ETCO_2$. (C) Cardiovascular collapse: exponential decrease in $ETCO_2$ with a normal waveform. (D) CO_2 rebreathing due to breathing system dysfunction: increased inspired CO_2 and $ETCO_2$. (E) Nonrebreathing system with low TV or leakage around the endotracheal tube: narrowed or absent alveolar plateau with decreased $ETCO_2$.

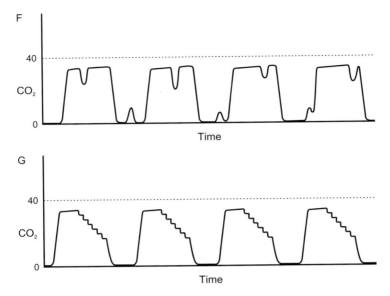

Figure 6.7(F–G). Variations in the normal capnograph. (F) Spontaneous ventilatory efforts during mechanical ventilation: clefts at various locations during inspiration and expiration. (G) Cardiogenic oscillations: small, regular step-like depressions at the end of the expiratory phase.

Table 6.2. Factors increasing the gradient between arterial and end-tidal CO_2

Increased alveolar dead space
• Hypoperfusion (reduced CO/pulmonary blood flow for any reason)
• Pulmonary embolism (air or thrombus)
• Obstructive pulmonary disease
• Excessive lung inflation
Increased anatomic dead space
• Shallow breathing (reduced TV for any reason)

exhausted CO_2 absorbent may result in inspiration or rebreathing of expired CO_2. This will appear on the capnograph as an increased baseline and the monitor will display increased end-tidal and inspired CO_2 (see Figure 6.7D). With a Mapleson (nonrebreathing) system, an inadequate fresh gas flow rate may result in a similar effect. Evidence of inspired CO_2 and observation of the abnormal capnographic waveform should prompt an immediate investigation of breathing system function.

Narrow or nonexistent plateaus with lowered $ETCO_2$ values may be observed in small patients with low TVs when nonrebreathing systems are used (see Figure 6.7E). In this situation, a rapid RR may actually result in some rebreathing of expired CO_2 despite adequate fresh gas flow rates. A leak around the endotracheal tube will produce a similar waveform pattern to that illustrated in Figure 6.7E.

In patients that are being mechanically ventilated, spontaneous ventilatory efforts appear as small notches or clefts on the capnograph at various points during inspiration and expiration (see Figure 6.7F). Observation of this pattern may indicate a need to reevaluate ventilator settings.

Cardiogenic oscillations appear as small, regular, tooth-like humps at the end of the expiratory phase and are related to changes in intrathoracic pressure associated with each cardiac cycle (see Figure 6.7G) These are rarely of any clinical significance, but many capnometers will report an erroneously high RR and a variable, erroneously low $ETCO_2$. This pattern tends to be seen more commonly in small patients because of the greater size of the heart relative to the thoracic cavity.

The use of capnography for routine anesthetic monitoring in dogs and cats has increased dramatically in recent years. Small handheld mainstream units, either alone or in combination with pulse oximetry, offer the advantage of portability (such as the Tidal Wave®, Philips Respironics). Alternatively, mainstream or side-stream units are available as part of larger multiparameter veterinary-specific patient monitors with ECG, ABP, pulse oximetry, and temperature capabilities. Capnography is noninvasive, technically simple to perform, and far superior to other noninvasive methods of assessing ventilation (such as RR and subjective assessment of TV). In addition, it offers the added advantage of also evaluating elements of circulatory status and equipment function at the same time. For these reasons, capnography is recommended for anesthetic monitoring in all canine and feline patients wherever possible.

Monitoring thermoregulation

Thermoregulatory function is depressed by administration of anesthetic agents and development of hypothermia is common in anesthetized animals, especially with longer procedures. Significant hypothermia will decrease anesthetic requirements and delay recovery. If the patient shivers as a thermogenic response, oxygen consumption will be dramatically increased. Though less common, hyperthermia is also possible and usually occurs in large breed, thick-coated dogs under multiple layers of drapes that are exposed to some form of active warming device. Since maintenance of normothermia during anesthesia is considered optimal, core body temperature must be monitored to document abnormalities and guide the use of warming devices.

The easiest way to measure temperature is to use a simple handheld rectal thermometer that can be inserted intermittently (usually every 20–30 minutes) to obtain readings. Alternatively, since patient access is often limited when animals are draped in for surgical procedures, an esophageal or rectal thermistor can be inserted and left in place. A cable attaches the thermistor to a monitor that continuously displays a digital temperature reading. Most multiparameter patient monitors used for evaluation of cardiopulmonary function also include a temperature probe.

Monitoring other parameters

Monitoring anesthetic depth, circulation, oxygenation, ventilation, and thermoregulation, as discussed above, should be considered standard in all canine and feline patients. In addition, there are a number of other parameters that should be monitored in selected patients or circumstances. A brief overview of these is provided below.

Renal function

Renal function is usually evaluated as part of the routine preanesthetic evaluation by assessing creatinine, blood urea nitrogen, and/or urine specific gravity. In healthy animals anesthetized for routine procedures, additional renal monitoring during anesthesia is usually not necessary. However, in patients with preexisting renal disease or hemodynamic instability, or patients that will be anesthetized for very long procedures, monitoring urine output using a closed collection system may be indicated.

Laboratory values

In addition to the tests routinely performed prior to anesthesia to determine the patient's physical status and anesthetic risk, repeating specific laboratory tests during and after anesthesia may be indicated in a variety of patients and procedures. Patients with preexisting blood loss, hemorrhage associated with surgery, or shock for any reason should have serial assessments of [Hb], packed cell volume, or hematocrit during anesthesia to track losses and response to volume administration. Measurement of total protein or total solids is commonly done concurrently. Serial lactate evaluations may also be useful as indicators of perfusion in these patients.

Decreases in colloidal osmotic pressure (COP) are common in critically ill animals and will be exacerbated by general anesthesia. Serial evaluation of COP in selected patients may be indicated to guide fluid therapy in selected anesthetized patients.

Patients with derangements in glucose homeostasis (i.e., diabetes or insulinomas) may require frequent reassessments of blood glucose (BG) during anesthesia to guide therapy and maintain glucose within an acceptable range. Neonatal patients, even if otherwise healthy, are predisposed to hypoglycemia and BG should be evaluated during and/or after anesthesia for all but the shortest procedures.

In critically ill animals, evaluation of acid–base status, serum electrolytes, and coagulation during anesthesia may also be indicated in a variety of scenarios.

Neuromuscular blockade

Neuromuscular function should be monitored using a nerve stimulator whenever a peripheral-acting muscle relaxant is administered.

Gastroesophageal reflux

Gastroesophageal reflux (GER) occurs commonly in anesthetized dogs and cats but is usually clinical inapparent (i.e., silent reflux). Potential adverse side effects of GER include aspiration of refluxed gastric contents and postanesthetic esophageal dysfunction. Measuring esophageal pH using a flexible pH sensing probe is a practical method to detect changes in pH associated with silent reflux. This will alert the anesthetist to the problem so that gastric and esophageal lavage and suction can be performed.

Endotracheal tube cuff inflation pressure

Endotracheal tubes with high-volume, low-pressure cuffs designed for use in humans are commonly used in dogs and cats. In human patients it is recommended that the pressure exerted by the cuff against the lateral wall of the trachea be maintained at approximately $25-30\,cm\,H_2O$. Higher pressures may be associated with ischemic damage to tracheal mucosa and lower pressures may not be effective at preventing aspiration. In veterinary medicine, cuff pressures are commonly assessed indirectly by closing the pop-off valve and squeezing the breathing bag to determine the airway pressure at which an audible leak is appreciated. Additional air is then added to the cuff as required. A more direct and quantitative approach involves using a portable handheld manometer that can be connected to the cuff inflation port to actually measure and maintain pressure within the cuff (Posey® Cufflator, Posey Respiratory Therapy, Arcadia, CA).

Managing common anesthetic complications

The preceding section has covered principles of monitoring anesthetic depth, circulation, oxygenation, ventilation, and thermoregulation in some detail. While it may seem obvious, it warrants mentioning once again that in order to do this effectively and optimize the standard of patient care, a trained individual dedicated to monitoring and managing anesthesia is necessary.

Traditionally, there has been a common misconception that anesthetic morbidity is rare in otherwise healthy patients presented for routine procedures that receive appropriate doses of anesthetic drugs. This myth was perpetuated by the fact that objective equipment-based evaluations were not commonly performed in general practice. In other words, because parameters such as ABP and $ETCO_2$ were not routinely measured, morbidities such as hypotension and hypoventilation went unrecognized in many patients. As anesthetic monitoring standards continue to evolve, however, it has become increasingly obvious that this is simply not the case. Veterinarians who routinely monitor these parameters recognize that hypotension and hypoventilation, for example, are in fact commonly observed during anesthesia. A retrospective study based on the records of approximately 100 healthy dogs and cats anesthetized for routine elective surgery using a variety of common anesthetic protocols in a general practice found the incidence of hypotension to be approximately 26%. It is likely that the incidence of hypoventilation in the same population is at least as high, if not higher.

While using objective, accurate monitors for assessment of circulation, oxygenation, and ventilation is the first step toward minimizing anesthetic morbidity, the clinician must also know how to respond when abnormalities are detected. The following section

Table 6.3. Drugs used to manage abnormalities of HR and rhythm

Drug	Intravenous dose	Indication
Atropine	0.02–0.04 mg/kg	Bradycardia
Glycopyrrolate	0.005–0.01 mg/kg	Bradycardia
Lidocaine	Dog: 2–4 mg/kg bolus followed by 40–80 mcg/kg/min infusion Cat: 0.5–1 mg/kg over 5 minutes	Ventricular dysrhythmias
Procainamide	Dog: 3–6 mg/kg bolus followed by 10–40 mcg/kg/min infusion Cat:?	Ventricular dysrhythmias
Diltiazem	0.05–0.15 mg/kg SLOW IV followed by 1–5 mcg/kg/min infusion if required	Supraventricular dysrhythmias
Verapamil	0.05–0.15 mg/kg SLOW IV	Supraventricular dysrhythmias
Esmolol	0.25–0.5 mg/kg SLOW IV followed by 50–200 mcg/kg/min infusion	Supraventricular dysrhythmias

?, dose unknown or not recommended.

provides guidelines for selected common complications encountered during anesthesia in dogs and cats.

Bradycardia and bradyarrhythmias

There is no single trigger for HR below which it is considered unacceptable and above which it is considered adequate. The significance of a single HR value in the absence of other monitored parameters and contextual information is minimal. The patient's ideal HR is the one at which circulatory function is optimal. It is up to the clinician to make this judgment based on other measured parameters, such as ABP and cardiac rhythm, and some key assumptions regarding the individual animal and the drugs administered.

Generally, HR values <50 beats per minute in dogs and <100 beats per minute in cats are likely to be associated with cardiovascular impairment and warrant consideration. In certain circumstances, and depending on other monitored parameters, HR values above these levels may also be cause for concern.

Sinus bradycardia may be due to drug-induced increases in vagal tone, vagally mediated reflexes, hyperkalemia, excessive anesthetic depth, or hypothermia. If treatment is warranted, increases in vagal tone usually respond to anticholinergic administration (see Table 6.3 for doses). In the case of excessive anesthetic depth or significant hypothermia, anticholinergic administration is often ineffective and treatment should focus on correcting the underlying cause (i.e., decreasing anesthetic depth and/or actively warming the patient). In some cases, reversal of anesthetic drugs, if possible, may be indicated to restore HR to an acceptable level.

In anesthetized patients, the decision to treat sinus bradycardia with an anticholinergic may be impacted by the animal's ABP. Patients that are bradycardic and hypotensive (see section on hypotension below) will almost certainly benefit hemodynamically from

A

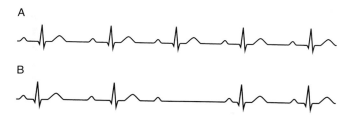

B

Figure 6.8. (A) First-degree AV block: prolongation of the P-R interval. (B) Type I second-degree AV block: progressive lengthening of the P-R interval followed by a blocked P wave.

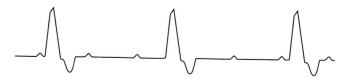

Figure 6.9. Third-degree AV block.

treatment because increasing HR will increase CO, which will increase ABP. In patients that are bradycardic but remain normotensive, the decision to administer an anticholinergic usually depends on the magnitude of bradycardia and the presence of concurrent bradyarrhythmias. Patients that are bradycardic and hypertensive are not likely to benefit hemodynamically from anticholinergic administration, and increasing HR in this situation may only serve to increase myocardial work in the face of increased afterload.

Bradyarrhythmias such as first and second atrioventricular (AV) block occur fairly frequently in healthy anesthetized dogs and cats due to administration of vagotonic drugs (opioids, alpha$_2$ agonists) (see Figure 6.8). The decision to treat these abnormalities once again depends on their impact on CO and will be a function of block frequency and the effective ventricular rate. Sporadic or intermittent second-degree AV block may not require treatment if a reasonable effective HR and ABP are maintained. Conversely, if blockade becomes more frequent and is associated with hypotension, anticholinergic administration is likely warranted. Note that in the case of hyperkalemia, bradycardia and AV block may not respond to an anticholinergic. In this situation, treatments to lower serum potassium levels should be initiated and, in the face of life-threatening dysrhythmias, 10% calcium gluconate should be administered (0.5–1.0 mL/kg administered slowly intravenously [IV] over 2–5 minutes).

In some canine patients, preexisting AV nodal disease may be present. In cases of high grade second-degree or third-degree AV block, bradycardia will be evident during the preanesthetic physical examination and should prompt a thorough ECG evaluation and cardiac workup prior to anesthesia (see Figure 6.9). These patients should not be anesthetized without a pacemaker as the ventricular rhythm may be suppressed by any anesthetic protocol, and bradycardia will not be responsive to anticholinerigic administration.

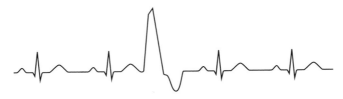

Figure 6.10. Premature ventricular complex.

Tachycardia and tachyarrhythmias

In many cases, tachycardia can be just as detrimental to circulatory function as brady-cardia. Generally, HR values >160 beats per minute in dogs and >200 beats per minute in cats are likely to be associated with some degree of cardiovascular impairment. In certain circumstances, and depending on other monitored parameters, HR values below these thresholds may also be cause for concern.

Sustained sinus tachycardia is associated with decreased SV and CO, which may lead to decreased ABP and perfusion. In anesthetized dogs and cats, sinus tachycardia may be a result of anesthetic drugs (ketamine, thiobarbiturates, anticholinergics, beta adrenergic agonists, etc.), inadequate anesthetic depth, hypercapnea, hypokalemia, hyperthermia, hypovolemia, anemia, hyperthyroidism, pheochromocytoma, and anaphylaxis. Obviously, treatment must be directed at the potential underlying cause. If anesthetic depth is inadequate, titrating additional injectable or inhalant anesthetic may be indicated. Alternatively, supplemental opioid or lidocaine administration may reduce the sympathetic response to noxious stimulation. If hypovolemia is suspected, volume resuscitation with crystalloids and/or colloids is indicated. Less commonly, a beta adrenergic blocking drug such as esmolol (see Table 6.3 for doses) may be indicated to control tachycardia in animals with hyperthyroidism or pheochromocytoma.

Isolated or sporadic ventricular premature complexes are not uncommon in healthy anesthetized dogs and cats and rarely require pharmacological intervention as their impact on CO is minimal (Figure 6.10). Patients with acid–base imbalance, electrolyte abnormalities (hypokalemia), hypoxemia, trauma, sepsis, shock, or primary myocardial disease may develop sustained, paroxysmal, or polymorphic ventricular tachycardia (VT). VT is a serious dysrhythmia and usually warrants treatment when it occurs in anesthetized patients. Identification and correction of contributing factors (such as hypoxema, hypokalemia, hypovolemia, etc.), where possible, is crucial. While direct current cardioversion is used to treat VT in humans, pharmacological treatment remains the most common approach in veterinary patients. Lidocaine is the first-line therapy and procainamide is indicated for refractory cases (see Table 6.3 for doses).

Isolated atrial or junctional premature complexes are also commonly observed in otherwise healthy patients during anesthesia and are usually of minimal hemodynamic significance (Figure 6.11). Sustained supraventricular tachycardia (SVT) or atrial fibrillation (AF) may negatively impact CO and circulatory status if the rate is high (Figure 6.12). Electrical cardioversion is the most effective treatment for acute onset SVT or AF in humans but may not be possible in many clinical veterinary settings. As with other

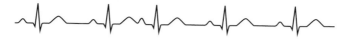

Figure 6.11.   Premature atrial complex.

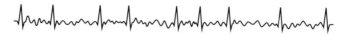

Figure 6.12.   Atrial fibrillation.

dysrhythmias, a thorough evaluation of potential underlying causes is indicated. In anesthetized dogs and cats, pharmacological interventions focus on converting SVT back to a normal rhythm or, in the case of AF, on lowering the ventricular response rate to improve SV and CO. Drugs used mostly commonly for acute management of these dysrhythmias are calcium channel blockers (diltiazem and verapamil) and beta adrenergic blockers (esmolol) (see Table 6.3 for doses). Note that in patients with underlying systolic dysfunction (such as dilated cardiomyopathy) both these classes of drugs must be used cautiously due to their potential negative inotropic effects. In this situation, it is prudent to start with the lowest possible dose and carefully titrate upward while monitoring circulatory status.

Hypotension

As stated above, hypotension is among the most commonly encountered anesthetic complications in dogs and cats and can only be recognized if ABP is actually measured. Hypotension is usually defined as a MAP <60 mm Hg and values in the 60–70 mm Hg range often trigger alterations to anesthetic management to prevent a further downward trend. If using a Doppler system to measure ABP, hypotension is defined as a SAP <80 mm Hg and values in the 80–90 mm Hg range may similarly precipitate adjustments to the anesthetic plan. Remember that in cats or other small patients, the Doppler may underestimate SAP by approximately 15 mm Hg and this should be taken into consideration when evaluating Doppler values in these patients. Sustained decreases in ABP below these levels may be associated with impaired perfusion and possible ischemic organ damage so every effort should be made to avoid hypotension whenever possible.

MAP is the product of CO and SVR. Thus any factor that decreases one or both of these determinants can result in hypotension. Common scenarios that may decrease CO include bradycardia, hypovolemia, and impaired myocardial contractility. Impaired contractility may be a function of primary cardiac disease, anesthetic drug-induced myocardial depression, sepsis, or systemic inflammatory response syndrome (SIRS). Common causes of reduced SVR include anesthetic-induced vasodilation, sepsis, and SIRS.

Many commonly used anesthetic agents can cause hypotension even when appropriate doses are administered. Isoflurane and sevoflurane are the two most popular inhalant anesthetics currently used in veterinary practice and both have the potential to cause significant, dose-dependent myocardial depression and vasodilation when administered to otherwise healthy patients. Acepromazine, due to its alpha adrenergic blocking effects, also causes vasodilation and may precipitate hypotension especially when used in combination with an inhalant. In compromised patients, the adverse effects of these agents are even more profound. Consequently, a balanced anesthetic protocol is advocated as this will minimize the required doses of these agents and reduce the risk of hypotension.

If hypotension or a trend toward hypotension is documented, potential causes must be considered so that treatment can be directed accordingly. Efforts should be made to optimize oxygenation and ventilation in hypotensive patients. The following outlines a reasonable approach to hypotension in most situations:

(1) Evaluate anesthetic depth and consider reducing it. Less inhalant anesthetic results in less myocardial depression and vasodilation, which in turn may improve ABP. In otherwise healthy patients this approach is often all that is necessary to restore ABP to acceptable levels. Even small adjustments to the vaporizer setting can have a significant impact. In some cases, the addition of supplemental agents that lack significant vasodilatory or myocardial depressant effects may facilitate lowering the vaporizer even further.

(2) Evaluate HR and consider augmenting it. As discussed above, bradycardia can contribute to lowered CO and hypotension. Consider anticholinergic administration (atropine or glycopyrrolate) if the patient is both hypotensive and bradycardic. Caution is warranted as rebound tachycardia may occur and be just as detrimental to CO as bradycardia (though it is usually short-lived). Note that it is not rational to administer an anticholinergic as a treatment for hypotension if the patient has a normal HR or is tachycardic. Please refer to Table 6.3 for doses.

(3) Evaluate circulatory volume and consider augmenting fluid administration. The average rate for IV crystalloid administration during anesthesia in normovolemic dogs and cats is approximately 10 mL/kg/hour. While administering IV boluses of crystalloids to normovolemic, but hypotensive, anesthetized patients has been advocated as a strategy to improve ABP, emerging evidence suggests this may not be beneficial and may even induce deleterious side effects related to hemodilution. In animals that are actually volume deficient due to dehydration, blood loss, or third-space losses, however, volume resuscitation must be initiated to restore preload and CO. This may require administration of crystalloids, synthetic colloids, and/or blood products.

(4) Evaluate myocardial function and consider augmenting cardiac contractility. If the first three strategies have failed to improve ABP or if the patient has documented or suspected myocardial dysfunction, therapy with a positive inotrope is indicated to improve SV and CO. Ephedrine is commonly used in patients that are otherwise healthy but experiencing anesthetic-induced hypotension. It tends to be less effective in the face of acidosis or reduced blood volume. Ephedrine stimulates both alpha- and beta adrenergic receptors and can be administered as a bolus, making it convenient for routine use. Dilution of the standard 50 mg/mL solution to 5 mg/mL makes accurate dosing in small patients feasible. Dobutamine and dopamine are also frequently used for their inotropic properties but their short half-lives mandate that they

Table 6.4. Drugs used to manage hypotension

Drug	Intravenous dose	Indication
Atropine	0.02–0.04 mg/kg	Hypotension due to bradycardia
Glycopyrrolate	0.005–0.01 mg/kg	Hypotension due to bradycardia
Ephedrine	0.05–0.2 mg/kg	Hypotension due to anesthetic-induced depression of myocardial contractility
Dobutamine	2–15 mcg/kg/min CRI (start low and titrate up to effect)	Hypotension due to depression of myocardial contractility and/or bradycardia
Dopamine	2–10 mcg/kg/min CRI (start low and titrate up to effect)	Hypotension due to depression of myocardial contractility and/or bradycardia
Epinephrine	0.05–0.3 mcg/kg/minute CRI (start low and titrate up to effect)	Hypotension due to profound vasodilation
Norepinephrine	0.05–0.3 mcg/kg/min CRI (start low and titrate up to effect)	Hypotension due to profound vasodilation
Phenylephrine	0.5–3 mcg/kg/min CRI (start low and titrate up to effect)	Hypotension due to profound vasodilation
Vasopressin	0.5–0.8 U/kg	Hypotension due to profound vasodilation

CRI, continuous rate infusion.

are administered via continuous infusion. These tend to be the drugs of choice in animals with hemodynamic instability or organic cardiac disease. The availability of a syringe pump greatly facilitates administration of drugs via continuous infusion. Please refer to Table 6.4 for doses.

(5) Evaluate vasomotor tone and consider augmenting SVR. In patients that are massively vasodilated and hypotensive, such as those with anaphylaxis, severe acidosis, sepsis, and SIRS, it may be appropriate to administer a vasopressor to increase SVR to a point where ABP can sustain reasonable perfusion. These patients are usually refractory to the other treatment strategies outlined above. Commonly used vasopressors include epinephrine, norepinephrine, and phenylephrine. Vasopressin may be used to treat vasodilatory shock in some situations. If ABP is overshot, the resulting vasoconstriction has the potential to sacrifice organ blood flow so this therapy requires intensive monitoring. Please refer to Table 6.4 for doses.

Hypertension

Hypertension is a much less frequent complication than hypotension in anesthetized dogs and cats. In healthy patients, MAP values >120 mm Hg or SAP values >160 mm Hg may be seen in response to noxious stimulation at lighter planes of anesthesia. This should be addressed by administration of additional anesthetic and/or analgesic agents. In general, the use of balanced anesthetic protocols will reduce the incidence of this complication.

Systemic hypertension may be a feature of certain diseases such as hyperadrenocorticism, hyperthyroidism, renal disease, or pheochromocytoma. These animals may have elevated ABP prior to anesthesia or, alternatively, they may be normotensive at presentation but experience acute hypertensive episodes during anesthesia. In situations where alpha adrenergic blockade (usually with phenoxybenzamine) has been initiated prior to anesthesia, beta adrenergic blockade with a drug like esmolol may be useful to treat tachyarrhythmias and acute hypertension during anesthesia.

Patients with chronic hypertension may also develop hypotension during anesthesia, especially with inhalant anesthetics, and may require support of ABP. In these patients, hypotension may compromise tissue perfusion to an even greater extent, as normal autoregulatory mechanisms no longer function at low pressures. Consequently, it may be prudent to maintain MAP in the 80–100 mm Hg range if possible.

Hypoxemia

Hypoxemia is a serious anesthetic complication with life-threatening consequences if not promptly recognized and treated. It is defined as a PaO_2 value <60 mm Hg or an SaO_2/SpO_2 value <90%. In some situations, PaO_2 values in the 60–80 mm Hg range and SaO_2/SpO_2 values in the 90–95% range may warrant consideration if they reflect a downward trend in oxygenation. In anesthetized animals, hypoxemia may not be accompanied by abnormalities in other monitored parameters, but in its terminal stages bradycardia or bradyarrhythmias may become evident.

In general, there are four major mechanisms of hypoxemia to consider: (1) decreased FiO_2 below 0.21, (2) hypoventilation if the patient is breathing room air (i.e., $FiO_2 = 0.21$), (3) ventilation–perfusion (V/Q) mismatch, and (4) shunt (also called venous admixture; V/Q ratio = 0).

The patient's response to administration of supplemental oxygen may vary depending on which of the four mechanisms is implicated. Inadequate FiO_2 and hypoventilation are both readily corrected by administration of oxygen. V/Q mismatch will show a variable response, while true shunt will show a minimal response. Table 6.5 lists causes of hypoxemia in anesthetized dogs and cats classified according to these mechanisms, realizing that in many cases a particular clinical scenario may involve more than one.

In healthy anesthetized patients the most common causes of hypoxemia are anesthetic machine or breathing system malfunction, hypoventilation (if the animal is breathing room air), inadvertent pop-off valve closure, endobronchial intubation, aspiration of gastric contents, and inappropriate use of nitrous oxide. These are, for the most part, entirely preventable. The importance of understanding the function and operation of the breathing system and anesthetic machine cannot be overstated. Confirming proper function prior to starting a case and ongoing monitoring of system function during the case are essential. Hypoventilation in anesthetized patients that are inspiring room air is common and can be prevented by monitoring ventilation and providing supplemental oxygen. Applying the principles of sound airway management will minimize the risk of

Table 6.5. Causes of hypoxemia in anesthetized dogs and cats

Cause	Mechanism	Comment
Delivery of excessive concentrations of nitrous oxide	Inadequate FiO_2	A minimum FiO_2 of 0.3 (i.e., delivery of 70% nitrous oxide) is recommended for patients with normal pulmonary function; nitrous oxide should not be used in patients with preexisting pulmonary dysfunction
Inadequate RR and/or TV in patients inspiring room air	Hypoventilation	Injectable anesthesia where oxygen is not supplemented (i.e., $FiO_2 = 0.21$) is associated with increased risk of hypoxemia; inhalant anesthesia, where the patient is inadvertently disconnected from the anesthetic machine, may result in hypercapneic hypoxemia if not detected
Sustained apnea in patients with patent airways receiving 100% oxygen	V/Q mismatch	Reduced V/Q; onset of hypoxemia is delayed if oxygen continues to be delivered at a high FiO_2
Endobronchial intubation	V/Q mismatch	Reduced V/Q secondary to inadvertent intubation of a bronchus
Pleural space disorders (pleural effusion, pneumothorax) and pulmonary disease (pneumonia, pulmonary edema, neoplasia)	V/Q mismatch	Reduced V/Q
Pulmonary embolism	V/Q mismatch	Increased V/Q (dead space)
Airway obstruction (mucous plugs, aspirated gastric material, kinked endotracheal tube, anatomical abnormalities)	Hypoventilation, V/Q mismatch, and Shunt	Hypercapnea may contribute in patients with airway obstruction inspiring room air; reduced V/Q is a major mechanism; V/Q = 0 is possible with complete obstruction
Closed pop-off valve or obstructed breathing system	Shunt	Reduced V/Q due to increased airway pressures and apnea; progressive decreases in venous return occur simultaneously and cardiovascular collapse will follow if not recognized

endobronchial intubation and aspiration of gastric contents. Finally, vigilant monitoring of fresh gas flows is necessary in all patients, but especially in those where the anesthetic protocol includes nitrous oxide.

In patients with pleural space disease, pulmonary parenchymal disease, pulmonary thromboembolism, or right-to-left shunts hypoxemia is common even in animals that are intubated and inspiring 100% oxygen. If the underlying cause can be addressed then oxygenation should improve. In animals where the underlying cause is not immediately correctible, advanced ventilatory strategies, circulatory support, and intensive monitoring may be indicated. Such management techniques are beyond the scope of this chapter.

When hypoxemia occurs during anesthesia, the following outlines a reasonable approach to management. The order in which these steps are carried out will vary depending on the clinical situation.

(1) Ensure adequate FiO_2 in patients connected to anesthetic machines. Confirm the oxygen supply (i.e., check the source) and ensure the flow meter is registering a flow rate. If nitrous oxide is being used, discontinue it and provide 100% oxygen.

(2) Provide supplemental oxygen to patients inspiring room air to counteract the effect of hypoventilation. In patients that are not intubated, oxygen delivery via a face mask may counteract hypoxemia due to hypoventilation; however, endotracheal intubation is recommended in most situations. Patients that are already intubated but not receiving oxygen should be connected to a breathing system and anesthetic machine. Ventilation should be evaluated using capnometry or blood gas analysis.

(3) Evaluate airway patency and reintubate if necessary. If the patient is not intubated, place an endotracheal tube and provide supplemental oxygen as above. If the patient is already intubated, assess tube patency by direct observation and by delivering positive pressure ventilation (PPV) with an Ambu bag or anesthetic machine and breathing system. If there is any doubt about tube patency, remove the tube and reintubate with a new one. Provide supplemental oxygen and evaluate ventilation using capnometry or blood gas analysis.

(4) Confirm correct endotracheal tube placement in intubated patients. Consider the possibility of esophageal intubation and reintubate if necessary. Consider the possibility of endobronchial intubation and, if there is any doubt, deflate the cuff and carefully back the tube out until the tip can be palpated at the thoracic inlet. If the tube is excessively long it should be removed and a tube of appropriate length inserted. Provide supplemental oxygen and evaluate ventilation using capnometry or blood gas analysis.

(5) Ensure proper breathing system function in patients that are connected to an anesthetic machine. Ensure that the pop-off is fully open and that airway pressures are not increased. Ensure that the patient has not become disconnected from the machine. Ensure that the breathing system is not obstructed.

(6) Assess the pleural space and perform thoracocentesis if indicated. Patients with significant pneumothorax or pleural effusion will benefit from thoracocentesis to improve V/Q matching. In some patients a thoracostomy tube should be placed to facilitate repeated thoracic drainage.

(7) Provide PPV. In patients where the cause of V/Q mismatch cannot be readily discerned and/or corrected, institution of PPV may improve V/Q matching.

(8) Evaluate cardiovascular function and consider inotropic support to improve pulmonary blood flow. In patients where the cause of V/Q mismatch cannot be readily discerned and/or corrected and cardiovascular function is questionable, administration of dobutamine or dopamine may improve V/Q matching.

(9) Evaluate hemoglobin concentration and consider blood product administration if indicated. Though anemia will not result in hypoxemia per se, it can significantly reduce CaO_2 and impair DO_2. If there is no concurrent gas exchange abnormality, PaO_2 or SaO_2/SpO_2 will remain within normal limits in this situation.

Hypoventilation and hypercapnia

Hypercapnia secondary to hypoventilation is one of the most commonly encountered anesthetic complications in dogs and cats. While the definition of what constitutes significant hypercapnia in otherwise normal patients remains debatable, the most frequently cited threshold is a $PaCO_2$ >60 mm Hg. This corresponds to an $ETCO_2$ value of approximately 55 mm Hg, assuming a normal $PaCO_2$–$ETCO_2$ gradient. Though mild hypercapnia is well tolerated in most patients that are receiving supplemental oxygen, those with intracranial pathology may experience a potentially dangerous increase in cerebral blood flow and intracranial pressure. For this reason, it is currently recommended that $PaCO_2$ be maintained between 30 and 32 mm Hg in these patients. Remember that in animals that are breathing room air, hypoventilation/hypercapnia may also result in hypoxemia.

Since pathological increases in CO_2 production (such as malignant hyperthermia) are extremely rare, causes of hypercapnia during anesthesia are either a result of: (1) hypoventilation, (2) rebreathing of previously exhaled CO_2 or, less commonly, (3) uptake of CO_2 from the pressurized peritoneum or thoracic cavity during laparoscopy or thoracoscopy. Hypoventilation is very common because all anesthetics depress ventilatory drive to some degree. Opioids, injectable anesthetics (such as propofol and thiopental), and inhalant anesthetics (such as isoflurane and sevoflurane) in particular cause potent dose-dependent hypoventilation. These effects are often exacerbated in animals that are obese or brachycephalic. Patient positioning or instrumentation that results in increased diaphragmatic pressure (such as the Trendelenburg position or placement of large retractors in the cranial abdomen) may also have adverse effects.

Rebreathing of CO_2 causing hypercapnia can occur in animals with normal V_A if there is a problem with the breathing system. Exhausted carbon dioxide absorbent or incompetent one-way valves in circle systems, or inadequate fresh gas flow rates in Mapleson systems are potential causes. Both of these are readily identified using capnography, as discussed previously.

While $ETCO_2$ is commonly used as a surrogate for $PaCO_2$, it is important to remember that a normal $ETCO_2$ value may not always be associated with normal $PaCO_2$. Potential causes for increases in the $PaCO_2$–$ETCO_2$ gradient have been discussed previously. In situations where capnometry is not available, assessments of ventilation can only be based on RR and qualitative impressions of TV, and these are often misleading. It is important to recognize that adequate SpO_2 values (>95%) in patients inspiring 100% oxygen in no way rule out the possibility of hypoventilation/hypercapnia.

When hypercapnia is observed in anesthetized patients based on $PaCO_2$ or $ETCO_2$ values, the following constitutes a reasonable approach to management:

(1) Determine if the patient is inspiring CO_2 and, if so, troubleshoot breathing system function. Evaluate the capnographic waveform and check to see if the monitor is

registering inspired CO_2. If inspired CO_2 is noted and the patient is connected to a circle system, do the following: (a) evaluate the integrity and function of the one-way valves and make the necessary adjustments, and/or (b) evaluate the activity of the carbon dioxide absorbent and replace it if necessary. With exhausted absorbent, increases in inspired CO_2 may be less dramatic and can often be compensated for by increasing the fresh gas flow rate if it is not feasible to change the absorbent or switch to a new machine in the middle of the case. If inspired CO_2 is noted and the patient is connected to a Mapleson system, evaluate the fresh gas flow rate and increase it to ensure adequate CO_2 removal.

(2) Assess anesthetic depth and consider reducing it. Less inhalant anesthetic will result in less depression of the brain stem respiratory center and may improve ventilation. Reversal of administered opioids as a strategy to counteract hypoventilation during anesthesia is not recommended except in cases of overdose.

(3) Provide PPV. While apnea constitutes an absolute indication for PPV, this strategy is also recommended in any patient that is hypoventilating regardless of the RR. Patients receiving supplemental opioids during anesthesia, especially continuous infusions at moderate to high dose rates, usually require PPV. Adjustments to ventilator settings (RR, TV, and peak inspiratory pressure) are made based on $PaCO_2$ or, in patients with presumably normal $PaCO_2$–$ETCO_2$ gradients, on $ETCO_2$.

Hyperventilation and hypocapnia

Due to the depressant effects of anesthetic agents on the respiratory center, hyperventilation during anesthesia is much less common than hypoventilation. Note that RR often increases in patients at lighter planes of anesthesia but, because TV is shallow, these animals are often hypoventilating. Due to increased dead space ventilation, $ETCO_2$ will not accurately reflect $PaCO_2$ in this situation and may actually be normal or decreased.

The most common cause of hypocapnia in anesthetized dogs and cats is iatrogenic hyperventilation due to overzealous PPV. Side effects of hypocapnia include alkalemia and reductions in cerebral blood flow. Consequently, it is recommended to monitor ventilation using $PaCO_2$ or $ETCO_2$ and make appropriate adjustments to ventilator settings to maintain CO_2 within an appropriate range.

Hypothermia

Hypothermia is a frequent side effect of anesthesia in dogs and cats. Factors that contribute to hypothermia include small patient size (i.e., larger surface area/mass ratio), long duration of anesthesia, anesthetic-induced vasodilation, open body cavities (i.e., laparotomy or thoracotomy), use of cold surgical preparation solutions, and administration of cold IV fluids.

In addition to warming IV surgical preparation solutions and IV fluids, patients anesthetized for procedures lasting more than 20–30 minutes benefit from some form of active warming. The most effective and safest options include: (1) circulating hot water blankets, (2) forced air warmers (such as the BairHugger® System, Arizant Healthcare Inc., Eden Prairie, MN), and (3) conductive fabric warmers (such as the HotDog® Patient

Warming System, Augustine Temperature Management, Eden Prairie, MN). In particular, the latter option appears to be extremely effective at maintaining normothermia even in small animals anesthetized for extended periods of time. It is important to monitor patient temperature while using any of these warming modalities to ensure that patients do not become hyperthermic.

Hyperthermia

Hyperthermia during anesthesia, in the absence of active warming, is uncommon. While a malignant hyperthermia-like syndrome has been reported in dogs and cats, the genetic basis for such a syndrome has not been established and the condition remains extremely rare. Iatrogenic hyperthermia is possible if temperature is not monitored and warming devices are not adjusted accordingly during the procedure.

Postanesthetic hyperthermia may be observed in cats and appears to be associated with administration of drugs such as opioids (hydromorphone and morphine in particular) and possibly ketamine. This phenomenon appears to be transient, occurring between 1 and 5 hours after tracheal extubation and can occur in cats that are significantly hypothermic during anesthesia. Temperatures in excess of 40°C are not uncommon and extreme hyperthermia (>42°C) has been reported. These findings highlight the importance of temperature monitoring in the postanesthetic period to recognize these patients and provide active cooling if indicated. Decreasing the ambient room temperature, providing a fan to circulate air, cooling the footpads with water or alcohol, providing room-temperature IV fluids, or administering acepromazine in agitated patients should be considered if temperature is 40°C or above.

Revised from "Monitoring Anesthetized Patients" by Steve C. Haskins in Lumb and Jones' Veterinary Anesthesia and Analgesia, Fourth Edition.

Chapter 7

Acid–base balance and fluid therapy

William W. Muir, Helio S.A. de Morais, and
David C. Seeler

Introduction

Homeostasis requires maintenance of a relatively constant fluid volume and stable composition in all fluid compartments. The practice of anesthesia, even in American Society
of Anesthesiologists (ASA) Category I patients undergoing routine procedures, may
precipitate abnormalities in this balance. In patients presenting with critical illness, all
fluid compartments may be significantly affected, and serious, potentially life-threatening
derangements in acid–base balance may exist. These abnormalities will be further exacerbated by the administration of anesthetic agents if efforts to accurately diagnose
underlying conditions, quantify fluid and acid–base disorders, and institute appropriate
management strategies are not made.

The interplay between acid–base balance and fluid therapy is complex and injudicious
administration of parenteral fluids during the perianesthetic period can have a detrimental
effect on a patient's acid–base status. In this chapter, basic principles of acid–base
balance and fluid therapy will be presented as well as clinical guidelines for diagnosing
acid–base disorders and providing appropriate perianesthetic fluid therapy to canine and
feline patients.

Regulation of acid–base balance

Animals produce large quantities of acid through their metabolic processes every day
that must be either excreted or metabolized to maintain acid–base balance. Despite this
substantial production, the hydrogen ion concentration in body fluids is maintained at an
extremely low level (40 nEq/L). Because the hydrogen ion exists in such miniscule concentrations, even small variations will have significant effects. For example, a change in
hydrogen ion concentration from 35 to 45 nEq/L is associated with a change in pH of
only 0.1 units, but this represents a 22% increase in its concentration.

The importance of the hydrogen ion in maintenance of homeostasis is not a function
of its concentration in a particular fluid compartment but rather its impact on ionization.

Essentials of Small Animal Anesthesia and Analgesia, Second Edition. Edited by Kurt A. Grimm,
William J. Tranquilli, Leigh A. Lamont.
© 2011 John Wiley & Sons, Inc. Published 2011 by John Wiley & Sons, Inc.

This is most critical within the intracellular space. Virtually all small metabolic intermediate molecules, with very few exceptions, are ionized at physiological pH. This results in ion trapping, which minimizes diffusional loss and is crucial to the maintenance of cellular homeostasis. In addition, ionization of amino acid residues (especially histidine) on larger protein molecules (notably enzymes) determines the three-dimensional shape of the molecules and affects their binding characteristics and overall function.

Acid–base terminology

Hydrogen ion (H^+)   A single free proton released from a hydrogen atom; note that "bare" protons do not actually exist in solution as they react with surrounding water molecules; however, this symbolic notation continues to be used out of convenience.

Acid (HA)   A molecule containing hydrogen atoms that can release H^+.

Base (A^-)   An ion or molecule that can accept H^+.

pH   The logarithmic scale conventionally used to express H^+ concentration ($[H^+]$) in solutions; pH is related to $[H^+]$ (expressed as equivalents per liter) as follows:

$$pH = \log(1/[H^+]) = -\log[H^+]$$

For example, normal $[H^+]$ is 40 nEq/L; therefore:

$$\text{normal pH} = -\log[0.00000004] = 7.4$$

Strong acid   An acid that rapidly dissociates and releases large amounts of H^+ in solution; for example, hydrochloric acid ($HCl \rightarrow H^+ + Cl^-$).

Weak acid   An acid that dissociates incompletely, releasing limited H^+ in solution; for example, carbonic acid ($H_2CO_3 \rightarrow H^+ + HCO_3^-$).

Strong base   A base that reacts rapidly with H^+ removing it from solution; for example, hydroxide ($OH^- + H^+ \rightarrow H_2O$).

Weak base   A base that binds weakly with H^+ in solution; for example, bicarbonate ($HCO_3^- + H^+ \rightarrow H_2CO_3$).

Acid dissociation constant (K_a)   The equilibrium constant for dissociation reactions that provides a quantitative measure of the strength of an acid in solution

pK_a   The logarithmic scale conventionally used to express K_a values where $pK_a = -\log K_a$; in general, weak acids have large pK_a values while strong acids have small pK_a values.

Henderson–Hasselbach equation   An equation derived from K_a, which describes the amount of H^+ available to react with bases:

$$pH = pK_a + \log\{[A^-]/[HA]\}$$

Respiratory or volatile acid   Acid that is excreted by the lungs, usually refers specifically to carbon dioxide (CO_2); however, CO_2 is not technically an acid (according to the Brønsted definition) because it lacks H^+ and cannot be a proton donor, thus, CO_2 is thought of as having the potential to create an equivalent amount of carbonic acid (H_2CO_3).

Metabolic or fixed acid   All acids produced by the body that are not excreted by the lungs (i.e., any acid other than CO_2/H_2CO_3), often referred to by their anions (e.g., lactate, phosphate, sulfate, acetoacetate, or β-hydroxybutyrate) instead of their acids (i.e., lactic acid, phosphoric acid, sulfuric acid, acetoacetic acid, and β-hydroxybutyric acid, respectively), which may be a source of confusion.

Acidosis   An abnormal process or condition that would lower arterial pH if there were no secondary changes in response to the primary etiologic factor.

Alkalosis   An abnormal process or condition that would raise arterial pH if there were no secondary changes in response to the primary etiologic factor.

Acidemia   Low blood pH; the result of acidosis.

Alkalemia   High blood pH; the result of alkalosis.

Systems responsible for maintaining hydrogen ion concentration

Regulation of $[H^+]$ in body fluids to prevent acidemia or alkalemia involves three primary mechanisms: (1) the chemical acid–base buffer systems in body fluids, (2) the respiratory center, and (3) the kidneys. The chemical buffer system responds to changes in $[H^+]$ within a fraction of a second and has a large capacity to bind H^+ until other systems can respond and definitively re-establish acid–base balance. The second line of defense is the respiratory system, which acts within minutes to eliminate volatile acid (i.e., CO_2) from the body via hyperventilation. The third line of defense is the kidneys and they are ultimately responsible for excretion of fixed acids and for initiating compensatory changes in plasma HCO_3^- concentration in the presence of respiratory acid–base disorders.

Chemical buffering to regulate acid–base balance

A buffer is defined as any substance that can reversibly bind H^+ and a buffer solution consists of a weak acid and its conjugate base. A generic buffer reaction is represented as follows:

$$H^+ + A^- \leftrightarrow HA$$

Free H^+ combines with the anionic base (A^-) to form a weak acid (HA), which can either remain in this state or dissociate back to A^- and H^+ depending on the $[H^+]$. A particular buffer is most effective when the local pH is within 1 pH unit of its pK_a (Table 7.1).

Chemical buffer systems are located throughout the body in a range of fluids and tissues as shown in Table 7.1. The three most important chemical buffers are the bicarbonate, phosphate, and protein buffering systems.

Bicarbonate buffer system   The bicarbonate system is responsible for approximately 80% of extracellular fluid (ECF) buffering, and contributes between 10% and 15% to total chemical buffering capacity. The system consists of a water solution containing H_2CO_3 (a weak acid) and its conjugate base, HCO_3^- (usually as the sodium salt $NaHCO_3$). The entire system may be represented as follows:

$$CO_2 + H_2O \leftrightarrow H_2CO_3 \leftrightarrow H^+ + HCO_3^- + Na^+ \leftrightarrow NaHCO_3$$

Table 7.1.   The major body buffer systems

Location	% of TBW	Local pH	Buffer	Buffer pK_a	Comment
Extracellular buffer systems					
Interstitial fluid	25	7.4	Bicarbonate	6.1	Important for metabolic/fixed acids
			Interstitial Proteins	6.4–7.9[a]	Not important; concentration too low
			Phosphate	6.8	Not important; concentration too low
Plasma	8	7.4	Bicarbonate	6.1	Important for metabolic/fixed acids
			Plasma proteins:		
			Albumin	6.4–7.9[a]	Minor buffer
			Globulins	6.4–7.9[a]	Not important
			Phosphate	6.8	Not important; concentration too low
Urine	<1	5.5–7.0	Phosphate	6.8	Responsible for most of "titratable acidity"
			Ammonia	9.2	Important buffer due to formation of ammonium
Intracellular buffer systems					
ICF	67	7.0–7.4	Intracellular proteins:		
			Oxyhemoglobin	6.7	Important for respiratory/ volatile acid
			Deoxyhemoglobin	7.9	
			All others	6.4–7.9[a]	Important buffers
			Phosphate	6.8	Important buffer

TBW, total body water.
[a] The imidazole ring of histidine has a pKa of 6.4–7.0 while the α-amino group has a pKa of 7.4–7.9.

The formation of H_2CO_3 from CO_2 and H_2O is catalyzed by the enzyme carbonic anhydrase, which is abundantly located in alveolar and renal tubular epithelial cells and in red blood cells. The H_2CO_3 then ionizes weakly to form very small amounts of H^+ and HCO_3^-. The second component of the system, $NaHCO_3$, ionizes almost completely, forming large amounts of HCO_3^- and Na^+.

Based on the low pK_a value of 6.1 and the limited concentrations of the two principle elements of the system (H_2CO_3 and HCO_3^-), it would be reasonable to assume that the bicarbonate system lacks significant buffering power. However, because the system is "open at both ends" (i.e., both pCO_2 and $[HCO_3^-]$ can be adjusted via respiratory and renal mechanisms, respectively), the effectiveness of the bicarbonate buffer system is greatly increased.

Phosphate buffer system   The phosphate buffer system is not important in the ECF but does play a major role in buffering renal tubular fluid and intracellular fluid (ICF). The main components of the system are H_3PO_4 (phosphoric acid, a triprotic weak acid) and its conjugate bases, $H_2PO_4^-$, HPO_4^{2-} and PO_4^{3-} (dihydrogen phosphate, hydrogen phosphate, and phosphate, respectively, usually in the form of sodium salts). At physiological pH values, the prevailing two species are $H_2PO_4^-$ and HPO_4^{2-}.

While the pK_a for the phosphate buffer system is 6.8, making it a potentially significant buffer in the ECF, its concentration here is only a fraction of the concentration of the bicarbonate buffer, so its contribution to ECF buffering is negligible.

In contrast, this system plays a key role in urine because phosphate is greatly concentrated in renal tubules and tubular fluid has a lower pH than ECF, making it an ideal fluid compartment for this buffer. The phosphate system is also important in the ICF for similar reasons (i.e., high concentrations are available and ICF pH is very close to 6.8).

Protein buffer system   Proteins constitute the most plentiful buffers in body fluids. While plasma proteins, notably albumin, make a modest contribution to ECF buffering, it is the contribution of intracellular proteins, which is by far the most important. Approximately 60–70% of the body's total chemical buffering capacity occurs in the ICF and most of this is attributed to proteins. This is a function of the high concentration of protein found in cells and the fact that most protein buffers have pK_a values fairly close to that of ICF. The most important protein-dissociable group is the imidazole ring of histidine (pK_a 6.4 to 7.0), while α-amino groups (pK_a 7.4–7.9) also play an important secondary role.

Hemoglobin is a key intracellular protein buffer. Because it is confined to red blood cells, it is also often classified as a blood buffer along with plasma proteins. Hemoglobin is responsible for more than 80% of the nonbicarbonate buffering capacity of whole blood while albumin makes up most of the other 20%. This is because hemoglobin is present in about twice the concentration and contains about three times the number of histidine residues per molecule compared to albumin.

Deoxyhemoglobin is a more effective buffer than oxyhemoglobin and this accounts for about 30% of the Haldane effect (the greater ability of deoxyhemoglobin to form carbamino compounds accounts for the other 70%). This means that oxygen unloading actually improves buffering capacity at exactly the location where additional H^+ is being produced by dissociation of H_2CO_3 to facilitate CO_2 transport as HCO_3^-.

Other factors impacting intracellular buffering   While the previous discussion has referred to the ECF and ICF as two totally distinct compartments, it is important to recognize that changes in $[H^+]$ are effectively communicated between them. Transfer of key elements across cell membranes has a significant impact on buffering and is facilitated by three major processes.

First, due to its high lipid solubility, CO_2 crosses cell membranes easily where it dissolves in H_2O to form $H_2CO_3^-$, which then dissociates to H^+ and HCO_3^-. Due to the bicarbonate system's ineffectiveness at buffering CO_2 (i.e., volatile acid) in the ECF, almost all buffering of respiratory acidosis and alkalosis occurs intracellularly.

Second, cell membranes contain various proton–cation antiporters, which facilitate entry of H^+ into cells in exchange for other cations, such as Na^+ and K^+, to maintain electroneutrality. The delivered H^+ are then buffered by the phosphate and protein buffer systems. More than half of buffering for metabolic acidosis and about one-third of buffering for metabolic alkalosis occurs intracellularly.

Finally, the presence of the HCO_3^-/Cl^- antiporter (or chloride pump) facilitates the movement of HCO_3^- produced from the dissociation of H_2CO_3 out of the cell in exchange for Cl^-. This is referred to as the chloride shift.

The isohydric principle Chemical buffer systems do not operate independently but work together in equilibrium with each other. Because there is only one $[H^+]$ in a given compartment, anything that changes the balance of one buffer system will affect the balance of all the others. This is known as the isohydric principle. Clinically, this means that measuring the concentrations of any one acid–base pair will provide a picture of overall acid–base balance in the body. Conventionally, the components of the bicarbonate system (i.e., H_2CO_3 measured as pCO_2, and HCO_3^-) are measured because they are accessible and easily determined. Blood gas machines measure pH and pCO_2 directly and the $[HCO^{3-}]$ is then calculated using the Henderson–Hasselbalch equation.

Respiratory regulation of acid–base balance

The second line of defense against acid–base abnormalities involves the respiratory system, which is able to excrete volatile acid (CO_2) and control $[H^+]$ by initiating changes in ventilation. Ventilatory changes occur rapidly and have profound effects on $[H^+]$. Changes in alveolar ventilation are inversely proportional to changes in arterial pCO_2 (P_aCO_2) and directly proportional to total body CO2 production. Changes in P_aCO_2, in turn, are inversely proportional to pH according to the Henderson–Hasselbach equation. Therefore, a decrease in alveolar ventilation will cause an increase in P_aCO_2 and a decrease in pH, while an increase in alveolar ventilation will cause a decrease in P_aCO_2 and an increase in pH.

Not only does alveolar ventilation impact pH, but the reverse also occurs. A decrease in pH will stimulate ventilatory drive while an increase in pH will inhibit it. Thus, the respiratory system operates as a typical negative feedback loop to maintain P_aCO_2 and therefore $[H^+]$ within a narrow range. Peripheral and central chemoreceptors sense changes in P_aCO_2, the respiratory center of the medulla integrates this information, and the muscles of respiration respond accordingly. This type of acid–base regulation is referred to as physiological buffering because it is an open system, as opposed to chemical buffering, which is a closed system. In general, the overall buffering capacity of the respiratory system is one to two times greater than the buffering power of all ECF chemical buffers combined.

Renal regulation of acid–base balance

While the lungs are responsible for elimination of volatile acid (CO_2), the kidneys serve as the primary means by which fixed, metabolic acids are eliminated from the body. Despite the fact that the amount of fixed acid produced daily is far, far smaller than the amount of CO_2 produced, the renal system is critical as there is no other mechanism for excretion of these acids. Quantitatively, even more important than excretion of fixed acids is the kidneys' ability to reabsorb bicarbonate, thereby conserving the primary buffer system of the ECF. The kidneys accomplish these two goals through three fundamental processes: (1) active secretion of H^+ into the tubular lumen, (2) indirect reabsorption of filtered HCO_3^- into tubular cells and ultimately the blood, and (3) production of new HCO_3^- in tubular cells involving the phosphate and ammonia buffer systems.

The first two mechanisms are interrelated in that the process of active H^+ secretion into the renal tubular lumen ultimately results in reabsorption of HCO_3^-. The cellular mechanisms of H^+ secretion depend on the location within the kidney. In the proximal tubules, the thick ascending loop of Henle and the early distal tubule, H^+ is secreted via secondary active transport. In the intercalated cells, H^+ is secreted by primary active transport.

In both cases secreted H^+ combines with filtered HCO_3^-, forming H_2CO_3, which dissociates into CO_2 and H_2O. The CO_2 diffuses easily into the tubular cell where it recombines with H_2O under the influence of carbonic anhydrase to generate a new H_2CO_3 molecule, which in turn dissociates into HCO_3^- and H^+. The HCO_3^- is then transported across the basolateral membrane by either $Na^+–HCO_3^-$ cotransport or $Cl^-–HCO_3^-$ exchange. Under normal circumstances, each time an H^+ is formed in a tubular cell an HCO_3^- is also formed and ultimately released back into the blood. Therefore, it can be said that HCO_3^- and H^+ "titrate" each other in the tubules.

In acidosis, there is excess H^+ relative to HCO_3^- but only a small part of this can be excreted in the ionic form, as urine pH has a lower limit of approximately 4.5. Consequently, excretion of large amounts of urine H^+ is accomplished by combining it with phosphate and ammonia buffers in the tubular lumen. This buffering actually results in the formation of "new" (i.e., not previously filtered) HCO_3^-, which ultimately enters the blood. The ammonia system is quantitatively more important than the urinary phosphate system. In the proximal tubular cells, glutamine is metabolized to form ammonium and HCO_3^-. The ammonium is secreted into the tubular lumen while the new HCO_3^- is transported back across the basolateral membrane. In the collecting tubules, H^+ is secreted into the tubular lumen as described previously, but now it combines with ammonia, which is readily able to diffuse across the luminal membrane. The result is ammonium, which is much less diffusable and becomes trapped in the urine, thereby providing a means of H^+ excretion. For each ammonium excreted, a new HCO_3^- is formed and added back to the blood.

Clinically, it is possible to quantify net renal acid excretion by determining HCO_3^- excretion, the amount of new HCO_3^- added to the blood (which is calculated by measuring urinary ammonium concentration), and urinary titratable acid. Titratable acid refers to the rest of the non-HCO_3^-, nonammonium buffer excreted in the urine (i.e., mainly phosphate).

As secretion of H^+ into the tubular lumen is a key step in all aspects of renal acid–base balance, it is not surprising that this process is tightly regulated. Key factors that may increase or decrease H^+ secretion include changes in the following: pCO_2, $[H^+]$, ECF fluid volume, angiotensin II levels, aldosterone levels, and potassium levels.

Temperature effects on acid–base balance

Evaluations of acid–base balance in a clinical setting typically involve measurement of ECF components simply because blood is an easily accessible fluid. However, it has been suggested that the intracellular environment is, in fact, the key compartment due to the phenomenon of ion trapping. There are two competing theories that seek to explain the regulation of intracellular pH across variations in temperature, the alpha-stat hypothesis, and the pH-stat hypothesis. While an in-depth discussion of these theories is not possible here, a brief definition of each is provided as they are relevant to the clinical interpretation of blood gas values.

The alpha-stat hypothesis states that the degree of ionization (referred to as "alpha") of the imidazole groups of intracellular proteins remains constant despite changes in temperature. In other words, the ideal intracellular pH is the pH of neutrality (i.e., the state where $[H^+] = [OH^-]$) and this pH will vary with changes in temperature. If the alpha-stat theory is correct, then blood gas values should not be corrected for the patient's body temperature.

The pH-stat theory states that the intracellular pH should be kept constant despite changes in temperature. If the pH-stat theory is correct, then temperature-corrected blood gas values should be used for interpretation. It should be noted that all blood gas analyzers are set to 37°C and all measurements are performed at this temperature. When other patient temperatures are entered the computer in the machine uses various correction formulae to calculate the so-called corrected values.

While both approaches continue to be used in clinical practice, the reality is, with significant variations in patient temperature, we simply do not fully understand the complexity of effects on cellular metabolism, vascular function, and respiration. Therefore, until definitive evidence is produced, both corrected and uncorrected blood gas values are of questionable utility in patients with significant deviations from 37°C.

The traditional approach to acid–base analysis

Any approach to clinical acid–base analysis must accurately identify the presence of an abnormality, quantify its magnitude, and offer insight into the nature and underlying cause. Acid–base physiology and analysis has a long history with over a hundred years of research and new additions to the literature every day. Newer approaches tend to build on or are modifications of previous approaches, so it is not surprising that the evolution of acid–base theory has led to considerable confusion for students and clinicians alike.

The first method that evolved is now referred to as the traditional or bicarbonate-based approach. It emerged from the work of Henderson and Hasselbach in the early 1900s and focuses on pCO_2 and HCO_3^- as key elements. This approach is responsible for much of the conventional acid–base terminology that is still commonly found in textbooks and continues to be used in many clinical situations. Consequently, a brief discussion of the traditional approach and related terminology will be included here.

Table 7.2.   Causes of acid–base abnormalities in dogs and cats classified according to the traditional approach

Metabolic acidosis	Metabolic alkalosis

• Diarrhea
• Renal tubular acidosis
• Dilutional acidosis (rapid 0.9% NaCl administration)
• Carbonic anhydrase inhibitors
• Ammonium chloride administration
• Cationic amino acid administration
• Hypoadrenocorticism
• Lactic acidosis
• Uremic acidosis
• Diabetic ketoacidosis
• Hyperphosphatemia
• Intoxication
  – ethylene glycol
  – salicylates
  – metaldehyde
	• Vomiting of stomach contents
	• Gastric suctioning
	• Thiazide or loop diuretics
	• Posthypercapneic alkalosis
	• Primary hyperaldosteronism
	• Hyperadrenocorticism
	• Oral administration of $NaHCO_3^-$
	• Oral administration of other organic anions
	• Refeeding syndrome
	• High dose penicillin derivative antibiotics
	• Severe potassium or magnesium deficiency

Respiratory acidosis	Respiratory alkalosis

• Airway obstruction
  – For example, aspiration, mass, tracheal collapse
• Central respiratory depression
  – For example, drug induced, neurological disease
• Neuromuscular disease
  – For example, myasthenia gravis, tetanus
• Increased CO_2 production with impaired ventilation
  – For example, heat stroke, malignant hyperthermia, cardiac arrest
• Restrictive extrapulmonary disorders
  – For example, diaphragmatic hernia, pleural space disease
• Intrinsic pulmonary disease
  – For example, pneumonia, pulmonary thromboembolism
• Ineffective mechanical ventilation
• Marked obesity (Pickwickian syndrome)
	• Hypoxia
	  – For example, severe hypotension, severe anemia, congestive heart failure
	• Pulmonary parenchymal disease
	  – For example, pneumonia, pulmonary thromboembolism
	• Centrally mediated hyperventilation
	  – For example, liver disease, hyperadrenocortism
	• Systemic inflammatory response syndrome
	• Exercise, excitement, pain, anxiety
	• Overzealous mechanical ventilation

Simple acid–base disorders

A simple acid–base disorder is one where there is a single primary etiologic disturbance. According to the traditional approach, there are four simple acid–base disorders to consider: (1) respiratory acidosis, (2) metabolic acidosis, (3) respiratory alkalosis, and (4) metabolic alkalosis. Respiratory disorders are caused by abnormal processes that alter pCO_2 levels, while metabolic disorders are caused by abnormal processes that alter $[HCO_3^-]$. A list of common causes of the four primary acid–base disorders in dogs and cats classified according to this approach can be found in Table 7.2.

Secondary or compensatory acid–base changes usually occur in response to most primary acid–base abnormalities in an effort to restore [H⁺] to normal. In simple acid–base disorders, these compensatory responses are predictable and a stepwise analysis is conducted according to Figure 7.1. With primary metabolic abnormalities, respiratory compensation involves either hyper- or hypoventilation. In most cases, the respiratory response occurs rapidly and is complete within hours, assuming the metabolic disturbance remains stable. With primary respiratory abnormalities, the compensatory response is biphasic. Acutely, the metabolic response is limited to chemical buffering, which may have a very modest impact on [HCO₃⁻]. With more chronic respiratory disorders, the kidneys respond and are able to excrete or reabsorb HCO₃⁻ as appropriate. This renal response is slow to be initiated and takes 2–5 days to reach its maximum potential.

The degree of expected compensation for acid–base disorders varies among species. In clinical canine patients, guidelines derived from healthy experimental dogs are commonly used and are presented in Table 7.3. There is limited data available for evaluating compensatory responses in cats but experimental evidence based on a small number of animals suggests cats do not appear to initiate a ventilatory response to metabolic acidosis. Consequently, extrapolation of canine values to feline patients may be misleading and cannot be recommended.

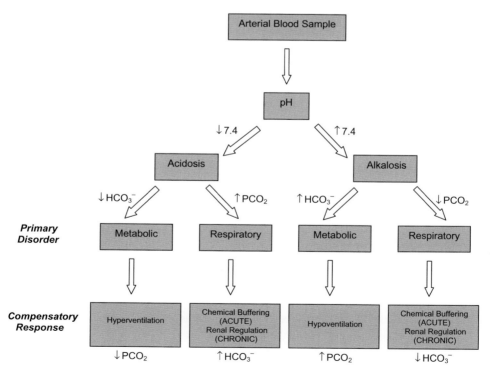

Figure 7.1.   Analysis of simple acid–base disorders according to the traditional approach.

Table 7.3. Expected compensatory changes to primary acid–base disorders in dogs according to the traditional approach

Primary disorder	Expected compensation
Metabolic acidosis	↓P_aCO_2 of 0.7 mm Hg per 1 mEq/L ↓HCO_3^- 3
Metabolic alkalosis	↑P_aCO_2 of 0.7 mm Hg per 1 mEq/L ↑HCO_3^- 3
Respiratory acidosis (acute)	↑HCO_3^- of 0.15 mEq/L per 1 mm Hg ↑P_aCO_2 2
Respiratory acidosis (chronic)	↑HCO_3^- of 0.35 mEq/L per 1 mm Hg ↑P_aCO_2 2
Respiratory alkalosis (acute)	↓HCO_3^- of 0.25 mEq/L per 1 mm Hg ↓P_aCO_2 2
Respiratory alkalosis (chronic)	↓HCO_3^- of 0.55 mEq/L per 1 mm Hg ↓P_aCO_2 2

Mixed acid–base disorders

A mixed acid–base disorder is present when there are two or more primary etiologic disturbances present simultaneously. Mixed disorders may be additive (such as respiratory and metabolic acidosis) or offsetting (such as respiratory alkalosis and metabolic acidosis) with regard to their effects on pH. A triple disorder is an example of a complex acid–base disorder where a respiratory disturbance further complicates concurrent metabolic acidosis and metabolic alkalosis. With the traditional approach, differentiating a mixed acid–base disorder from a simple disorder and its compensatory response is accomplished by evaluating the magnitude of the compensation as discussed above and shown in Table 7.3. If the compensatory response is not within the range expected for the primary disorder then a mixed disorder is diagnosed. Caution must be exercised when evaluating the appropriateness of metabolic compensation to a primary respiratory disorder as it will depend on the chronicity of the respiratory abnormality, which may be difficult to ascertain clinically.

In general, the possibility of a mixed acid–base disorder should be suspected if one or more of the following are observed: (1) the presence of a normal pH with abnormal PCO_2 and/or [HCO_3^-], (2) a pH change in a direction opposite that predicted for the known primary disorder, and (3) pCO_2 and [HCO_3^-] changing in opposite directions.

Mixed acid–base disorders are more difficult to decipher than simple disorders and a diagnosis must be made in the context of the patient's clinical signs and other diagnostic information. In most cases, the clinical significance of the acid–base perturbations will be a function of the underlying cause(s), which should become the focus of treatment.

Limitations of the traditional approach

While intuitively appealing and relatively simple in nature, the traditional bicarbonate-based approach remains essentially descriptive. In the mid-1960s, a group of researchers expanded on this concept in an attempt to better quantify and predict the nature of various acid–base disturbances. This approach, using acid–base maps or nomograms, became known as the Boston approach and these nomograms are still found in many textbooks. Unfortunately, the Boston/traditional approach has significant limitations. It fails to take into account the influence of nonbicarbonate buffer systems (i.e., plasma proteins and phosphate) as well as the effect of serum electrolytes (notably Na^+, K^+, and Cl^-). Also, it incorrectly assumes that both pCO_2 and HCO_3^- are independent variables when in fact only pCO_2 is independent.

Consequently, the traditional approach is unable to provide insight into complex mixed acid–base disorders and can actually be misleading in certain circumstances. Metabolic acidosis, in particular, poses significant problems for the traditional approach. This abnormality has been reported to be the most common acid–base disturbance in dogs and cats and accompanies such diverse conditions as sepsis, trauma, renal failure, and endocrine emergencies. In these settings, the traditional approach is not helpful. While it still retains a place in clinical acid–base analysis, its use should be reserved for patients with simple acid–base disorders and normal serum albumin and phosphate concentrations.

Alternative approaches to acid–base analysis

An increasing appreciation for the frequency and complexity of clinical acid–base disorders meant that better approaches for clinical assessment were sought. Highlights in the evolution of acid–base theory include the base excess approach, the anion gap approach, and the strong ion approach and its various modifications.

The base excess approach to acid–base analysis

The base excess approach (also referred to as the Copenhagen approach) was described by Sigaard-Andersen in the late 1950s as an attempt to better distinguish the relative contributions of the respiratory and metabolic components while still remaining faithful to the traditional concepts. The base deficit or excess (BDE) was defined as the amount of acid per unit volume that must be added to achieve a normal pH at a P_aCO_2 of 40 mm Hg using whole blood. This approach was later modified in the 1960s to use only serum base excess and the parameter became known as the standardized base excess (SBE). Like the Boston group, the Copenhagen group generated data based on large numbers of human patients, leading to the development of SBE nomograms to facilitate clinical acid–base assessment. Most modern automated blood gas analyzers report an SBE value calculated from this human data. While a canine SBE nomogram has been developed using this approach, it is rarely used because commercial blood gas analyzers are programmed specifically for human blood. In a broader sense, this approach has also met with criticism because the SBE parameter represents the net effect of all metabolic acid–base abnormalities. In the case of coexisting metabolic acidosis and alkalosis, for example, SBE alone may fail to identify any acid–base abnormality as these two disturbances could apparently cancel each other out.

The anion gap approach to acid–base analysis

The anion gap approach was developed in 1975 by Emmit et al. and has proven to be a useful tool in the analysis of certain mixed acid–base disorders. The anion gap (AG) is calculated clinically as the difference between the major cations and anions that are commonly measured in plasma as shown below:

$$AG = ([Na^+]+[K^+])-([Cl^-]+[HCO_3^-])$$

In reality, because electroneutrality must be maintained, there is no actual difference between the total number of cations and anions in plasma, so what the AG really represents is the difference between unmeasured cations and anions. Since changes in unmeasured cations of the magnitude necessary to impact AG do not occur clinically, AG is essentially a tool used to estimate the concentration of unmeasured anions.

Under normal circumstances, plasma proteins make up the majority of the unmeasured anions represented by the AG, and normal AG values are approximately 12–24 mEq/L in dogs and 13–27 mEq/L in cats. In metabolic acidosis, calculation of the AG may be useful in identifying the underlying cause, as different pathological states will impact the AG differently.

In the case of organic acidosis, fixed acids such as lactic acid or ketoacids are added to plasma where they rapidly dissociate into their anions (which are not measured as part of a typical biochemical profile) and H^+ (which is buffered by HCO_3^-). The net effect is a decrease in measured anions (i.e., HCO_3^-) with no change in Cl^-, leading to an increased AG. These types of acidosis are therefore classified as increased AG or normochloremic metabolic acidosis. In contrast, the loss of HCO_3^- that may accompany gastrointestinal fluid loss or renal tubular acidosis is associated with Cl^- retention so the AG doesn't change. Consequently, these types of acidosis are classified as normal AG or hyperchloremic metabolic acidosis. Causes of metabolic acidosis classified according to the AG approach are shown in Table 7.4.

Table 7.4. Causes of metabolic acidosis in dogs and cats classified according to the AG approach

Metabolic acidosis
Normal AG (hyperchloremia)
• Diarrhea
• Renal tubular acidosis
• Dilutional acidosis (rapid 0.9% NaCl administration)
• Carbonic anhydrase inhibitors
• Ammonium chloride administration
• Cationic amino acid administration
• Hypoadrenocorticism
Increased AG (normochloremia)
• Lactic acidosis
• Uremic acidosis
• Diabetic ketoacidosis
• Hyperphosphatemia
• Intoxication
– Ethylene glycol
– Salicylates
– Metaldehyde

A significant factor that confounds interpretation of the AG is hypoalbuminemia. Since albumin is the major unmeasured anion in the normal state, the presence of hypoalbuminemia will decrease the AG and obscure the presence of anions, which would otherwise increase it. In other words, a patient with concurrent lactic acidosis and hypoalbuminemia may have a normal calculated AG and this would be clinically misleading. In dogs, the AG can be adjusted for changes in protein concentration by using the following formula:

$$AG_{alb\ adj} = AG + 4.2(3.77 - [\text{albumin measured in g/dL}])$$

While not as substantial as the effect of albumin, phosphate can also impact the AG. In dogs, the AG can be adjusted for both albumin and phosphate by using the following formula:

$$AG_{alb\ phos\ adj} = AG + 4.2(3.77 - [\text{albumin measured in g/dL}])$$
$$+ (2.52 - 0.58[\text{phosphorous measured in mg/dL}])$$

While the AG is a useful tool in certain situations it remains limited in its ability to elucidate complex mixed acid–base disorders. Attempts to optimize its usefulness have been explored in humans and have led to the concept of the delta ratio or the delta gap. Both of these parameters attempt to relate the change in AG to the change in $[HCO_3^-]$, each from their respective reference values. Neither the delta ratio nor the delta gap has been studied in dogs or cats.

The strong ion approach to acid–base analysis

In 1983, Stewart published his now widely accepted model of acid–base physiology, which has been referred to by various names including the Stewart approach, the quantitative approach, the physicochemical approach, and the strong ion approach. According to Stewart there are three independent determinants of acid–base balance: (1) pCO_2, (2) the difference between strong cations and strong anions (strong ion difference or SID), and (3) the total concentration of weak acids (A_{TOT}). As is the case with the traditional approach, the pCO_2 variable is the primary determinant of the respiratory component of plasma pH. The SID and A_{TOT} variables provide independent measures of the metabolic component of plasma pH. Therefore, according to the strong ion approach, there are four possible primary metabolic acid–base disorders instead of only two with the traditional approach. Metabolic acidosis is caused by a decrease in SID or an increase in A_{TOT}, while metabolic alkalosis is caused by an increase in SID or a decrease in A_{TOT}. Please refer to Table 7.5 for common metabolic acid–base disorders classified according to the strong ion approach.

SID

Strong ions (also known as nonbuffer ions) are defined as any ion that is completely dissociated at physiological pH and include Na^+, K^+, Ca^{2+}, Mg^{2+}, and Cl^-, as well as

Table 7.5. Causes of metabolic acid–base abnormalities classified according to the strong ion approach

SID acidosis ($\downarrow$ SID)	SID alkalosis ($\uparrow$ SID)
Dilution acidosis ($\downarrow$ Na$^+$)	**Concentration alkalosis ($\uparrow$ Na$^+$)**
• With hypervolemia	• Pure water loss
– Severe liver disease	– Water deprivation
– Congestive heart failure	– Diabetes insipidus
– Nephrotic syndrome	• Hypotonic fluid loss
• With normovolemia	– Vomiting
– Psychogenic polydipsia	– Nonoliguric renal failure
– Hypotonic fluid infusion	– Postobstructive diuresis
• With hypovolemia	**Hypochloremic alkalosis ($\downarrow$ Cl$^-_{corr}$)**
– Vomiting	• Gain of Na$^+$ relative to Cl$^-$
– Diarrhea	– Isotonic or hypertonic
– Hypoadrenocorticism	NaHCO$_3^-$ administration
– Third space loss	• Loss of Cl$^-$ relative to Na$^+$
– Diuretic administration	– Vomiting of stomach contents
Hyperchloremic acidosis ($\uparrow$ Cl$^-_{corr}$)	– Thiazide or loop diuretics
• Loss of Na$^+$ relative to Cl$^-$	
– Diarrhea	
• Gain of Cl$^-$ relative to Na$^+$	
– Fluid therapy (0.9% NaCl, 7.2% NaCl, KCl-supplemented fluids	
• Cl$^-$ retention	
– Renal failure	
– Hypoadrenocorticism	
Organic acidosis ($\uparrow$ unmeasured strong ions)	
• Uremic, keto- or lactic acidosis	
• Toxicities	
– Ethylene glycol	
– Salicylate	
A$_{TOT}$ acidosis ($\uparrow$ A$_{TOT}$)	**A$_{TOT}$ alkalosis ($\downarrow$A$_{TOT}$)**
Hyperalbuminemia	**Hypoalbuminemia**
• Water deprivation	• Decreased production
Hyperphosphatemia	– Chronic liver disease
• Translocation	– Acute phase response to inflammation
– Tumor cell lysis	– Malnutrition/starvation
– Tissue trauma/rhabdomyolysis	• Extracorporeal loss
• Increased intake	– Protein-losing nephropathy
– Phosphate-containing enemas	– Protein-losing enteropathy
– Intravenous phosphate	• Sequestration
• Decreased loss	– Inflammatory effusions
– Renal failure	– Vasculitis
– Urethral obstruction	
– Uroabdomen	

unmeasured ions such as lactate, β-hydroxybutyrate, acetoacetate, and sulfate. The SID is a term used to describe the difference between the sum of strong cations and the sum of strong anions. It is usually represented by the following equation (where $[A^-]$ refers to all unmeasured strong anions):

$$SID = ([Na^+]+[K^+]+[Ca^{2+}]+[Mg^{2+}])-([Cl^-]+[A^-])$$

Under physiologically normal conditions, the SID of plasma is approximately 40–44 mEq/L and this difference is balanced by the negative charge on HCO_3^- and A_{TOT}. Under pathological conditions, additional strong anions accumulate and $[A^-]$ becomes clinically significant, indicating organic acidosis. The SID may be calculated by measuring as many strong ions as possible and summing their charges. This original definition has now come to be known as the apparent SID (SID_{app}), which distinguishes it from the effective SID (to be discussed later). With the capability to routinely measure lactate concentrations in the clinical setting, some recommend the addition of [lactate] to the SID_{app} calculation as follows:

$$SID_{app} = ([Na^+]+[K^+]+[Ca^{2+}]+[Mg^{2+}])-([Cl^-]+[lactate])$$

In fact, because Na^+ and Cl^- are quantitatively the most important strong ions, SID_{app} is often further simplified in clinical situations as follows:

$$SID_{app\ simpl} = [Na^+]+[Cl^-]$$

Concentration of weak acids (A_{TOT})

Stewart used the term A_{TOT} to reflect the sum of all weak acids in both the dissociated and undissociated states (i.e., A^- plus HA) according to the law of conservation of mass. The major contributors to A_{TOT} are albumin, globulins, and inorganic phosphate, and these weak acids are also sometimes referred to as buffer ions. Changes in the concentrations of any of these, either directly or through changes to plasma free water content, will affect pH.

Simplifications of the strong ion approach

The strong ion approach provides a sound mechanistic framework to explain why plasma pH changes in any setting and successfully integrates electrolyte and acid–base physiology. Unfortunately, Stewart's equations are mathematically complex and thus not easily applicable to the clinical setting. Consequently, a number of simplified modifications have been developed to facilitate clinical use of Stewart's strong ion approach.

The effective SID modification

Some 10 years after Stewart published his strong ion theory, Figge et al. proposed a modification to Stewart's approach, which attempts to quantify the effects of unmeasured strong anions using a parameter that he referred to as the strong ion gap (SIG). The term effective SID (SID_{eff}) was proposed to represent the contribution of weak acids.

Therefore, unmeasured strong anions (i.e., the SIG) can be estimated by subtracting the SID_{eff} (calculated using formulas involving the weak acids HCO_3^-, albumin, and phosphate) from the SID_{app} (calculated according to the equation presented previously). Despite its potential usefulness in humans, Figge's formulas for calculation of SID_{eff} are complex and have not been evaluated in dogs and cats, so this approach is not currently feasible in veterinary medicine. The general concept of the SIG, however, has been revisited by others and will be discussed again below.

The base excess modification

In 1993, Fencl et al. published an additional modification of the Stewart approach that resurrected the concept of SBE and combined this with principles of the strong ion theory. The so-called Fencl–Stewart approach uses a set of equations to estimate the magnitude of effect of changes in SID and A_{TOT} on the SBE value reported by blood gas analyzers. Equations for four distinct parameters have been proposed that can be calculated based on routine laboratory measurements: (1) the albumin effect or SBE_{Alb}, (2) the phosphate effect or SBE_{Phos}, (3) the free water effect or SBE_{FW} (based on sodium), and (4) the chloride effect or SBE_{Cl}. With the availability of lactate analyzers, a fifth parameter, the lactate effect or SBE_{Lact}, can also be calculated. A sixth effect, the unmeasured strong ion effect or SBE_{XA}, can then be calculated by subtracting the sum of the individual SBE effects from the reported SBE value or $SBE_{reported}$ (see Table 7.6). Some authors use different terminology and refer to the SBE_{XA} as the base excess gap (BEG). Values of SBE_{XA} less than $-5\,mEq/L$ are suggestive of an increase in unmeasured strong anions.

Table 7.6. Formulas for calculating contributions of key parameters according to the base excess modification of the strong ion approach

SBE effect (in mEq/L)	Formulas
Effects relating to A_{TOT}:	
(1) SBE_{Alb}	$3.7([Alb_{normal\ ref}] - [Alb_{measured}])$ in g/dL
	$0.37([Alb_{normal\ ref}] - [Alb_{measured}])$ in g/L)
(2) SBE_{Phos}	$1.8([Phos_{normal\ ref}] - [Phos_{measured}])$ in mmol/L
	$0.58([Phos_{normal\ ref}] - [Phos_{measured}])$ in mg/dL
Effects relating to SID:	
(3) SBE_{FW}	Dogs $0.25([Na^+_{measured}] - [Na^+_{normal\ ref}])$ in mEq/L
	Cats $0.22([Na^+_{measured}] - [Na^+_{normal\ ref}])$ in mEq/L
(4) SBE_{Cl}	$[Cl^-_{normal\ ref}] - [Cl^-_{corr}]$ in mEq/L,
	where $Cl^-_{corr} = [Cl^-_{measured}] \times ([Na^+_{normal\ ref}]/[Na^+_{measured}])$
(5) SBE_{Lact}	$-1[Lact_{measured}]$ in mmol/L
(6) SBE_{XA} (also known as BEG)	$SBE_{reported} - (SBE_{Alb} + SBE_{Phos} + SBE_{FW} + SBE_{Cl} + SBE_{Lact})$

See text for additional definitions.
$Alb_{normal\ ref}$, midpoint of the albumin reference range; $Alb_{measured}$, patient's albumin concentration; $Phos_{normal\ ref}$, midpoint of the phosphorous reference range; $Phos_{measured}$, patient's phosphorous concentration; $Na^+_{normal\ ref}$, midpoint of the sodium reference range; $Na^+_{measured}$, patient's sodium concentration; $Cl^-_{normal\ ref}$, midpoint of chloride reference range; Cl^-_{corr}, corrected chloride; $Cl^-_{measured}$, patient's chloride concentration; $Lact_{measured}$, patient's lactate concentration.

Table 7.7. Summary of metabolic acid–base influences identified by the base excess modification of the strong ion approach

Acidifying influences	Individual SBE effect
Hyperalbuminemia	↓ SBE_{Alb}
Hyperphosphatemia	↓ SBE_{Phos}
Free water excess (Hyponatremia)	↓ SBE_{FW}
Hyperchloremia	↓ SBE_{Cl}
Hyperlactatemia	↓ SBE_{Lact}
Increased unmeasured strong anions	↓ SBE_{XA} (<−5 mmol/L is clinically significant)
Alkalinizing influences	**Individual SBE effect**
Hypoalbuminemia	↑ SBE_{Alb}
Free water deficit (hypernatremia)	↑ SBE_{FW}
Hypochloremia	↑ SBE_{Cl}

This approach facilitates identification of various metabolic acid–base influences and allows their contribution to the overall SBE to be estimated (see Table 7.7). This approach provides the clinician with a more complete picture of a patient's acid–base status because it takes into consideration more contributing factors. Though there are presently no controlled studies evaluating the accuracy of these formulas in dogs and cats, there is anecdotal evidence to suggest that this approach is helpful in understanding complex acid–base disorders in these species.

The simplified SIG modification

As discussed previously, the SIG represents the difference between all unmeasured strong cations and anions. While SIG is undoubtedly a useful concept, calculation of this parameter using Figge's formulas for SID_{eff} (discussed previously) remains mathematically challenging and is not clinically applicable to dogs and cats. Fortunately, a simplification of the SIG (SIG_{simpl}) incorporating the AG has been developed that is useful in these species. The SIG_{simpl} offers a more accurate approach to identifying unmeasured strong anions in plasma than does the AG because the AG is not specific to strong ions. Unlike SIG_{simpl}, the uncorrected AG also includes the effects of nonvolatile buffer ions such as albumin, globulins, and phosphate. Since albumin is the most important of these buffers in plasma, it is included in the formula for calculation of the SIG_{simpl}. In dogs at a plasma pH of 7.4, the calculation is as follows:

$$SIG_{simpl} = [albumin_{measured} \text{ in } g/dL] \times 4.9 - AG$$

In cats at a plasma pH of 7.35, the calculation is as follows:

$$SIG_{simpl} = [albumin_{measured} \text{ in } g/dL] \times 7.4 - AG$$

An increase in unmeasured strong anions is suspected when the SIG_{simpl} is less than −5 mEq/L. In patients with significant hyperphosphatemia, however, the AG should be corrected for phosphorous (refer to section on AG) prior to calculating the SIG_{simpl}. While controlled studies in dogs and cats evaluating the SIG_{simpl} have not been published at this time, this approach appears very promising as a clinical tool for acid–base analysis in these species.

Regulation of fluid balance

Fluid therapy is a supportive measure used commonly in the management of fluid, electrolyte, and acid–base disorders in veterinary medicine. As is the case with other symptomatic treatment modalities, it is always necessary to identify and correct the underlying cause if normal fluid balance is to be definitively restored. The ability to design an appropriate fluid therapy plan for a patient requires at least a basic understanding of the applied physiology of body fluids.

Fluid balance terminology

Total body water (TBW)   The sum of body water comprises approximately 60% of body weight.

ICF compartment   The sum of body water contained within cells; comprises approximately 40% of body weight or approximately 67% of TBW.

ECF compartment   The sum of body water not contained within cells; comprises approximately 20% of body weight or approximately 33% of TBW.

Interstitial fluid compartment   A subcompartment of the ECF containing body water located in the spaces surrounding cells; comprises approximately 15% of body weight, 25% of TBW, or 75% of the ECF.

Intravascular fluid (plasma) compartment   A subcompartment of the ECF containing body water located within blood vessels; comprises approximately 5% of body weight, 8% of TBW, or 25% of the ECF.

Blood volume   The sum of plasma water volume and red cell volume; comprises approximately 8–9% of body weight in dogs (i.e., 80–90 mL/kg) and 6–7% of body weight in cats (i.e., 60–70 mL/kg).

Transcellular fluid compartment   A subcompartment of the ECF containing cerebrospinal fluid, gastrointestinal fluid, bile, glandular secretions, respiratory secretions, synovial fluid, and renal tubular fluid; comprises approximately 1% body weight.

Electrolyte   A substance that dissociates in solution to form electrically charged particles or ions; usually expressed in millimoles per liter or milliequivalents per liter.

Osmosis   The process whereby water moves down a concentration gradient across a semipermeable membrane.

Osmotic pressure   The pressure required to prevent water from moving down a concentration gradient across a semipermeable membrane .

Osmole (Osm)   A unit of osmotic pressure equivalent to 1 mol of any nondissociable substance.

Osmolarity   The number of osmoles per kilogram of solvent; expressed as milliosmoles per kilogram.

Osmolality   The number of osmoles per liter of solution; expressed as milliosmoles per liter; in biologic fluids, there is a negligible difference between osmolality and osmolarity.

Ineffective osmole   An osmole that is able to cross fluid compartment membranes and therefore cannot generate osmotic pressure; for example, urea.

Effective osmole   An osmole that is unable to cross fluid compartment membranes and therefore generates osmotic pressure; for example, glucose.

Tonicity   A measure of the effective osmolality of a solution; the tonicity of a solution may be less than the measured osmolality if both effective and ineffective osmoles are present.

Colloid osmotic pressure (COP)   The component of total osmotic pressure in plasma contributed by colloids measured using an oncometer; also known as oncotic pressure.

Fluid and electrolyte distribution

Though it is convenient to compartmentalize body fluids as outlined in the definitions above, in reality the water and solutes in these spaces are in dynamic equilibrium across cell membranes, capillary endothelium, and other specialized lining cells. Electrolytes are not distributed evenly across the major compartments as membrane permeability varies for different solutes. Approximate electrolyte concentrations in each of the three major fluid compartments are shown in Table 7.8. In pathological states, fluid volumes and electrolyte concentrations may fluctuate dramatically and changes to one compartment will invariably impact the others.

Hypotonic fluid loss refers to loss of water in excess of solute, which causes water to shift from the intracellular space into the interstitial space and ultimately into the intravascular space. Thus the osmolality of the ECF is increased relative to the ICF. Hypotonic fluid loss is characterized clinically by signs of dehydration including dry, tacky mucous membranes and decreased skin turgor.

Hypertonic fluid loss refers to loss of solute in excess of water that causes water to move out of the intravascular and interstitial spaces and into cells via an osmotic gradient. Clinically, this is characterized by decreased perfusion and hypovolemia.

Isotonic fluid loss refers to loss of water and solute in comparable proportions so there are no osmotically mediated shifts in water between the ICF and ECF. Clinical signs of

Table 7.8.   Approximate distribution of electrolytes across fluid compartments (milliequivalents per liter)

Ion	Plasma	Interstitial fluid	ICF
Na^+	142	145	13
K^+	5	4	155
Ca^{2+}	5	3	2
Mg^{2+}	2	2	35
Cl^-	106	115	2
HCO_3^-	24	30	10
Phosphates	2	2	113
Sulfates	1	1	20
Protein	16	1	60

isotonic fluid loss, if of sufficient magnitude, may also result in hypoperfusion and hypovolemia.

Considerations for perianesthetic fluid therapy

The act of inducing and maintaining anesthesia, even in a healthy animal, will disrupt the normal mechanisms of fluid balance to some extent. In a dehydrated or hypovolemic patient, this disruption can have serious consequences both during and after anesthesia. Fluid therapy is recommended as a supportive measure in anesthetized dogs and cats for the following reasons: (1) to establish and maintain venous access, (2) to counteract physiological changes associated with anesthetics, (3) to replace insensible fluids lost during anesthesia, and (4) to correct fluid losses caused by preexisting disease or trauma and to replace ongoing losses associated with the procedure (often surgery).

Patient status

Prior to inducing anesthesia it is optimal if the patient's fluid balance is normal or as close to normal as possible. In healthy animals presenting for elective procedures this is usually not an issue. In compromised patients, however, there may be one or more fluid disturbances present that may or may not be related to the original presenting complaint. It is imperative that these are recognized and addressed by initiating an appropriate fluid therapy plan. Some fluid disturbances may require immediate and aggressive intervention while many chronic or longstanding abnormalities are best corrected more gradually. The following discussion highlights some of the most common fluid balance abnormalities encountered in dogs and cats.

Hypovolemia

Hypovolemia is documented in a wide range of trauma and disease states and may be a result of (1) fluid loss from the intravascular space specifically (e.g., hemorrhage), (2) fluid loss from multiple fluid compartments (e.g., dehydration), or (3) relative fluid deficiency caused by a decrease in vascular tone (e.g., anesthetic-induced vasodilation in animals with otherwise normal fluid balance). The most serious consequence of hypovolemia is decreased cardiac preload, resulting in diminished cardiac output (CO), inadequate tissue perfusion, and impaired oxygen delivery. The term shock is used to describe global impairment of tissue perfusion and oxygenation.

Depending on the severity and nature of the fluid deficit, hypovolemia may be effectively managed with crystalloids, synthetic colloids, blood products, or a combination of all of these. With acute hemorrhage, loss of up to 30% of the blood volume can typically be managed with crystalloids with or without colloids, while loss of 50% of blood volume will likely require blood component therapy in addition to the above options. Specific strategies for fluid resuscitation of the hypovolemic patient vary depending on the cause (e.g., hemorrhage vs. nonhemorrhage) and the time frame (e.g., acute vs. chronic).

Anemia

Anemia may occur in the absence of any changes in plasma volume (e.g., with red blood cell destruction), or it may be accompanied by hypovolemia (e.g., with severe hemorrhage). In both cases, adequate oxygen delivery to tissues can potentially be compromised. In the chronically anemic, normovolemic animal with normal cardiovascular function, compensatory increases in CO and changes in the affinity of hemoglobin for oxygen are initiated to maintain oxygen delivery. In anemic animals with concurrent cardiovascular dysfunction, this ability to compensate is diminished. The administration of anesthetic agents to an otherwise compensated, chronically anemic animal may also precipitate decompensation, as both injectable and inhalant anesthetics depress the cardiovascular system. In animals that are both anemic and hypovolemic, as in the case of severe hemorrhage, the impact on oxygen delivery in the acute setting may be profound.

While most texts recommend "considering" administration of a blood product when hematocrit drops below 20–25% in dogs and 18–20% in cats, it is not possible to identify a single hemoglobin or hematocrit "trigger" for any species. The decision to initiate red blood cell transfusion can only be made on a case-by-case basis and must take into account all physiological factors related to the patient as well as any procedural factors such as whether or not a major surgery is planned.

Hypoproteinemia

Hypoproteinemia (usually hypoalbuminemia) results in a decrease in COP, which favors the movement of fluid out of the intravascular and into the interstitial compartment. The administration of intravenous crystalloids increases hydrostatic pressure and, in the face of low COP, the potential for capillary leakage and development of tissue edema is enhanced. This is especially problematic in patients with critical illness as they are predisposed to development of both hypoalbuminemia and increased capillary permeability associated with inflammatory conditions. Management of fluid balance in hypoproteinemic states may involve small volumes of crystalloids, synthetic colloids, and other albumin-containing fluids such as stored plasma, fresh frozen plasma (FFP), and possibly human serum albumin. In critically ill animals, it is generally recommended that serum albumin concentrations be maintained >1.5–2.0 g/dL (15–20 g/L).

Hyponatremia

Hyponatremia is defined as a serum sodium concentration <140 mEq/L in dogs and <149 mEq/L in cats. Clinical signs may be subtle or absent in chronic disorders characterized by slower decreases in sodium and plasma osmolality. Typically, concentrations <125 mEq/L result in early signs of toxicity while concentrations <120 mEq/L are associated with severe signs such as seizures or cerebral edema. Treatment of hyponatremia should focus on identifying and managing the underlying disease and, only if necessary, increasing serum sodium concentration and plasma osmolality. Isotonic crystalloids, synthetic colloids, and occasionally hypertonic saline are treatment options. Rapid increases in sodium can result in osmotic myelination syndrome or myelinosis, which can occur one to several days after therapy. In patients without neurological deficits, serum sodium concentration should not increase more than 0.5 mEq/L/h (note that this refers to the patient's reported sodium concentration, not the rate of supplementation). In patients exhibiting signs of cerebral edema, serum sodium concentrations may be corrected more quickly (at 1–2 mEq/L/h) until neurological symptoms resolve and then decreased again to 0.5 mEq/L/h. In most cases, the target serum sodium concentration is 120–125 mEq/L.

Hypernatremia

Hypernatremia is defined as a serum sodium concentration >155 mEq/L in dogs and >162 mEq/L in cats. Increases in sodium concentrations >170 mEq/L result in early signs of toxicity while concentrations >180 mEq/L are associated with severe neurological deficits. Treatment of hypernatremia must focus on correction of the underlying problem and other fluid balance abnormalities. Isotonic and hypotonic crystalloids are treatment options. Rapid correction can result in acute cerebral edema, which may manifest as seizures or coma. In general, when serum sodium is >165–170 mEq/L, correction should proceed slowly and serum sodium concentration should not decrease more than 0.5 mEq/L/h depending on the inciting cause and concurrent fluid balance.

Hypokalemia

Hypokalemia in both dogs and cats is defined as a serum potassium concentration <3.6 mEq/L and is documented more often in cats. Clinical signs of hypokalemia include muscle weakness, cardiac arrhythmias, hypotension, and renal insufficiency with associated metabolic acidosis. It is important to recognize that the class I antiarrhythmic agents (e.g., lidocaine, procainamide) will be ineffective when administered to a hypokalemic patient. It is generally recommended that the maximal rate of potassium supplementation (typically as potassium chloride) is 0.5 mEq/kg/h, although higher rates may be employed (i.e., up to 1 mEq/kg/h) if the deficit is severe and the patient can be closely monitored. Note that in order to accomplish these rates of administration, the solutions infused will have high potassium concentrations and therefore high osmolality. Consequently, administration though a central line may be indicated.

Hyperkalemia

Hyperkalemia is defined as a serum potassium concentration >5.5 mEq/L in the dog and >5.0 mEq/L in the cat. Clinical signs include muscle weakness and cardiac arrhythmias with the most severe abnormalities associated with urinary system pathology. Animals with moderate hyperkalemia (6–7 mEq/L) are more likely to develop arrhythmias during anesthesia even if they have not exhibited abnormal electrocardiographic abnormalities earlier. Management strategies for hyperkalemia may include infusion of crystalloids in cases of circulatory collapse; administration of calcium chloride or calcium gluconate to temporarily restore the gradient between resting and threshold membrane potentials and stabilize cardiac electrical activity; dextrose with regular insulin to facilitate movement of potassium into cells while avoiding hyperglycemia; and sodium bicarbonate to treat acidemia.

Hypocalcemia

Hypocalcemia is defined as a total serum calcium concentration <2.0 mmol/L (8 mg/dL) in both dogs and cats. Ionized calcium should also be measured where possible and normal values are typically 50% of total serum calcium. Clinical signs of hypocalcemia may include tetany, seizures, hyperthermia, and cardiac arrhythmias. Cardiac electrical abnormalities may manifest as a prolonged QT interval and/or ventricular arrhythmias. Treatment involves calcium gluconate supplementation infused slowly over 10–30 minutes while monitoring the electrocardiogram followed by a maintenance infusion if necessary in critically ill patients. Fluid therapy with a crystalloid is typically indicated to manage fluid balance and counteract hyperthermia.

Hypercalcemia

Hypercalcemia is defined as a fasting serum calcium concentration >3.0 mmol/L (12 g/dL) in both dogs and cats. It is most commonly associated with neoplastic lesions, toxin ingestion, or hyperparathyroidism. Clinical signs may include muscle weakness, seizures, and less commonly cardiac arrhythmias. Potential rhythm disturbances include bradycardia, prolonged PR interval, wide QRS complexes, and shortened QT interval. Management of hypercalcemia is dependent on the underlying cause and surgery for neoplasia or parathyroidectomy should be performed if indicated. Lowering serum calcium prior to anesthesia and surgery is recommended where possible. Strategies to accomplish this may involve crystalloids, phosphorus binding agents, furosemide, prednisone, salmon calcitonin, and sodium bicarbonate.

Hypoglycemia

Hypoglycemia is defined as a blood glucose concentration <65 mg/dL (3.5 mmol/L) in both dogs and cats. Clinical signs will vary depending on whether blood glucose levels fall rapidly or slowly. Rapid declines are associated with dilated pupils, tachycardia, tremors, vocalization, and intense hunger. Slower declines may result in hypothermia, visual impairment, weakness, ataxia, depression, somnolence, seizures, and bradycardia. Obviously in the anesthetized patient these signs will be absent and, unless blood glucose is being monitored, hypoglycemia may go undetected. Hypoglycemia is most often recognized in neonates, patients with insulinomas, or patients with portosystemic shunts. Management of hypoglycemia will depend on the clinical setting but may involve 50% Karo corn syrup (ACH Food Companies Inc.,Cordova, TN) applied to the gums, intravenous dextrose boluses, or 2.5–5% dextrose infusions.

Hyperglycemia

Moderate hyperglycemia is commonly documented in dogs and cats that are stressed or diabetic. In cases of diabetic ketoacidosis glucose concentrations are usually >300 mg/dL (17 mmol/L) while in hyperglycemic hyperosmolar syndrome concentrations may be >600 mg/dL (33 mmol/L) with effective serum osmolality >320–330 mOsm/L. Treatment strategies for these life-threatening conditions are complex and require intensive monitoring over an extended period of time. Therapies typically include crystalloids with electrolyte supplementation, sodium bicarbonate, insulin, and dextrose.

Metabolic acidosis or alkalosis

Metabolic acid–base disorders should be addressed by correcting the underlying cause where possible and stabilizing fluid balance with a crystalloid (either an acidifying or alkalinizing solution as appropriate) along with other types of fluids if indicated.

Dehydration

Dehydration refers to a net loss of fluid from the body. Depending on the underlying cause the fluid lost may be hypotonic, isotonic, or hypertonic. Therefore, dehydration may impact the intravascular, interstitial, and intracellular compartments to varying degrees. The magnitude of dehydration is often estimated clinically based on history and physical exam findings and categorized as a percentage (usually as <5%, 5–6%, 6–8%, 8–10%, 10–12%, and >12% dehydration). Patients estimated to have >12% dehydration are considered to be in shock. The dehydration replacement volume required (in liters) can be estimated by multiplying this percentage (expressed as a decimal) by the patient's body weight (in kilograms). The fluid therapy plan for managing dehydration will depend on the magnitude of the deficit, the time frame, and a variety of other factors specific to the clinical situation. Crystalloids are the mainstay of treatment in most cases, along with electrolyte supplementation as indicated.

Preexisting disease states

Fluid balance has the potential to be altered in almost any disease state characterized by organ system or endocrine dysfunction, and fluid therapy plans will vary widely depending on the underlying condition.

Cardiovascular disease   Fluid balance is absolutely critical in patients with cardiac dysfunction as the failing heart is unable to deal with fluid deficits or excesses. The goal of the fluid therapy plan is to optimize fluid balance and cardiovascular function and it must take into account the following: (1) the type of cardiac disease (i.e., systolic vs. diastolic dysfunction), (2) the severity of the dysfunction (i.e., compensated vs. decompensated disease), (3) the presence of other concurrent abnormalities affecting fluid balance (such as hypovolemia, anemia, dehydration, electrolyte disturbances, etc.), and (4) the nature of any planned procedures (such as invasive surgery).

Renal disease   Because the kidneys play a key role in maintaining fluid and acid–base homeostasis, fluid balance in the patient with chronic renal disease or acute renal injury will invariably be compromised. Urine constitutes the primary sensible fluid loss in the normal state and derangements in urine production (either increases or decreases) are hallmarks of renal failure. The goal of fluid therapy in these patients is to restore fluid balance if possible and prevent further renal injury that may result from hypoperfusion.

Hemostatic disorders   Common hemostatic disorders in dogs and cats include immune-mediated hemolytic thromobocytopenia, disseminated intravascular coagulation, von Willebrand's disease, rodenticide toxicity, and hepatic failure. In all cases of these, fluid balance should be corrected and electrolyte and acid–base abnormalities addressed. Vitamin K may be indicated in cases of chronic hepatic disease or rodenticide toxicity, while FFP is often administered to supply coagulation factors and control potential hemorrhage. Tranfusion of cellular blood components (packed red blood cells [PRBCs] or fresh whole blood) may be indicated in anemic animals, while transfusion of platelet-containing products (fresh whole blood or platelet-rich plasma) may be indicated in animals with significant thrombocytopenia.

Endocrine disease   Common endocrine diseases that impact fluid balance in dogs and cats include diabetes insipidus, diabetes mellitus, hyperadrenocorticism, hypoadrenocorticism, hyperthyroidism, and hypothyroidism. In all cases, assessment of fluid, electrolyte, and acid–base balance should be a part of the initial diagnostic evaluation and the fluid therapy plan must address all of these abnormalities in the context of the patient's specific disease.

Considerations for fluid delivery and administration

As the practice of veterinary medicine has become increasingly sophisticated, so has the evolution of fluid therapy in canine and feline patients. While the subcutaneous or intraosseous routes may have advantages in certain clinical situations, the intravenous route has emerged as the route of choice for parenteral fluid therapy in a wide range of patients. Fluids administered intravenously should be warmed to 37°C before being infused, especially if they will be administered rapidly and/or in large volumes.

Intravenous access may be obtained using one of the following types of catheters: (1) winged needle catheters, (2) over-the-needle catheters, (3) through-the-needle catheters, and (4) catheters placed with the aid of an introducer and guide wire. Catheter selection depends on the indication for fluid administration, the type and volume of fluid required, the planned site of catheter placement (peripheral vs. central vein), the planned duration of catheter placement, the size of the patient, the experience of the operator, the availability of catheter products, and cost.

Common catheter materials include polyethylene, polyurethane, silicone elastomer, and polyvinyl chloride (PVC). These vary in their reactivity, stiffness, and thrombogenicity. Over-the-needle catheters are used extensively in routine clinical practice because they are easy to insert into canine and feline peripheral veins, are cost effective, and are well-suited for situations where fluid therapy needs are short term (i.e., usually less than 72 hours). For dogs and cats, standard over-the-needle catheter sizes range from 24 to 14 gauge, with 22, 20, and 18 gauge being used most commonly.

If rapid volume administration is indicated, it is important to place the largest-diameter catheter possible. The maximal rate of fluid flow increases as the radius of the catheter lumen is increased. For catheters less than 14 gauge in diameter, this relationship is linear, but for larger catheters the flow rate increases geometrically with size and is proportional to the lumen of the radius raised to the fourth power (r^4).

There are many different types of fluid administration sets available. Most have one or more injection or connection ports that facilitate simultaneous infusion of multiple compatible solutions through a single catheter. All sets use an in-line drip chamber to visualize and estimate the rate of flow. Depending on the brand, drip sizes are calibrated so that 1 mL equals 10, 15, 20, or 60 drops. If an automated fluid pump is not available, the number of drops per minute required to deliver a particular volume over a particular time period can be calculated according to the following formula:

$$Drops/minute = (total\ infusion\ volume \times drops/mL\ of\ drip\ set)/$$
$$total\ infusion\ time\ in\ minutes$$

The drip rate can then be set manually using the in-line roller clamp to control the rate of flow in the drip chamber. Electronic fluid pumps are now commonly found in many veterinary practices and ensure more accurate fluid delivery. The use of a fluid pump or syringe pump is recommended in very small patients that may be easily overhydrated or in patients with critical illness requiring intensive fluid therapy.

Assessing fluid balance and monitoring response to therapy

As there is no single quantitative method to definitively measure fluid balance in a particular compartment, fluid therapy plans are by necessity empirical. Consequently, it is important to gather as much information as possible about the patient, make an informed assessment, devise a rational plan, and be prepared to modify the plan based on the response of the patient.

The most basic way to assess fluid balance involves evaluation of physical parameters including heart rate, respiratory rate, pulse pressure, capillary refill time, mucous membrane color and moisture, skin turgor, mentation, and extremity color and temperature. It is important to note that abnormalities in these parameters may not be sensitive indicators of hypovolemia so other data should be collected where possible.

Central venous pressure (CVP) is a measure of the hydrostatic pressure within the intrathoracic vena cava and reflects the interplay between intravascular blood volume, cardiac function, venous compliance, and intrathoracic pressure. Due to the simplicity and availability of CVP monitoring, and despite numerous limitations, this technique is commonly used to guide fluid therapy in critically ill patients.

Mean arterial blood pressure (ABP) is related to CO and systemic vascular resistance (SVR) as follows:

$$Mean\ ABP = CO \times SVR$$

So while ABP is related to CO, it is not a specific measure of intravascular volume. In the initial stages of acute blood loss, for example, the sympathetic nervous system (if intact) responds rapidly and dramatically to augment myocardial function and initiate vasoconstriction such that ABP may remain normal. Therefore, an isolated ABP measurement may be misleading unless interpreted as part of the overall picture.

CO provides an actual assessment of volume instead of a pressure measurement used as a surrogate for volume. While not feasible in routine cases and not without limitations, CO monitoring is valuable in selected critically ill patients requiring fluid resuscitation.

Performing baseline and serial assessments of packed cell volume (PCV) and total solids (TS) is essential in patients with significant blood loss and/or fluid shifts requiring volume resuscitation. Here again a one-time measurement may be misleading, and reassessment at regular intervals (sometimes as often as every 15–20 minutes) during the initial resuscitation phase may be indicated to evaluate ongoing losses and response to therapy.

While not useful in evaluating intravascular volume at the time of presentation, measurement of urine output in conjunction with urine specific gravity is valuable when managing fluid balance over longer time periods (i.e., at hourly intervals or more). When renal function is otherwise normal, urine output of less than 1 mL/kg/h suggests decreased glomerular filtration due to renal hypoperfusion resulting from hypovolemia and/or dehydration. With intravenous fluid therapy, expansion of intravascular volume will occur and urine volume will increase accordingly.

Blood lactate concentration has emerged as a useful indicator of perfusion during volume resuscitation in dogs and cats. With inadequate oxygen delivery to tissues, cells revert to anaerobic metabolism and lactate production increases. While there are other potential causes of hyperlactatemia that should be ruled out, the most common is hypoperfusion and tissue hypoxia. Normal blood lactate concentrations are <2.0 mmol/L in dogs and <1.46 mmol/L in cats. In dogs, concentrations in the 3–5 mmol/L range represent a mild increase, concentrations in the 5–8 mmol/L represent a moderate increase, and concentrations >8 mmol/L represent a severe increase. Restoration of adequate perfusion during volume resuscitation will result in a reduction in blood lactate levels.

Evaluations of acid–base status using blood gas analysis and serum electrolyte concentrations should be carried out frequently in the traumatized or critically ill patient as acid–base balance, electrolyte balance, and fluid balance are all inextricably linked. An effective fluid therapy plan will need to address all of these derangements. Clinical approaches to acid–base balance and an overview of common electrolyte abnormalities in dogs and cats have been discussed previously in this chapter.

In normal animals, changes in intravascular and interstitial fluid volumes occur in parallel; however, in diseased states, the distribution pattern of fluid may be affected. Colloid osmometry is the technique used to measure COP clinically. This allows the clinician to distinguish between decreased COP versus increased hydrostatic pressure as a cause for intravascular fluid loss or edema formation. The COP of whole blood in normal dogs is approximately 20 mm Hg, while the COP of plasma is approximately 17.5 mm Hg. The COP of whole blood in normal cats is approximately 25 mm Hg, while the COP of plasma is approximately 20 mm Hg.

Types of fluids

Fluids available for intravenous use in small animal patients may be broadly classified into three different categories: (1) crystalloids, (2) colloids, and (3) blood products.

Crystalloids

This is the most commonly administered type of fluid. A crystalloid solution consists of a sodium or dextrose base dissolved in water. Depending on the particular type of crystalloid, various other electrolytes and/or buffers may also be added. If the electrolyte composition of the solution approximates that of plasma, then the solution is referred to as a balanced electrolyte solution (BES). Crystalloids may be further classified into four subtypes: (1) replacement solutions, (2) maintenance solutions, (3) hypertonic solutions, and (4) free water solutions. The composition and important properties of selected crystalloids is provided in Table 7.9.

Replacement solutions

These solutions are used to replace water and electrolyte deficits due to hypovolemia and/or dehydration. They are all isotonic with Na^+ concentrations similar to that of ECF. Consequently, their distribution is limited to the ECF only and fluid distribution occurs in proportion to the intravascular and interstitial compartment volumes. This means that only 20–25% of the volume of an intravenously infused replacement crystalloid will remain within the intravascular space 1 hour later.

In the emergency phase of volume resuscitation, rates of administration of up to 90 mL/kg/h in dogs and 60 mL/kg/h in cats (i.e., approximately one blood volume per hour) may be indicated. During this phase the patient must be reassessed at intervals of 5–10 minutes and the fluid rate adjusted as indicated. Once the endpoints of the emergency phase have been achieved, then the rehydration phase can commence to address deficits in the interstitial compartment using less aggressive rates of administration.

In anesthetized dogs and cats, replacement crystalloid solutions are recommended for administration in most routine cases. The standard recommended rate of BES administration in anesthetized dogs and cats is approximately 10–20 mL/kg/h. In patients with particular fluid balance disturbances, other rates and/or types of fluid may be indicated.

Commonly used replacement solutions in dogs and cats include the BESs Plasma-Lyte® 148 and Plasma-Lyte® A (Baxter, Deerfield, IL), Normosol® R (Hospira, Lake Forest, IL), and lactated Ringer's. All of these contain one or more buffers (acetate, gluconate, or lactate) and are therefore referred to as alkalinizing solutions. Sodium chloride 0.9% is a nonbalanced electrolyte replacement solution and is also referred to as an acidifying solution. Please refer to Table 7.9 for more information about specific replacement solutions.

Maintenance solutions

These solutions are designed to meet the water and electrolyte requirements of patients that are unable to maintain adequate fluid and electrolyte intake. They are

Table 7.9. Composition of selected crystalloids

Fluid	Na⁺	K⁺	Ca²⁺	Cl⁻	Mg²⁺	Glucose (g/L)	Buffer (mEq/L)	Cals/L	pH	mOsm/L	Classification
7% NaCl	1199	0	0	1199	0	0	0	0	5.0	2400	Hypertonic
5% NaCl	855	0	0	855	0	0	0	0	5.0	1711	Hypertonic
3% NaCl	513	0	0	513	0	0	0	0	5.0	1026	Hypertonic
Plasma-Lyte M in 5% dextrose[a]	40	16	5	40	3	50	12 acetate / 12 lactate	180	5.0	377	Maintenance
Plasma-Lyte 56 in 5% dextrose[a]	40	13	0	40	3	50	16 acetate	170	5.0	363	Maintenance
Normosol M in 5% dextrose[a]	40	13	0	40	3	50	16 acetate	170	5.0	363	Maintenance
0.9% NaCl	154	0	0	154	0	0	0	0	5.0	308	Replacement; not balanced
Plasma-Lyte 148	140	5	0	98	3	0	27 acetate / 23 gluconate	17	5.5	294	Replacement; BES
Plasma-Lyte A	140	5	0	98	3	0	27 acetate / 23 gluconate	17	7.4	294	Replacement; BES
Normosol R	140	5	0	98	3	0	27 acetate / 23 gluconate	18	6.4	294	Replacement; BES
2.5% dextrose in 0.45% NaCl[a]	77	0	0	77	0	25	0	85	4.5	280	Maintenance[a]
Lactated Ringer's	130	4	3	109	0	0	28 lactate	9	6.5	273	Replacement; BES
5% dextrose	0	0	0	0	0	50	0	170	4.0	252	Free water
0.45% NaCl	77	0	0	77	0	0	0	0	5.0	154	Maintenance[b]

[a] Potassium supplementation required.
[b] Potassium and dextrose supplementation required.
BES, balanced electrolyte solution.

269

usually hypotonic but isosmotic, with lower Na^+ and Cl^- concentrations and higher K^+ and dextrose concentrations compared to replacement solutions. Consequently, they are rarely infused at rates greater than those required to meet the patient's maintenance needs. Maintenance fluid requirements for hospitalized dogs and cats can be estimated using the following formula:

$$\text{Total Maintenance Volume} / \text{Day (mL)} = 1.2\,[70 \times \text{BW(kg)}^{0.75}]$$

This works out to between 27 and 84 mL/kg/day in patients ranging from 90 to 1 kg, respectively. Therefore, the widely quoted estimate of approximately 60 mL/kg/day will overestimate maintenance requirements in large dogs while underestimating requirements in small dogs and cats.

Common commercially available maintenance solutions in dogs and cats include Plasma-Lyte 56, Plasma-Lyte M, and Normosol M. Since it may not be economical in many practices to keep commercially prepared solutions on hand, maintenance solutions can be prepared in house by diluting a BES replacement solution with either sterile water or 5% dextrose in a 1:1 ratio and supplementing with potassium chloride at 20–25 mEq/L.

Hypertonic solutions

Hypertonic saline solutions (usually 5% or 7% NaCl) are used occasionally in dogs and cats during the emergency phase of volume resuscitation to rapidly increase intravascular volume. Administration of intravenous hypertonic saline initiates a transient fluid shift, lasting up to about 30 minutes, from the interstitial compartment into the intravascular compartment. This has the potential to improve CO, ABP, and perfusion until definitive volume replacement can be delivered. The recommended maximum dose and rate for 7% NaCl is 4–7 mL/kg in dogs and 2–4 mL/kg in cats given at 1 mL/kg/min.

Free water solutions

Five percent dextrose in water (D_5W) contains no electrolytes and, once the dextrose is metabolized, only free water remains. It is not considered as a replacement solution, as true pure water deficits are not common and infusion of large volumes of D_5W may lead to dilution of serum electrolytes and formation of edema. Consequently, D_5W is used most often as a vehicle for infusion of other medications or to provide free water in severe cases of severe hypernatremia.

Colloids

Colloids are suspensions of high molecular weight (MW) particles that do not readily leave the intact intravascular space. Colloid administration increases COP and intravascular volume directly and, because they are negatively charged, also draws Na^+ and therefore water from the interstitium, which increases intravascular volume further.

Colloid solutions are indicated to provide rapid intravascular volume expansion or to improve COP in patients with low serum albumin concentrations. Colloids are often classified as either synthetic or biologic. The biologic colloids are a subset of blood products that are able to exert COP including plasma, albumin, and whole blood. These are discussed later under the section on blood products.

Synthetic colloids

Synthetic colloids are polydisperse solutions with molecules ranging in size from a few thousand to several million Daltons. The quoted MW for a particular product represents the average MW of the molecules in that solution. Synthetic colloids may be delivered as small boluses (5 mL/kg in dogs or 2.5 mL/kg in cats) given to effect over a time span ranging from several minutes (in the case of hypovolemic shock) to several hours (if managing interstitial edema, hypoproteinemia, etc.). Numerous veterinary references cite a 20–30 mL/kg/day maximum dosage, and this is based on concerns that higher dosages will adversely impact coagulation. The composition and important properties of selected synthetic crystalloids is provided in Table 7.10.

Commonly used synthetic colloids in dogs and cats include the dextrans (Dextran 70), the hetastarches (HESpan [B. Braun Medical Inc., Irvine, CA] and Hextend [Hospira]), the gelatins (Gelofusine [B. Braun Australia Pty. Ltd., Castle Hill, NSW, Australia] and Haemaccel [Intervet/Schering-Plough Animal Health, Walton, Milton Keynes, Buckinghamshire, UK]), pentastarch (Pentaspan, Bristol-Myers Squibb Canada, Montreal, Canada), and tetrastarch (Voluven, Hospira).

Blood products

Blood products may be indicated to replace deficits in red blood cells, plasma proteins, intravascular volume, platelets, and/or coagulation factors. The blood products most frequently used in small animal practice include: (1) fresh or FFP, (2) fresh or stored whole blood, and (3) PRBCs. Platelet-rich plasma, platelet concentrate, cryoprecipitate, and 25% serum albumin may also be indicated in specific clinical situations. Of these, the albumin-containing solutions (whole blood, plasma, serum albumin) are classified as biologic colloids due to their ability to impact COP, while whole blood and PRBCs are referred to as cellular blood products.

Plasma

Plasma is separated from whole blood and either used as fresh or FFP. FFP contains plasma proteins and coagulation factors (if used within several hours of thawing), but no platelets. Albumin accounts for about 80% of plasma's colloidal activity. Because it equilibrates with the interstitial compartment more rapidly and to a greater extent than the synthetic colloids, very large volumes of plasma are required to impact plasma COP. Consequently, synthetic colloids are usually preferred over plasma if increasing COP is the primary clinical objective.

Table 7.10. Physicochemical properties and composition of selected synthetic colloids

Fluid	Mean MW (kDa)	Molar substitution	Colloid (g/L)	Na$^+$	K$^+$	Ca^{2+}	Cl$^-$	Buffer (mEq/L)	pH	mOsm/L	COP (mmHg)
6% hetastarch in 0.9% NaCl (HESpan)	600	0.7	60	154	0	0	154	0	5.5	309	32.7 ± 0.2
6% hetastarch in BES (Hextend)	670	0.75	60	143	3	5	124	28 lactate	5.9	307	37.9 ± 0.1
6% dextran 70 in 0.9% NaCl	70	N/A	60	154	0	0	154	0	5.1–5.7	310	61.7 ± 0.5
10% pentastarch in 0.9% NaCl (Pentaspan)	200	0.5	100	154	0	0	154	0	5.0	326	32 ± 1.4
4% succinylated fluid gelatin (Gelofusine)	30	N/A	40	154	0.4	0.4	125	0	7.4	279	34
3.5% urea cross-linked gelatin (Haemaccel)	35	N/A	35	145	5.1	6.3	145	0	7.2–7.3	310	25.6–28.6
6% tetrastarch (Voluven)	130	0.4	60	154	0	0	154	0	4.0–5.5	308	37.1 ± 0.8
Hemoglobin-based oxygen carrier (Oxyglobin, OPK Biotech LLC., Cambridge, MA)	200	N/A	130	150	4	0	118	27 lactate	7.8	300	43.3 ± 0.1

Whole blood

Whole blood transfusion is indicated in any situation characterized by loss of both red blood cells and plasma volume. Fresh whole blood is preferred over stored blood if clotting factors and platelets are specifically indicated, as these components deteriorate within 24 hours of collection.

PRBCs

One unit of PRBCs contains the cells plus the small amount of plasma and anticoagulant that remains after the plasma has been removed from one unit of whole blood. When used as a monotherapy, PRBCs are indicated for treatment of anemia only but they are commonly transfused in combination with plasma, crystalloids, and/or synthetic colloids in management of whole blood loss.

Revised from "Acid–Base Physiology" by William W. Muir and Helio S. A. de Morais; and "Fluid, Electrolyte, and Blood Component Therapy" by David C. Seeler in Lumb and Jones' Veterinary Anesthesia and Analgesia, Fourth Edition.

Chapter 8

Anesthesia management of dogs and cats

Richard M. Bednarski

Introduction

Successful anesthetic management of dogs and cats requires an understanding of basic physiology and pharmacology integrated with various clinical competencies relating to anesthesia and pain management. The approach to anesthetic management should always be systematic and follow a stepwise plan as outlined in Table 8.1. In some situations, a standardized form may be useful to organize relevant patient-related data (Figure 8.1). Similarly, the details of the anesthetic plan can also be itemized in a standardized worksheet (Figure 8.2).

At first glance, this approach may seem unnecessarily complicated and impractical. In reality, though, experienced veterinarians work through this process every day. They simply are able to move through the steps very quickly and efficiently when dealing with young, healthy patients presenting for routine elective procedures. By adopting this approach or something similar for every animal requiring anesthesia, the process will become second nature. Then, when presented with more challenging and complex cases, the veterinarian will be better equipped to identify the key issues and formulate a rational plan.

Rather than attempting to address all of the steps outlined in Table 8.1, this chapter will focus primarily on considerations for drug protocol and clinical technique selection. The other steps are covered elsewhere in this text and the reader is referred to chapters addressing patient evaluation, physiology, pharmacology, airway management, equipment, monitoring, fluid therapy, pain management techniques, and anesthesia for special procedures or diseases for more detailed information.

Drug protocol selection

Based on Table 8.1, it is apparent that drug protocol selection constitutes only one component of the overall anesthetic management picture. While selection of an inappropriate drug protocol may undoubtedly contribute to a poor outcome, the reverse is not

Essentials of Small Animal Anesthesia and Analgesia, Second Edition. Edited by Kurt A. Grimm, William J. Tranquilli, Leigh A. Lamont.

PREANESTHETIC PATIENT EVALUATION FORM

CASE NUMBER	123456	PATIENT NAME	Spot Smith

HISTORY

Signalment

				Significant Historical Findings?

Age 10 months   Sex F intact

Breed Lab X   Weight 19.6 kg

Presenting complaint and/or reason for anesthesia:

Elective ovariohysterectomy

Significant Historical Findings?

YES _____ NO X

If YES, describe:

Concurrent Medications?

YES _____ NO X

If YES, describe:

Previous Anesthesia?

YES _____ NO X

If YES, describe:

PHYSICAL EXAMINATION

Cardiovascular System

HR 110 bpm   Rhythm normal sinus

Quality strong   mm/CRT pink, <2 seconds

Abnormal Cardiac Auscultation?

YES _____ NO X

If YES, describe:

Respiratory System

RR 24 brpm   Effort normal

Abnormal Pulmonary Auscultation?

YES _____ NO X

If YES, describe:

Thermoregulatory System

Temp 38.3°C

Pain Assessment

Preexisting Pain Present?

YES _____ NO X

If YES, describe:

Other Body Systems

Neuro NSF   Renal NSF

Hepatic NSF   GI NSF

LABORATORY TEST RESULTS

Hct	0.42	Na^+		Creatinine	1.1	ALT	48	Urine SG	
Hb		K^+		BUN		ALP		Other	
WBC		Cl^-		Glucose	87	AST			
Platelets		Ca^{2+}		CK		PT/PTT			
T. Protein	71	Amyl/Lip		Lactate		Fibrinogen			

ADJUNCTIVE TEST RESULTS

ECG?

YES _____ NO X

If YES, describe:

Thoracic Radiographs?

YES _____ NO X

If YES, describe:

Abdominal Radiographs?

YES _____ NO X

If YES, describe:

Ultrasound?

YES _____ NO X

If YES, describe:

Other?

YES _____ NO X

If YES, describe:

ASA CLASSIFICATION OF PHYSICAL STATUS

(I)   II   III   IV   V   E

SUMMARY OF PATIENT PROBLEMS AS THEY RELATE TO ANESTHESIA

Healthy patient presenting for elective procedure.

No anesthetic-related complications anticipated.

Figure 8.1. Preanesthetic patient evaluation form. NSF, no significant findings.

Table 8.1. Systematic approach to anesthetic management of dogs and cats

Step	Details
1. Evaluation of the patient	Integrate all patient-related information including: • Signalment • History • General inspection and temperament • Complete physical examination • Pain assessment • Interpretation of laboratory tests • Interpretation of other diagnostic tests Determine physical status based on above
2. Review of the planned procedure	Integrate all relevant procedural information including: • Level of invasiveness • Expected intensity of pain • Potential complications • Duration • Requirements for patient positioning
3. Preparation of the patient	Initiate stabilization procedures, if required, to address: • Pain • Dehydration • Hypovolemia • Anemia • Electrolyte and/or acid–base disturbances • Pneumothorax, pleural effusion • Cardiac dysrhythmias • Other decompensated disease states Institute appropriate preanesthetic fasting interval
4. Formulation of anesthetic and pain management plan	Generate a comprehensive plan based on the above, including: • Selection of drug protocol – Preanesthetic agents – Induction agents – Maintenance agents – Supplemental anesthetic agents – Analgesic agents – Other drugs for supportive care • Selection of clinical anesthetic techniques and equipment – Injectable drug delivery • IV catheters and accessories – Airway management • Endotracheal tubes and accessories – Inhalant anesthetic delivery • Anesthetic machine • Breathing system – Local, regional anesthetic/analgesic techniques • Drugs, needles, nerve locator, and so on • Selection of patient monitoring techniques and equipment – Anesthetic depth – Basic cardiopulmonary parameters – Arterial blood pressure • Oscillometric, Doppler, or direct system – End-tidal carbon dioxide • Capnometer

Table 8.1. (*Continued*)

Step	Details
	– Hemoglobin saturation • Pulse oximeter – Electrocardiogram (ECG) • ECG monitor – Core body temperature • Thermometer – Airway inhalant anesthetic and oxygen concentrations • Airway gas monitor – Arterial blood gas parameters • Blood gas analyzer – Others • Selection of supportive care techniques and equipment – Fluid and electrolyte therapy • Fluids and accessories • Fluid pumps, syringe pumps – Thermoregulatory support • Circulating water blanket, forced air warmer, conductive fabric warmer – Mechanical ventilation • Ventilator – Other pharmacological support • Drugs, syringe pumps, etc.
5. Implementation of the plan	Execute the plan as outlined above and initiate the following: • Monitoring of the patient – Documentation of monitored parameters – Interpretation of monitored parameters and trends – Recognition of significant abnormalities • Management of patient-related complications – Initiation of interventions and/or provision of supportive care where appropriate • Management of equipment-related complications – Recognize and troubleshoot equipment malfunctions • Management of the patient at recovery – Airway management – Management of pain – Management of excitement/dysphoria – Management of hypothermia – Recognition and management of other complications – Provision of continued monitoring and supportive care • Record keeping – Documentation of all information related to the case
6. Retrospective evaluation	Complete an objective evaluation of the anesthetic and pain management plan and its outcome

ANESTHETIC PLAN WORKSHEET

CASE NUMBER 123456		PATIENT NAME Spot Smith		WEIGHT 19.6 kg	
PRE-ANESTHETIC PERIOD					
Stabilization/Correction/Evaluation of Preexisting Abnormalities Required?					
YES _____		NO X _____			
If YES, outline plan:					
Preanesthetic Drugs		Dosage (mg/kg)	Dose (mg)	Volume (mL)	Route
Sedative	Acepromazine	0.05 mg/kg	0.98 mg	0.1 mL	IM
Opioid	Hydromorphone	0.1 mg/kg	1.96 mg	0.98 mL	IM
Anticholinergic					
Dissociative					
Other					
ANESTHETIC PERIOD					
Anesthetic Drugs					
Injectable Induction		Dosage (mg/kg)	Dose (mg)	Volume (mL)	Route
Injectable Agent(s)	Thiopental	10 mg/kg	196 mg	7.8 mL to effect	IV
Inhalant Induction		% Delivered	O$_2$ Flow (mL/kg/min)	O$_2$ Flow (mL/min)	Route
Inhalant Agent	NA				
Injectable Maintenance		Dosage (mg/kg)	Dose (mg)	Volume (mL)	Route
Injectable Agent(s)	NA				
Inhalant Maintenance		% Delivered	O$_2$ Flow (mL/kg/min)	O$_2$ Flow (mL/min)	Route
Inhalant Agent	Isoflurane	3% initially; ↓ to 1–2% to effec	50 mL/kg/min; ↓ to 20 mL/kg/min	1 L/min initially; ↓ to 400 mL/min	Circle system
Supplemental Analgesia		Dosage (mg/kg)	Dose (mg)	Volume (mL)	Route
Local Anesthetic	NA				
Opioid					
Other					
Fluid Therapy		Rate (mL/kg/hour)	Rate (mL/hour)	Drip Rate (dr/s)	Route
Crystalloid	Plasmalyte 148	10 mL/kg/h	196 mL/h	0.54 dr/s	IV
Colloid				(10 drop/mL drip	
Blood Product				set)	
Monitoring Techniques					
ECG___ X Oscillometric BP___ X Doppler BP____ Direct BP___ _					
Pulse Oximetry____ X Capnometry___ X Temperature___ X Other_____					
POSTANESTHETIC PERIOD					
Postanesthetic Drugs		Dosage (mg/kg)	Dose (mg)	Volume (mL)	Route
Opioid	Hydromorphone	0.05 mg/kg	0.98 mg	0.49 mL	IV
NSAID	Carprofen	4 mg/kg	78.4 mg	1.57 mL	SC
Sedative					
Other					

Figure 8.2.   Anesthetic plan worksheet.

necessarily true. The selection of a perfectly reasonable drug protocol does not ensure that complications will not occur. Regardless of the drugs selected, vigilant monitoring of the anesthetized patient is required and supportive interventions need to be initiated when indicated.

Numerous drugs are available to today's practitioner and they may be combined and delivered in many ways. It is not necessary for most veterinarians to have all of these drugs at their disposal, and the use of many different drug protocols does not necessarily imply superior anesthetic care. However, familiarity with only a single anesthetic technique will, at best, limit the veterinarian's ability to perform all of the diagnostic and surgical procedures common in today's modern practice and, at worst, may compromise the care of certain patients.

Balanced anesthesia

Anesthetic protocols involving single drugs have largely been abandoned in favor of protocols that incorporate multiple drugs from different classes to achieve unconsciousness, analgesia, and muscle relaxation. This approach is referred to as balanced anesthesia. Most balanced anesthetic protocols have four different phases: (1) preanesthesia, (2) induction, (3) maintenance, and (4) recovery. Ultimately, the selection of drugs and clinical techniques for each of these phases will depend on patient-related factors, procedure-related factors, drug availability, personal experience, and cost. The four phases of anesthetic management will be discussed in general terms below and a summary of key patient- and procedure-related factors will follow.

Preanesthetic medication

Almost all patients will benefit from the administration of a preanesthetic drug or drug combination prior to induction with an injectable or inhalant anesthetic. The goals of successful preanesthetic medication in dogs and cats are summarized in Box 8.1. In healthy dogs and cats, most preanesthetic medications are usually administered via the intramuscular (IM) or subcutaneous (SC) routes 15–20 minutes prior to induction of anesthesia. This reduces stress and anxiety in the animal and facilitates restraint for intravenous (IV) catheter placement. In patients with special needs where an IV catheter is already in place, the IV route may also be used for preanesthetic administration.

In most young to middle-aged healthy dogs and cats, preanesthetic medication usually involves a combination of a sedative and an analgesic. In patients requiring moderate to profound levels of sedation, the phenothiazine acepromazine or the alpha$_2$ adrenergic agonist dexmedetomidine are the most commonly used options. In geriatric, debilitated, or hemodynamically unstable patients, or in any patient where sedation requirements are less, the benzodiazepine midazolam may be used instead. Opioids are routinely included as part of the preanesthetic medication in patients, even those that are not painful and/or will not be subjected to painful procedures. Synergism between the opioid and sedative results in superior sedation and reduces anesthetic requirements for induction and maintenance. The most commonly used opioids for preanesthetic medication in dogs and cats include the pure agonists, hydromorphone, oxymorphone, and morphine; the agonist–antagonist butorphanol; and the partial agonist buprenorphine. In patients where heavy sedation is not a priority and/or sedative administration is contraindicated, an opioid alone is often administered.

The anticholinergics atropine or glycopyrrolate have been commonly included in preanesthetic protocols in dogs and cats to prevent bradycardia and/or limit salivary secretions. The need for routine preemptive administration of anticholinergics in the

Box 8.1. Goals of the preanesthesia phase in dogs and cats.

Minimize patient stress and anxiety

- Facilitates restraint
- Enhances safety for patient and handler

Decrease requirements for injectable and inhalant anesthetics

- Smoothes induction, maintenance, and recovery phases
- Provides better cardiopulmonary stability

Enhance perioperative pain management

- Provides preemptive analgesic effect
- Reduces intra- and postoperative analgesic requirements

Decrease autonomic reflex activity

- Provides a more stable plane of anesthesia
- Results in less arrhythmogenic potential

---

preanesthetic period has been questioned in recent years as anesthetic drug protocols and monitoring standards have evolved. As is the case with any drug, the decision to use an anticholinergic should be based on an understanding of its advantages and disadvantages and should be made on a case-by-case basis.

Nonsteroidal anti-inflammatory drugs (NSAIDs) such as carprofen, meloxicam, deracoxib, firocoxib, and tepoxalin are common components of pain management plans for dogs and cats undergoing surgical procedures and are often administered prior to anesthesia. While they do not contribute to preanesthetic sedation and do not appear to have significant anesthetic-sparing effects, injectable NSAIDs (i.e., carprofen or meloxicam) may be given along with other preanesthetic medications 15–20 minutes prior to induction of anesthesia. Alternatively, they may also be injected at the time of recovery if intraoperative hypotension and/or hemostasis is/are a concern.

A flowchart outlining the thought process for designing preanesthetic protocols in dogs and cats can be found in Figure 8.3. Dosages for commonly used preanesthetic drugs from each of the three main categories (sedatives, opioids, and anticholinergics) are provided in Tables 8.2 and 8.3. For more detailed information on the pharmacology, indications, and contraindications of all of these drugs, please refer to Chapter 2.

Induction of anesthesia

The goals of optimal anesthetic induction in dogs and cats are summarized in Box 8.2. The transition from the conscious to the anesthetized state is usually accomplished by the administration of one or more injectable drugs. In specific situations,

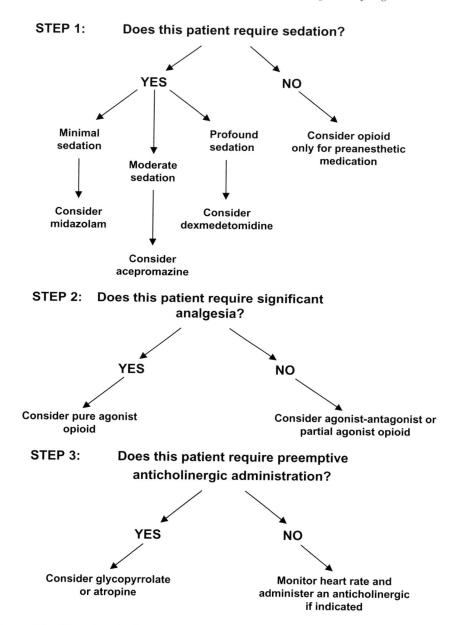

Figure 8.3. Steps in selecting preanesthetic medications in dogs and cats.

induction with an inhalant agent such as isoflurane or sevoflurane administered via a face mask or in an induction chamber may also be indicated. Inhalant inductions are not recommended for routine use because it is difficult to precisely control the delivered concentration of drug, and pollution of the local atmosphere with anesthetic vapor is significant.

Table 8.2. Common preanesthetic medications[a] in dogs

Drug	IM, SC dose in mg/kg	IV dose in mg/kg
Sedatives:		
Midazolam[b]	0.1–0.3	0.1–0.2
Acepromazine[c]	0.02–0.1	0.01–0.05
Dexmedetomidine[d]	0.005–0.01	0.001–0.005
Opioids:		
Hydromorphone	0.05–0.1	0.05–0.1
Oxymorphone	0.05–0.1	0.05–0.1
Morphine	0.3–1.0	0.3–0.5 *slowly*
Butorphanol	0.2–0.4	0.2–0.4
Buprenorphine	0.005–0.02	0.005–0.01
Anticholinergics:		
Atropine	0.04	0.02
Glycolyrrolate	0.01	0.005

[a] Refer to Figure 8.1 for suggestions on how to combine drugs from each of the three categories; an injectable NSAID (carprofen, meloxicam) may also be administered as part of the preanesthetic medication if indicated.
[b] The maximum total dose is often capped at approximately 7 mg to prevent overdosing large breed dogs.
[c] The maximum total dose is often capped at approximately 3 mg to prevent overdosing large breed dogs.
[d] The maximum total dose is often capped at approximately 0.5 mg to prevent overdosing large breed dogs.

Table 8.3. Common preanesthetic medications[a] in cats

Drug	IM dose in mg/kg	IV dose in mg/kg
Sedatives:		
Midazolam	0.1–0.2	0.1–0.2
Acepromazine	0.05–0.2	0.02–0.05
Dexmedetomidine	0.01–0.03	0.003–0.01
Opioids:		
Hydromorphone	0.05–0.1	0.05–0.1
Oxymorphone	0.05–0.1	0.05–0.1
Morphine	0.1–0.3	0.1–0.3 *slowly*
Butorphanol	0.2–0.4	0.2–0.4
Buprenorphine	0.005–0.02	0.005–0.01
Anticholinergics:		
Atropine	0.04	0.02
Glycolyrrolate	0.01	0.005

[a] Refer to Figure 8.1 for suggestions on how to combine drugs from each of the three categories; an injectable NSAID (carprofen, meloxicam) may also be administered as part of the preanesthetic medication if indicated.

Box 8.2.   Goals of the anesthetic induction phase in dogs and cats.

Facilitate a smooth, rapid transition to general anesthesia

- Avoids or minimizes excitement (stage 2 of anesthesia)
- Provides adequate muscle relaxation for endotracheal intubation if indicated
- Provides a suitable duration of action to allow completion of the procedure or transfer to the maintenance phase

Maintain adequate cardiopulmonary stability

Injectable induction protocols may use either the IM or IV route. The IM route is technically straightforward and may be preferred in certain situations where large numbers of relatively young, healthy patients are being anesthetized for short routine procedures (e.g., spay/neuter programs in animal shelters). In most cases, higher total doses of drug are required with this route, and there is no possibility to titrate to effect. While the IV route usually requires placement of a catheter, it offers the advantage of dosing to effect and is usually associated with more rapid inductions and recoveries. Since IV access is recommended for most patients undergoing general anesthesia anyway, catheter placement prior to induction is simply good practice. For these reasons, IV induction protocols are preferred for most dogs and cats requiring general anesthesia.

Injectable IM induction agents commonly used in dogs and cats include ketamine combinations, tiletamine–zolazepam (Telazol®, Pfizer Animal Health, New York), and alphaxalone-CD. There are numerous IM protocols that have been reported for general anesthesia in dogs and cats and most combine the preanesthetic medication and the induction agent(s) in a single IM injection. Most of these cocktails involve various combinations of dissociatives, benzodiazepines, alpha$_2$ agonists, and opioids. A few selected protocols are presented in Tables 8.4 and 8.5, though this list is by no means exhaustive.

Injectable IV induction agents commonly used in dogs and cats include ketamine, Telazol, propofol, thiopental, etomidate, and alphaxalone-CD. Other supplemental drugs may also be administered concurrently and are referred to as coinduction agents. In the case of ketamine, this practice is well recognized, as a benzodiazepine (diazepam or midazolam) is almost always coadministered to counteract ketamine-induced muscle rigidity and potential seizure activity. Though not mandatory, coinduction agents can also be used with propofol, thiopental, etomidate and alphaxalone-CD to minimize their dose requirements. This benefits patients by smoothing out the induction phase and reducing the potential for adverse cardiopulmonary side effects. Diazepam, midazolam, and lidocaine (in dogs only) are the most commonly used coinduction agents in small animals. The combination of a coinduction agent with propofol, thiopental, etomidate, or alphaxalone-CD tends to be most useful in patients that are not profoundly sedated after the preanesthetic period and where higher doses of IV induction drug are anticipated.

Table 8.4.   Selected IM anesthetic protocols[a] for dogs

Combination	IM Dose in mg/kg[b]	Comments
Dexmedetomidine Ketamine Opioid	0.005–0.01 3–6 See Table 8.2	May administer dexmedetomidine and opioid first and follow with ketamine 10 minutes later
Telazol Opioid	2–10 See Table 8.2	Telazol is reconstituted according to the label instructions and the opioid is added in separately
Dexmedetomidine Telazol Opioid	0.005–0.01 2–4 See comment	To reduce injection volume, Telazol may also be reconstituted as follows: 2.5 mL dexmedetomidine plus 2.5 mL butorphanol (10 mg/mL) *or* 2.5 mL hydromorphone (2 mg/mL) *or* 2.5 mL morphine (15 mg/mL) The combination is then dosed at 0.02–0.04 mL/kg

[a] Recovery times may be prolonged with any dissociative-based IM protocol.
[b] Lower end of dose range will result in heavy sedation/immobilization, while the higher end will produce general anesthesia of variable duration.

Note that if midazolam has been given IM as part of the preanesthetic medication, it may be appropriate to reduce or eliminate the dose of benzodiazepine given IV as a coinduction agent. Dosages for commonly used injectable and inhalant induction and coinduction drugs in dogs and cats can be found in Tables 8.6 and 8.7. For more detailed information on the pharmacology, indications, and contraindications of all of these drugs, please refer to Chapter 2.

In debilitated and/or hemodynamically unstable patients, induction with an opioid (usually fentanyl, remifentanil, oxymorphone, or hydromorphone) in combination with a benzodiazepine (midazolam or diazepam) given in alternating IV increments to effect often produces a smooth induction and facilitates transfer to the maintenance phase of anesthesia. This approach will be discussed in more detail in an upcoming section.

Maintenance of anesthesia

Goals of the anesthetic maintenance phase in dogs and cats are summarized in Box 8.3. Unless an IM injectable induction protocol has been used, most procedures lasting more than 15 minutes will require the administration of additional anesthetic agents to extend or maintain anesthesia. This can be accomplished with either injectable or inhalant anesthetics. Any of the IV injectable agents listed in the previous section can be used in smaller "top-up" doses given to effect if the duration of anesthesia only needs to be extended for a few minutes. Repeated redosing with thiopental is not recommended, as redistribution sites may become saturated, leading to a prolonged recovery.

Table 8.5.   Selected IM anesthetic protocols[a] for cats

Combination	IM Dose in mg/kg[b]	Comments
Dexmedetomidine Ketamine Opioid	0.01–0.02 5–10 See Table 8.3	May administer dexmedetomidine and opioid first and follow with ketamine 10 minutes later
Telazol Opioid	2–10 See Table 8.3	Telazol is reconstituted according to the label instructions and the opioid is added in separately
Dexmedetomidine Telazol Opioid	0.005–0.01 2–4 See comment or Table 8.3	To reduce injection volume, Telazol may also be reconstituted as follows: 2.5 mL dexmedetomidine plus 2.5 mL butorphanol (10 mg/mL) *or* 2.5 mL hydromorphone (2 mg/mL) *or* 2.5 mL morphine (15 mg/mL) The combination is then dosed at 0.02–0.04 mL/kg
Xylazine Telazol Ketamine Opioid	1–2 5–10 4–8 See Table 8.3	To reduce injection volume, Telazol may be reconstituted as follows: 4 mL of ketamine (100 mg/mL) plus 1 mL of xylazine (100 mg/mL) The combination is then dosed at 0.04–0.08 mL/kg and the opioid is added in separately
Dexmedetomidine Telazol Ketamine Opioid	0.002–0.004 2–4 1–3 See Table 8.3	To reduce injection volume, Telazol may be reconstituted as follows: 4 mL of ketamine (100 mg/mL) plus 1 mL of dexmedetomidine (0.5 mg/mL) The combination is then dosed at 0.02–0.04 mL/kg and the opioid is added in separately
Ketamine Midazolam Opioid	8–10 0.2–0.3 See Table 8.3	
Alphaxalone-CD Opioid	10–12 See Table 8.3	May not be suitable for invasive surgical procedures

[a] Recovery times may be prolonged with any dissociative-based IM protocol.
[b] The lower end of the dose range will result in heavy sedation/immobilization while the higher end will produce general anesthesia of variable duration.

If longer-duration injectable maintenance is required, propofol is considered the drug of choice and can be administered as a continuous rate infusion (CRI) for extended periods of time. After appropriate preanesthetic medication and IV induction, propofol CRI doses for anesthetic maintenance in dogs and cats range from 0.2 to 0.8 mg/kg/min and are often supplemented with ketamine, midazolam, dexmedetomidine, and/or opioids as indicated.

Most contemporary small animal veterinary hospitals are equipped with inhalant anesthetic machines, so the most common means of maintaining anesthesia in dogs and

Table 8.6.   Anesthetic induction and co-induction agents in dogs

Injectable induction drugs[a]	IV dose in mg/kg
Propofol	2–10
Thiopental	5–15
Midazolam[b]/ketamine	0.1–0.4/3–10
Telazol	2–8
Etomidate	0.5–2
Alphaxalone-CD	1–3
Coinduction drugs	IV dose in mg/kg
Midazolam[b]	0.1–0.4
Lidocaine	2–4
Inhalant induction agents	Delivered for induction (%)
Sevoflurane (MAC 2.3%)	4–5
Isoflurane (MAC 1.3%)	2.5–3.5
Possible combinations of above[c]	
Propofol alone	Lidocaine/propofol
Thiopental alone	Lidocaine/thiopental
Telazol alone	Lidocaine/telazol
Etomidate alone	Lidocaine/etomidate
Alphaxalone-CD alone	Lidocaine/alphaxalone-CD
Midazolam/ketamine	Lidocaine/midazolam/ketamine
Sevoflurane alone	Midazolam/lidocaine/propofol
Isoflurane alone	Midazolam/lidocaine/thiopental
Midazolam/propofol	Midazolam/lidocaine/etomidate
Midazolam/thiopental	Midazolam/lidocaine/alphxalone-CD
Midazolam/etomidate	Midazolam/sevoflurane
Midazolam/alphaxalone-CD	Midazolam/isoflurane

[a] The lower end of dose range is usually feasible if preanesthetic medication has been administered or coinduction agents are to be included.
[b] Can substitute diazepam at the same dose.
[c] It is usually recommended to administer the coinduction agent(s) and immediately titrate the primary induction drug to effect.

cats is to use isoflurane or sevoflurane. For longer and/or more invasive procedures, it is also common practice to supplement inhalant anesthesia with other drugs during the maintenance phase to reduce inhalant requirements once preanesthetic medications have worn off. This may be accomplished in several ways, including the use of local and regional anesthetic or analgesic techniques, or the administration of supplemental systemic drugs such as hydromorphone, oxymorphone, morphine, fentanyl, remifentanil, lidocaine, ketamine, midazolam, and dexmedetomidine. These techniques will be discussed again later in this chapter.

Recovery from anesthesia

The ideal anesthetic recovery should be rapid, complete, and stress free for the patient. In selected cases, drug reversal may be indicated to hasten recovery. Commonly used reversible drugs include dexmedetomidine (reversed with atipamezole), midazolam and diazepam (reversed with flumazenil), and opioid agonists (reversed with pure antagonists

Table 8.7. Anesthetic induction and coinduction agents in cats

Anesthetic/coinduction drug[a]	IV dose in mg/kg
Propofol	4–10
Thiopental	5–15
Midazolam[b]/ketamine	0.1–0.3/3–10
Telazol	2–8
Etomidate	0.5–2
Alphaxalone-CD	2–5
Coinduction drugs	IV dose in mg/kg
Midazolam[b]	0.1–0.3
Inhalant anesthetic agents	Delivered for induction (%)
Sevoflurane (MAC 2.6%)	4.5–5.5
Isoflurane (MAC 1.6%)	3–4

Possible combinations of above[c]

Propofol alone	Isoflurane alone
Thiopental alone	Midazolam/propofol
Telazol alone	Midazolam/thiopental
Etomidate alone	Midazolam/etomidate
Alphaxalone-CD alone	Midazolam/ alphaxalone-CD
Midazolam/ketamine	Midazolam/sevoflurane
Sevoflurane alone	Midazolam/isoflurane

[a] The lower end of the dose range is usually feasible if preanesthetic medication has been administered or coinduction agents are to be included.
[b] Can substitute diazepam at the same dose.
[c] It is usually recommended to administer the coinduction agent(s) and immediately titrate the primary induction drug to effect.

Box 8.3. Goals of the anesthetic maintenance phase in dogs and cats.

- Maintain an adequate level of unconsciousness, analgesia, and muscle relaxation throughout
- Maintain adequate cardiopulmonary stability
- Facilitate adjustment of anesthetic depth if indicated
- Ensure a predictable, smooth recovery

such as naloxone or the agonist–antagonist butorphanol). In other situations, supplemental sedation may be required with low doses of dexmedetomidine, acepromazine, or midazolam to prevent or treat dysphoria or agitation. In all cases, management of pain must be a priority and the most commonly used postanesthetic analgesics are opioids and NSAIDs. Occasionally, adjunctive analgesic agents may also be indicated as part of the pain management plan. Please refer to Tables 8.8 and 8.9 for injectable and oral postoperative analgesic dosage recommendations.

It is important to remember that patient monitoring and provision of supportive care does not stop with the termination of anesthetic drug delivery. All patients will benefit from inspiration of supplemental oxygen in the immediate recovery phase to counteract

Table 8.8.   Injectable postoperative analgesics in dogs and cats

Drug	Dogs (mg/kg)	Cats (mg/kg)
Opioids:		
Hydromorphone	0.05–0.2 IM, SC 0.05–0.1 IV	0.05–0.1 IM, SC, IV
Oxymorphone	0.05–0.2 IM, SC 0.05–0.1 IV	0.05–0.1 IM, SC, IV
Morphine	0.3–1.0 IM, SC 0.3–0.5 IV *slowly* 0.1–0.2 IV loading dose followed by 0.1–0.3 IV CRI/h	0.1–0.3 IM, SC or IV *slowly*
Butorphanol	0.2–0.4 IM or IV	0.2–0.4 IM or IV
Buprenorphine	0.005–0.02 IM 0.005–0.01 IV	0.005–0.02 IM 0.005–0.01 IV

Fentanyl[a]	0.002–0.003 IV loading dose
	  followed by 0.001–0.01 IV
	  CRI/h
		0.002–0.003 IV loading dose
		  followed by 0.001–0.01 IV
		  CRI/h

NSAIDs		
Carprofen	4.0 IM, SC, IV q 24 h	1.0 IM, SC, IV *once only*
Meloxicam	0.2 IM, SC, IV loading dose then reduce to 0.1 q 24 h	0.1–0.2 SC

[a] Also may be delivered via the transdermal route at 0.002–0.005 mg/kg/h.

hypoxemia. In healthy patients anesthetized for short procedures, this may be considered optional, but in patients with airway abnormalities or impairment of oxygenation and/or ventilation, supplemental oxygen should be provided. Pulse oximetry is particularly useful for detecting hypoxemia in patients during the transition from >90% to 21% inspired oxygen concentrations.

The patient should be closely observed until it can maintain sternal recumbency and vital signs monitored until they return to normal. In patients that are critically ill or hemodynamically unstable, intensive monitoring and supportive care for an extended period of time may be indicated. Other postanesthetic complications that may be encountered include hypothermia, hyperthermia, airway obstruction, and aspiration of regurgitated gastroesophageal contents.

Drug selection: patient-related factors

Many of the patient-related factors that need to be considered are discussed elsewhere in this text and the reader is referred to Chapters 11 through 17 for more information. A few special considerations are presented below as they relate to drug selection.

Species differences: cats versus dogs

As a generalization, cats tend to require higher dosages of sedatives on a per kilogram basis than do dogs to achieve a comparable clinical effect. This is due largely to their higher body surface area (BSA)/mass ratio but also reflects species variation in central

Table 8.9. Oral postoperative analgesics in dogs and cats

Drug	Dogs (mg/kg)	Cats (mg/kg)
NSAIDs:		
Carprofen	4.0 PO q 24 h	1.0 PO *once only (variable duration)*
Meloxicam	0.2 PO then reduce to 0.1 q 24 h	0.1–0.2 SC *once only per U.S. label*
Deracoxib	3.0–4.0 PO q24 h for 5–7 days *or* 1.0–2.0 PO q 24 h chronically	Not established
Firocoxib	5.0 PO q 24 h	Not established
Tepoxalin	10–20 PO then reduce to 10 q 24 h	Not established
Opioids:		
Morphine[a]	1.5–3.0 PO q 12 h	Not recommended
Codeine	0.5–2.0 PO q 6 h	0.2–0.5 PO q 6 h
Oxycodone	0.1–0.3 q 8–12 h	Not recommended
Adjunctive Analgesics:	5–10 PO q 8–12 h	5–10 PO q 8–12 h
Tramadol	2–10 PO q 8–12 h	2–10 PO q 8–12 h
Gabapentin	3–5 PO q 24 h	3–5 PO q 24 h

[a] Sustained-release product (MS Contin, Purdue Pharma L.P., Stamford, CT).

nervous system receptor densities. When dosed on the basis of BSA instead of body weight, clinically effective dosages for dexmedetomidine and acepromazine tend to be similar in both dogs and cats. This is the same explanation for why large and giant breed dogs require lower doses on a per kilogram basis compared to small and toy breeds.

While midazolam usually produces a mild sedative or calming effect in dogs, the response in cats is unpredictable. Administration of midazolam to young, healthy cats alone or with an opioid may cause excitation and actually make the patient less tractable. In older and/or debilitated cats, however, the combination of a benzodiazepine and opioid may produce a desirable calming effect without significant adverse cardiopulmonary side effects.

Regarding opioids, it has traditionally been felt that cats are more prone to excitatory responses when pure agonist opioids such as morphine and hydromorphone are administered to pain-free patients in the preanesthetic period. Consequently, opioids are most often administered to young, healthy cats in combination with a sedative such as acepromazine or dexmedetomidine in the preanesthetic period. Note that this excitatory response is usually not evident when appropriate doses of pure agonist opioids are administered to feline patients that are debilitated and/or painful as a result of a disease, injury, or surgical procedure.

Young, healthy patients

It is important to recognize that published drug doses for most sedatives, injectable anesthetics, and inhalant anesthetics are based on studies involving young, healthy animals of normal body weight. There are numerous drugs and drug combinations that are suitable for use in this patient population and examples can be found in Tables 8.2–8.7. As a generalization, most of these patients will benefit from a balanced anesthetic protocol that incorporates a sedative–analgesic combination administered as preanesthetic medication, an injectable anesthetic(s) for induction, and an inhalant agent for maintenance of anesthesia. Routine preemptive use of an anticholinergic (i.e., atropine or glycopyrrolate) as part of the preanesthetic medication is somewhat controversial and is becoming less frequent in small animal clinical practice. Many anesthesiologists now advocate a "wait and see" approach, whereby cardiovascular parameters are closely monitored and an anticholinergic is administered when or if indicated. Pain management needs will vary widely in this patient population and the pain management plan should be formulated on a case-by-case basis.

Aggressive patients

The temperament of the patient plays a significant role in anesthetic drug selection. Animals that are simply frightened or anxious often respond favorably to conventional sedative–analgesic protocols when provided with a safe, quiet place to rest while the drugs take effect. Patients that are truly aggressive or vicious, however, may not be adequately sedated with conventional drug combinations to permit safe handling. In these patients, an IM dexmedetomidine–opioid combination at or above the higher end of the recommended dose range is usually effective (see Tables 8.2 and 8.3). In some cases, a dissociative-based protocol administered IM may be necessary to provide adequate sedation and immobilization (see Tables 8.4 and 8.5). In general, acepromazine–opioid and especially midazolam–opioid combinations are not reliable sedatives in extremely aggressive dogs or cats. In most situations, the goal of IM drug administration in an aggressive patient is to facilitate safe handling and completion of a thorough physical examination, and allow additional anesthetic drugs to be titrated IV to effect if necessary.

Geriatric patients

In general, geriatric animals tend to be more susceptible to the depressant effects of sedatives and anesthetics than do younger patients. For this reason, doses of sedatives can often be markedly decreased or eliminated altogether in these patients. Depending on the animal's temperament, opioids and benzodiazepines often produce adequate sedation–analgesia without causing appreciable depression of cardiopulmonary function. The incorporation of opioids with or without benzodiazepines will also reduce the required doses of injectable and inhalant anesthetic agents and improve cardiopulmonary stability. In geriatric patients that are debilitated, depressed, or hemodynamically unstable, the combination of an opioid (fentanyl, remifentanil, hydromorphone, or oxymorphone) with a benzodiazepine (midazolam or diazepam) titrated IV to effect may be adequate to induce general anesthesia and facilitate smooth transfer to an inhalant agent. The decision to include an anticholinergic (i.e., atropine or glycopyrrolate) should be made on a case-by-case basis.

Neonatal or pediatric patients

Neonatal and pediatric patients are classified as dogs and cats that are less than 12 weeks of age. Like geriatric patients, neonates are more susceptible to the depressant effects of sedatives and anesthetics than are young to middle-aged adults. In addition, they are more likely to develop hypothermia and/or hypoglycemia so strategies to avoid and/or manage these complications must be in place. Short-acting and/or reversible drugs are particularly useful and low doses of opioids, benzodiazepines, dissociatives, propofol, and inhalants are commonly used. Acepromazine and dexmedetomidine are rarely indicated. This is one of the few circumstances where preemptive administration of an anticholinergic is almost always recommended to counteract bradycardia and maintain cardiac output.

Breed-related anesthetic concerns

Myths and misconceptions regarding specific breed-related sensitivities to various anesthetic agents or techniques are commonplace in veterinary medicine and among breeders. Despite the volume of information that can be found on breed websites and in the lay literature, very few of these popular opinions have ever been substantiated by any scientific evidence. In reality, there are only a few breed-specific anesthetic concerns that are truly noteworthy.

Greyhounds and thiobarbiturates   It is generally recommended that thiobarbiturates (e.g., thiopental) be avoided in greyhounds and other sighthounds due to the potential for prolonged and rough recoveries. Any other injectable or inhalant agent (see Table 8.6) may be used as an alternative for induction of anesthesia depending on other patient-related and procedure-related factors.

Brachycephalic dogs and upper airway obstruction   Anatomical abnormalities of the upper airway are common in brachycephalic breeds, notably the English bulldog, and result in a constellation of symptoms commonly referred to as brachycephalic airway syndrome. Due to the potential for airway obstruction in the perianesthetic period these dogs constitute an increased anesthetic risk even if otherwise healthy. In addition, many brachycephalic breeds seem to have a high resting vagal tone so routine preemptive administration of an anticholinergic may be warranted. Drug selection in these patients should involve an injectable anesthetic agent(s) to facilitate rapid induction and prompt endotracheal intubation. Mask inductions with inhalant agents are not appropriate in these patients.

Boxers and acepromazine   Some Boxer dogs may have an increased response or an exaggerated vasovagal response to acepromazine. While controlled studies have not been performed, there are anecdotal reports of cardiovascular collapse in apparently healthy Boxer dogs administered standard doses of acepromazine. For this reason, many anesthesiologists advise caution when using acepromazine in this breed and some advocate avoiding it altogether.

Trauma patients or hemodynamically unstable patients

As is the case with any patient, correction of preexisting abnormalities prior to proceeding with anesthesia will be associated with better outcomes. IV access should be secured initially and all sedative, analgesic, and anesthetic drugs should be administered IV. For the most part, potent sedatives with significant adverse cardiopulmonary effects such as acepromazine and dexmedetomidine are contraindicated. Many traumatized or hemodynamically unstable patients are tachycardic at presentation and anticholinergics are rarely indicated. Pure agonist opioids and benzodiazepines form the basis of most anesthetic protocols for these patients and are supplemented with low doses of injectable and/or inhalant agents. Vigilant cardiopulmonary monitoring is mandatory and aggressive supportive interventions are often necessary. Example induction and maintenance protocols for this population of patients can be found in Tables 8.10 and 8.11.

Preexisting disease(s)

Patients with preexisting disease conditions commonly require anesthesia for reasons that may or may not be related to their disease process. The cardiovascular, pulmonary, hepatic, renal, gastrointestinal, endocrine, or central nervous systems may be affected and multiple disease conditions affecting multiple organ systems are not uncommon.

Table 8.10.   Induction protocols for patients with trauma and/or hemodynamic instability

Drugs	IV dose in mg/kg
Pure agonist opioids	
Fentanyl	0.005–0.01
Remifentanil	0.006–0.012
Hydromorphone	0.05–0.1
Oxymorphone	0.05–0.1
Benzodiazepines	
Midazolam[a]	0.1–0.3
Lidocaine	2–4 (dogs only)
Injectable anesthetics	
Low dose propofol	1–3
Low dose ketamine	3–5
Low dose etomidate	0.3–1
Possible combinations of above	
Opioid/midazolam[b]	
Opioid/midazolam/low dose propofol	
Opioid/midazolam/lidocaine/low dose propofol	
Opioid/midazolam/low dose ketamine	
Opioid/midazolam/lidocaine/low dose ketamine	
Opioid/midazolam/low dose etomidate	
Opioid/midazolam/lidocaine/low dose etomidate	

[a] Can substitute diazepam at the same dose.
[b] Repeat in alternating increments to effect until intubation is possible; for all other combinations, administer opioid and coinduction agent and then titrate propofol, ketamine, or etomidate IV to effect.

Table 8.11. Anesthetic maintenance protocols for patients with trauma and/or hemodynamic instability

Drugs	IV CRI dose in mg/kg/h
Inhalant anesthetics	
Low dose isoflurane	Delivered to effect
Low dose sevoflurane	Delivered to effect
Pure agonist opioids	
Fentanyl[a,d]	0.005–0.05
Remifentanil[b,d]	0.006–0.06
Benzodiazepine	
Midazolam	0.2–0.4
Local anesthetic	
Lidocaine[c]	3–12 (dogs only)
Dissociative	
Ketamine	0.1–1
Possible combinations of above	
Low dose inhalant with one or more supplemental agents	
Fentanyl or remifentanil with one or more nonopioid supplemental agents	

[a] Usually following a loading dose of 0.002–0.003 mg/kg IV.
[b] Usually following a loading dose of 0.003–0.004 mg/kg IV.
[c] Usually following a loading dose of 1–2 mg/kg IV; reduce CRI to low end of dose range after 1 hour.
[d] Lower CRI rates are used to supplement analgesia and reduce inhalant requirements while higher rates will produce profound analgesia suitable for surgery; ventilatory support is required at higher dose rates.

Depending on the disease state, the reserve capacity of one or more organ systems may be compromised, making these patients more susceptible to adverse side effects associated with anesthetic drug administration. General anesthesia also carries the risk of causing decompensation of a previously compensated disease state. Selection of an appropriate drug protocol must involve a basic understanding of the disease, pathophysiology, and pharmacological knowledge of how specific drugs will impact the organ system in question. Profound depression of the central nervous and cardiopulmonary systems may occur with the administration of sedatives and high doses of injectable and inhalant anesthetics, but specific recommendations will vary depending on the type of disease.

Drug selection: procedure-related factors

The indications for administration of sedative, analgesic, and anesthetic drugs in dogs and cats are numerous and diverse. An understanding of the procedure to be performed, including its level of invasiveness and potential for inducing pain, as well as its duration, will have a significant impact on drug protocol and clinical technique selection.

Level of invasiveness of procedure

Noninvasive procedures requiring patient cooperation   This category includes diagnostic procedures such as radiographs and ultrasound, and therapeutic procedures such as bandage changes. A sedative–analgesic combination, similar to what would be used for preanesthetic medication, is usually sufficient to perform these quick procedures. In certain patients, though, general anesthesia with injectable and/or inhalant anesthetics may be indicated. Even though pain may not be present, it is usually recommended that an opioid be included in the protocol to synergize with the sedative and optimize the level of sedation. IV catheter placement is usually not indicated for routine sedation–analgesia but may be advisable in compromised patients where adverse side effects are more likely. Like IM preanesthetic medications, these combinations are usually administered 15–20 minutes prior to the planned procedure and the animal is left in a quiet place undisturbed while the drugs take peak effect. In other situations, IV administration may be preferred if the patient is amenable to this. Lower doses are typically indicated if the IV route is utilized and peak effect will be attained within 2–5 minutes. The duration of action will vary depending on the combination, the dose, and the route of administration, but most will last between 45 minutes and 2 hours. The use of dexmedetomidine offers the advantage of reversibility with atipamezole, which facilitates a prompt and predictable recovery. In most cases, it is not necessary to reverse the opioid. The decision to coadminister an anticholinergic with the sedative–analgesic combination should be made on a case-by-case basis.

Guidelines for selecting sedative–analgesic combinations are essentially the same as for selecting preanesthetic medications and can be found in Figure 8.3. Dosage recommendations are also similar to those used for preanesthetic medication (see Tables 8.2 and 8.3). Depending on the temperament of the animal and the planned procedure, doses for sedation–analgesia that are at or above the higher end of the recommended preanesthetic range may be indicated if the animal is not going to proceed to general anesthesia.

Minimally invasive procedures requiring general anesthesia   This category includes procedures such as computed tomography (CT) scans, magnetic resonance imaging (MRI), dental cleanings, and endoscopies. In dogs and cats, these procedures typically require a level of patient relaxation and cooperation not possible with sedation–analgesia only, and general anesthesia is usually indicated. Even though these procedures may be short and relatively noninvasive, it is important to remember that every time a patient undergoes general anesthesia, regardless of the procedure being performed, monitoring of anesthetic depth and cardiopulmonary function is mandatory. In most cases, a balanced anesthetic protocol is recommended, usually with some form of preanesthetic medication. Even though pain is not a major component of most of these procedures, opioids are often included in the preanesthetic medication to improve sedation and reduce requirements for induction and maintenance drugs. IV catheterization is recommended in most cases and decisions regarding airway management and other types of supportive care, such as fluid therapy, depend largely on the length of the procedure and risks associated with the patient and procedure. Dosages for preanesthetic, induction, and maintenance drugs can be found in Tables 8.2–8.7.

Invasive surgical procedures associated with mild to moderate pain   This category includes surgical procedures such as castrations, minor lumpectomies, and minor tooth extractions. These procedures will require general anesthesia with additional consideration given to perioperative pain management. A given surgical procedure, such as an ovariohysterectomy, may cause mild, moderate, or severe pain depending on the surgeon performing the procedure, the presence of preexisting pain unrelated to the procedure, and the individual animal's pain tolerance. These factors must be taken into consideration when designing a pain management plan, and if there is ever any question, the patient should be given the benefit of the doubt.

Placement of an IV catheter, endotracheal intubation, and provision of fluid therapy are usually recommended for all but the shortest of procedures. Selection of drugs for the preanesthetic, induction, and maintenance phases will depend on patient-related factors and the length of the procedure. For procedures associated with mild to moderate pain only, administration of an agonist–antagonist (e.g., butorphanol) or a partial agonist (e.g., buprenorphine) opioid is usually sufficient. For procedures with the potential to cause at least moderate pain it is advisable to consider a pure agonist opioid (e.g., hydromorphone, oxymorphone, or morphine). In addition to the opioids, NSAIDs are also commonly used to manage perioperative pain, assuming there is no contraindication for their use. The NSAID may be given preemptively or during the recovery phase and additional doses are often administered for several days postoperatively. Local and regional anesthetic or analgesic techniques may be appropriate in some cases and should be included where possible. Guidelines for selecting sedative–analgesic combinations can be found in Figure 8.3 and dosage recommendations for preanesthetic, induction, and maintenance agents can be found in Tables 8.2–8.7.

Invasive surgical procedures associated with moderate to severe pain   This category includes anesthesia for any major surgical procedure, or anesthesia of a patient with significant preexisting pain due to disease, injury, or trauma. All of the considerations listed in the preceding section are also relevant here; however, the anesthetist must recognize the need to proactively and aggressively manage pain throughout the pre-, intra-, and postoperative periods. A multimodal approach to pain management that incorporates various analgesic drugs and techniques is the best way to accomplish this.

As a generalization, the agonist–antagonist or partial agonist opioids (e.g., butorphanol and buprenorphine) are usually not appropriate choices for the management of moderate to severe pain in most patients. Pure agonist opioids (e.g., morphine, hydromorphone, oxymorphone, and fentanyl) are the opioids of choice for perioperative pain management in these cases and they can be administered in a variety of ways, including intermittent IM, SC, or IV injections; CRIs; epidural administration; or transdermal administration. Opioids are a required component of the preanesthetic medication in this patient population and supplemental doses are often administered throughout the procedure if it is prolonged. Opioids are also used in the immediate postoperative period and are usually continued for at least the first 24 hours after surgery. In some cases, postanesthetic opioid requirements may persist for days or even weeks.

In addition to opioids, other supplemental agents such as lidocaine and ketamine are commonly employed during the maintenance phase. Please refer to Table 8.12 for dosages and potential combinations. Local and regional anesthetic and analgesic techniques are also common adjuncts to general anesthesia. Please refer to Box 8.4 for a list

Table 8.12.   Supplemental systemic analgesics for use during the maintenance phase of anesthesia

Drugs	IV dose in mg/kg
Pure agonist opioids	
Hydromorphone	0.05–0.1 q 4 hours
Oxymorphone	0.05–0.1 q 4 hours
Fentanyl[a,e]	CRI at 0.002–0.05/h
Remifentanil[b,e]	CRI at 0.003–0.06/h
Morphine[c]	CRI at 0.1–0.3/h (usually dogs only)
Local anesthetic	
Lidocaine[d]	CRI at 3–12/h (dogs only)
Dissociative	
Ketamine	CRI at 0.1–1/h
Possible combinations of above for use with an inhalant or propofol CRI	
Opioid only	
Lidocaine only	
Opioid/lidocaine	
Opioid/lidocaine/ketamine	
Opioid/ketamine	

[a] Usually following a loading dose of 0.002–0.003 mg/kg IV.
[b] Usually following a loading dose of 0.003–0.004 mg/kg IV.
[c] Usually following a loading dose of 0.1–0.2 mg/kg *slow* IV.
[d] Usually following a loading dose of 1–2 mg/kg IV; reduce CRI to low end of dose range after 1 hour.
[e] Lower CRI rates are used to supplement analgesia and reduce inhalant requirements while higher rates will produce profound analgesia suitable for surgery; ventilatory support is required at higher dose rates.

Box 8.4.   Local and regional anesthetic and analgesic techniques commonly performed in dogs and cats.

- Epidural anesthesia–analgesia
- Mandibular and maxillary (dental) nerve blocks
- Paw blocks for onychectomy in cats
- Brachial plexus blocks
- Proximal hind limb nerve blocks (femoral, peroneal)
- Continuous local anesthetic infiltration
- Interpleural anesthesia
- Intercostal nerve blocks
- IV regional anesthesia
- Proximal forelimb nerve blocks (radial, median, ulnar, musculocutaneous)

of common techniques in dogs and cats. If not contraindicated, an NSAID is often included in the pain management plan and may be continued for several days postoperatively (see Tables 8.9 and 8.10).

Length of procedure

Short procedures lasting less than 15 minutes   This category is arbitrarily classified as any general anesthetic procedure, surgical or otherwise, that lasts less than 15 minutes.

Preanesthetic medication with a sedative–analgesic combination is still recommended for most patients presenting for short procedures as it will reduce injectable anesthetic requirements. Short-acting and/or reversible drugs are useful preanesthetics as they will not significantly prolong recovery. Analgesic needs will vary depending on the patient and the procedure and have been discussed in preceding sections. Preanesthetic medications are usually given IM or SC but may be given IV if the patient is amenable to this. Most of the injectable anesthetic agents (thiopental, propofol, ketamine–benzodiazepine, etomidate, Telazol, alphaxalone-CD) are appropriate for induction and maintenance for very short periods (i.e., 5–15 minutes). Consequently, transfer to an inhalant anesthetic is usually not indicated. In select patients, a mask or chamber induction with isoflurane or sevoflurane followed by a very brief maintenance phase may be appropriate, but this approach is not recommended for routine use. While the IV route is preferred for administration of injectable anesthetics for reasons discussed previously, the IM route utilizing a dissociative-based protocol may be an option if the patient is not tractable. Remember that the recovery phase will be significantly longer if the IM route is utilized. For recommendations on preanesthetic medications, induction drugs, and analgesic drugs, please refer to Tables 8.2–8.7.

In almost all situations, it is recommended to place an IV catheter prior to induction with an IV anesthetic. Endotracheal intubation may be considered optional in otherwise healthy patients anesthetized for very short procedures, but patients with high-risk airways (e.g., brachycephalic dogs) should always be intubated. Even if intubation is not part of the anesthetic plan, the anesthetist must be prepared to place an endotracheal tube immediately in the event of a complication. This means that access to appropriately-sized endotracheal tubes, a laryngoscope, and a means of positive pressure ventilation (i.e., an Ambu bag or anesthetic machine and breathing system) must be readily available.

In most cases where fluid balance is otherwise normal, IV fluid therapy during the procedure itself may not be indicated. In animals with fluid balance abnormalities, however, a fluid therapy plan addressing the patient's needs is a mandatory part of the anesthetic plan, even for short-duration anesthesia. Instrumenting the patient with numerous pieces of monitoring equipment may not be practical for procedures lasting less than 15 minutes and may in fact delay the start of the procedure. However, monitoring anesthetic depth and basic cardiopulmonary parameters is always mandatory, and the inclusion of one or two key pieces of monitoring equipment such as pulse oximetry, noninvasive blood pressure measurement, or capnometry (if the patient is intubated) is helpful.

It is important to remember that patients anesthetized with injectable drugs are breathing room air (i.e., 21% oxygen) unless they are provided with a supplemental source of oxygen. In this situation, hypoventilation is much more likely to result in desaturation and hypoxemia compared to situations where the patient is intubated and is inspiring close to 100% oxygen. For anesthetized patients inspiring room air, pulse oximetry may be particularly useful in detecting hypoxemia before the patient becomes clinically cyanotic. Treatment in this situation may involve provision of supplemental oxygen via a face mask or, if the patient is bradypneic or apneic, immediate endotracheal intubation and positive pressure ventilation with 100% oxygen.

Intermediate procedures lasting 15–60 minutes This category includes any general anesthetic procedure, surgical or otherwise, that lasts between 15 minutes and 1 hour. Considerations for preanesthetic medication, induction, and pain management are essentially the same as those discussed above. Compared to short-duration procedures, the main difference here is that additional drugs need to be administered after induction to extend the maintenance phase of anesthesia. In most cases, this is most often accomplished by transferring the patient to an inhalant anesthetic such as isoflurane or sevoflurane. Alternatively, maintenance with an injectable drug such as propofol administered as a CRI is also possible. IV catheterization and endotracheal intubation should be performed in all of these patients. Patients receiving total IV anesthesia with a propofol CRI for greater than 15 minutes should also be intubated to protect the airway. Provision of supplemental oxygen is also recommended, as hypoventilation is common and may result in hypoxemia if patients are inspiring room air. All patients anesthetized for more than 15–20 minutes will benefit from routine IV fluid therapy and those patients with preexisting fluid balance abnormalities will require more aggressive management.

As with all cases, basic monitoring of anesthetic depth and cardiopulmonary parameters is standard. In addition, application of monitoring equipment such as capnometry, arterial blood pressure measurement, pulse oximetry, electrocardiography, and body temperature will provide additional information that will facilitate optimal case management. Complications such as hypotension and hypoventilation occur commonly even in young, healthy patients that are administered reasonable doses of standard anesthetic agents. An understanding of the principles of patient monitoring and the operation of routine monitoring equipment facilitates recognition and correction of abnormalities before they become life threatening.

Long procedures lasting more than 60 minutes This category includes any general anesthetic procedure, surgical or otherwise, that lasts greater than 1 hour. Considerations for preanesthetic medication, induction, and pain management are essentially the same as those discussed above. With long-duration procedures, the selection of an appropriate anesthetic agent for the maintenance phase becomes increasingly important. For most patients requiring long-duration anesthesia, inhalant agents such as isoflurane and sevoflurane are the drugs of choice for maintenance as they will still result in rapid and predictable recoveries. IV catheterization, endotracheal intubation, and IV fluid therapy are standard requirements, and other supportive interventions may be indicated for certain patients and/or clinical situations.

While monitoring of anesthetic depth and cardiopulmonary function is necessary for all patients undergoing general anesthesia, the level of monitoring care provided becomes increasingly important as the length of the procedure increases. Monitoring modalities such as capnometry, arterial blood pressure measurement, pulse oximetry, electrocardiography, and body temperature are routinely indicated. Additional modalities that may be useful in specific cases include airway gas analysis, blood gas analysis, central venous pressure measurement, cardiac output measurement, and neuromuscular blockade assessment.

Record keeping

The anesthetic record is a legal document that is part of the patient's permanent medical record. It allows the anesthetist to document trends during the case and make informed management decisions. It also facilitates retrospective evaluation of the anesthetic and pain management plan so that appropriate changes can be made for future cases if necessary.

Revised from "Dogs and Cats" by Richard M. Bednarski in Lumb and Jones' Veterinary Anesthesia and Analgesia, Fourth Edition.

Chapter 9

Anesthesia and immobilization of small mammals

*Paul A. Flecknell, Claire A. Richardson,
Aleksandar Popovic, Rachael E. Carpenter, and
David B. Brunson*

Introduction

Anesthesia of small mammals provides some unique challenges to veterinary anesthetists. In addition to the usual factors to be considered when selecting an anesthetic plan, the potential interactions between the anesthetic and the particular research protocol needs to be weighed when working in laboratory animal medicine. It is important to discuss the proposed anesthetic regimen with the research group concerned and try to indicate any specific pharmacological properties of the anesthetic that are likely to be relevant.

Laboratory mammal anesthesia

General considerations

The majority of laboratory animals will be young, healthy adults, although in some circumstances animals with concurrent disease will be encountered. Laboratory veterinarians should be able to provide information on the health status of the animals and the incidence of clinical and subclinical disease. Most facilities require that animals undergo a period of acclimatization, usually for 1–2 weeks, prior to their use in research procedures. This provides an excellent opportunity for habituation to handling and restraint. It also provides time for the anesthetist and the animal care staff to assess the behavior and temperament of animals, perform a general clinical examination, and obtain background data such as growth rate and food and water consumption. This information is of considerable value when assessing postoperative recovery. Some basic biologic data for common rodents and rabbits are provided in Table 9.1.

Essentials of Small Animal Anesthesia and Analgesia, Second Edition. Edited by Kurt A. Grimm, William J. Tranquilli, Leigh A. Lamont.
© 2011 John Wiley & Sons, Inc. Published 2011 by John Wiley & Sons, Inc.

Table 9.1. Physiological data for rodents and rabbits

	Mouse	Rat	Rabbit	Guinea pig	Hamster	Gerbil
Adult body weight (g)	25–40	300–500	2000–6000	700–1200	85–150	85–150
Body temperature (°C)	37.5	38	38	38	37.4	39
Respiratory rate (breaths/min)	80–200	70–115	40–60	50–140	80–135	90
Heart rate (beats/min)	350–600	250–350	135–325	150–250	250–500	260–300

Source: Flecknell P.A., Richardson C.A., Popovic A. 2007. Laboratory animals. In: *Lumb and Jones' Veterinary Anesthesia and Analgesia*, 4th ed. W.J. Tranquilli, J.C. Thurmon, and K.A. Grimm, eds. Ames, IA: Blackwell Publishing, p. 766.

Anesthetic or analgesic administration may cause discomfort, irritation, and/or ulceration of the skin, mucous membranes, vascular endothelium, or muscles due to low or high pH, temperature (straight from the refrigerator) and/or administered by an inappropriate route (e.g., pentobarbital by intramuscular [IM] route).

Intravenous (IV) injection or placement of IV catheters for anesthetic administration in conscious rodents may be challenging even for experienced clinicians. The use of physical restraint (e.g., restraint tubes) or volatile anesthetics for induction may provide the desired restraint to facilitate this task.

Anesthetic delivery systems

A major advantage of using volatile anesthetics in small mammals is the ease of administration using an anesthetic induction chamber. Ideally, chambers of different sizes should be available (e.g., for animals weighing less than 100 g and for animals weighing up to 1 kg). To reduce the period of involuntary excitement during induction, the chamber should be filled rapidly with the maximum safe induction concentration of the agent. After loss of consciousness, the animal can then be removed from the chamber, and maintained by using a face mask, at a reduced concentration of agent. Providing effective gas scavenging when a face mask is being used can be difficult, but several systems are available commercially that assist with this, for example, the double-mask system.

Anesthesia can also be induced by face mask, and this can be a rapid and convenient technique when using sevoflurane in rats and mice. Volatile anesthetics generally provoke a breath-holding response in rabbits that is often associated with violent struggling unless preanesthetic agents are given. After sedation, the animal should be observed carefully during administration of the anesthetic, and the mask removed briefly if breath holding occurs.

Some laboratory animal units are only equipped to provide compressed air as the anesthetic carrier gas, and this is inadvisable. All of the currently available agents produce some degree of respiratory depression, but hypoxia can be prevented by delivery in oxygen. During recovery from anesthesia, oxygen should continue to be provided until the animal has begun to regain consciousness. If this is not done, then severe hypoxia can occur in some individuals.

Injectable agents

One noteworthy difference relating to the use of injectable anesthetics in small rodents in comparison to dogs and cats is the difficulty of IV access. This results in anesthetic combinations often being administered as single injections by the intraperitoneal (IP), subcutaneous (SC), or IM route, rather than IV, to effect. Although this is a simple and rapid means of producing anesthesia, it has inevitable consequences in relation to the safety of certain anesthetic agents, especially those in which the anesthetic dose is close to the lethal dose. Since there is considerable variation between different strains of rodents in their response to anesthetic agents, anesthetic combinations that either have a broad safety margin or are wholly or partially reversible are preferred when available.

The high metabolic rate of small mammals can result in relatively high dose rates of some anesthetic agents being required to achieve unconsciousness. When coupled with the relative lack of efficacy of agents such as ketamine, this can lead to very high doses being administered (e.g., 100 mg/kg ketamine). Since the drug formulations for veterinary use are normally optimized to give convenient volumes for a dog or a cat, the volume of drug to be injected can be high and, if given IM, can damage tissue and cause pain on injection. Anesthetic combinations that are most widely used in rodents and rabbits are discussed below, and suggested dose rates are listed in Table 9.2.

Ketamine cannot be recommended as the sole anesthetic agent in rodents and rabbits, but when combined with adjunctive drugs such as acepromazine, dexmedetomidine, or opioids, varying planes of anesthesia can be produced. Combinations with tranquilizers often produce only light anesthesia, which is insufficient for surgical procedures, whereas combinations with alpha$_2$ agonists such as dexmedetomidine and xylazine may produce surgical anesthesia. In contrast, in rabbits, combinations of ketamine with acepromazine and diazepam often produce surgical planes of anesthesia.

The use of dexmedetomidine or xylazine with ketamine has the advantage that the sedative–analgesic component of the combination can be reversed with alpha$_2$ antagonists such as atipamezole. Since this anesthetic combination produces cardiovascular and respiratory depression, in addition to other systemic effects such as hyperglycemia and diuresis, it is common to administer the antagonist. Reversing the alpha$_2$ agonist will, of course, reduce the level of postoperative analgesia provided, so that additional agents (e.g., carprofen or buprenorphine) should be administered.

In guinea pigs, the effects of ketamine and xylazine and/or dexmedetomidine are more variable, and surgical anesthesia may not be produced. In all species, if the plane of anesthesia is insufficient, then administering additional doses of the combination may have unpredictable effects. It is preferable to administer a low concentration of an inhalant anesthetic to deepen anesthesia. This same approach can be used to prolong the period of surgical anesthesia. As an alternative, the surgical site can be infiltrated with local anesthetic. As in other species, it is inadvisable to administer atropine routinely when using high doses of alpha$_2$ agonists. Severe hypertension causing mortality has been reported in rats.

Tiletamine in combination with zolazepam (Telazol®, Pfizer Animal Health, New York) has been recommended as an anesthetic for use in rodents and rabbits. As with ketamine–benzodiazepine combinations, the depth of anesthesia produced is not always

Table 9.2. Anesthetic and related drugs for use in rodents and rabbits[a]

Drug	Dose rate	Effect	Anesthesia duration (min)	Sleep time (min)
Anesthetic and related drugs for use in mice				
Fentanyl–fluanisone and diazepam	0.3 mL/kg IM + 5 mg/kg IP	Surgical anesthesia	30–40	120–240
Fentanyl–fluanisone and midazolam[b]	10 mL/kg IP	Surgical anesthesia	30–40	120–240
Ketamine and medetomidine	75 mg/kg + 1 mg/kg IP	Surgical anesthesia	20–30	60–120
Ketamine and xylazine	80 mg/kg + 10 mg/kg IP	Surgical anesthesia	20–30	60–120
Tiletamine–zolazepam	80–100 mg/kg IM	Immobilization		60–120
Tribromoethanol	240 mg/kg IP	Surgical anesthesia	15–45	60–120
Anesthetic and related drugs for use in rats				
α-Chloralose	50–65 mg/kg IP	Light anesthesia	480–600	Nonrecovery only
Chloral hydrate	400 mg/kg IP	Light/surgical anesthesia	60–120	120–180
Fentanyl–fluanisone and diazepam	0.3 mL/kg IM + 2.5 mg/kg IP	Surgical anesthesia	20–40	120–240
Fentanyl–fluanisone and midazolam[b]	2.7 mL/kg IP	Surgical anesthesia	20–40	120–240
Ketamine and medetomidine	75 mg/kg + 0.5 mg/kg IP	Surgical anesthesia	20–30	120–240
Ketamine and xylazine	75 mg/kg + 10 mg/kg IP	Surgical anesthesia	20–30	120–240
Tiletamine–zolazepam	40–50 mg/kg IP	Light anesthesia	15–25	60–120
Urethane	1000 mg/kg IP	Surgical anesthesia	360–480	Nonrecovery only
Anesthetic and related drugs for use in rabbits				
Alphaxalone–alphadolone	6–9 mg/kg IV	Light anesthesia	5–10	10–20
Fentanyl–fluanisone and diazepam	0.3 mL/kg IM + 2 mg/kg IP or IV	Surgical anesthesia	20–40	60–120
Fentanyl–fluanisone and midazolam[b]	0.3 mL/kg IM + 2 mg/kg IM or IV	Surgical anesthesia	20–40	60–120
Ketamine and acepromazine	50 mg/kg IM + 1 mg/kg IM	Surgical anesthesia	20–30	60–120
Ketamine and medetomidine	15 mg/kg SC + 0.25 mg/kg SC	Surgical anesthesia	20–30	90–180

(Continued)

Table 9.2. *(Continued)*

Drug	Dose rate	Effect	Anesthesia duration (min)	Sleep time (min)
Ketamine and xylazine	35 mg/kg IM + 5 mg/kg IM	Surgical anesthesia	20–30	60–120
Propofol	10 mg/kg IV	Light anesthesia	5–10	10–15
Thiopentone	30 mg/kg IV	Surgical anesthesia	5–10	10–15
Anesthetic and related drugs for use in guinea pigs				
Alphaxalone–alphadolone	40 mg/kg IP	Immobilization		90–120
Fentanyl–fluanisone and diazepam	1 mL/kg IM + 2.5 mg/kg IP	Surgical anesthesia	45–60	120–180
Fentanyl–fluanisone and midazolam[b]	8 mL/kg IP	Surgical anesthesia	45–60	120–180
Ketamine and medetomidine	40 mg/kg + 0.5 mg/kg IP	Moderate anesthesia	30–40	90–120
Ketamine and xylazine	40 mg/kg + 5 mg/kg IP	Surgical anesthesia	30	90–120
Anesthetic and related drugs for use in hamsters				
Fentanyl–fluanisone and midazolam[b]	4 mL/kg	Surgical anesthesia	20–40	60–90
Ketamine and medetomidine	100 mg/kg + 0.25 mg/kg IP	Surgical anesthesia	30–60	60–120
Ketamine and xylazine	100–200 mg/kg + 10 mg/kg IP	Surgical anesthesia	30–60	90–150
Anesthetic and related drugs for use in gerbils				
Fentanyl–fluanisone and midazolam[b]	8 mL/kg	Surgical anesthesia	20	60–90
Ketamine and medetomidine	75 mg/kg + 0.5 mg/kg IP	Medium anesthesia	20–30	90–120
Ketamine and xylazine	50 mg/kg + 2 mg/kg IP	Immobilization		20–60

[a] Note that considerable between-strain variation occurs, so dose rates should be taken only as a general guide.
[b] Dose (in milliliters per kilogram) of a mixture of one part Hypnorm (fentanyl–fluanisone) plus two parts water for injection, and one part midazolam (5-mg/mL initial concentration).
Source: Flecknell P.A., Richardson C.A., Popovic A. Laboratory animals. In: *Lumb and Jones' Veterinary Anesthesia and Analgesia*, 4th ed. W.J. Tranquilli, J.C. Thurmon, and K.A. Grimm, eds. Ames, IA: Blackwell Publishing, p. 775.
IM, intramuscularly; IP, intraperitoneally; IV, intravenously; SC, subcutaneously.

sufficient to enable surgical procedures. Combining the mixture with xylazine increases anesthetic depth, but the effects are still variable.

Etorphine–methotrimeprazine (Immobilon, VetaPharma Ltd. Sheburn-in-Elmet, LEEDS, UK), fentanyl–fluanisone (Hypnorm, VetaPharma Ltd.), and fentanyl–droperidol (Innovar-Vet, Shering-Plough Animal Health, Union, NJ) have been used in rodents and rabbits. All of these agents produce immobility and profound analgesia when used alone, but also cause significant respiratory depression. Fentanyl–fluanisone, when combined with midazolam or diazepam, produces surgical anesthesia in all species. Attempts to develop similar mixtures with the other commercially available neuroleptanalgesic combinations have been less successful.

Fentanyl–fluanisone–midazolam has the advantage that it can be mixed and administered as a single injection, but the active components must be diluted with sterile water before being combined. The mixture is stable for several weeks, but on occasion can crystallize. If this is noted, the mix should be discarded. The fentanyl component can be reversed by using naloxone, but this also reverses all analgesic effects of the combination. It is preferable to reverse the fentanyl with a mixed agonist–antagonist such as butorphanol, nalbuphine, or the partial agonist buprenorphine. This reverses any respiratory depression, although full recovery may be prolonged because of the sedative effects of the midazolam and fluanisone. Flumazenil will reverse the midazolam, but its relatively short half-life means that resedation can occur.

In rabbits, the combination is best administered separately, fentanyl–fluanisone initially to produce sedation, analgesia, and peripheral vasodilation. This makes placement of an IV catheter, for example, in the marginal ear vein, simple and enables slow IV administration of the midazolam to produce the desired effects.

In rats, rabbits, and guinea pigs, mixtures of potent opioids (e.g., fentanyl or sufentanil) can be combined with dexmedetomidine or other alpha$_2$ agonists to produce surgical anesthesia. In some instances, the addition of a benzodiazepine improves the degree of muscle relaxation. These combinations have the advantage that they can be completely reversed by using specific antagonists.

Thiobutabarbital (Inactin, Sigma-Aldrich Corp., St. Louis, MO) has been extensively used to provide medium- to long-term anesthesia in rats. It is considered to have minimal effects on the cardiovascular system; in many respects, however, it resembles other barbiturates, producing reduction in cardiac output and organ blood flows.

Urethane is a hypnotic agent that produces long-lasting and stable anesthesia with minimal cardiovascular and respiratory system depression. Urethane provides good narcosis and muscle relaxation, but the analgesic component may not be adequate. It is commonly used in terminal experiments for central and peripheral neural function studies where reflex responses need to be preserved. When administered IP, the most common route used, it has profound endocrine and metabolic effects, producing superficial damage and necrosis of intra-abdominal organs and massive leakage of plasma into the peritoneal cavity. The onset of the aforementioned effects is rapid. Similar effects have not been observed when urethane was administered SC, IV, or intra-arterially. Urethane is carcinogenic and potentially mutagenic; therefore, it should only be used if other suitable alternatives are not available and only for non-recovery studies.

Chloralose is used to provide long-lasting anesthesia, particularly in studies in which maintenance of cardiovascular responses is required. Chloralose is a hypnotic, and the anesthesia depth produced may be insufficient to enable surgical procedures to be undertaken. Induction and recovery from chloralose are very prolonged, so the agent is normally used only for terminal procedures. To avoid problems associated with a prolonged onset of action, anesthesia is often induced using another agent (e.g., isoflurane). Following IV cannulation and any other surgical procedures, chloralose is then administered.

Although now rarely used, chloral hydrate, because of its minimal effects on the cardiovascular system, is still used to anesthetize laboratory animals. It is also used in neuropharmacology studies, because it is thought to have a reduced likelihood of interacting with other compounds. It produces medium-duration anesthesia. The anesthesia depth varies between different strains of rodent and can be sufficient for surgical procedures to be undertaken. In some strains of rat, chloral hydrate can cause postanesthetic ileus, which can be fatal. Using a dilute solution of chloral hydrate (36 mg/mL) can reduce the incidence of ileus.

Tribromoethanol (Avertin, Aldrich Chemical Co., Milwaukee, WI) is a hypnotic that produces surgical anesthesia in rats and mice that lasts approximately 15–20 minutes. It has become extremely popular for anesthesia of mice for embryo transfer and for the production of transgenic animals, and has been reported to be safe and effective. However, if improperly prepared or poorly stored, tribromoethanol can cause gastrointestinal disturbances. More recently, it has been reported that tribromoethanol can cause low-grade peritoneal irritation, even when correctly prepared and stored. In view of these potential adverse effects, tribromoethanol is better replaced with other anesthetic combinations.

Monitoring and intraoperative care

It is particularly important to provide high standards of perioperative care with laboratory animals, since not only can problems such as hypothermia prolong recovery, they cause widespread physiological effects that may interfere with particular research objectives. As in veterinary clinical practice, one staff member may need to act as both anesthetist and surgeon, so detailed clinical monitoring may be lacking. Use of electronic monitoring devices can therefore be of considerable value. The type of monitoring used should be selected based on the species, duration of anesthesia, type of surgery, and assessment of the risk of complications or emergencies.

Small size is correlated with a rapid heart rate (>300 beats per minute) that may exceed the upper limits of some monitors, and the low signal strength may not be detectable. In addition, small body size limits such procedures as invasive blood pressure monitoring and makes most noninvasive devices ineffective. Some equipment is now available that can function despite these problems, and routine electronic monitoring is becoming increasingly commonplace.

Assessment of respiratory function

Clinical observation of respiratory rate and pattern is relatively straightforward, but can be complicated by placement of surgical drapes, especially in small rodents. In these smaller species, the anesthetic circuit will not normally contain a reservoir bag, so observation of bag movements cannot be used to monitor respiration. Unfortunately, many electronic monitors do not respond to the relatively small respiratory movements and low tidal volumes, especially when used with animals weighing less than 200 g. In these small mammals, direct observation of respiratory rate and pattern may be the only option available.

In common with other species, the pattern, rate, and depth of anesthesia vary both with anesthetic depth and with the anesthetic regimen used. With inhalant anesthetics and the majority of injectable regimens, respiratory rate falls. Typical respiratory rates during anesthesia are 50–100 breaths per minute for small rodents and 30–60 breaths per minute for rabbits. Since many of these animals show a very marked stress-related tachypnea prior to induction, assessment of the degree of respiratory depression should either be based on estimates of normal resting rate (Table 9.1) or established by observing the animals preoperatively when undisturbed. A reduction to less than 50% of the estimated normal respiratory rate should cause concern. Gradual changes in rate, rather than a sudden reduction, are more usual, so keeping an anesthetic record is advisable.

The adequacy of oxygenation and pulse rate can be assessed by using a pulse oximeter, but the high heart rates in rodents may exceed the upper limits of the monitor. A monitor with an upper limit of at least 350 beats per minute is needed, and successful operation may also depend on the type of probe used. It is advisable to try several instruments, probes, and probe positions to find the most reliable combination. In the authors' experience, a signal can usually be obtained from the hind foot in rodents or the base of the tail. In rabbits, the toe, tail, tongue, and ear are also useful. In particular, the use of an angled probe placed in the mouth has proven particularly reliable.

End-tidal carbon dioxide is difficult to measure in small mammals. The gas volume sampled by side-stream capnographs may be very large in relation to the animal's tidal volume, and mainstream capnographs usually introduce too much dead space into the anesthetic-breathing circuit. In rabbits, equipment designed for pediatric use in people usually functions well.

Maintenance of an airway may be assisted by placement of an endotracheal tube, but the small size of many laboratory species makes this technically difficult. Rabbits can be intubated by using either an otoscope to visualize the larynx or a blind technique. Prior to intubation, the animal should breathe 100% oxygen for 1–2 minutes. Uncuffed endotracheal tubes should be used to maximize the airway internal diameter (ID); a 3–3.5-mm-diameter tube is usually suitable for a 3–4-kg rabbit. Tubes with a diameter of less than 2.5 mm are required for very small rabbits (<800 g), and these should be purchased from specialty suppliers.

When an otoscope is used the rabbit is positioned on its back. The mouth is opened and its tongue pulled forward into the gap between the incisors and premolars. Care must be used not to injure the tongue on the edges of the incisors. The otoscope speculum should be inserted into the gap between the teeth on the opposite side of the mouth to the tongue and advanced until the end of the soft palate or the larynx is visible. In some animals, the epiglottis will be positioned behind the soft palate, hiding the larynx from view. To expose the larynx, an introducer is used to reposition the epiglottis and soft

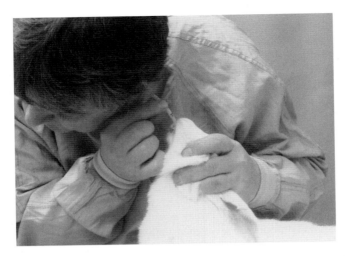

Figure 9.1.   Intubation of a rabbit by using the "blind technique." The rabbit is in sternal recumbency, and oxygen is administered for at least 2 minutes prior to intubation. To intubate, the endotracheal tube is placed in the rabbit's mouth to the level of its larynx. On inspiration, the endotracheal tube is gently advanced into the larynx in the direction of the loudest breath sounds.
Source: Flecknell P.A., Richardson C.A., Popovic A. 2007. Laboratory animals. In: *Lumb and Jones' Veterinary Anesthesia and Analgesia*, 4th ed. W.J. Tranquilli, J.C. Thurmon, and K.A. Grimm, eds. Ames, IA: Blackwell Publishing, p. 778.

palate. The larynx should then be sprayed with local anesthetic. The introducer is then advanced through the otoscope speculum, through the larynx, and into the trachea. The otoscope is removed and the endotracheal tube threaded onto the introducer and into the trachea. The introducer is then withdrawn.

To place a tube using the blind technique, the rabbit is positioned in sternal recumbancy, with its head and neck extended upward (Figure 9.1). The endotracheal tube is introduced into the gap between the incisors and premolars and advanced into the pharynx. When the larynx is reached, some increase in resistance is felt. The tube can then be advanced into the larynx and trachea. Successful placement is usually accompanied by a slight cough. In some cases, the tube passes into the esophagus and will need to be withdrawn and repositioned. Passage of the tube is often assisted by gently rotating it through 45° as it is advanced into the larynx. The tube position can be monitored by listening at the end of the tube. If breath sounds can be heard, the tube should be in the pharynx or the trachea. As an alternative to intubation, a laryngeal mask can be used. This technique is easier to master than endotracheal intubation, but manual or mechanical ventilation may not be effective. If only oxygen supplementation is required, a nasal catheter can be passed and positioned in the back of the pharynx.

Intubation of small rodents is made easier if a specialized apparatus is used. A technique using a modified otoscope speculum to visualize the larynx and an over-the-needle catheter as the endotracheal tube is relatively easy to master. Although a variety of other methods have been described, the modified otoscope enables rapid, atraumatic intubation and is supplied together with an instructional video.

After intubation, animals can be maintained on an appropriate anesthetic circuit; for example, a purpose-made low dead space T-piece for small rodents, or a pediatric T-piece or unmodified Bain's circuit for rabbits.

Assessment of cardiovascular function

Clinical monitoring of the cardiovascular system is difficult in small rodents because of their size. Peripheral pulses are difficult or impossible to palpate, and heart rate is frequently greater than 250 beats per minute. In rabbits and guinea pigs, the chest can be auscultated or palpated, but this is difficult in smaller rodents. An esophageal stethoscope can be used in rabbits.

When using electronic monitoring equipment, the upper rate limits (e.g., 250 or 300 beats per minute) are often exceeded, and some instruments will not detect the low-amplitude electrocardiographic signal.

Other clinical assessments, such as use of capillary refill time, are practical. In all species, assessment of the color of the mucous membranes enables some assessment of peripheral perfusion and oxygen saturation of hemoglobin.

Arterial blood pressure can be measured by using noninvasive systems in larger rabbits or by using pediatric-sized cuffs or specially designed veterinary equipment. Blood pressure can be measured in this way in rats, using a tail cuff, but special apparatus is required. Invasive blood pressure monitoring is possible in all species, but surgical exposure of the vessel is needed in rodents, which tends to limit the use of this technique to nonrecovery procedures. In rabbits, an over-the-needle catheter can be placed in the central ear artery.

Blood volume in all of these species is approximately 70 mL/kg of body weight, so small rodents will have very low total blood volumes (e.g., 2 mL for a 30-g mouse). It is therefore critically important to minimize blood loss by careful hemostasis and to monitor blood loss by accurate weighing of swabs and assessing other losses at the surgical site.

Thermoregulation

Small mammals have an increased surface area/body weight ratio that results in rapid cooling during anesthesia. Maintaining body temperature and careful monitoring to ensure this is being achieved effectively are important. Hypothermia can cause delayed recovery from anesthesia and, if severe, can cause cardiac arrest. Rectal temperature should be monitored with an electronic thermometer. The probe size of less expensive instruments is usually appropriate for animals weighing 250 g or more, but specialized instruments are needed for very small rodents (e.g., mice and hamsters). To reduce loss, the area of fur shaved during preparation of the surgical site should be minimized, and use of skin disinfectants should be limited to the minimum necessary to maintain asepsis.

Animals should be placed on a heating pad maintained at 37–39°C. It is important that measures to maintain body temperature are continued into the postoperative period.

Emergencies

All of the measures for coping with anesthetic emergencies applicable to companion animals can be used in laboratory species, but as with many other techniques, small body size can limit or complicate some of these procedures.

To assist ventilation if an animal has not been intubated, its head and neck should be extended, the tongue pulled forward, and the chest gently squeezed between the anesthetist's thumb and forefinger. If the tongue is difficult to grasp, it can be rolled forward using a cotton swab.

When an animal has been intubated, respiration can be assisted relatively easily. Attempting to assist ventilation by using a face mask is usually unsuccessful, but in small rodents a soft piece of rubber tubing can be placed over the nose and mouth, and the lungs inflated by gently blowing down the tube.

As mentioned earlier, since total blood volume is low in small rodents, every effort should be made to minimize blood loss and avoid overhydration. If fluid therapy is required, this can be delivered via an over-the-needle catheter in the tail vein of rats, the medial tarsal vein in guinea pigs, or the marginal ear vein, cephalic vein, or jugular vein in rabbits.

If whole blood is required, then a suitable donor may be available in the research facility. All of the commonly available fluid products can be administered safely to small mammals and other laboratory species. In smaller rodents in which IV access is not practicable, IP or SC administration of warmed electrolyte solutions can slowly replace fluid deficits, but will be of minimal benefit if rapid hemorrhage is occurring. In these smaller species, placement of an intraosseous catheter can provide an alternative route for fluid replacement.

If cardiac arrest occurs, external cardiac massage and emergency drugs such as epinephrine can be used when attempting resuscitation.

Postoperative care

If possible, a separate recovery area should be provided, because this makes it easier to provide an optimal environment during this period. It also encourages individual attention and special nursing, if those are required. Most of the commonly used anesthetics will continue to cause some degree of respiratory depression in the immediate postoperative period. In addition to continuing to monitor respiratory function, care must be taken that respiratory obstruction does not occur. Small rodents and rabbits may attempt to hide and push into the corner of a recovery cage, and this can result in airway obstruction. Also, when allowed to recover in a group, rodents may huddle together, which can decrease oxygen availability for the animals at the bottom of the group. Although recovery is often more rapid after use of inhalational agents, significant hypoxia (oxygen saturation of less than 90%) can occur, and this should be prevented by maintaining the animal in an oxygen-enriched environment, either by using a face mask or by delivering oxygen into the incubator until respiratory function is judged to be appropriate.

It is important that measures to maintain normal body temperature are continued in the recovery period. This can often be achieved by allowing animals to recover in a pen or cage in a recovery room (maintained at a high ambient temperature, with supplemental heating of the cage as necessary) or inside an incubator. A temperature of 25–30°C is needed for adult animals and 35–37°C for neonates. If an incubator is unavailable, heating pads and lamps should be provided. Since small mammals can be heated rapidly, care must be taken not to overheat or burn the patient, and a thermometer should be placed next to the animal to monitor the temperature in its immediate environment.

During recovery from anesthesia, animals should be provided with bedding, such as synthetic sheepskin. If this is not available, then towels or a blanket should be used. Sawdust or wood shavings are unsuitable because this type of bedding will often stick to an animal's eyes, nose, and mouth. Tissue paper is often provided as bedding for small rodents, but it is relatively ineffective because animals usually push it aside during recovery from anesthesia and end up lying in the bottom of a plastic cage soiled with urine and feces.

Drinking water should be available, but care must be taken that this not be spilled or placed in a bowl that the animal may drown in. If the animal's skin becomes wet, it will lose heat rapidly. Small rodents are usually accustomed to using water bottles, so this is rarely a problem, but it can present difficulties with rabbits, guinea pigs, ferrets, and larger species.

It may also be necessary to provide fluid therapy postoperatively. This can be given by IV infusion in larger animals, but it is most convenient in small rodents to give warmed (37°C) SC or IP dextrose/saline at the end of surgery (Table 9.3).

Food should be provided for most laboratory species immediately after they regain consciousness and are at a minimal risk of aspiration. A mash made by soaking pelleted diet in warm water is often rapidly consumed by small rodents, providing both additional fluid as well as food intake.

Pain assessment

If analgesics are administered appropriately, then it is essential that attempts are made to assess the severity of postoperative pain. Only when this is done can one determine whether an appropriate dose of analgesic has been administered. Pain assessment is also essential to judge whether an appropriate type of analgesic has been selected, when to repeat dosing, and when to discontinue therapy.

Table 9.3. Volumes of fluid for administration to rodents and rabbits

Route	Mouse	Rat	Rabbit	Guinea pig	Hamster	Gerbil
Intraperitoneal (mL)	2	5	50	20	3	2–3
Subcutaneous (mL)	1–2	5	30–50	10–20	3	1–2

Volumes are suggested rates for adult animals. All fluids should be warmed to body temperature prior to administration.
Source: Flecknell P.A., Richardson C.A., Popovic A. 2007. Laboratory animals. In: *Lumb and Jones' Veterinary Anesthesia and Analgesia*, 4th ed. W.J. Tranquilli, J.C. Thurmon, and K.A. Grimm, eds. Ames, IA: Blackwell Publishing, p. 781.

Unfortunately, assessing pain in many species is difficult. At present, the only practical option may be to judge the likely pain intensity based on the type of surgery and skill of the surgeon and use this to formulate an analgesic protocol (critical anthropomorphic approach). As with anesthesia selection, the aims of the particular research project should be considered when selecting the analgesic plan.

Analgesic efficacy clearly varies considerably between different strains of rodents, and this reinforces the need for pain scoring systems. At the time of writing, pain scoring schemes have been developed for rats, following abdominal surgery. In this species, back arching, contraction of the abdominal muscles, staggering and falling (not related to anesthetic recovery), and twitching of the skin overlying the back and abdomen all appear to be pain related. If more than one or two back arches, abdominal contractions, or staggers are seen in a 5-minute period, then additional analgesia may be required. Illustrative material is available from www.digires.co.uk. In mice, similar behaviors have been noted, as has a reduction in normal activities such as climbing, but these behaviors have not yet been developed into a formal pain scoring system.

Some rabbits also show abdominal contractions after laparotomy, but changes in postoperative behavior in this species appear to be much more variable and to be markedly inhibited in some animals by the presence of an observer. Virtually no information is available regarding pain-associated behavior in guinea pigs, hamsters, or gerbils.

In rats, and probably other small rodents, analgesic efficacy can be assessed retrospectively by evaluating food and water intake and body weight. Body weight, food intake, and water intake decreases after many types of surgery in several different strains of rat, and administration of analgesics reduces this effect. However, changes are not always consistent, particularly in juvenile animals.

Pain alleviation

Since all of the analgesic agents available for use in animals and people have been developed and tested for safety and efficacy in laboratory animals, likely effective doses can be suggested for most agents. However, the assessments of efficacy made during drug development are often based on tests that rely on acute painful stimuli (e.g., brief noxious heat or pressure). These differ from clinical pain. The dose rates suggested in Table 9.4 are based on clinical experience, published data that incorporated a means of assessing postoperative pain, or data from analgesimetric assays, such as the late-phase formalin test, that are believed to be more relevant to clinical pain.

Nonsteroidal anti-inflammatory drugs   All of the nonsteroidal anti-inflammatory drugs (NSAIDs) available for use in animals can be administered to laboratory species. The general considerations related to their use in other species apply equally to laboratory species; however, since most laboratory animals undergoing surgery are young, healthy adults, concerns related to preexisting disease are often minimal. Of the agents available, the oral preparation of meloxicam is of particular value because it is highly palatable to many small rodents, particularly if added to a favorite foodstuff. The duration of action of NSAIDs in rodents and rabbits is uncertain, but carprofen and meloxicam appear to have duration of at least 8 and possibly 24 hours.

Table 9.4. Suggested analgesic doses for rodents and rabbits

Analgesic	Mouse	Rat	Rabbit	Guinea pig	Hamster	Gerbil
Buprenorphine	0.1 mg/kg SC per 6–12 hours	0.01–0.05 mg/kg SC per 6–12 hours	0.01–0.05 mg/kg SC	0.05 mg/kg SC	0.1 mg/kg SC	0.1 mg/kg SC
Butorphanol	2 mg/kg SC per 4 hours	2 mg/kg SC per 4 hours	0.1–0.5 mg/kg SC	2 mg/kg SC	?	?
Carprofen	10 mg/kg SC	5 mg/kg SC	4 mg/kg SC once daily or 1.5 mg/kg PO daily	2.5 mg/kg	?	?
Flunixin	2.5 mg/kg SC twice daily	2.5 mg/kg SC twice daily	1.1 mg/kg SC twice daily	?	?	?
Meloxicam	5 mg/kg SC per 4 hours	1–2 mg/kg SC or 4 mg/kg PO	0.2 mg/kg SC daily	?	?	?
Morphine	2–5 mg/kg SC	2–5 mg/kg SC per 4 hours	2–5 mg/kg SC or IM per 4 hours	2–5 mg/kg SC or IM per 4 hours	?	?
Oxymorphone	?	0.2–0.3 mg/kg SC	0.1–0.2 mg/kg IM or IV	?	?	?
Pethidine	10–20 mg/kg SC or IM per 2–3 hours	10–20 mg/kg SC or IM per 2–3 hours	10 mg/kg SC or IM per 2–3 hours	10–20 mg/kg SC or IM	?	?

Dose rates are based largely on uncontrolled clinical trials and a limited range of procedures, and so are likely to be subject to revision. A "?" indicates that information is insufficient to make a firm recommendation of an appropriate dose.

Source: Flecknell P.A., Richardson C.A., Popovic A. 2007. Laboratory animals. In: *Lumb and Jones' Veterinary Anesthesia and Analgesia*, 4th ed. W.J. Tranquilli, J.C. Thurmon, and K.A. Grimm, eds. Ames, IA: Blackwell Publishing, p. 767.

IM, intramuscularly; IV, intravenously; PO, per os (orally); SC, subcutaneously.

Opioids   These are effective at alleviating postoperative pain, but some species-specific side effects have been reported. Opioids may also cause sedation or excitement, with their effects varying considerably in different animal species. The effects on behavior also depend on the drug dose that has been administered. Morphine sedates rats, but produces excitement in mice and, at high doses, a characteristic elevated and rigid tail (the Straub tail response). Although an effective analgesic, buprenorphine use in some strains of rat in some research institutes has been reported to cause pica, manifested as compulsive eating of bedding material. This is most severe when inappropriately high drug doses are administered, but can also be seen at lower dose rates. Although the problem can be prevented by housing the animals on grid floors, it may represent abdominal discomfort or nausea so an alternative analgesic should be used for that particular strain of animal. This side effect does not occur consistently, and, in view of the prolonged duration of action and safety of buprenorphine, this analgesic is often considered the opioid analgesic of choice in rats and other laboratory species.

Effective pain control

Whatever the analgesic plan, it is important to administer sufficient drug to relieve pain effectively and assess patients frequently. Preoperative administration of analgesics before elective surgery is advocated. In addition to providing more effective pain relief, it may also reduce the dose of anesthetic required. Experience with small rodents and rabbits has shown that the use of buprenorphine in this way enables the concentration of isoflurane or halothane needed for surgical anesthesia to be reduced by 25–50%. Care should be taken when using injectable anesthetics administered IP or IM. As discussed earlier, in these circumstances the dose of anesthetic cannot be adjusted to meet individual requirements, and it is clear that opioids can potentiate the effects of anesthetic drugs. When using neuroleptanalgesics, the opioid component will provide analgesia that can conveniently be partially reversed with the administration of buprenorphine or butorphanol. The latter opioid provides better reversal, but has a short duration of action, so either an additional dose should be given, or it should be combined with a NSAID.

As in other species, combinations of different agents (multimodal approach) can be particularly effective: for example, local nerve block at the time of a thoracotomy, coupled with the administration of systemic opioids and NSAIDs, followed by repeated administration of opioids and NSAIDs, as required. As the degree of pain subsides, the opioids can be reduced and pain controlled solely with NSAIDs.

Anesthesia of neonatal rodents

Neonatal rodents can be safely and effectively anesthetized with inhalant anesthetics, such as isoflurane or sevoflurane. The majority of injectable anesthetics may be associated with a high mortality, but fentanyl–fluanisone has been used in neonatal and juvenile rats.

Hypothermia is still used as an anesthetic technique for neonates in some research laboratories. The technique remains controversial, but mortality is low when this approach is used. This approach should be used only when alternative methods have been shown to be unsuitable. Reducing body temperature to around 4–5°C by placing newborn rodents in a refrigerator or on crushed ice immobilizes them and slows their cardiac and respiratory function to virtually undetectable levels. At these temperatures, nerve conduction is slowed or completely blocked, so that it is assumed that surgery can be performed without the animals experiencing pain or distress.

Rodents and rabbits

Small rodents and rabbits do not vomit, so there is generally no need to withhold food or water prior to anesthesia. Withholding food from small rodents for prolonged periods can be detrimental because it can predispose them to hypoglycemia. Rabbits and guinea pigs are more likely to develop postoperative gastrointestinal disturbances if food is withheld. In anesthetized guinea pigs, small quantities of food are often found in the mouth, but this is not prevented by withholding food.

Since anesthesia of rodents is often induced by using an anesthetic chamber or by using an injection of drugs by the IP or SC routes, preanesthetic medication is not often given. In rabbits, induction with a volatile agent delivered via a face mask may be considered, but a sedative agent (e.g., dexmedetomidine, diazepam, or acepromazine) should be administered because animals often find this procedure stressful. Even when volatile agents are not used, sedatives or tranquilizers can have significant benefits because rabbits are easily stressed when handled and restrained. Administration of the drug before removal from the animal's cage or pen is advisable. Suitable agents are listed in Table 9.5.

When only immobilization is required, rather than anesthesia, high doses of some of the agents listed in Table 9.5 may be effective, but often low doses of anesthetic combinations (e.g., ketamine–dexmedetomidine) are more useful. Preanesthetic medication with an analgesic may be advisable in all of these species, as part of a perioperative pain management regimen, and dose rates of suitable analgesics are listed in Table 9.4.

As in other species, atropine or glycopyrrolate can be administered to reduce bronchial and salivary secretions, although this is rarely needed in rodents that are free of respiratory infection. However, these agents may be useful to block vagal inhibition of sinus heart rate caused by some surgical procedures (e.g., handling of the viscera or carotid cannulation that may involve direct vagal manipulation). It is advisable to use glycopyrrolate in rabbits because atropine is often relatively ineffective in this species.

The IP route of administration is the easiest for small rodents, because larger amounts of fluids may be administered. However, errors during administration by this route are quite common (e.g., intravisceral, SC, or administration into the adipose tissue). Such errors may cause organ damage or delayed onset of action of the anesthetic agent. Injections are usually made into the left lower abdominal quadrant. Rodents are restrained in dorsal recumbency, as shown in Figure 9.2.

Most of the commercially available analgesic and anesthetic agents are available in high concentrations, so that only very small volumes would be required for injection in

Table 9.5. Preanesthetic agents for use in rodents and rabbits

Drug	Species	Dose rate	Effect
Acepromazine	Rat, guinea pig	2.5mg/kg IP or SC	Sedation, but still active
	Mouse, hamster, gerbil	3–5mg/kg IP or SC	Sedated, often immobilized
	Rabbit	1mg/kg SC or IM	Sedation, often immobilized, some analgesia
Acepromazine + butorphanol	Rabbit	0.5mg/kg + 1.0mg/kg IM or SC	
Atropine	Mouse, hamster, gerbil, rat, guinea pig	40mcg/kg SC or IM	Reduced bronchial and salivary secretions, inhibits vagal responses, ineffective in many rabbits
Diazepam	Mouse, hamster, gerbil, guinea pig	5mg/kg IP	Sedation
	Rat	2.5mg/kg IP	
	Rabbit	1–2mg/kg IM	
Glycopyrrolate	Rabbit	0.01mg/kg IV or 0.1mg/kg SC or IM	Reduced bronchial and salivary secretions, inhibits vagal responses
Innovar-Vet (fentanyl–droperidol)	Rabbit	0.22mL/kg IM	Sedation and analgesia; often sufficiently immobilized for minor surgical procedures
Hypnorm (fentanyl–fluanisone)	Mouse	0.5mL/kg IM	Sedation and analgesia; often sufficiently immobilized for minor surgical procedures
	Hamster	1.5mL/kg IM	
	Guinea pig	0.4mL/kg IM	
	Mouse, hamster, gerbil, rat, guinea pig	0.5mL/kg SC or IP	
	Rabbit	0.3–0.5mL/kg SC or IM	
Medetomidine	Mouse, hamster, rat	30–100mcg/kg SC or IP	Sedation and some analgesia, immobilized at higher dose rates
	Rabbit	100–500mcg/kg SC or IP	
Midazolam	Mouse, hamster, gerbil, guinea pig	5mg/kg IP	Sedation
	Rat	2.5mg/kg IP	
	Rabbit	1–2mg/kg IM	
Xylazine	Mouse, hamster, rat	5mg/kg SC or IM	Sedation and some analgesia, immobilized at higher dose rates
	Rabbit	2.5mg/kg SC or IM	

Source: Flecknell P.A., Richardson C.A., Popovic A. 2007. Laboratory animals. In: *Lumb and Jones' Veterinary Anesthesia and Analgesia.* 4th ed. W.J. Tranquilli, J.C. Thurmon, K.A. Grimm, eds. Ames, IA: Blackwell Publishing, p. 767.
IM, intramuscularly; IP, intraperitoneally; IV, intravenously; SC, subcutaneously.

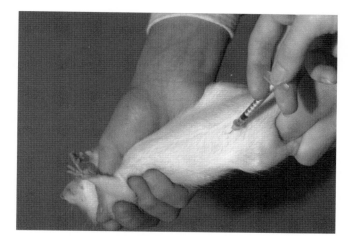

Figure 9.2.   IP injection of a rat. The rat is restrained in dorsal recumbency by an assistant. An injection is made into its lower right abdominal quadrant.
Source: Flecknell P.A., Richardson C.A., Popovic A. 2007. Laboratory animals. In: *Lumb and Jones' Veterinary Anesthesia and Analgesia*, 4th ed. W.J. Tranquilli, J.C. Thurmon, and K.A. Grimm, eds. Ames, IA: Blackwell Publishing, p. 769.

small rodents. Precise dosing is easier if insulin syringes are used. Alternatively, a commercial preparation can be diluted to provide a more accurately administered volume. For IV administration, butterfly or over-the-needle catheters with or without extension sets may be used for initial induction and anesthetic maintenance by infusion.

Hamsters

Animals can be held in both hands, immobilizing the head to avoid being bitten. Alternatively, grasp the loose skin around the neck and back region firmly. The saphenous vein may be used for IV administration. For other routes, see Table 9.6.

Gerbils

Gerbils are generally easy to handle and can be scooped into the palm of a hand. Alternatively, they can be picked up gently at the base of the tail, but grasping the distal end of the tail might detach skin. Gerbils dislike being picked up and turned onto their backs. The lateral tail or saphenous veins may be used for IV administration. For other routes of administration, see Table 9.6.

Guinea pigs

Guinea pigs are easily lifted by grasping them gently around the thorax and shoulders with one hand while supporting the hind quarters with the other hand. Aural, saphenous, or penile veins (only under anesthesia) may be used for IV administration.

Table 9.6.   Routes of injection for rodents and rabbits

Injection site	Species	Location	Needle size (gauge)	Precautions
Intramuscular	Rodents	Quadriceps or posterior thigh muscles	25–27	Muscle mass is very small, avoid sciatic nerve
	Rabbits	Quadriceps, dorsal lumbar, or posterior thigh muscles	24–27	Avoid sciatic nerve
Intravenous	Mice and rats	Lateral tail or saphenous vein	24–28	
	Rabbits	Marginal ear vein, cephalic or saphenous vein	23–25	Use a local anesthetic cream (EMLA Cream, AstraZeneca LP. Wilmingotn, DE) prior to injection
Subcutaneous	Rodents	Interscapular or inguinal region	21–25	Highly viscous liquids may cause discomfort and are difficult to inject
	Rabbits	Interscapular or flanks	21–25	

Source: Flecknell P.A., Richardson C.A., Popovic A. 2007. Laboratory animals. In: *Lumb and Jones' Veterinary Anesthesia and Analgesia*, 4th ed. W.J. Tranquilli, J.C. Thurmon, and K.A. Grimm, eds. Ames, IA: Blackwell Publishing, p. 770.

Mice

Mice are not as easily habituated to restraint as are other rodents, and there are great variations between different strains. Some are relatively docile and easy to catch, whereas others may be extremely active. Mice are usually grasped by the base of the tail and lifted from the cage. When placed on a nonslip surface such as a cage lid or laboratory coat, they can be grasped by the loose skin overlying the animal's back, with the tail restrained between the operator's fingers. This form of restraint is particularly suitable for IP, IM, and SC administration of drugs.

Rats

The easiest and most humane way to lift a rat is with one hand supporting the hind quarters and the other hand supporting the head, with the thumb under the foreleg and mandible. Rats can be grasped using the loose skin overlying the neck and back, if necessary.

Rabbits

Gently approach the rabbit in the cage or floor pan and grasp the skin of the neck and back firmly, supporting the abdomen and hind legs with the other hand. When carrying rabbits, the head is kept between the arm and the chest of the handler. Wrapping the rabbit in a towel or a purpose-designed restraint device may facilitate handling and is particularly helpful when performing IV injections.

Anesthetic considerations for other nondomesticated and exotic mammals

Chinchillas

Chinchillas are easily removed from their cages by grasping them by the base of the tail and lifting them off their feet. Anesthesia can be induced with sevoflurane or isoflurane. Midazolam (5 mg/kg) plus ketamine (15–20 mg/kg) administered IM produces relaxation and analgesia for up to 2 hours and may facilitate induction of anesthesia. Thiopental in dilute solution can be administered IV to effect for minor surgical procedures. Epidural anesthesia has been used for cesarean section because the lumbosacral fossa is easily located and is comparatively large. Epidural anesthesia techniques are similar to those used for dogs and cats and can be achieved with local anesthetics such as lidocaine. In a 2004 study, an IM combination of midazolam (1.0 mg/kg), medetomidine (0.05 mg/kg), and fentanyl (0.02 mg/kg) was compared with the IM injection of either xylazine (2.0 mg/kg) with ketamine (40.0 mg/kg) or medetomidine (0.06 mg/kg) with ketamine (5.0 mg/kg) to assess combination anesthetic actions in chinchillas. The xylazine–ketamine and medetomidine–ketamine combinations provided longer surgical tolerance, but overall the midazolam–medetomidine–fentanyl combination was preferred because it induced less cardiopulmonary depression and achieved good anesthesia with the potential for complete reversal.

Squirrels

Squirrels can be anesthetized with isoflurane or sevoflurane administered into an induction chamber. Ketamine (10–20 mg/kg) is the most commonly used injectable anesthetic in gray and fox squirrels. It provides adequate immobilization for physical examination and diagnostic procedures. A combination of medetomidine and ketamine has also been used to immobilize squirrels.

Prairie dogs

In prairie dogs, ketamine (100 to 150 mg/kg) plus xylazine (20 mg/kg) administered IV produces 1.5–2.0 hours of satisfactory surgical anesthesia. Xylazine can be administered 10 minutes prior to ketamine or may be given at the same time. For longer periods of anesthesia, inhalant anesthetics can also be administered via a mask or following endotracheal intubation. Because prairie dogs are obligate nasal breathers, they need to only have their nose in the mask for induction and maintenance of inhalant anesthesia. Visualization of the larynx is difficult without the use of a modified otoscope or laryngoscope. If all that is required is a short period of sedation, a lower dose of ketamine (40 mg/kg) can be combined with acepromazine (0.4 mg/kg) and administered IM. Butorphanol (2 mg/kg SC) or buprenorphine (0.02 mg/kg SC) may be used to produce analgesic effects in prairie dogs.

Marmots

Marmots are similar to prairie dogs and have been successfully anesthetized with combinations of xylazine–ketamine, medetomidine–ketamine, and xylazine–Telazol.

Agoutis

Agoutis are large, excitable, agile rodents that can injure themselves or handlers if not carefully restrained. Ketamine alone (25–35 mg/kg) has been used to immobilize agoutis. Ketamine can be coadministered with analgesics or sedative–analgesics for painful procedures. Inhalant anesthetics (isoflurane or sevoflurane) delivered via a face mask or by endotracheal tube produce good surgical anesthesia following ketamine immobilization.

Nutria

The coypu (nutria) is difficult to restrain for IV injection. They have no readily accessible superficial veins. Endotracheal intubation can be performed in anesthetized animals with a slightly flexible tube containing a curved stylet. Intubation can be performed without visualization of the laryngeal opening. Animals weighing 3–5 kg require a 5-mm endotracheal tube. Upon insertion, apnea may occur. Following intubation, anesthesia can be maintained with any inhaled anesthetic. Ketamine (10–20 mg/kg) plus 2 mg of xylazine have been assessed together in 4–5-kg nutria for tail amputation surgery. Prolonged anesthesia was produced by 20 mg/kg of ketamine, whereas 10 mg/kg was insufficient for surgery. Administration of medetomidine (0.1 mg/kg IM) plus ketamine (5 mg/kg IM) induces rapid anesthesia in nutria. Immobilization lasts for approximately 40–60 minutes. Atipamezole (0.5–0.7 mg/kg IM) will awaken animals within 5–10 minutes of administration. The atipamezole dose should be four- to fivefold the dose of medetomidine. Atropine (0.1 mg/kg) is effective as a preanesthetic to decrease salivary secretions.

Voles

Voles have been anesthetized for nearly 3 hours with pentobarbital at an IP dose of 0.06 mg/g of body weight. Surgical anesthesia can be induced for 15–20 minutes in meadow voles with a 0.06–0.09 mg/g dose of pentobarbital injected IM. In recent years, the use of IM or IP pentobarbital for anesthesia has been supplanted with injectable combinations and the use of inhalant anesthetics in most rodent species.

Bats

Bats should be handled with thick leather gloves to prevent one from being bitten. Bats harbor a number of viruses that can cause human illnesses and even death. Therefore, sedation and anesthesia are recommended if extensive handling is necessary. Fruit bats (*Eidolon helvum*) have been sedated with a phenothiazine tranquilizer (chlorpromazine, 2.5 mg/100 g IM). After the tranquilizer has taken effect, the bat can be mounted on a restraining board with wings extended and an inhalant anesthetic administered by mask.

Other methods of chemical restraint include xylazine (2–3 mg/kg IM) administration, which will provide 30–40 minutes of sedation. Ketamine can be given IM at a dose of 10–20 mg/kg along with this dose of xylazine to provide more complete immobilization with muscle relaxation and a quiet recovery. Medetomidine (50 mcg/kg IM) has also been combined with ketamine (5 mg/kg IM) for short-term immobilization. Telazol (tiletamine–zolazepam) may be a good alternative for injectable immobilization at an IM dose of 8–10 mg/kg. IP pentobarbital injection at a dose of 0.05 mg/g of body weight has been used in a number of genera of bats (*Rhinolophus, Hipposideros, Tadarida, Molussus, Eptesicus, Chilonycteris,* and *Artibeus*) to implant electrodes surgically on the round window of the cochlea or in the brain. Smaller doses (0.03–0.045 mg/g) have been used for *Myotis lucifugus* and *Pleocotus townsendii.*

Isoflurane or sevoflurane delivered by mask or into an induction chamber can be safely used to anesthetize bats. Following mask induction, *megachiropterous* can be intubated (2–3 mm ID) to maintain anesthesia. When intubating bats, care must be taken to avoid lacerations from teeth and direct contact with saliva. IV access is feasible via the brachial vessels overlying the distal humerus.

Armadillos

There are 10 living genera of armadillos. *Dasypus novemcinctus*, the most common, weighs 4–5 kg as an adult. Armadillos should be caught close to the base of the tail to avoid the hind claws. Because armadillos can incur a large oxygen debt, they may lie completely still without breathing for long periods. Armadillos also have the ability to recover spontaneously from repeated episodes of ventricular fibrillation. Anesthetics may be administered into the subcarpal tissues or the paraspinal muscles by inserting a needle between two bands slightly to one side of the midline. The site should be disinfected to avoid risk of abscess formation. IV injections can be made into the two prominent superficial femoral veins. The femoral vein is the only accessible superficial vein that can be easily catheterized.

Neuroleptanalgesic combinations (e.g., fentanyl–droperidol, 0.20–0.25 mL/kg IM) appear to produce sufficient depression and analgesia for surgery. Longer procedures have been performed with slow IV infusion of thiopental. Infused over a period of 1 hour, 5 mL of 0.5% solution is adequate and safe for most adults. The usual dosage is 5–6 mg/kg/h. Alternatively, pentobarbital (25 mg/kg IV) has been administered via the superficial femoral vein. Half the dose is given rapidly, followed by the remainder to effect. Apnea and breath holding are not reported to be a problem with this technique.

Telazol (8.5 mg/kg IM), xylazine (1 mg/kg) with ketamine (7.5 mg/kg), and medetomidine (75 mcg/kg) with ketamine (7.5 mg/kg) have been evaluated for their anesthetic actions following IM administration. All three combinations induced anesthesia within 5 minutes. Armadillos were immobilized for approximately 45 minutes, with recovery requiring 2–3 hours. When atipamezole was used to antagonize medetomidine, recovery was shortened to 15 minutes or less.

Inhalation anesthesia with isoflurane or sevoflurane is easily achieved with an induction chamber. Premedication with atropine (total dose, 0.1 mg IM) can be used to diminish secretions. A soft polyethylene endotracheal tube 4–8 mm ID is easily placed through the laryngeal opening with the use of a laryngoscope. Following intubation, anesthesia may be maintained with inhalant anesthesia.

Mink

A metal or clear plastic tube is convenient for restraining mink. The dimensions of the tubes will vary according to the size of the mink being restrained. One end of the tube is covered with hardware cloth, with the other remaining open. The mink is inserted head first into the tube. Vaccinations or other injections can be administered SC or IM on the inner surface of the hind leg while the animal is restrained. Anesthesia has been induced via isoflurane or sevoflurane administration. Maintenance of anesthesia by use of rebreathing or nonrebreathing delivery systems is preferred. In field situations, mink and polecats have been successfully immobilized and anesthetized with a combination of ketamine (10 mg/kg IM) and medetomidine (0.20 mg/kg IM) for radiotransmitter implantation. Induction was achieved in less than 4 minutes, and immobilization lasted from 28 to 54 minutes. Older reports indicate that reserpine (0.036–0.05 mg) can be administered orally in feed to render the mink less nervous and excitable. Apparently, there is a wide margin of safety with few cumulative toxic effects.

Ferrets

Ferret anesthesia is commonly induced with sevoflurane or isoflurane in an induction chamber. Atropine (0.04 mg/kg) can be administered either SC or IM prior to induction. To maintain anesthesia, inhalants are then delivered via a mask or through an endotracheal tube. Injectable mixtures for producing short periods of anesthesia in ferrets include ketamine (26 mg/kg IM) plus acepromazine (0.22 mg/kg IM); ketamine alone (20–30 mg/kg IM) to produce light surgical anesthesia for 40–60 minutes; alphaxalone/alphadalone (12–15 mg of total steroid/kg IM), which is a 3:1 mixture of alphaxalone with alphadolone acetate, to produce 15–30 minutes of light anesthesia; and Telazol at a dose of 5–10 mg/kg IM. A mixture of Telazol (250 mg tiletamine and 250 mg zolazepam) solubilized in 4 mL of ketamine (400 mg) and 1 mL of 10% xylazine (100 mg/mL) designed for use in exotic cats can be used in ferrets and feral cats at a dose of 0.03–0.04 mL/kg IM. This mixture has been used for castrations, declawing, and intra-abdominal surgery. Medetomidine (0.1 mg/kg IM) can also be combined with ketamine (5 mg/kg IM) to induce a short period of anesthesia in ferrets.

Skunks

In general, rapid-acting volatile anesthetics such as isoflurane or sevoflurane are preferred for anesthetizing skunks. For small skunks, a transparent plastic disposable bag is an ideal container for induction with sevoflurane or isoflurane. Anesthesia is induced while the skunk is in the bag. Once immobilized, the skunk is removed and the bag is discarded. This procedure should be performed in a well-ventilated room to minimize human exposure to anesthetic gases and skunk musk. The best age for removal of the scent glands in skunks appears to be 5–6 weeks of age, when the skunk's weight is about 2 lb.

An anesthetic technique for wild skunks caught in traps using a 9-ft. pole syringe has been described. The operator stands at a distance while making an IM injection and thus facilitates handling without exposure to musk or possibly being bitten. The immobilizing combination of ketamine (16 mg/kg IM) plus xylazine (8 mg/kg IM) has been effective in skunks. Anesthesia is usually induced in less than 3 minutes, with immobilization lasting approximately 30 minutes. Skunks are less likely to expel musk if the operator is slow and deliberate. Skunks that expel musk usually direct it at the pole syringe when the drug is injected.

Stoat and weasel

Stoat (*Mustela erminea*) and weasel (*Mustela nivalis*) are extremely fierce and difficult to handle. They will bite through thick leather gloves and, if held tightly, may be asphyxiated. A satisfactory and nontraumatic method of inducing anesthesia is to place these animals in an induction chamber attached to the end of the cage by means of a removable slide. Isoflurane or sevoflurane is then introduced into the box via the fresh gas line from the vaporizer. Safe induction concentrations range from 2.5% to 4.0%. Once the animal is unable to right itself, it can be removed from the chamber and inhalant anesthesia maintained at lower concentrations by using a face mask or via delivery through an endotracheal tube. The intubation technique is similar to that used for ferrets. Light surgical anesthesia can be maintained with 1.5–2.0% concentrations of isoflurane or 2–3% sevoflurane. Alternately, medetomidine (0.1 mg/kg IM) plus ketamine (5 mg/kg IM) has been used to immobilize stoats with variable success.

Badgers

Badgers (*Taxidea taxus*), which have a ferocious disposition, have been successfully immobilized with ketamine. The average effective dose is 20 mg/kg IM, and repeated smaller doses are sometimes administered. Complete recovery occurs in 90–180 minutes, depending on the total dose administered. A number of studies have evaluated anesthetic combinations in badgers in comparison with ketamine alone (20 mg/kg). The addition of midazolam with lower doses of ketamine (10–15 mg/kg) did not improve anesthesia, nor did the combination of medetomidine (80 mcg/kg) with only 5 mg/kg of ketamine. The combination of butorphanol, medetomidine, and ketamine however, appeared to improve overall muscle relaxation and anesthesia. Following immobilization with either ketamine (15–25 mg/kg IM) plus xylazine (0.5–1.0 mg/kg) or Telazol (8–12 mg/kg) plus xylazine (0.5–1.0 mg/kg), anesthesia can be maintained with isoflurane or sevoflurane delivered through a mask or endotracheal tube.

Wild procyonids

Members of this family include the ring-tailed cat, raccoon, coatimundi, mountain coati, lesser panda, and giant panda. Anesthetic techniques used in these species are primarily based on experience gained in the immobilization and anesthesia of raccoons. These anesthetic techniques would appear applicable for most procyonids. IV anesthesia is not practical because of difficulty in restraining these species. Ketamine or Telazol have been used extensively and are made more efficacious when supplemented with an alpha$_2$ agonist (e.g., xylazine or dexmedetomidine). A phenothiazine (acepromazine) or benzodiazepine (diazepam) tranquilizer can also be combined with ketamine. When ketamine has been used alone at a dose of 20–30 mg/kg IM, induction takes 3–7 minutes, and recovery can be expected to occur in 45–90 minutes. A combination of a lower dose of ketamine (10 mg/kg IM) with xylazine (2 mg/kg IM) or other alpha$_2$ agonist is more often used to immobilize wild procyonids today. Induction occurs in 3–5 minutes after IM injection. Anesthesia appears adequate, lasts for 15–20 minutes, and can be prolonged by administering one-quarter to one-half of the original combination dose IM or by the administration of isoflurane or sevoflurane via a face mask or an endotracheal tube.

Telazol has been used in a variety of procyonids for chemical restraint and short, minor surgical procedures. A dose of 10 mg/kg IM induces anesthesia lasting for 20–60 minutes. With this dose, reflexes (including the palpebral, corneal, pinnal, pharyngeal, and laryngeal) should persist.

Marsupials

Possums and gliders belong to several marsupial families. Of these marsupials, the most common species in captivity is the sugar glider. These small marsupials are best anesthetized with sevoflurane or isoflurane in a chamber or by mask. Inhalants can be administered via a closed system or via a mask once an opossum is adequately sedate. For prolonged procedures, thiopental can be given for induction of anesthesia and intubation, followed by administration of isoflurane or sevoflurane. For smaller possum species, as for sugar gliders, chamber induction with a fast-acting inhalant anesthetic (isoflurane or sevoflurane) is the preferred technique, but depression of the central nervous system may be difficult to assess when possums are stressed (enter into a physiological sleep) and become nonresponsive to external stimuli.

Alternatively, ketamine (20 mg/kg IM) alone or Telazol (5 to 6 mg/kg IM) alone can be used. Ketamine (20–25 mg/kg IM) and fentanyl–droperidol (0.75 to 1.0 mL/kg IM) have both been used to immobilize opossums satisfactorily for handling. In another report, surgical anesthesia was achieved in possums with 5 mg/kg IM of xylazine combined with ketamine at 20–30 mg/kg IM. Koalas have also been immobilized safely and rapidly with alphaxalone–alphadolone (Althesin) at doses of 3–6 mg/kg IM or 1–2 mg/kg IV.

Insectivora

Hedgehogs and other insectivores, such as tenrecs, shrews, and moles, are easily anesthetized with isoflurane or sevoflurane in oxygen in an induction chamber or box. Anesthesia can be maintained with the inhalant delivered via a face mask or endotracheal tube at a concentration ranging from 0.5% to 1.5% for isoflurane and from 2.5% to 3.5% for sevoflurane. Hedgehogs can be intubated relatively easily. The most commonly used injectable anesthetic is ketamine (5–20 mg/kg IM), alone or in combination with diazepam (0.5–2.0 mg/kg IM), xylazine (0.5–1.0 mg/kg IM), or medetomidine (100 mcg/kg IM). Telazol can also be effective at a dose of 1–5 mg/kg IM.

Hypothermia is a real threat because of the hedgehog's small body size. Fluids can be given IV or SC in the loose tissue beneath the spines. SC fat may account for up to 50% of the hedgehog's body weight and can cause delayed absorption of fluids and anesthetics when injected in this tissue. IM injections require a needle length sufficient to extend through fatty SC tissues. Either buprenorphine (0.01 mg/kg) or butorphanol (0.2–0.4 mg/kg IM or SC) can be administered to provide analgesic therapy following surgery.

Revised from "Laboratory Animals" by Paul A. Flecknell, Claire A. Richardson, and Aleksandar Popovic; and "Exotic and Zoo Animal Species" by Rachael E. Carpenter and David B. Brunson in Lumb and Jones' Veterinary Anesthesia and Analgesia, Fourth Edition.

Chapter 10

Local anesthetics and regional analgesic techniques

Roman T. Skarda and William J. Tranquilli

Introduction

Local anesthetics are a group of chemically related compounds that reversibly bind sodium channels and block impulse conduction in nerve fibers. The interruption of neural transmission in sensory afferent nerves or tracts by a local anesthetic drug after local tissue infiltration, regional nerve blocks, or epidural or intrathecal (subarachnoid) injection uniquely and most effectively prevents or reduces pain or nociceptive input during and after surgery. Analgesia in the desensitized area is not only complete by such techniques, but it also removes the immediate secondary (central) sensitization to pain and reduces the central facilitation of the nociceptive pathway.

The use of a local anesthetic is essential if surgery is to be performed in a conscious patient and the pain associated with trauma and inflammation is to be relieved. The use of a local anesthetic technique before surgery may also benefit patients by avoiding general anesthesia or reducing the amount of general anesthetic. Sustained analgesia into the recovery period is a great benefit to patients when a local anesthetic with a longer anesthetic effect is used. Knowledge of the clinical pharmacology of individual local anesthetics enables the achievement of effective and safe neural blockade. Local anesthetic techniques discussed herein have their own particular rate of onset, duration, and risk of complication.

Electrophysiology

The conduction of impulses in excitable membranes requires a flow of sodium ions through selective sodium channels into the nerve in response to depolarization of the nerve membrane. Mammalian voltage-gated sodium channels consist of one large alpha subunit that contains four homologous domains (D_1–D_4), each with six putative α-helical transmembrane segments (S_1–S_6) and one or two smaller auxiliary beta subunits. Under resting conditions, sodium ions are at a higher concentration outside than inside the nerve, and a voltage difference across the axonal membrane, known as resting potential,

Essentials of Small Animal Anesthesia and Analgesia, Second Edition. Edited by Kurt A. Grimm, William J. Tranquilli, Leigh A. Lamont.
© 2011 John Wiley & Sons, Inc. Published 2011 by John Wiley & Sons, Inc.

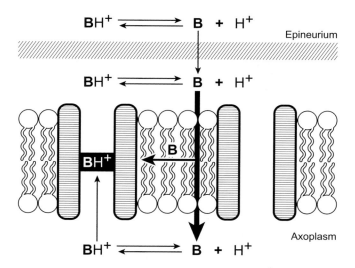

Figure 10.1. Site of action of amino-ester and amino-amide local anesthetics. The uncharged base form diffuses most readily across the lipid barriers and interacts at the intermembrane portion of the sodium channel. The charged form (BH^+) gains access to a specific receptor via the axoplasmic surface of the sodium channel pore. Modified from Carpenter and Mackey, p. 414, with permission.

of 270 mV exists. When the nerve is stimulated, the permeability of the membrane to sodium ions increases transiently, and sodium passes through the membrane by way of sodium-selective ionic channels that exist in various conformations (i.e., resting, open, or inactivated), depolarizing the plasma membrane. During depolarization, the action potential moves in obligatory fashion along the axon, allowing for impulse propagation along the nerve membrane. After a few milliseconds, the membrane repolarizes as a result of inactivation or "closing" of the sodium channels. During repolarization, the membrane is no longer permeable to sodium ions, but potassium channels open, and potassium ions flow down their electrochemical gradient out of the cell.

Mechanisms of action

The precise mode of action of local anesthetic drugs is unknown, but perhaps the combination membrane-expansion and specific-receptor theory is most accepted. In this theory, the quaternary ammonium compounds (amides) and ester local anesthetics first pass through the cell membrane as the uncharged base (B) to reach the intracellular site where the uncharged base is protonated and the charged cation (conjugated acid, BH+) binds to the receptor and "plugs" the channel (Figure 10.1). Perhaps best accepted is the idea that local anesthetics bind to sodium-selective ionic channels in nerves, inhibiting the sodium permeability that underlies action potential and depolarization of the cell membrane. Electrical transmission through a myelinated axon stops when enough concentration of the anesthetic is applied to bathe at least three consecutive nodes of Ranvier.

Frequency-dependent block

Local anesthetics may differ in their ability to bind to sodium channels, depending on the channel status. Open ion-conducting and inactivated sodium channels have a greater local anesthetic affinity than resting, nonconducting sodium channels. Repetitive stimulation of nerve fibers increases the binding affinity of the receptor site for local anesthetics and facilitates the development of neural blockade, a phenomenon called use-dependent or frequency-dependent block, or phasic block.

Other mechanisms of action

Local anesthetics will bind to many different sites that may contain a variety of different sodium channels. The sodium channels in the heart, brain, and axons are not identical. However, if local anesthetics achieve a sufficient tissue concentration, they will affect all excitable membranes, including those that exist in the heart, brain, and neuromuscular junction. The molecular mechanisms by which local anesthetics produce epidural or spinal (subarachnoid) analgesia may include local anesthetic binding to sodium and potassium channels within the dorsal and ventral horns and binding to neural calcium channels, which causes hyperpolarization of cell membranes. Alterations in membrane calcium ion (Ca^{2+}) may be responsible for deformation or expansion of the cell membrane and thus the transmission or conduction of nerve impulses. Local anesthetics may inhibit substance P binding and evoke increases in intracellular calcium (Ca^{2+}), and potentiate γ-aminobutyric acid (GABA)-mediated chloride currents by inhibiting GABA uptake.

Antimicrobial activity

Additional and sometimes controversial benefits of local anesthetics, which are routinely administered before minor skin surgery and for postoperative pain relief, include both a potent antimicrobial effect and improved wound healing. Administration of 1%, 2%, and 4% lidocaine demonstrates a dose-dependent inhibition of growth for all strains of bacteria tested (e.g., *Staphylococcus aureus*, *Escherichia coli*, *Pseudomonas aeruginosa*, and *Enterococcus faecalis*) and no change in the susceptibility of the bacteria to lidocaine by the addition of epinephrine. Likewise, administration of 2% and 5% lidocaine and 1% prilocaine demonstrates a powerful antimicrobial effect on various bacteria, including *E. coli*, *S. aureus*, *P. aeruginosa*, and *Candida albicans*. In contrast, 0.25% and 0.5% bupivacaine shows poor antimicrobial effectiveness, and ropivacaine has no antimicrobial effect on such microorganisms.

Chemical structure

All local anesthetics contain an aromatic ring at one end of the molecule and an amine at the other, separated by a hydrocarbon chain (Table 10.1). The aromatic end is derived from benzoic acid or aniline and is lipophilic. The amine end is derived from ethyl alcohol or acetic acid and is hydrophilic. Substitution of alkyl groups on the aromatic ring or amine end increases lipid solubility and potency.

Chirality

In general, local anesthetics are supplied commercially as racemic mixtures of both R-(+) and S-(−) optical stereoisomers. Differences in structure result in various pharmacodynamic and pharmacokinetic actions. Ropivacaine is provided as the hydrochloride of the pure S-(−) enantiomer. It is associated with a reduced incidence of both cardiovascular and central nervous system (CNS) toxicity, a concern with use of racemic bupivacaine. In addition, epidural ropivacaine is similar to bupivacaine in onset, depth, duration, and extent of sensory blockade, although motor block is less intense and briefer.

Levobupivacaine is a pure S-(−) enantiomer similar to ropivacaine, and is also less toxic than bupivacaine, which is attributable to a lesser affinity for brain and myocardial tissue than either that of the R-(+) enantiomer or racemic bupivacaine.

Chemical grouping

The clinically useful local anesthetic drugs essentially segregate into amino esters and amino amides, based on the chemical link between the aromatic moiety and the hydrocarbon chain (Table 10.1). Amino esters have an ester link, and the amino amides have an amide link, respectively. The nature of linkage (ester vs. amide) has a notable effect on the chemical stability and the route of metabolism. Ester-linked local anesthetics include cocaine, benzocaine, procaine, chloroprocaine, and tetracaine. Most esters are readily hydrolyzed by plasma cholinesterase and have short half-lives when stored in solution without preservatives. Amide-linked local anesthetics include lidocaine, prilocaine, dibucaine, etidocaine, mepivacaine, bupivacaine, levobupivacaine, ropivacaine, and articaine. The amide agents are very stable, cannot be hydrolyzed by cholinesterase, and rely on enzymatic degradation in the liver. The amide structure of articaine is similar to that of other local anesthetics but contains an additional ester group, which is quickly hydrolyzed by esterases, shortening its duration of action. Ropivacaine and levobupivacaine are synthesized as single S-(−) optical isomers. Other local anesthetics exist as racemates or have no asymmetrical carbons.

The clinical action of local anesthetics may be described by their lipid solubility, anesthetic potency, speed of onset, duration of action, and tendency for differential block. These properties do not sort independently and their relevancy to each other can be compared in Table 10.2.

Differential nerve blockade

Controversy still surrounds the differential susceptibility of nerve fibers to local anesthetics and its relation to selective functional deficit. It is apparent that differential block of impulses in nerve fibers exists, varying among anatomical features (different peripheral nerves, fiber diameter, presence or absence of myelination, and surrounding tissue),

Table 10.1. Trade names, chemical structure, and main clinical uses of ester-linked and amide-linked local anesthetic agents

Drug name	Trade name	Chemical structure	Main clinical use
Amides			
Lidocaine	Xylocaine Lignocaine	$NHCOCH_2N(C_2H_5)_2$ (2,6-dimethylphenyl)	Infiltration, nerve blocks, intra-articular, epidural
Prilocaine	Citanest	$NHCOCHNHCH_2CH_2CH_3$ with CH_3 (methylphenyl)	Infiltration, nerve blocks, epidural
Etidocaine	Duranest	$NHCOCHN$ with CH_2CH_3, CH_2CH_3, $CH_2CH_2CH_3$ (2,6-dimethylphenyl)	Infiltration, nerve blocks, epidural
Mepivacaine	Carbocaine	CH_3—N—CONH (piperidine, 2,6-dimethylphenyl)	Infiltration, nerve blocks, intra-articular, epidural
Bupivacaine	Marcaine	$(CH_2)_3CH_3$—N—CONH (piperidine, 2,6-dimethylphenyl)	Infiltration, nerve blocks, epidural, subarachnoid
Levobupivacaine	Chirocaine	CH_3, CH_3, NH—C(=O)—(piperidine N—CH_2CH_2CH_2CH_3)	Infiltration, nerve blocks, epidural, subarachnoid

330

Drug	Trade name	Structure	Indications
Ropivacaine	Naropin	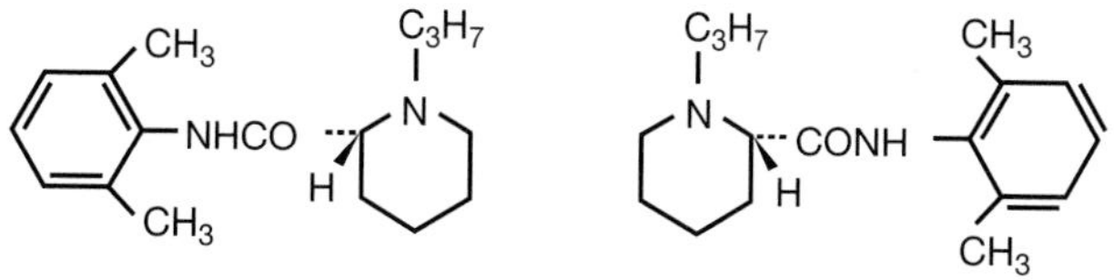 (structure)	Infiltration, nerve blocks, epidural, subarachnoid
Articaine	Ultracain Carticain	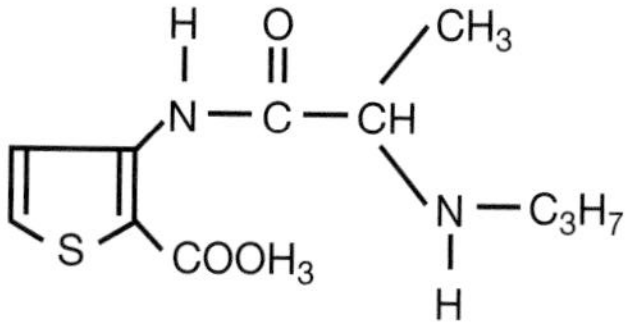 (structure)	Infiltration, nerve blocks, intravenous, regional anesthesia, epidural
Esters			
Cocaine		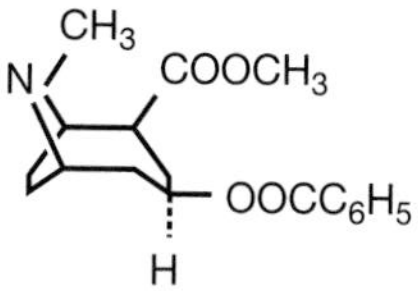 (structure)	Topical
Benzocaine	Americaine	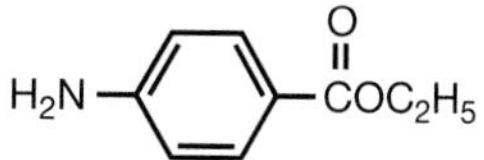 (structure)	Topical
Procaine	Novocain	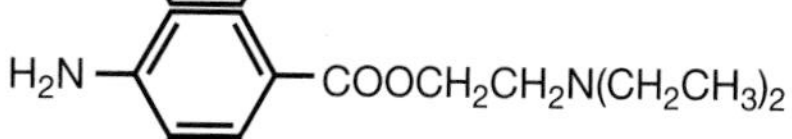 (structure)	Infiltration, nerve blocks, epidural
Chloroprocaine	Nesacaine	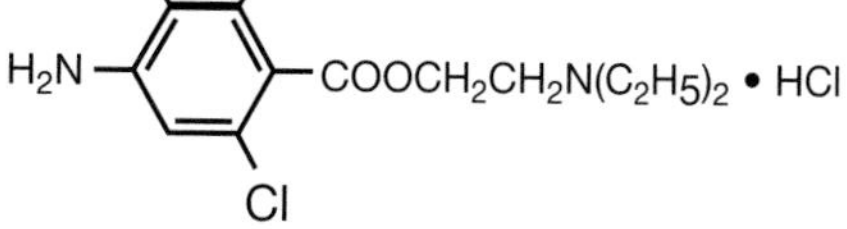 (structure)	Infiltration, nerve blocks, epidural
Tetracaine	Pontocaine Amethocaine	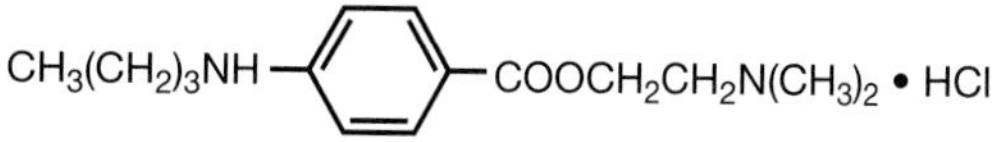 (structure)	Topical, subarachnoid

Selected chemical labels visible in structures:

- Ropivacaine: C_3H_7, NHCO, CH_3, CH_3
- Articaine: C_3H_7, CH_3, O, $N-C-CH$, $N-C_3H_7$, H, COOCH$_3$, S, COOH$_3$
- Cocaine: CH_3, N, COOCH$_3$, OOCC$_6$H$_5$, H
- Benzocaine: O=COC$_2$H$_5$, H$_2$N
- Procaine: COOCH$_2$CH$_2$N(CH$_2$CH$_3$)$_2$, H$_2$N
- Chloroprocaine: COOCH$_2$CH$_2$N(C$_2$H$_5$)$_2$ • HCl, Cl, H$_2$N
- Tetracaine: CH$_3$(CH$_2$)$_3$NH, COOCH$_2$CH$_2$N(CH$_3$)$_2$ • HCl

331

Table 10.2. Physical, chemical, and biologic properties of currently available local anesthetic agents

Drug	Lipid solubility	Relative anesthetic potency[a]	pK_a	Plasma protein binding (%)	Onset of action	Duration of action (min)
Ester linked						
Low potency, short duration						
Procaine	1	1	8.9	6	Slow	45–60
Chloroprocaine	1	1	9.1	7	Fast	30–60
High potency, long duration						
Tetracaine	80	8	8.6	80	Slow	60–360
Amide linked						
Intermediate potency, short duration						
Articaine	52	4	7.8	65	Fast	30–45
Intermediate potency and duration						
Lidocaine	3.6	2	7.86	65	Fast	60–120
Mepivacaine	2	2	7.7	75	Fast	90–180
Prilocaine	1	2	7.7	55	Fast	120–180
Intermediate potency, long duration						
Ropivacaine	14	6	8.07	95	Intermediate	180–480
High potency, long duration						
Bupivacaine	30	8	8.1	95	Intermediate	180–480
Levobupivacaine	31.1	ND	8.09	>97	Intermediate	180–480
Etidocaine	140	6	7.74	95	Fast	180–480

[a] The potency given is relative to procaine.
ND, not determined.

different local anesthetics, critical duration of drug exposure (absorption, distribution, and elimination of drug from the site of injection), and different animal species (e.g., frogs, rats, cats, and people). Sensory and motor fibers have a characteristic neurophysiological profile, motor and sensory function, and conduction-block susceptibility (Table 10.3).

In situ studies

Local anesthetics block nociceptive fibers (small unmyelinated C fibers and myelinated A-δ fibers) more readily and before other sensory and motor fibers (large myelinated A-γ, A-β, and A-α fibers) (Table 10.3). Local anesthetics block small-diameter myelinated or unmyelinated fibers at a lower concentration than is required to block large fibers of the same type. This is probably attributable to the longer action potentials and the discharge at higher frequencies of smaller fibers.

Differential brachial plexus blockade

Brachial plexus block in dogs produces more rapid onset of motor block when compared with sensory block after the administration of bupivacaine (0.375% with 5 mg/mL

Table 10.3. Classification of nerve fibers and order of blockade

	Fiber type				
	A-α	A-β	A-γ	A-δ	B	C
Function	Somatic motor	Touch, pressure	Proprioception	Fast pain, temperature	Vasoconstriction, preganglionic sympathetic	Slow pain, postganglionic sympathetic polymodal nociceptors
Myelin	Heavy	Moderate	Moderate	Light	Light	None
Diameter (μM)	12–20	5–15	3–6	2–5	1–3	0.4–1.5
Priority of blockade	←5	←4	←3	←2	←1	→2
Signs of blockade	Loss of motor function	Loss of sensation to touch and pressure	Loss of proprioception	Pain relief, loss of temperature sensation	Increased skin temperature	Pain relief, loss of temperature sensation

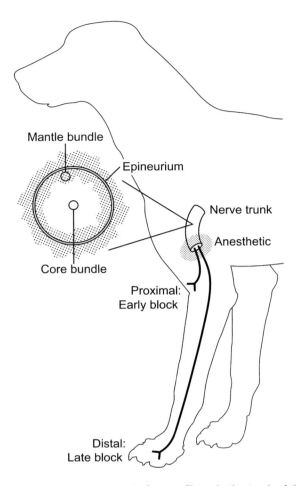

Figure 10.2. Somatosensory arrangement of nerve fibers in the trunk of the brachial plexus of the dog. Nerve fibers in the mantle or peripheral bundles innervate primarily motor fibers of the proximal limb, whereas nerve fibers in the core or center bundles innervate for the most part the sensory fibers of the distal foot. The concentration gradient that develops during initial diffusion of local anesthetic into the nerve trunk causes onset of anesthesia to proceed from proximal to distal. Recovery from anesthesia also proceeds from proximal to distal because of absorption of local anesthetic into the circulation surrounding the nerve trunk.

epinephrine, 4 mg/kg) (9.7 vs. 26.2 minutes, mean values). This phenomenon is explained by the somatotopical arrangement of nerve fibers such that the motor fibers would be located at the periphery of the nerve trunk (mantle bundles) and the sensory fibers in the center (or core) (Figure 10.2). Consequently, if sufficient analgesic drug is applied to produce motor blockade, the diffusion of the analgesic or its transport into the nerve by the local blood supply will first affect the motor fibers.

Differential epidural and spinal blockade

In general, progression of epidural and spinal anesthesia is related to the diameter, myelination, and conduction velocity of affected nerve fibers. Exposure of mixed-nerve trunks within the spinal vertebral column to a sufficient concentration of an analgesic drug might cause a loss of sensation in this order: pain, heat and cold, touch, proprioception, and skeletal muscle tone. Recovery of sensation is expected to be in the reverse order.

Autonomic small unmyelinated C fibers and myelinated B fibers seem to be readily desensitized after epidural or spinal administration of local anesthetics. Spinal anesthesia is generally characterized by preganglionic sympathetic nerve blockade (B fibers) that extends further than sensory block (A-δ fibers), and sensory block extends further than somatic motor block (A-α fibers).

Sensory anesthesia sufficient for surgery usually cannot be obtained without motor impairment. Adequate sensory analgesia with little or no motor blockade can be achieved with the epidural administration of low concentrations of bupivacaine or ropivacaine combined with opioids and/or alpha$_2$ agonists. Epidural blockade may be able to differentiate between sympathetic, somatic, and central pain in patients with chronic pain.

Factors influencing efficacy

A variety of factors can influence the quality of regional anesthesia, including local anesthetic dose, site of administration, additives such as epinephrine or hyaluronidase, pH adjustment and carbonation, baricity, temperature, mixtures of local anesthetics, and altered physiology (such as pregnancy).

Dose of local anesthetic

A greater dose (volume and/or concentration) will facilitate overall efficacy, thereby decreasing the delay of onset of action and increasing both the likelihood of successful anesthesia and its duration. The potential of systemic toxicity by inadvertent intravenous (IV) injection or neurotoxicity precludes the routine administration of large doses of local anesthetic.

All local anesthetics can be neurotoxic, particularly in concentrations and doses larger than those used clinically. Large-scale surveys, using histopathologic, electrophysiological, behavioral, and neuronal cell models, indicate that lidocaine and tetracaine seem to have a greater potential for neurotoxicity than does bupivacaine at clinically relevant concentrations.

Volume of local anesthetic

Generally, a larger volume of local anesthetic will produce a faster and denser block. An exception to this rule is articaine, which readily penetrates tissues and produces anesthesia in approximately 2 minutes, irrespective of the volume injected. The necessity of a larger injected volume of anesthetic solution for a high rate of complete sensory block can be minimized during plexus blocks in dogs if an adequate concentration of a local anesthetic agent (e.g., 1% mepivacaine or 0.375% bupivacaine) is precisely administered at multiple injection sites covering all major nerves of the brachial plexus.

Concentration of local anesthetic

A higher concentration of local anesthetic will also produce a faster and denser block. Increasing the concentration of lidocaine and bupivacaine during phasic ("use dependent") inhibition of sodium currents increases the rate of binding but has no effect on unbinding sodium channels. In general, the chance for successful desensitization and anesthesia decreases when the concentration is lowered. One study suggests that lumbar epidural anesthesia with 10 mL of 2% lidocaine in humans produces more intense blockade of large-diameter and small-diameter sensory nerve fibers than that with 20 mL of 1% lidocaine. Similarly, administration of 0.75% ropivacaine into the lumbar epidural space of dogs produces a higher rate of complete anesthesia than does 0.5% ropivacaine of similar volume (0.22 mL/kg).

Injection site

In general, the fastest onset (within 3–5 minutes) and shortest duration (1 hour) of anesthesia is usually produced after subcutaneous and intrathecal injections of 2% lidocaine or mepivacaine hydrochloride solution, followed in order of increasing onset time for minor nerve blocks (5–10 minutes), major nerve blocks, and epidural anesthesia (10–20 minutes).

Additives

Vasoconstrictors

As a general rule, the addition of a vasoconstrictor to a local anesthetic agent, such as epinephrine, allows for decreased local perfusion, delayed rate of vascular absorption of local anesthetic, and therefore increased intensity and prolonged anesthetic activity. Lumbar epidural anesthesia, using 10 mL of 1% lidocaine with epinephrine 1:200,000 produces a more intense block of both large-diameter and small-diameter sensory nerve fibers than that achieved with lidocaine alone.

The usual concentration of epinephrine is 5 mcg/mL or 1:200,000 (1 mg/200 mL of saline), which may be obtained by adding 0.1 mL of 1:1000 (0.1 mg) epinephrine to 20 mL of local anesthetic solution. Alternatively, 1:1000 epinephrine may be diluted with preservative-free normal saline. The maximum safe concentration of epinephrine is 1:50,000; concentrations less than 1:200,000 are less effective. Market preparations of local anesthetics that contain epinephrine 1:200,000 have a lower pH (to slow oxidation of the epinephrine) than do plain solutions; for example, 2% lidocaine without and with epinephrine 1:200,000 has a pH of 6.78 and 4.55; and 0.5% bupivacaine without and with epinephrine (1:200,000) has a pH of 6.04 and 3.73, respectively. The low pH of the epinephrine preparations will potentially decrease the amount of free protonated anesthetic base available for diffusion through the axonal membrane, thereby slowing the onset of action.

Epinephrine effects depend on the injection site and the local anesthetic, but, in general, it reduces the potential toxicity of local anesthetics by causing vasoconstriction and thus preventing higher blood concentrations. Acidic epinephrine-containing local anesthetic solutions can decrease the pH at the site of injection, depending on the buffer demand of the injectate and the buffer capacity of the tissue. Epinephrine should not be added to local anesthetics intended for nerve blocks that have an erratic blood supply and for intravenous regional anesthesia (IVRA) with use of a tourniquet because it can cause nerve ischemia and prolonged blockade. Epinephrine often causes tissue necrosis along wound edges. Norepinephrine and phenylephrine appear to have no clinical advantage over epinephrine.

Hyaluronidase

Hyaluronidase depolymerizes hyaluronic acid, the tissue cement or ground substance of the mesenchyme, aiding in the spread of a local anesthetic injection. The increased permeability of tissues may enhance systemic absorption (and toxicity) but shortens the duration of anesthetic effects because more drug is available in base form. The addition of 5 IU of hyaluronidase/mL of 1% lidocaine with 1:200,000 epinephrine solution in a standard dose and technique for ophthalmic surgery (2 mL as retrobulbar injection for intraocular anesthesia, 2 mL for upper-eyelid anesthesia, and 4 mL for extraorbital facial nerve blockade) reportedly does not increase the systemic absorption and cerebrospinal fluid (CSF) concentration of lidocaine in dogs. However, administration of hyaluronidase does not seem to enhance the efficacy of newer local anesthetics with improved spreading power (e.g., articaine and ropivacaine). Administration of 2% articaine or 1% ropivacaine produces a faster onset of anesthesia and less pain on injection than does administration of 1% bupivacaine.

pH adjustment and carbonation

The pH of the local anesthetic solution affects the local distribution of the anesthetic. Extracellular increase of bicarbonate increases the cross-membrane pH gradient, the intracellular concentration of the ionized local anesthetic, and local anesthetic effects. The addition of sodium bicarbonate to procaine, chloroprocaine, mepivacaine, or lidocaine will shorten the onset of nerve block, enhance the density of block, and prolong the duration of block in isolated nerve preparations. This is likely because the amount of nonionized base increases, which enhances diffusion of the local anesthetic through axonal membranes and ion trapping due to the increased cross-membrane pH gradient.

The efficacy of alkalinization depends on the local anesthetic and regional block techniques. The addition of sodium bicarbonate for median nerve block in humans decreases the pain on injection and increases the rate of onset of motor block, but has no effect on duration of sensory anesthesia. Similarly, adjusting the pH of 1% lidocaine or 0.25% bupivacaine with sodium bicarbonate to 7.4 has little effect on duration of anesthesia after injection into the infraorbital foramen or abdominal musculature. Alkalinization produces the best results with 2% lidocaine and 0.5% bupivacaine for epidural block, with 2% lidocaine for axillary brachial plexus block, and with 2% mepivacaine for sciatic and femoral nerve blocks. Bicarbonate has minimal effects when added to ropivacaine.

Local anesthetic solutions may deteriorate over time with the addition of bicarbonate. Solutions of lidocaine and 2-chloroprocaine readily alkalinize to near physiological pH without precipitation. Mepivacaine 1.5% precipitates above neutral pH within 20 minutes. Bupivacaine and etidocaine precipitate after the addition of small amounts of sodium bicarbonate and cannot be alkalinized to physiological pH. Mixtures should be used within 20 minutes of their preparation.

Baricity

This is defined as the calculated ratio of the density of a solution to the density of CSF. One of the most important physical properties affecting the spread of local anesthetic solutions and level of analgesia achieved after intrathecal administration of a local anesthetic is its density relative to the density of CSF at 37°C.

Density is the weight of a unit volume of solution (grams per milliliter) at a specific temperature, whereas the specific gravity (SG) is the calculated ratio of the density of a solution (x) to the known density of water (y), (SG = x/y). The density of a drug in solution cannot be determined from a simple formula because it depends on the physical state of that substance in solution. The density of intrathecal agents is usually compared with the density of the CSF. At room temperature, most glucose-free drugs are isobaric with respect to CSF, but as drugs warm to body temperature they become relatively hypobaric. The densities of 2% lidocaine and 0.5% and 0.75% bupivacaine, for example, are slightly less than that of normal range of CSF in humans and therefore can be considered slightly hypobaric. Continued dilution of 0.75% bupivacaine with water produces increasingly hypobaric solutions. Hypobaric solutions have a baricity less than that of CSF and will migrate to nondependent areas during and immediately after the injection. Glucose-free 0.5% bupivacaine acts as a hypobaric solution, which produces a higher level of analgesia in the nondependent side compared with the dependent side in patients positioned laterally. The unpredictability of extent of spinal block provided by spinal bupivacaine (0.5%) and tetracaine (0.5%) may be related to individual variations in CSF densities. Patients with higher CSF densities demonstrate a higher spinal block after administration of bupivacaine (0.5%, 3 mL).

Dextrose and hypertonic saline-containing local anesthetic solutions (e.g., tetracaine in 10% glucose and dibucaine in 5% hyperbaric saline) have an SG greater than that of CSF. They will migrate from the site of injection to dependent areas. Hyperbaric solutions are created by combining local anesthetics (e.g., 0.5% bupivacaine or 0.5% ropivacaine) with an equal volume of 10% dextrose, producing final drug and dextrose concentrations of 0.25% and 5%, respectively.

Temperature

The cooling of mammalian nerves *in vitro* slows the conduction velocity and increases the susceptibility to local anesthetic inhibition of transmission. The potency of local anesthetics increases *in vitro* and *in vivo* with cooling in some instances but not in others. Inhibition of C fibers (as assessed by galvanic skin potentials) is marginally faster when ice-cold lidocaine (1%) is used compared with room-temperature lidocaine (1%) for median nerve blocks in volunteers. Cooling of lidocaine increases its pK_a and the relative amount of the protonated (active) form within lipid, thereby potentiating the anesthetic effect. On the other hand, a decrease in temperature from 37 to 20°C decreases the uptake of lidocaine in mammalian sciatic nerve by 45%. It is unlikely that cooling of local anesthetics (5°C) before injection of small volumes (5 mL) will be of any effect under clinical conditions because of rapid warming of the local anesthetic by the surrounding tissue, preventing the nerve itself from growing cold.

Pregnancy

Pregnant women with lidocaine (1%)-induced median nerve block at the wrist have a greater decrease in sensory nerve action potential than do nonpregnant women, indicating that pregnancy increases median nerve susceptibility to lidocaine desensitization. Similarly, isolated vagus nerves removed from pregnant rabbits are more susceptible to bupivacaine-induced conduction block than are nerve fibers from nonpregnant animals. Progesterone administration to nonpregnant rabbits replicates the increased local anesthetic susceptibility of pregnancy. Distention of the lumbar epidural venous plexus during pregnancy may displace the local anesthetic solution to more cranial regions of the spinal canal. Therefore, to prevent excessive cranial spread of anesthesia, a reduced dose of epidural and spinal anesthetics during pregnancy is recommended.

Drug disposition

Local anesthetics, as the name implies, are deposited at or near the desired site of action. In general, local anesthetics are injected near a nerve bundle. Intraneural injection is painful and may cause nerve damage. The factors that determine the distribution of local anesthetic near the injection site are illustrated in Figure 10.3. Most clinically used local anesthetics are weak bases and are supplied as mildly acidic hydrochloride salts to improve solubility and stability. In solution, local anesthetics exist as nonionized base (B) and ionized cation (BH⁺). The nonionized anesthetic (B) diffuses across the tissue barriers and into the axonal nerve membrane, where membrane stability and neural blockade occur. Nonspecific binding of anesthetic in connective tissue, fat, and muscles and absorption of anesthetic into the vascular and lymph systems reduce the mass (volume × concentration) of the anesthetic available at the neural tissue. Once absorbed into the bloodstream, the local anesthetic is distributed to the lungs, where a significant part (20–30%) is absorbed, depending mainly on the physicochemical properties of the local anesthetic. After back diffusion of the anesthetic from the lung into the blood, the anesthetic is distributed to systemic tissues (e.g., brain, heart, and liver) and is metabolized in the liver to compounds that are primarily excreted by the kidney and bile.

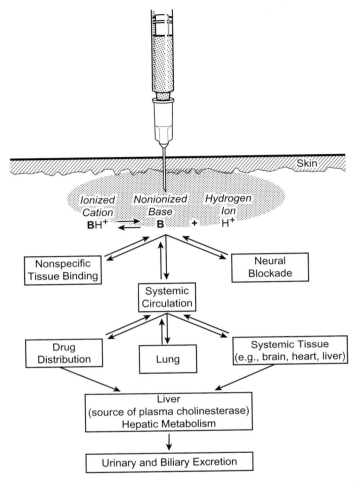

Figure 10.3.   Factors that determine the diffusion of local anesthetic near the site of injection and within the body. The nonionized base of the anesthetic (B) diffuses into the axon and nonspecific tissues. Nonspecific tissue binding and absorption into the bloodstream reduce the mass of drug available to diffuse into neural tissue.

Absorption

Systemic absorption of local anesthetics is determined primarily by the drug dose (volume or concentration), duration of effect at the site of action, vascularity of the injection site, and use of a vasoconstrictor. Local anesthetic solutions generally are ineffective when applied to the intact skin.

Topical application of local anesthetics includes transdermal patches, creams, and iontophoretic delivery systems. Proparacaine is the topical local anesthetic most commonly used in veterinary medicine. After application of a lidocaine patch (Lidoderm Patch, Endo Pharmaceuticals, Chadds Ford, PA) a sufficient amount of 5% lidocaine penetrates the human intact skin to produce analgesia in patients with neuropathic pain associated with postherpetic neuralgia and in patients with postthoracotomy and post-mastectomy pain, but less than the amount necessary to produce a complete sensory block. A single patch (10 × 14-cm adhesive bandage) contains 700 mg of lidocaine, which is used in a 12-hour-on and 12-hour-off period to minimize systemic absorption.

The eutectic mixture of 2.5% lidocaine and 2.5% prilocaine (e.g., EMLA® Cream, AstraZeneca Pharmaceuticals LP, Wilmington, DE) contains 25 mg of lidocaine and 25 mg of prilocaine per each gram or milliliter, which has a sufficiently high concentration of readily available anesthetic base and high water content to penetrate the intact skin and produce reliable cutaneous anesthesia for a wide range of applications in people (e.g., venipuncture in children, radial artery cannulation in adults, and laser treatment) and for venipuncture in dogs, cats, rabbits, and rats. In humans, EMLA preparation is applied as a thick layer under an occlusive dressing, and maximum depth of analgesia of approximately 5 mm is achieved for 30 minutes after a 90-minute application and for a 60-minute period after a 120-minute application of the cream. In general, the depth of cutaneous analgesia in people ranges from 1 to 6 mm and is believed to be time dependent (1–4 hours).

Amethocaine cream 1 g (5% wt/wt) applied for 30 or 60 minutes on the dorsum of the hand produces good analgesia for venous cannulation similar to analgesia produced by 5% EMLA Cream (2.5 g) applied for 30 or 60 minutes. In comparison to the gel preparation, a 30-minute application of the amethocaine-patch system provides profound topical anesthesia of human skin that lasts longer than a 60-minute application of EMLA (3–6 hours vs. 20 minutes).

ELA-Max Cream (PD-Rx Pharmaceuticals Inc., Oklahoma City, OK) is designed to produce analgesia of the skin to reduce venipuncture pain in 20–30 minutes in children without the use of an occlusive dressing. The preparation contains 4% lidocaine, which is liposome encapsulated to enable fast penetration into the stratum corneum. It remains in the epidermis after absorption and minimizes the rapid metabolism of lidocaine. ELA-Max Cream lacks the active ingredient of prilocaine, which has been associated with methemoglobinemia (MHG) in infants. Accordingly, ELA-Max Cream may be more suitable for use in cats susceptible to methemoglobin (MHb) formation.

Numby Stuff® patches (Iomed Inc., Salt Lake City, UT), which consist of 2% lidocaine and 1:100,000 epinephrine, are percutaneously administered through iontophoretic drug administration by using a battery generator to deliver a small electrical current (4 mA) through two small electrodes. Each application device delivers 1 mL of the anesthetic to a depth of up to 10 mm in 10 minutes, giving a transient blanching and tingling of the skin

Transdermal local anesthesia achieved by iontophoresis reduces the pain of IV injection of hyperosmolar saline. This technique involves the use 0.5 mL of lidocaine (2–4%) with or without epinephrine 1:50,000 and a current intensity of 0.1–0.2 mA/cm^2 at the anode and placement of the cathode on the dorsal surface of the forearm for 10 minutes.

Although veterinary use of Lidoderm patches, ELA-Max Cream, Numby Stuff patches, and transdermal local anesthesia by iontophoresis is minimal to date, potential uses include local analgesia for small wound repair, venipuncture, or catheter placement (IV and epidural).

Distribution

Distribution of local anesthetic at the injection site depends on the volume of local anesthetic injected, inclusion of a vasoconstrictor or hyaluronidase in the local anesthetic solution, and the specific drug employed. The SG (baricity) of the solution relative to the SG of the CSF influences distribution within the CNS.

The distribution of amino-ester local anesthetics (e.g., procaine, chloroprocaine, and tetracaine) in body tissues is limited because of their rapid enzymatic hydrolysis by nonspecific plasma pseudocholinesterases. Amide-type local anesthetics (e.g., lidocaine, mepivacaine, prilocaine, bupivacaine, levobupivacaine, etidocaine, and ropivacaine) are widely distributed after IV bolus injection or a fast rate of vascular absorption. Their pharmacokinetic properties are usually described by a two- or three-compartment model.

In blood, all amide-linked local anesthetics are partially protein bound, primarily to α_1-acid glycoprotein (AAG) and, to a lesser extent, to albumin. In general, protein binding of local anesthetics is positively correlated with the degree of ionization in the physiological pH range and the drug's potency. Plasma protein binding of local anesthetics ranges from 6% for the least potent and short-acting procaine to 95% for the more potent and longer-persisting bupivacaine, etidocaine, and ropivacaine (Table 10.2)

Free drug concentration in plasma, not the protein-bound concentration of drug, governs tissue concentrations. The effect of serum protein binding on lidocaine distribution into the brain and CNS in dogs after IV lidocaine administration indicates that free or unbound fraction of lidocaine is an important determinant of lidocaine entry into the brain and CSF. Protein binding of lidocaine in dogs that receive a loading dose (2 mg/kg) and a maintenance infusion (50 mcg/kg/h) of lidocaine is associated with increased protein binding and only slight increases of free plasma concentrations of lidocaine.

In dogs, the concentration of lidocaine bound to AAG varies considerably, and is higher in dogs with inflammatory disease. Local anesthetic protein binding approaches saturation only at very high drug concentrations, primarily after prolonged infusion of a long-acting local anesthetic (e.g., ropivacaine or levobupivacaine) and local anesthetic–opioid combination to provide prolonged postoperative analgesia. The slow rise in total plasma concentration with increasing duration of infusion of ropivacaine and levobupivacaine appears to be the predominant reason for rare complications related to systemic toxicity produced by these drugs.

Biotransformation and excretion

The liver and lungs are major sites for plasma clearance of local anesthetics. Metabolism converts relatively lipid-soluble local anesthetics into more water-soluble metabolites.

For esters, the primary step is ester hydrolysis, catalyzed by nonspecific plasma cholinesterases. The rate of plasma hydrolysis is rapid, yielding half-lives measured in seconds, and is inversely related to toxicity (chloroprocaine [most rapid] > procaine > tetracaine [least rapid]).

Procaine and benzocaine are metabolized to paraaminobenzoic acid (PABA), a breakdown product responsible for allergic reactions and anaphylaxis in some human patients. The majority of the PABA is excreted unchanged or as conjugated product in the urine. Chloroprocaine and tetracaine are metabolized similarly, but not to PABA. Cocaine is an atypical ester in that it undergoes either ester hydrolysis or *N*-demethylation to norcocaine and then ester hydrolysis and significant hepatic metabolism and urinary excretion. Cocaine is rarely used in veterinary medicine, although it can be abused for stimulation of horses before a race. Ester metabolism can, theoretically, be slowed by reduced cholinesterase activity during pregnancy and long-term cholinesterase inhibition via poisons, thereby prolonging the clearance of ester anesthetics and increasing the potential for toxicity.

The amino-amide local anesthetics undergo nearly exclusive metabolism by the liver and hepatic degradation, which requires conjugation with glucuronic acid. Cats glucuronidate drugs to a lesser extent than dogs, making cats more prone to develop toxic side effects when given amide local anesthetics.

The order of clearance of amides is prilocaine (most rapid) > etidocaine > lidocaine > mepivacaine or ropivacaine > bupivacaine (least rapid). Lidocaine undergoes oxidative *N*-dealkylation by cytochrome $P450_{3A4}$. Mepivacaine, etidocaine, bupivacaine, and ropivacaine also undergo *N*-dealkylation and hydroxylation. They are further conjugated with glucuronide before they are excreted from the body via the urine or bile. Prilocaine undergoes hydrolysis to *o*-toluidine, a compound that can oxidize hemoglobin to MHb.

Since all amide local anesthetics are metabolized by the liver, drug clearance is highly dependent on hepatic blood flow, hepatic extraction, and enzyme function. Clearance of amide local anesthetics can be reduced or prolonged by factors that decrease hepatic blood flow, such as β-adrenergic or H_2-receptor blockers, by hypotension during regional and general anesthesia, or by heart or liver failure.

Local anesthetic toxicity

When careful technique and appropriate dose are used, local anesthetics are relatively free of harmful side effects. However, local anesthetics may cause severe toxic reactions after unintentional IV administration, vascular absorption of an excessive dose (large volume or high concentration) of the local anesthetic agent, or ingestion of topical local anesthetic preparations.

Doses of local anesthetics, especially those for cats and small dogs, should always be carefully calculated and reduced in sick animals. For example, in healthy dogs and cats, the dose of lidocaine should not exceed 10 and 4 mg/kg, respectively, to prevent toxicity. Repeated applications, the application of higher than the recommended doses, or impaired elimination may all contribute to increasing blood concentration of local anesthetics. Potential damage may also occur from chemical contamination of the local anesthetic solution, allergic reactions, or MHG, or from neural ischemia produced by local pressure or hypotension. The systemic toxicity of local anesthetics involves primarily the CNS and the cardiovascular system.

CNS toxicity

In general, toxic and lethal doses of local anesthetic drugs produce signs of CNS excitation, leading ultimately to convulsive activity followed by CNS depression (unconsciousness and coma) with eventual respiratory arrest and cardiovascular collapse. Acute CNS toxicity occurs at lower doses than those required to produce acute cardiovascular system toxicity.

As the plasma concentration of the drug increases, humans experience a predictable sequence of signs and symptoms, such as numbness of tongue, light-headedness, visual disturbance, muscle twitching, unconsciousness, and convulsions, which may progress to coma, respiratory arrest, cardiovascular depression, and death. In small animals, low concentrations of local anesthetics produce sedation, whereas higher concentrations produce seizures, probably because of selective depression of inhibitory fibers in the subcortical area (amygdala), with subsequent spread, leading to grand mal seizures. Muscle twitching and convulsions are usually the first signs of local anesthetic toxicity observed in dogs and cats. More potent local anesthetics consistently produce seizures at lower blood concentrations and lower doses than do the less potent local anesthetics.

In awake dogs, the mean cumulative dose of serially and rapidly administered IV local anesthetics to produce convulsions is 4.0 mg/kg tetracaine, 5.0 mg/kg bupivacaine, 8.0 mg/kg etidocaine, and 22 mg/kg lidocaine, indicating a relative CNS toxicity of tetracaine, bupivacaine, etidocaine, and lidocaine of about 1:1.2:2:4.

In cats, procaine (the least potent CNS depressant, less lipid soluble and less protein bound) produces seizures at 35 mg/kg IV, whereas bupivacaine (one of the most potent CNS depressants, highly lipid soluble and highly protein bound) induces convulsions at approximately 5 mg/kg IV. IV-administered lidocaine at a dose of 11.7 ± 4.6 mg/kg causes seizures in cats. Increased arterial PCO_2 (68 to 81 mm Hg) and decreased pH reportedly decrease the convulsive dose of procaine, lidocaine, and bupivacaine by approximately 50% in cats. The toxic effects of local anesthetics within the CNS are enhanced by increased cerebral blood flow, by increased concentration of ionized drug in the brain, or by the direct excitatory effect on subcortical structures.

Cardiovascular toxicity

Since an alarming editorial in 1979 about cardiac arrest in humans following regional anesthesia with etidocaine and bupivacaine, ropivacaine and, recently, levobupivacaine were developed as alternative long-acting amide local anesthetics with less potential for cardiovascular toxicity.

Local anesthetic cardiovascular toxicity may result from direct electrophysiological and mechanical effects on the heart or the peripheral circulation and from local anesthetic actions on the autonomic nervous system. The use of lower concentrations can result in CNS excitation, with increased heart rate, arterial blood pressure, pulmonary artery pressure, and cardiac output. With larger toxic blood concentrations, the systemic effects are characterized by decreased heart rate, arterial blood pressure, pulmonary artery pressure, and cardiac output.

Results from animal studies demonstrate increased systemic toxicity associated with bupivacaine and etidocaine as compared with lidocaine, the most extreme of which include severe CNS and cardiovascular reactions, eventually leading to hemodynamic instability, cardiovascular collapse, and death. Local anesthetics bind and inhibit cardiac sodium channels. Bupivacaine binds more readily and for a longer duration to cardiac sodium channels than does lidocaine. The bupivacaine S-(−) isomer binds cardiac sodium channels less readily than does the R-(+) isomer, forming the basis for the development of levobupivacaine and ropivacaine.

Toxicosis after ingestion or topical application

Topical local anesthetic preparations containing lidocaine, benzocaine, tetracaine, and dibucaine, which are in many prescription and nonprescription products, such as ointments, teething gels, suppositories, and aerosols, can be hazardous to animals if ingested. Ingestion of topical benzocaine preparations or spray before endotracheal intubation has produced varying degrees of vomiting, cyanosis, dyspnea, respiratory depression, prolonged sedation, hypotension, cardiac arrhythmias, tremors, seizures, and even death in dogs and cats. Likewise, digestion of ointments and creams containing 0.5% and 1.0% dibucaine hydrochloride, which may not be considered dangerous by pet owners, has produced salivation, vomiting, hypothermia, bradycardia, hypotension, weakness, seizures, dysrhythmia, and death in dogs and cats. Between 1995 and 1999 the National Animal Poison Control Center (NAPCC) recorded over 70 cases of toxicosis induced by either ingestion or the inappropriate use of lidocaine, benzocaine, or dibucaine in a variety of animals, including dogs, cats, and ferrets. The clinical signs included salivation, vomiting, hypothermia, depression, tremors, weakness, bradycardia, hypotension, and seizures.

Local toxicity

Neurotoxicity

When properly used, local anesthetics rarely produce local neurotoxic effects or localized tissue damage. Neurotoxicity of local anesthetics can be demonstrated *in vitro* by the collapse of growth cones and neuritis in cultured neurons. Comparison of seven local anesthetics in a study on growing neurons of the freshwater snail demonstrates neurotoxicity in this order: procaine = mepivacaine (least neurotoxic) < ropivacaine = bupivacaine < lidocaine < tetracaine < dibucaine (most neurotoxic).

Myotoxicity

All clinically used local anesthetics are myotoxic, with a drug-specific and dose-dependent rate of toxicity that worsens with serial or continuous administration. Some reports indicate that single and repeated injections of clinical doses of mepivacaine or bupivacaine produce skeletal muscle damage in rats. The administration of bupivacaine and ropivacaine induces Ca^{2+} release of the sarcoplasmic reticulum and simultaneously inhibits Ca^{2+} reuptake into the sarcoplasmic reticulum, suggesting an important mechanism in observed myotoxicity. Although skeletal muscle damage from local anesthetics is not a major clinical problem, case reports have been published of local anesthetic-induced myotoxicity in humans after local and regional anesthesia, peripheral nerve blocks, retrobulbar injections, and trigger-point infiltration for treatment of myofascial pain.

MHG

MHG or increased concentration of MHb in the blood is defined as an altered state of hemoglobin whereby the ferrous form of iron (Fe^{2+}) is oxidized to the ferric state (Fe^{3+}), which increases oxygen affinity for hemoglobin (as seen with MHG) and reduces oxygen release at tissues. In addition, oxidative denaturation of hemoglobin can cause Heinz body formation, which can lead to erythrocyte lysis. MHG can cause hypoxia, cyanosis, or even death.

A number of local anesthetic agents, most notably benzocaine and prilocaine, and less often procaine and lidocaine, are implicated as causative agents. Benzocaine induces MHG in several species, whereas lidocaine may increase MHG in cats and people. It appears that these agents do not directly produce MHG, but rather a metabolite, *o*-toluidine, is responsible.

An intense chocolate brown-colored blood and central cyanosis unresponsive to the administration of 100% oxygen suggest the diagnosis of MHG. MHb concentrations of 15% or more cause a brown discoloration to the blood, which is visible on a white paper towel. Laboratory confirmation is by blood co-oximetry, indicating an MHb concentration of greater than 15% (1–2% is normal).

The clinical consequences of MHG are related to the blood concentration of MHb. In humans, dyspnea, nausea, and tachycardia occur at an MHb concentration of >30%, whereas lethargy, stupor, and deteriorating consciousness occur as the MHb concentration approaches 55%. Acquired toxic MHG has been induced with benzocaine topical anesthetics (spray, cream, and ointment). Peak MHb concentrations are directly related to the total dose of benzocaine or prilocaine administered.

MHG has been induced by the nasal, oropharyngeal, and dermal applications of benzocaine in sheep, dogs, and cats. A 2-second spray of benzocaine (estimated dose, 56 mg) to the mucous membranes of the nasopharynx of dogs, cats, monkeys, rabbits, and miniature pigs produces MHb concentrations ranging from 3.5% to 38%, 15–60 minutes after drug administration.

Benzocaine is combined with butamben and tetracaine in a topical anesthetic spray (Cetacaine, Cetylite Industries, Inc., Pennsauken, NJ) that has been commonly used to desensitize the larynx before intubation. Cats are at an increased risk for developing MHG and Heinz body anemia with benzocaine-containing products, including Cetacaine. Because of the susceptibility of cats, ferrets, or other exotic animals to MHG, the topical use of Cetacaine should be avoided.

Allergic reactions

Although allergic reactions to local anesthetics may occur, they are uncommon and often misdiagnosed after accidental IV injection of local anesthetics. True anaphylaxis or life-threatening allergic immune reaction is mediated by immunospecific antibodies (immunoglobulins E or G) that interact with mast cells, basophils, or the complement system to liberate vasoactive mediators and recruit other inflammatory cells. Such reactions have been documented with amino ester local anesthetics (e.g., procaine), particularly those that are metabolized directly to PABA, which is a common allergen. Anaphylaxis to amide local anesthetics (e.g., lidocaine) is much less common. Some reaction may result from hypersensitivity to a preservative (e.g., methylparaben, whose chemical structure is similar to that of PABA). Allergic reactions of dogs and cats treated with amide-linked local anesthetics are very rare.

Anaphylactoid-adverse drug reactions may mimic anaphylaxis, characterized by bronchospasm, upper airway edema, vasodilatation, increased capillary permeability, and cutaneous wheal and flare. Rapid cardiopulmonary intervention with airway maintenance, epinephrine administration, and volume expansion is essential to avoid a fatal outcome.

Treatment of adverse reactions

When local anesthetic-induced convulsions occur, hypoxia, hypercarbia, and acidosis can develop rapidly. Because these metabolic changes greatly increase the toxicity of local anesthetics, prompt therapy with oxygen administration by mask to a dyspneic patient and supporting ventilation (e.g., endotracheal intubation, oxygen supplementation, and positive-pressure ventilation) is indicated.

Anticonvulsant drug therapy is indicated if seizure activity interferes with ventilation or is prolonged. Diazepam or midazolam can be given IV in dogs and cats at 0.5–1 mg/kg in increments of 5–10 mg to effect, with minimal side effects. Thiopental or propofol (1–2 mg/kg IV) acts more rapidly but may produce greater cardiorespiratory depression than that produced with benzodiazepine therapy.

Acute hypotension may be treated with IV fluids (10 mL/kg/h) and vasopressors (phenylephrine, 0.5–5.0 mcg/kg/min, or norepinephrine, 0.02–0.2 mcg/kg/min). Caution must be exercised to avoid intravascular volume overload, which can produce pulmonary edema, pleural effusion, mucous membrane discoloration, pigmenturia, vomiting, and neurological abnormalities, particularly in small dogs and cats.

An IV bolus of epinephrine (1–15 mcg/kg) may be required in presence of myocardial failure. Guidelines for cardiopulmonary resuscitation should be followed when toxicity progresses to cardiac arrest. Animal studies suggest that lidocaine intoxication causes myocardial depression that can be successfully treated with continued advanced cardiac life support. In contrast, cardiotoxic effects associated with incremental overdosage of bupivacaine, levobupivacaine, or ropivacaine are not as easily treated by resuscitation efforts. The administration of epinephrine may lead to severe arrhythmias, including ventricular fibrillation, with a subsequent mortality rate from bupivacaine, levobupivacaine, ropivacaine, and lidocaine of approximately 50%, 30%, 10%, and 0%, respectively. Early bupivacaine overdose (inadvertent IV injection) and toxicity is best treated with a lipid-containing product (Lyposyn 20% Intravenous Lipid, Hospira, Inc., Lake Forest, IL) capable of absorbing bupivacaine and lowering bupivacaine plasma concentrations rapidly.

Even though the risk of cardiovascular toxicity of ropivacaine has not been completely eliminated, ropivacaine may offer clear advantages over bupivacaine, in that ropivacaine accumulates less sodium-channel blockade at physiological heart rates, dissociates from sodium channels more rapidly, is less cardiotoxic, and is more susceptible to treatment than is bupivacaine.

Ventricular dysrhythmias, including life-threatening ventricular tachycardia associated with local anesthetic toxicity in dogs, have been treated with bretylium tosylate (2–6 mg/kg IV). Procainamide and quinidine may be effective treatments for ventricular arrhythmias in dogs and cats. Lidocaine is generally contraindicated in patients with amide local anesthetic toxicity.

MHG is easily treated and rapidly reduced to hemoglobin by slow (over several minutes) IV administration of a 1% solution of methylene blue (methylthioninium chloride, 4 mg/kg in dogs and 1–2 mg/kg in cats). The dose can be repeated in dogs, but repeated administration of methylene blue in cats is controversial because of the risk of Heinz-body anemia and the aggravation of subsequent hemolysis without further lowering MHb content.

Tachyphylaxis

Tachyphylaxis, or the acute tolerance to local anesthetic agents, is defined as decreases in intensity, segmental spread, or duration after repeated administration of equal doses of an anesthetic. Various ester-type local anesthetics (e.g., cocaine, procaine, and tetracaine) and amide-type local anesthetics (e.g., lidocaine, mepivacaine, bupivacaine, etidocaine, and dibucaine) have been used at increasing doses to maintain a similar level of effect during surface anesthesia, nerve blocks, brachial plexus block, and epidural and subarachnoid anesthesia. The underlying mechanisms of tachyphylaxis are not well understood. Local alterations in disposition and absorption of local anesthetics (but not in structure [ester vs. amide] or the pharmacological properties of local anesthetics themselves [e.g., brief vs. long acting]), technique, mode of administration (intermittent vs. continuous), and pharmacodynamic processes (interactions at receptor sites) may all play a role in the development of tachyphylaxis.

Local and regional analgesic techniques: dogs

The popularity of local anesthetic-induced neural blockade in dogs has increased over the past several years. A major driving force behind this increased usage is acceptance of the concept of blocking multimodal pathways to control animals' pain and suffering. Unlike most general anesthetics, which block the perception of pain by inducing unconsciousness, local anesthesia and regional anesthesia completely block the transmission of noxious impulses in a region of the body of a conscious patient. Local and regional anesthesia also decreases the quantity of opioid and inhalation anesthetic required to obtain the desired plane of anesthesia intraoperatively. Topical anesthesia, infiltration anesthesia, field blocks, selected nerve blocks of the head (anesthesia of the maxilla, upper teeth, eye and orbit, mandible, and lower teeth), anesthesia of the foot and leg (ring block, brachial plexus block, and IVRA), multiple intercostal nerve blocks, lumbosacral epidural anesthesia, and continuous epidural anesthesia provide surgical analgesia and anesthesia in dogs that are considered at risk for inhalant or IV anesthesia. Continuous interpleural analgesia and epidural opioid analgesia can also be used to relieve postoperative pain following general anesthesia.

Topical anesthesia

Many local anesthetics are effective when placed topically on mucous membranes and may be used in the mouth, airway, esophagus, and genitourinary tract. Local anesthetics used topically include lidocaine (2–5%), proparacaine (0.5%), tetracaine (0.5–2.0%), butacaine (2%), and cocaine (4–10%). Preparations that are applied topically come in creams, ointments, jelly, powders, and aerosols. Injectable preparations of lidocaine (0.5–5.0%) with and without epinephrine can also be applied topically to mucous membranes (1–5%). Topical local anesthetic agents can relieve pain during cleaning or dressing of wounds, although their effect is highly variable. The lowest effective dose of topical anesthetic should always be used in order to prevent toxicity from excessive plasma concentrations. Time between application of topical anesthetics and onset of anesthesia is generally longer, and pain relief less, than that achieved with infiltration anesthesia. A 2–4% solution of lidocaine used for topical anesthesia on mucous membranes produces effects in approximately 5 minutes and lasts for 30 minutes.

Local instillation of proparacaine (0.5%), tetracaine (0.5–1.0%), butacaine (2%), piperocaine (2%), oxybuprocaine (0.4%), or cocaine (1–4%) into the conjunctival sac anesthetizes the cornea and conjunctiva for short procedures (e.g., removal of hypertrophied gland of the third eyelid). Proparacaine (0.5%) has been advocated as an excellent topical anesthetic for examination of a painful eye, removal of foreign bodies, sutures, obtaining conjunctival scrapings, and subconjunctival injections. Anesthesia occurs rapidly (1–6 minutes), lasts for 10–15 minutes after single instillation, and may last for up to 2 hours after repeated instillation without untoward effects (e.g., irritation or epithelial damage). A series of three to five instillations of one or two drops of proparacaine at approximately 1-minute intervals may be necessary to produce satisfactory anesthesia of the cornea and conjunctiva. Topical anesthesia is very safe, is simple to apply, and can be repeated, although dogs may resent the application of cold solutions. Data on vascular uptake and maximum blood concentration are not available, large interpatient variability should be expected, and potential for bacterial contamination exists.

Local anesthetic sprays (10% lidocaine or 14–20% benzocaine) anesthetize the mucosa up to a depth of 2 mm within 1–2 minutes after application. Anesthesia lasts for approximately 15–20 minutes. The movable nozzle of the spray can enable easy access to the site of application. Pressure on the nozzle with the forefinger delivers a specific quantity of the anesthetic each second (10 mg of lidocaine from a 10% lidocaine spray can). The average expulsion rate from a benzocaine (Cetacaine) spray is 200 mg/s.

Endotracheal tubes are frequently coated with local anesthetic jells but should not be lubricated with jelly containing 20% benzocaine hydrochloride. Topical sprays and ointments containing 14–20% benzocaine cause dose-dependent MHG. Preparations with over 8% benzocaine include Hurricane Spray (20%) (Beutlich Pharmaceuticals LP, Waukegan, IL), Hurricane Topical Anesthetic Gel (20%) and Liquid (20%) (Beutlich Pharmaceuticals), Camphophenique Sting Relief Formula (20%) (Bayer Health Care LLC. Morristown, NJ), Dermoplast Anesthetic Pain Relief (20%) (PrestigeBrands, Inc., Irvington, NJ), and Cetacaine Spray (14%) (Cetylite Industries, Inc., Pennsauken, NJ). Exposure of the tracheal mucosa to topical benzocaine oxidizes blood hemoglobin in dogs in proportion to the absorbed dose within 10 minutes. MHb cannot bind oxygen or carbon dioxide. Dogs are usually asymptomatic when concentrations of MHb are less than 20%, but show fatigue, weakness, dyspnea, and tachycardia at concentrations between 20% and 50%. Laryngeal sprays containing benzocaine should be used with caution, and if signs of cyanosis and respiratory distress develop, MHG should be considered. In general, benzocaine should be used sparingly and cautiously while continuously monitoring for cyanosis. Dogs at risk of hypoxia after using benzocaine topical anesthesia should receive oxygen and IV methylene blue (1.5 mg/kg) therapy.

One of the oldest forms of topical anesthesia is superficial cooling. Ethyl chloride can be used to freeze a small local area of skin for punctures, skin biopsy, or incision of small abscesses. Ethyl chloride is sprayed on the skin for 3–7 seconds from an inverted bottle and a distance of 10–20 cm, with the jet stream aimed so that it meets the skin at an acute angle to lessen the shock of impact. Surface anesthesia results from cooling (<4°C), which occurs during the evaporation process. Attempts to freeze large skin areas by using ethyl chloride are contraindicated because of the potential for frostbite. Ethyl chloride's brief action (<2 minutes), ability to produce a freezing sensation, and flammability when exposed to open flames and electric sparks (electrocauterization) limit its use. Inhalation of ethyl chloride should be avoided because it may produce narcotic and general anesthetic effects, or fatal coma with respiratory and cardiac arrest.

Pontocaine cream and a liposomal tetracaine preparation (0.5% tetracaine encapsulated into phospholipid vehicles) effectively penetrate human skin within 30–60 minutes of application, producing long-lasting (>4 hours) analgesia. The most clinically usable cream contains a 5% eutectic mixture of 2.5% lidocaine and 2.5% prilocaine (EMLA cream), which overcomes the human stratum corneum barrier within 1 hour of topical application without adverse effects. Lidoderm patches have been used to reduce pain associated with surgical incision in dogs.

Infiltration anesthesia

Infiltration of local anesthetics requires their extravascular placement by direct injection and may be the most reliable and safest of all the local anesthetic techniques. Lidocaine (0.5–2.0%) is the local anesthetic most often used for infiltration. Only sharp and sterile needles should be used. Local anesthesia can be produced by multiple intradermal or subcutaneous injections of 0.3–0.5 mL of local anesthetic solution by using a 2.5-cm, 22–25-gauge needle or by using a longer needle (3.75–5.0 cm) and slowly injecting local anesthetic while advancing the needle along the line of proposed incision (linear infiltration). Pain is minimal if the needle is advanced slowly into the first desensitized wheal and successive injections are made at the periphery of the advancing wheal. This technique assures that the dog senses only the initial needle insertion. Intradermal deposition of local anesthetic over a superficial abscess, cyst, or hematoma is a routine procedure. Infection along the filtration site will not occur if the needle has not entered the abscess. The amount of local anesthetic used for infiltration anesthesia depends on the size of the area to be anesthetized. Approximately 2–5 mg/kg of lidocaine or mepivacaine and 4–6 mg/kg of procaine without epinephrine may be used to diffuse into surrounding tissue from the site of injection and anesthetize the nerve fibers and endings. Large amounts of relatively dilute solutions are often infiltrated into operative sites. The lowest possible concentration of local anesthetic that will produce the desired effect should be administered. For example, an average dog (20 kg) will tolerate approximately 50 mL of 0.5% lidocaine without demonstrating signs of toxicity, whereas only 20–30 mL of 1% lidocaine or 10–15 mL of 2% lidocaine can be injected. The local anesthetic may be diluted in 0.9% sodium chloride solution (not with sterile water) to a 0.25% solution if a large volume of local anesthetic is needed for infiltration of a large operative area. The total dose of drug administered should be reduced by 30–40% in old dogs (>8 years) and sick or cachectic dogs in poor condition.

Continuous-infiltration anesthesia

This can be accomplished by the use of a continuous catheter-insertion system and a disposable infusion pump. A sterile multipore catheter is placed within the surgical incision (e.g., total ear canal ablation with lateral bulla osteotomy, forelimb amputation, or median and lateral thoracotomies) at the end of the surgical procedure. The catheter is connected to an elastomeric reservoir infusion pump, which is filled with local anesthetic (i.e., lidocaine, mepivacaine, or ropivacaine) to its full capacity (65, 100, 270, or 335 mL) to deliver the local anesthetic at a constant rate (0.5, 2.0, 4.0, or 5.0 mL/h) for several days. This technique is generally well tolerated, producing good postoperative analgesia for up to 50 hours, with no acute local anesthetic toxicity, hemodynamic instability, or breakthrough pain. Early signs of toxicity, such as nystagmus, restlessness, apprehension, and vomiting, are readily treated by removing the pump.

Field block

This technique can be used for anesthetizing large areas. First, intradermal or subcutaneous linear infiltration is produced around the lesion as previously described. Local anesthetic is then deposited in the deeper tissues by passing the needle through the desensitized skin far enough to infiltrate the deep nerves supplying the area (Figure 10.4).

Regional nerve blocks

Injection of local anesthetic solution into the connective tissue surrounding a nerve produces loss of sensation (sensory nerve block) and/or paralysis (motor nerve block) in the region supplied by the nerves (regional anesthesia). Smaller volumes (1–2 mL) of local anesthetic are needed to produce nerve blocks when compared with a field block, thereby reducing the danger of toxicity.

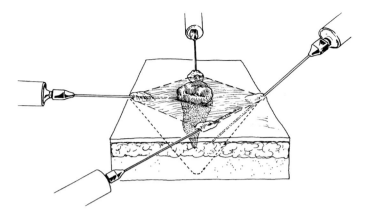

Figure 10.4.   Field block producing walls of anesthesia enclosing the surgical field.

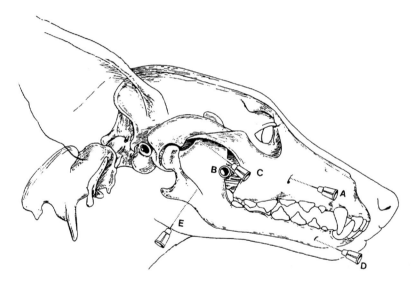

Figure 10.5.   Needle placement for producing nerve blocks on the head: infraorbital (A); maxillary (B); zygornatic, lacrimal, and ophthalmic (C); mandibular (E); and mental (D) nerves.

Regional anesthesia of the face

The administration of local anesthetic around the infraorbital, maxillary, ophthalmic, mental, and alveolar mandibular nerves provides valuable and practical advantages when combined with effective sedation or general anesthesia (Figure 10.5). Each nerve may be desensitized by injecting 1–2 mL of a 2% lidocaine hydrochloride solution by using a 2.5–5-cm, 20–25-gauge needle.

The infraorbital nerve is desensitized at its point of emergence from the infraorbital canal. The needle is inserted either intraorally or extraorally approximately 1 cm cranial to the bony lip of the infraorbital foramen. The needle is advanced to the infraorbital foramen, which can be found between the dorsal border of the zygomatic process and the gum of the upper canine tooth (Figure 10.5A). Successful injections desensitize the upper lip and nose, the roof of the nasal cavity, and the surrounding skin up to the infraorbital foramen.

The maxillary nerve must be desensitized to completely desensitize the maxilla, upper teeth, nose, and upper lip. The needle is placed percutaneously along the ventral border of the zygomatic process approximately 0.5 cm caudal to the lateral canthus of the eye and is advanced into close proximity of the pterygopalatine fossa (Figs. 10.5B). Local anesthetic is administered at the point where the maxillary nerve courses perpendicular to the palatine bone between the maxillary foramen and foramen rotundum.

Eye and orbit

Anesthesia of the eye and orbit is produced by desensitizing the ophthalmic division of the trigeminal nerve. General anesthesia for ophthalmic procedures has increased in popularity; however, retention of ocular reflexes during light and medium planes of general anesthesia in dogs can disturb the surgical field. Regional anesthesia, by anesthesia of ophthalmic nerves, produces immobility of the eye in addition to sensory anesthesia, and prevents the oculocardiac reflex, which can cause bradycardia, arrhythmias, and cardiac arrest as result of traction on the extrinsic muscles of the eye. A 2.5-cm, 22-gauge needle is inserted ventral to the zygomatic process at the level of the lateral canthus. The point of the needle should be approximately 0.5 cm cranial to the anterior border of the vertical portion of the ramus of the mandible. The needle is advanced medial to the ramus of the mandible in a mediodorsal and somewhat caudal direction until it reaches the lacrimal, zygomatic, and ophthalmic nerves at the orbital fissure. Deposition of 2 mL of local anesthetic at this site produces akinesia of the globe because of the proximity of the abducens, oculomotor, and trochlear nerves to the ophthalmic nerve. Motor block is assessed by cessation of the following eye movements: laterally, caused by the lateral rectus muscle (abducens nerve); and upward, downward, medially, and laterally, caused by the superior, inferior, medial, and lateral rectus muscles, respectively (oculomotor nerve). The superior oblique muscle rotates the eye downward and laterally (oculomotor nerve), whereas the inferior oblique muscle rotates the globe upward and laterally (trochlear nerve).

Retrobulbar or peribulbar anesthesia for local anesthesia of the eye runs the risk of direct subarachnoid injection, peribulbar hemorrhage, globe perforation, and intravascular injection. When performing retrobulbar anesthesia, the risk of puncturing the globe is minimal if a 7.5-cm, 20-gauge needle is inserted at the lateral canthus through the anesthetized conjunctiva and is advanced past the globe toward the opposite mandibular joint until the base of the orbit is encountered. When performing peribulbar anesthesia, the potential for puncturing ciliary and scleral blood vessels is minimal if a 5-cm curved needle (0.5 mm internal diameter) conformed to the roof of the orbit is inserted through the anesthetized conjunctival sac at the vertical meridian. Directing the needle away from the globe and toward the orbit also minimizes the risk of perforating the globe.

Injection of local anesthetic into the optic sheath can cause respiratory arrest attributable to the infiltration of local anesthetic into the subarachnoid space of the CNS. The pressure generated by injection into the optic nerve sheath or intrascleral injection is three or four times that produced by injection into the retrobulbar adipose tissue (135 vs. 35 mm Hg). Increased resistance encountered during retrobulbar block should serve as a warning, mandating redirection of the needle in order to prevent subarachnoid injection.

Lower lip

This can be desensitized by percutaneously inserting a 2.5-cm, 22–25-gauge needle rostral to the mental foramen at the level of the second premolar tooth. Approximately 1–2 mL of local anesthetic is deposited in close proximity to the mental nerve (Figure 10.5D).

Mandible and lower teeth

The mandible (including molars, premolars, canine, incisors, skin) and the mucosa of the chin and lower lip can be desensitized by injecting 1–2 mL of the local anesthetic in close proximity to the inferior alveolar branch of the mandibular nerve as it enters the mandibular canal at the mandibular foramen (Figure 10.5E). A 2.5-cm, 22-gauge needle is inserted at the lower angle of the jaw approximately 0.5 cm rostral to the angular process and is advanced 1–2 cm dorsally along the medial surface of the ramus of the mandible to the palpable lip of the mandibular foramen.

Intercostal nerve block

Intercostal nerve blocks may be used for relieving pain during and after thoracotomy, pleural drainage, and rib fractures, thereby minimizing the need for systemic analgesics that may depress respiration. They are not recommended for dogs with pulmonary diseases, which impair blood–gas exchange, or for dogs that cannot be observed for several hours after injection because of the potential for clinically delayed pneumothorax.

A minimum of two adjacent intercostal spaces both cranial and caudal to the incision or injury site are selectively blocked because of overlap of nerve supply. The site for needle placement is the caudal border of the rib near the intervertebral foramen (Figure 10.6). Approximately 0.25–1.0 mL of 0.25% or 0.5% bupivacaine hydrochloride per site, with or without epinephrine 1:200,000, is deposited. Small volumes and/or diluted local anesthetic solutions should be used as initial pain therapy so that the total dose does not exceed 3 mg/kg. Small dogs receive 0.25 mL/site, medium dogs 0.5 mL/site, and large dogs 1.0 mL/site. Postthoracotomy pain is generally controlled for 3–6 hours after successful block. Intercostal nerve block produces relatively high blood concentrations of local anesthetic for a given dose; therefore, the risk of toxic blood concentrations is greater.

Selective intercostal nerve block is easily performed because of the proximity of each nerve to its adjacent rib. The intercostal nerves can be visualized beneath the parietal

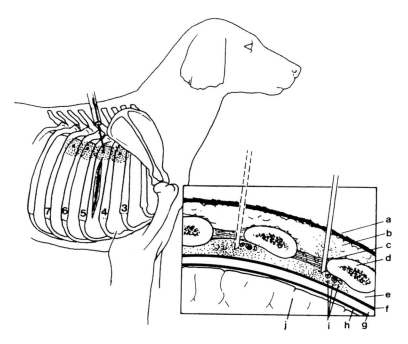

Figure 10.6. Needle placement for inducing intercostal nerve blocks. Inset: (a) skin; (b) subcutaneous tissue; (c) intercostal muscles; (d) rib; (e) subcostal space; (f) pleura costails and fascia; (g) interpleural space; (h) pleura pulmonalis; (i) intercostal artery, vein, and nerve; and (j) lung. Numbers 3–7 refer to the numbers of the ribs.

pleura during thoracotomy. This technique provides consistent analgesia and does not produce respiratory depression, with subsequent hypercarbia and hypoxemia.

Interpleural regional analgesia

Pain from rib fractures, metastasis to the chest wall, pleura, and mediastinum, mastectomy, chronic pancreatitis, cholecystectomy, renal surgery, abdominal cancer, and posthepatic neuralgesia can be reduced by intermittent or continuous administration of local anesthetic into the pleural space through a catheter. The mechanisms of pain relief produced by interpleural analgesia are not fully understood, but at least three different sites of actions have been hypothesized: (1) retrograde diffusion of local anesthetic through the parietal pleura, causing intercostal nerve block; (2) unilateral block of the thoracic sympathetic chain and splanchnic nerves; and (3) diffusion of the anesthetic into the ipsilateral brachial plexus, resulting in a parietal block.

The catheter is placed into the pleural space either percutaneously or prior to closure of a thoracotomy. Percutaneous placement of a catheter into the pleural space is difficult to perform on dogs with pleural fibrosis, because thickening of the pleura makes identification of the pleural space guesswork. The dog should be sedated, and the skin, subcutaneous tissues, periosteum, and parietal pleura over the caudal border of the rib should first be desensitized with 1–2 mL of 2% lidocaine solution, using a 2.5–5-cm, 20–22-gauge needle. A 5.0-cm, 17-gauge Huber point (Tuohy) needle is then used for catheter placement. The stylet is removed and the needle filled with sterile saline until a meniscus is seen at the needle's hub. The needle is then advanced until a clicking sensation is perceived as the needle tip perforates the parietal pleura or until the meniscus disappears when the needle tip enters the pleural space (hanging-drop technique).

The hanging-drop technique for the identification of the subatmospheric pleural pressure is not always reliable because the meniscus may also disappear when the needle passes through the intercostal muscles. Alternatively, a freely moving 10-mL glass syringe is attached to the needle. The syringe and needle are then advanced as a unit. On entering the pleural space, the plunger of the syringe is drawn inward by the negative pressure of the interpleural space. Some veterinarians place the catheter in the tissue plane superficial to the parietal pleura, close to or in the subcostal space, in order to produce a more effective block attributable to a decreased loss of local anesthetic through thoracic drainage tubes. A catheter (6–10-cm length of fenestrated medical grade silastic tubing, 2 mm inside diameter) can be introduced and advanced 3–5 cm beyond the needle tip with minimal resistance after the needle tip is placed subpleurally.

A technique has been developed to insert the catheter without disconnection to minimize the risk of pneumothorax. The technique involves the use of a Tuohy needle to which a Y-piece with a latex balloon and catheter is attached. The needle is inserted until the balloon collapses under the negative pressure of the pleural cavity; the catheter is then advanced as required. The needle is then carefully withdrawn over the catheter, and the catheter is left in place. Approximately 1–2 mg of bupivacaine/kg (0.5%, with or without 5 mcg of epinephrine/mL) is injected over 1–2 minutes following negative aspiration of air or blood through the catheter. The catheter is then cleared with 2 mL of physiological saline solution. Bolus interpleural bupivacaine is effective in relieving postthoracotomy pain for 3–12 hours. Complications, such as lung trauma, bleeding, and pneumothorax, are occasionally reported with the blind percutaneous insertion technique. The balloon technique is superior to other methods (i.e., loss-of-resistance technique, low-friction syringe-piston movement, and infusion technique). A catheter can be placed in the open chest by inserting the Tuohy needle through the skin over the rib at a site that is at least two intercostal spaces caudal to the incision while care is taken to retract the lung. The catheter is then passed through the needle and placed 3–5 cm subpleurally under direct vision. Local anesthetic is injected in the usual manner. The ventral tip of the catheter is best anchored by using one encircling suture in the intercostal space at the site of puncture.

Dogs that recover from lateral thoracotomy should be placed with the incision side down. Dogs that have had a sternotomy should be placed in sternal recumbency for approximately 10 minutes to allow the local anesthetic to pool near the incision and adjacent intercostal nerves. The external portion of the catheter should be anchored with tape, sutured to the skin, and covered with a nonocclusive-type dressing that allows air circulation.

The optimum total dose, concentration, or volume of interpleural bupivacaine in sick dogs have not been reported. Theoretically, one or two of the three branches of the phrenic nerve can be blocked, leaving the remaining branch(es) intact. Isolated contraction of the costal portion of the diaphragm without contraction of the crural portion may result in paradoxical respiration with negative intra-abdominal pressure. The catheter is usually removed 24 hours after thoracotomy when postoperative pain has normally decreased. Long-term use (over several weeks) of an interpleural catheter is possible if the catheter is subcutaneously tunneled.

Infection, tachyphylaxis, systemic toxicity, unilateral sympathetic block (evidenced as a Horner's syndrome and increased subcutaneous skin temperature of the affected side), pleural effusion, phrenic nerve paralysis or paresis, and catheter-related complications (e.g., intrapulmonary placement of catheter) can occur if the procedure is performed improperly. Pain relief is minimal in people and dogs with a misplaced catheter, loss of local anesthetic in the chest tube, excessive bleeding into the pleural space, or altered diffusion within the parietal pleura after mechanical irritation by the surgical procedure. Care must be taken to avoid the serious potential complication of pneumothorax.

Anesthesia of the foot and leg

Several techniques may be used to induce anesthesia of the foot and leg successfully: (1) infiltration of tissues around the limb by using local anesthetic solution (ring block); (2) intra-articular injection of local anesthetic; (3) infiltration of the brachial plexus with local anesthetic solution (brachial plexus block); (4) injection of local anesthetic into an accessible superficial vein in an extremity that is isolated from the general circulation by placing a tourniquet proximal to the injection site (IVRA); (5) perineural infiltration of sensory nerves in the limbs (nerve block); and (6) injection of local anesthetic solution into the lumbosacral epidural space to induce anesthesia of the hind legs.

Ring block   Local infiltration and field block around the distal extremity may be performed with a 2–5-cm, 22–23-gauge standard needle. Intradermal wheals around a superficial lesion and subcutaneous infiltration around the limb are performed by using a short (<3-cm) and fine (23–25-gauge) needle.

Intra-articular analgesia   Intra-articular morphine provides analgesia, as indicated by cumulative pain scores and measurement of pain threshold, but not to the same level as intra-articular bupivacaine. Intra-articular morphine (0.1 mg/kg) did not produce the bradycardia, respiratory depression, or hypotension that might be observed after systemic administration of morphine. Ongoing inflammation is apparently needed for intra-articular opioids to produce noticeable antinociceptive effects. Recent studies have suggested that intra-articular mepivacaine results in less chondrocyte toxicity than either bupivacaine or lidocaine.

Brachial plexus block   Brachial plexus block is suitable for operations on the front limb within or distal to the elbow. The technique should be done in well-sedated standing or laterally recumbent dogs. A 7.5-cm, 20–22-gauge needle is inserted medial to the shoulder joint and directed parallel to the vertebral column toward the costochondral junction (Figure 10.7). In larger dogs, approximately 10–15 mL of 2% lidocaine hydrochloride solution with 1:200,000 epinephrine is injected slowly as the needle is withdrawn, if no

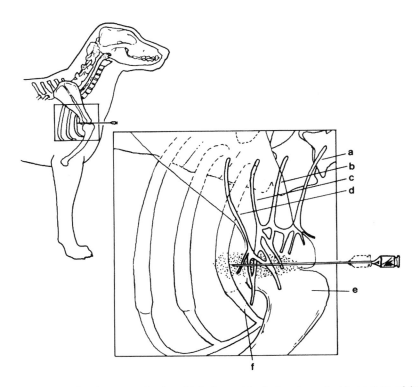

Figure 10.7.   Needle placement for brachial plexus block. Inset: ventral branches of (a) sixth, (b) seventh, (c) eighth cervical, and (d) first thoracic spinal nerves; (e) tuberosity of humerus; and (f) first rib.

blood is aspirated into the syringe, thereby placing the local anesthetic in close proximity to the radial, median, ulnar, musculocutaneous, and axillary nerves. Gradual loss of sensation and motor function occurs within 10–15 minutes. Anesthesia lasts for approximately 2 hours, and total recovery requires approximately 6 hours.

   A peripheral nerve stimulator can be used to accurately locate the radial, median, ulnar, musculocutaneous, and axillary nerves, thereby reducing the dose of local anesthetic for successful brachial plexus blockade in dogs. One electrode (the alligator clip on the positively charged lead wire [red plug]) from the nerve locator is attached to the skin, while the other electrode (the alligator clip on the negatively charged lead wire [black plug]) is attached to the proximal portion of the insulated needle (22 gauge × 4.25 in.). A 20-mL syringe containing the local anesthetic agent (2% lidocaine, 0.5% ropivacaine, or 0.5% bupivacaine, diluted with 0.9% sodium chloride solution to make a 0.375% concentration) is attached to a three-way stopcock, a fluid extension set, and the needle (Figure 10.8). As the needle is inserted medial to the scapulohumeral joint toward the costochondral junction of the first rib, medial to the scapula but outside the thorax, the nerve stimulator is turned on to 2 Hz and 1.0 mA. As the paw begins to twitch, the needle is precisely placed to obtain maximal twitch with as little current (<0.5 mA) as possible.

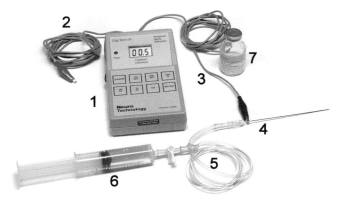

Figure 10.8. (1) Peripheral never-stimulator used as an aid in accurately locating nerves when performing nerve block procedures: The nerve locator is set at 2 Hz and low output (0.5 mA); the 0.5 mA current delivered to the patient is displayed; (2) the lead wire with red plug (+) and alligator clip for the patient's electrode; (3) the lead wire with black plug (−) and alligator clip for the needle; (4) Insulated needle (22 gauge, 4.25 in., 0.72 × 10.79 mm); (5) extension set; (6) 20-mL syringe with three-way stopcock, filled with (7) 0.2 ropivacaine hydrochloride.

At this point, the syringe is aspirated to ensure that it is not in a blood vessel, and 0.1–0.2 mL of the anesthetic is injected until the twitch disappears. The technique is repeated three or more times, by fanning the needle dorsal and ventral from the initial placement. Direct deposition of the local anesthetic on the nerves at a maximum dose of 1.5 mg/kg of lidocaine, ropivacaine, or bupivacaine will produce good brachial plexus blockade for up to 10 hours. Brachial plexus block is relatively simple and safe to perform and produces selective anesthesia and relaxation of the limb distal to the elbow joint. The relatively long waiting period (15–30 minutes) required to attain maximal anesthesia and some occasional failures to obtain complete anesthesia, particularly in fat dogs, are disadvantages of the technique.

IVRA   IVRA is a rapid and reliable method for producing short-term (<2 hours) anesthesia of the extremities. The clinical value of IVRA in humans is well established. The IVRA technique is also known as the Bier block. The technique is best accomplished in dogs by placing an IV catheter in an appropriate and accessible vein (e.g., the cephalic or lateral saphenous vein) distal to the tourniquet. The limb is first desanguinated by wrapping it with an Esmarch bandage. A rubber tourniquet is placed around the limb proximal to the Esmarch bandage. The tourniquet must be tight enough to overcome arterial blood pressure. Once the tourniquet is secured, the Esmarch bandage is unwrapped, and 2.5–5 mg/kg lidocaine is injected IV with light pressure. A period of 5–10 minutes is required to achieve maximum anesthesia before beginning the surgical procedure. Diluted concentrations (0.25% and 0.5%) of lidocaine produce adequate sensory blockade as long as the tourniquet is applied. By avoiding leakage and keeping the local anesthetic isolated in the limb, the incidence and severity of toxic symptoms are decreased and the percentage of successful blocks increased. Complications resulting from blood-flow deprivation to the limb do not usually occur if the procedure is limited to less than 60–90 minutes.

Once the tourniquet is removed, sensation returns within 5–15 minutes and residual analgesia remains for up to 30 minutes. The site and mechanism of local anesthetic action in IVRA are unclear but may involve desensitization of major nerve trunks and/or sensory nerve endings. Unlike the desensitization described in other nerve blocks, the onset of anesthesia and muscle paralysis begins distally and progresses proximally; thus, the local anesthetic should be injected as distally as possible in the limb. The blood-free surgery site is ideal for taking biopsy samples and removing a foreign body from the paws. Prolonged procedures (>90 minutes) may produce tourniquet-induced ischemia, which is associated with pain and increased blood pressure. Reversible shock occurs if the tourniquet is removed after 4 hours; and sepsis, endotoxemia, and death can occur if the tourniquet is applied for 8–10 hours. Bupivacaine should not be used because of the increased potential for cardiovascular collapse and death associated with its use IV.

Lumbosacral epidural anesthesia

This technique is noted for its simplicity, safety, and effectiveness, and is one of the most frequently used regional anesthetic techniques described for surgical procedures caudal to the umbilicus. Epidural anesthesia is frequently recommended for cesarean section.

The procedure is not difficult when performed by an experienced clinician. The epidural space is located between the inner and outer layers of the dura mater (Figure 10.9). It contains nerves (cauda equina), fat, blood vessels, lymphatics, and occasionally the end of the spinal cord with its surrounding meninges (arachnoid and dura mater). The subarachnoid space contains CSF. After a thorough surgical preparation, the local anesthetic solution is injected through a disposable 2.5–7.5-cm, 20–22-gauge spinal needle as a single dose or is injected through a catheter that is inserted at least 1.5–2.0 cm beyond the end of an 18- or 17-gauge Huber-point (Tuohy) or 18-gauge Crawford needle. A 2.5-cm, 22-gauge spinal needle is used for small dogs, a 3.8-cm, 20-gauge needle for medium-sized dogs, and a 7.5-cm, 18-gauge needle for large dogs. Important landmarks for needle placement are easily identified in most dogs. The iliac prominences on either side of the spine are palpated by using the thumb and middle finger of one hand (Figure 10.9). The spinous process of the seventh lumbar (L7) vertebra is located with the index finger. The lumbosacral (L7–S1) interspace should be palpated from both the cranial and caudal directions by moving the finger on the dorsal spinous processes of L6– L7 and S2–S1. This will help to avoid inadvertent placement of the needle into the L6–L7 interspace. The needle must be placed correctly on the midline and caudal to the L7 spinous process, and is inserted until a distinct popping sensation is felt as the needle point penetrates the interarcuate ligament. Tail movement may indicate that the needle has engaged nerve tissue. The epidural space is best identified by the loss-of-resistance test, using either an air-filled or a saline-filled syringe. Deliberate injection of 3–4 mL of air into the epidural space of dogs weighing 20–27 kg results in bubble formation that can persist for 24 hours. The bubbles, however, are not large or numerous enough to impede transfer of local anesthetic across the meninges and into the CSF, spinal roots, and cord, nor do they localize in any particular region (e.g., nerve roots); thus, subsequent injection of

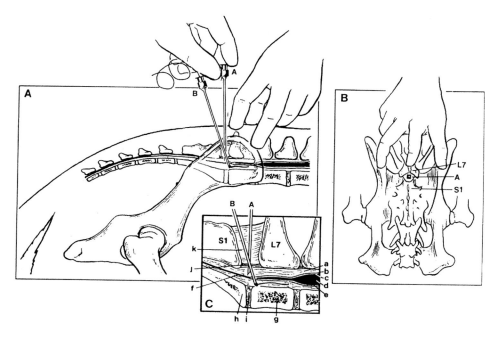

Figure 10.9. **A.** Aseptic needle placement, using sterile surgical gloves, into the lumbosacral epidural space of a dog (A) and catheter placement for continuous epidural anesthesia using a local anesthetic and/or analgesia using an opioid (B). **B.** Dorsal view. Palpation of the dorsal spinous process of the L7 vertebra and dorsoiliac wings. **C.** Inset: (a) epidural space with fat and connective tissue; (b) dura mater; (c) arachnoid membrane; (d) spinal cord; (e) CSF; (f) cauda equine; (g) seventh lumbar (L7) vertebra; (h) first sacral (S1) vertebra; (i) intervertebral disc; (j) interarcuate ligament (ligamentum flavum); and (k) interspinous ligament.

local anesthetic does not result in patchy anesthesia or inadequacies attributable to bubbles. Subcutaneous crepitation may be felt at the site of skin penetration if air has been injected outside the epidural space.

After the needle has been placed, the stylet is removed from the needle hub and the stylet is carefully examined for CSF or blood. Also, the needle (or catheter) should be carefully inspected for flow of CSF or blood before the local anesthetic is administered. If inadvertent subarachnoid puncture occurs, as indicated by the presence of CSF, the procedure may either be abandoned or the intended epidural dose reduced by at least 50%. The presence of blood indicates penetration of the ventral venous plexus, after which the needle should be repositioned epidurally. Obtaining CSF at the L7–S1 site is common, even though the subarachnoid space of dogs usually ends cranial to the lumbosacral interspace. The spinal cord and meninges in younger and smaller dogs and cats may occasionally extend into the lumbosacral vertebral junction.

A subarachnoid injection may be made if CSF is encountered, with the precaution that 1 mL of local anesthetic per 10 kg of body weight is then injected over a 1-minute period. The reduced dose should avoid total spinal anesthesia with cardiovascular and respiratory depression or collapse. If blood is encountered, the needle is withdrawn and cleansed, and another attempt is made to place it into the epidural space. Intravascular injection of local anesthetic can cause systemic toxicity, which is characterized by convulsions, cardiopulmonary depression, and the absence of regional anesthesia. Inadvertent subarachnoid administration of small amounts (2 mL) of fresh autologous blood aspirated from the venous plexus during attempted lumbar epidural puncture in dogs may cause pelvic limb spasm. If this occurs, most dogs recover rapidly and demonstrate no signs of meningeal irritation, long-term neurological sequelae, or neuropathological changes. To avoid excessive cranial advancement of neural blockade, it is also good practice to elevate the dog's head for approximately 5 minutes immediately after completion of the epidural administration of the anesthetic.

The shape and bevel orientation of the spinal needle affect the size of the dural defect. Large dural defects in humans may result in post-lumbar puncture headache attributable to a postulated increased CSF leak. Likewise, a bevel orientation parallel with rather than perpendicular to the dural fibers causes smaller dural defects (39,400 vs. 73,300 μm²), because the needle splits rather than cuts the longitudinal dural fibers. It is good practice to administer the calculated dose of local anesthetic at the body temperature of the dog and slow enough (over 45–60 seconds) to avoid causing pain.

Continuous epidural anesthesia   The indications, advantages, contraindications, and complications associated with continuous epidural anesthesia in dogs are similar to those of the single-injection method. Additional advantages of continuous epidural anesthesia are the ability to tailor the anesthesia duration to the length of operation and to maintain a route for injecting epidural opioids during surgery and postoperatively. For a more comprehensive discussion of this technique and its advantages and disadvantages the reader is referred to the fourth edition of *Lumb and Jones' Veterinary Anesthesia and Analgesia.*

Briefly, a Tuohy needle is placed into the epidural space between the L7 and S1 intervertebral space, similar to the single-injection epidural block technique. Catheterization is facilitated by first desensitizing the lumbosacral space with a small amount (2 mL) of 2% lidocaine. The Tuohy needle is inserted at a 15°–45° angle from the vertical position with the bevel directed cranially and is advanced until the epidural space has been entered. The three techniques previously discussed to confirm placement—hanging drop, loss of resistance to air, and loss of resistance to saline—may be more readily performed in dogs that are positioned in sternal rather than in lateral recumbency. Because the techniques may not always be ultimate proof that the needle has been placed epidurally, aspiration of the plunger before injection should verify whether a vein has been entered. At this point, catheters with a stylet are preferred. A slight resistance is usually encountered when the catheter passes through the tip of the Tuohy needle. Special markings on the catheter denote the distance the catheter has been advanced. The catheter is advanced at least two to three markings beyond the hub of the needle, which ensures that at least 2–3 cm of catheter has entered the epidural space. Flushing the needle with saline, rotating the needle, and advancing the catheter while slowly withdrawing the needle helps to thread the catheter into the epidural space. If these maneuvers fail, the needle and catheter should be withdrawn together. No attempt should be made to withdraw the catheter back through the needle, because this may sever the catheter. If this does occur, most authorities believe that no attempt should be made to retrieve a severed catheter. Wire-reinforced catheters have been inserted epidurally to the anterior lumbar (L4) or thoracic (T1) vertebrae with minimal resistance and without coiling, turning on themselves, kinking, or knotting.

Local anesthetic choice A variety of local anesthetics of different concentrations and doses have been used to produce a wide spectrum of epidural sensory and motor blockades. The selected local anesthetic and dosage (concentration and volume) depends on a patient's size, the desired extent of anesthesia, and the desired onset and duration of epidural anesthetic effect. A test dose of 0.5–1.0 mL of 2% lidocaine hydrochloride solution produces almost immediate dilation of the external anal sphincter, followed by relaxation of the tail and ataxia of pelvic limbs, within 3–5 minutes. Approximately 1 mL of 2% lidocaine per 4.5 kg of body weight will completely anesthetize the pelvic limbs and posterior abdomen caudal to the first lumbar (L1) vertebra within 10–15 minutes after administration. The flexor-pinch reflex of pelvic limbs will be absent in 5–10 minutes after injection. Clinical experience indicates that the disappearance of the toe reflexes is associated with surgical anesthesia from midthorax to coccyx sufficient for abdominal surgery. The latent period is prolonged to 20–30 minutes if 0.75% bupivacaine hydrochloride is administered and is attributable to the drug's low solubility and slow uptake by nervous tissue. Good anesthesia for abdominal and orthopedic surgeries caudal to the diaphragm is generally achieved by administering 1 mL/5 kg (maximum, 20 mL) of 2% lidocaine or 0.5% bupivacaine, both with freshly added 1:200,000 epinephrine.

A reduced volume of 2% lidocaine (1 mL/6 kg) is generally satisfactory for epidural anesthesia in dogs for cesarean section. The reason for the (approximately 25%) decrease in dose requirement during pregnancy is unclear. Several theories have been proposed: (1) distension of epidural veins, which decreases the size of the epidural space, and/or increase in the spread of local anesthetic; (2) hormonal changes, which influence proteins that affect membrane sensitivity; and (3) chronic exposure to progesterone, which alters the permeability of intercellular connective-tissue matrix, thereby facilitating diffusion of local anesthetics across the nerve sheath. It is rarely necessary to inject more than 3 mg of lidocaine/kg of body weight for epidural anesthesia during cesarean section in dogs.

The anesthesia duration obtained from the deposition of epidural local anesthetic drugs primarily depends on the drug selected, the dermatomal level of anesthesia, and the presence or absence of epinephrine (Table 10.4). Postoperative analgesia (after general anesthesia) lasts longer when epidural anesthesia is performed at the end of surgery, and is attributable to a diminished intensity of the painful stimulus. Epidural bupivacaine (0.75%) has induced surgical anesthesia for periods lasting from 4 to 6 hours. Surgical anesthesia caudal to the last rib is produced and gradually converted into a phase of postoperative analgesia lasting for 24 hours without affecting motor activity or cardiopulmonary function, if a combination of 0.7–1.0 mL/10 cm vertex–coccyx distance of 0.5% bupivacaine hydrochloride solution and 0.1 mg/kg of morphine hydrochloride is injected epidurally.

Table 10.4. Commonly used local anesthetic drugs and doses for peripheral and epidural block procedures in conscious dogs

Local anesthetic		Conc. (%)	Usual doses (mg/kg)		Toxic doses, IV (mg/kg)		Approximate onset of motor and sensory block (min)	Approximate duration of motor and sensory block (h)	Motor block
Generic name	Trade name (manufacturer)		With epinephrine	Without epinephrine	Convulsive	Lethal			
Ester linked									
Procaine	Novocaine (Withrop Laboratories)	1–2	8	6	36	100	10–15	0.5	±
Chloroprocaine	Nesacaine (Pennwalt)	1.0–1.5	8	6	–	–	7–15	0.5–1.0	±
Amide linked									
Lidocaine	Xylocaine (Astra Pharmaceutical Products)	0.5–2.0	7	5	11–20	16–28	10–15	1–2	+
Mepivacaine	Carbocaine (Breon Laboratories)	1–2	7	5	29	–	5–10	2.0–2.5	+
Bupivacaine	Marcaine (Breon Laboratories)	0.25–0.5	3	2	3.5–4.5	5–11	20–30	2.5–6.0	±
Ropivacaine	LEA 103 (Breon Laboratories)	0.5	5	3	4.9	–	5–15	2.5–4.0	+
Etidocaine	Duranest (Astra Pharmaceutical Products)	0.5–0.75	5	3	4.5	20	5–10	2–5	+++

Conc., concentration; IV, intravenous; ±, inconsistent motor nerve block; +, weak motor nerve block; +++, strong motor nerve block.

Table 10.5. Physiochemical properties and doses of opioids for epidural analgesia in dogs

Opioid	Molecular weight of base	pK^a (25°C)	Oil–water partition coefficient[a]	Dose (mg/ kg)	Approximate time for pain relief (min)	Approximate duration of analgesia (h)
Morphine sulfate	285	7.9	1.42	0.05–0.15	30–60	10–24
Meperidine hydrochloride	247	8.5	38.8	0.5–1.5	10–30	5–20
Methadone hydrochloride	309	9.3	116	0.05–0.15	15–20	5–15
Oxymorphone hydrochloride	301	–	–	0.05–0.15	20–40	10–22
Fentanyl citrate	336	8.4	813	0.001–0.01	15–20	3–5

[a] Octanol–pH 7.4 buffer partition coefficient.

The epidural administration of lidocaine (2%, 5 mg/kg with epinephrine 1:200,000), bupivacaine (0.5%, 1.25 mg/kg with epinephrine 1:200,000), and lidocaine (2%, 2.5 mg/ kg with epinephrine 1:200,0000) combined with bupivacaine (0.5%, 0.61 mg/kg with epinephrine 1:200,000) results in the combination achieving a shorter time to sphincter relaxation than does bupivacaine alone (23 ± 2 vs. 84 ± 23 seconds), longer analgesia than lidocaine alone (94 ± 8 vs. 54 ± 5 minutes), and longer muscle relaxation than either lidocaine (102 ± 8 vs. 59 ± 6 minutes) or bupivacaine (102 ± 8 vs. 57 ± 20 minutes).

Epidural opioid analgesia Providing long-term analgesia while inducing minimal systemic effects is an important objective in medical care. Epidurally administered opiates (e.g., morphine) provide lengthy analgesia caudal to the umbilicus with very few systemic side effects. A single epidural injection of 5 mg of morphine before major intra-abdominal surgery consistently reduces intraoperative and postoperative pain in people for at least 3 days.

Preservative-free preparations of morphine have not been associated with spinal cord histopathological changes. In contrast, parenterally administered morphine, which contains various preservatives (such as sodium bisulfite, metabisulfite, chlorbutanol, edetate disodium, formaldehyde, or phenol), has neurotoxic effects when placed directly on the spinal cord. Contraindications to epidural opioid analgesia are primarily associated with the epidural catheterization technique itself.

The presence of a large number of opiate receptors in the substantia gelatinosa of the dorsal horn of the spinal cord suggests that the administration of small doses of opioids into the epidural space should produce effective analgesia. The administration of epidural opioids offers the advantage of producing more profound and prolonged analgesia with significantly smaller doses and less sedation than the analgesia produced by comparable parenterally administered (intramuscular or IV) opioids. Epidural opioids relieve somatic and visceral pain by selectively blocking nociceptive impulses without interfering with sensory and motor function or depressing the sympathetic nervous system (selective spinal analgesia).

The physiochemical properties of opioids, particularly their lipid solubility, molecular weight, pK_a, and receptor-binding affinity, are important in determining their pharmacokinetic and pharmacodynamic properties and the onset and duration of analgesia (Table 10.5). Relatively hydrophilic morphine (oil–water partition coefficient, 1:42) remains in the CSF for longer periods, allowing rostral spread and analgesia distant from the site of injection (nonsegmental distribution of analgesia). The lumbosacral epidural administration of 0.1 mg of morphine/kg can produce adequate postthoracotomy analgesia in dogs.

Epidurally administered morphine is distributed by at least four different pathways: (1) transdural passage to the CSF and neural axis, (2) vascular uptake by epidural venous plexi and spinal radicular arteries, (3) lymphatic uptake, and (4) deposition into epidural fat. Pharmacodynamic studies evaluating the degree of analgesia and CSF and plasma drug concentrations of epidurally administered morphine support a spinal mechanism of action. These studies also indicate that rapid but short-lasting serum concentrations and delayed long-lasting CSF concentrations are often achieved with epidurally administered doses of morphine in dogs.

Potential side effects of epidural opioids include respiratory depression, dysphoria, urinary retention, delayed gastrointestinal motility, vomiting, rubbing of the face, and catheter-related problems such as catheter displacement, occlusion, and infection from chronic epidural catheterization.

The analgesic efficacy, duration of action, and adverse effects of epidurally administered morphine are dose related. The most serious adverse effect is respiratory depression, which is biphasic. Respiratory depression has been attributed to the absorption of morphine into epidural veins and subsequent circulatory redistribution to the brain (early depression), and cephalad movement of morphine in CSF to the brain stem (late respiratory depression). Severe respiratory depression should not occur when therapeutic doses (0.1 mg/kg) of morphine are administered epidurally.

Side effects are more common with intrathecal injection. Myoclonus and neuroexitation are very rarely observed complications in human patients after the epidural or IV administration of opioids. Similarly, involuntary muscle contractions in dogs, after either epidural or subarachnoid administration of preservative-free morphine, are extremely rare.

Nonopioid epidural analgesia Similar to morphine, the administration of alpha$_2$ agonists can produce a powerful effect on nociceptive processing by activating a dense population of alpha$_2$ receptors (i.e., α_{2A}, α_{2B}, α_{2C}, and α_{2D}) (heteroceptors) in the CNS and periphery. In addition, some alpha$_2$ agonists can also activate imidazoline receptors (I_1 and I_2) and produce direct effects on sensory transmission (e.g., xylazine). Spinally administered alpha$_2$ agonists mediate analgesia by activating presynaptic alpha$_2$ adrenoceptors, which are located on primary afferent C fibers terminating in the superficial laminae of the dorsal horn of the spinal cord. This activation induces G_0 proteins that decrease calcium influx, which results in a decreased release of neurotransmitters and/or neuropeptides (e.g., glutamate, substance P, neurotensin, calcitonin gene-related peptide, and vasoactive intestinal peptide), resulting in antinociception. Activation of the alpha$_2$ heteroceptors, which are located postsynaptically on wide-dynamic-range projection neurons targeted by primary afferent fibers in the dorsal horn, results in hyperpolarization of neurons via G_i protein-coupled potassium channels, producing postsynaptically mediated spinal analgesia similar to opioids' effects.

Ketamine has an analgesic action at many sites both centrally and peripherally. The mechanism of analgesic action of epidurally and intrathecally administered ketamine has not been clearly defined, and investigation into the contribution of supraspinal and/or spinal sites related to its analgesic and anesthetic action has not provided conclusive results. While reports regarding the efficacy of ketamine as a spinal analgesic are controversial, ketamine may block *N*-methyl-D-aspartate (NMDA) receptors and interact with subtypes of opioid, propionate, kainate, γ-aminobutyric acid receptors, and/or monoaminergic (serotonergic, noradrenergic, and dopaminergic) neural systems. Ketamine also inhibits voltage-gated sodium-ion and potassium-ion channels, thereby suppressing myelinated nerve conduction. Ketamine may reverse opioid tolerance by interacting with NMDA receptors, the nitric oxide pathway, and μ-opioid receptors. Evidence of the efficacy of ketamine for treatment of chronic pain in human patients has been reviewed and is considered moderate to weak. Epidural and intrathecal doses of 1–3 mg of ketamine/kg of body weight have shown analgesic efficacy while rapidly being distributed to the plasma and CSF (0.4 and 0.3 hours, respectively) from the epidural space of dogs.

Glucocorticoids (e.g., prednisone, prednisolone, and methylprednisolone) are most commonly administered by systemic routes, either oral or injectable, to relieve pain and reduce inflammation. Perineural injection, either to spinal nerve roots or to peripheral nerves, to alleviate pain caused by nerve root disease or peripheral neuropathies is common in human patients. As of this writing, recommendations or dosages for the use of epidural glucocorticoids in dogs and other small companion animals have not been developed.

Epidural opioids (e.g., morphine or oxymorphone) with local anesthetics (e.g., lidocaine, bupivacaine, or ropivacaine) or alpha$_2$ adrenoceptor agonists (e.g., xylazine, medetomidine, or dexmedetomidine) are administered to dogs before surgery to reduce general anesthetic requirements and provide intraoperative and postoperative pain control. Several investigators have reported additive or synergistic effects of epidurally administered opioids and local anesthetics in dogs. Although numerous local anesthetic/opioid combinations have been used, morphine with lidocaine or bupivacaine are most widely used. Epidural administration of morphine–bupivacaine provides longer-lasting analgesia than does morphine alone. The times for rescue-oxymorphone administration in dogs treated with either epidural morphine, bupivacaine, a morphine–bupivacaine combination, or saline were 5.4, 9.1, 24, and 2.6 hours, respectively.

Synergistic antinociceptive interactions have been observed between a variety of alpha$_2$ adrenoceptor and opioid receptor agonists. The epidural administration of alpha$_2$ adrenoceptor agonists alone or in combination with morphine has gained some degree of use in veterinary practice.

Adverse effects Adverse effects associated with epidural and subarachnoid anesthesia in dogs include (1) hypoventilation secondary to respiratory muscle paralysis, which is attributable to the spread of local anesthetic to the cervical spinal segments; (2)

hypotension, Horner's syndrome, and hypoglycemia caused by sympathetic blockade; (3) Shiff–Sherrington-like reflexes; and (4) muscular twitches, coma, convulsion, and circulatory depression caused by toxic plasma concentrations of local anesthetic. Improper injection technique can cause delay in onset of anesthesia, unilateral hind-limb paresis, partial anesthesia of the tail or the perineal region, and sepsis.

Reports about delayed hair regrowth after epidural analgesia in dogs, though controversial, have been difficult to confirm. In one study, hair regrowth was complete after 4 months, and there was no difference in hair length among groups, indicating that neither epidural analgesia nor scrubbing or clipping seemed to affect hair regrowth in at least the limited number of dogs in this study. Complications with epidural anesthetic techniques can be prevented in most instances by following several basic rules, which include careful selection of drugs and dosage, aspiration before injection (to assure that the tip of the needle is not in a blood vessel or subarachnoid space), and injection of test doses.

Absolute contraindications for epidural anesthetic techniques include infection at the lumbosacral puncture site, uncorrected hypovolemia, bleeding disorders, therapeutic or physiological anticoagulation, degenerative central or peripheral axonal diseases, and anatomical abnormalities that would make epidural anesthesia difficult. Bacteremia, neurological disorders, and minidose heparin therapy are relative contraindications. The benefits of epidural anesthesia often outweigh the risks.

Local and regional analgesic techniques: cats

Commonly used techniques in cats are topical anesthesia, local infiltration, nerve blocks (e.g., selective blockade of distal branches of nerves about the head, forelimb, and hind limb), brachial plexus block, IVRA, epidural anesthesia, and epidural analgesia. Because of restraint problems, local and regional anesthetic techniques are typically administered to heavily sedated or anesthetized cats. A number of local anesthetic drugs that vary in potency, toxicity, and cost are available for these purposes. Most commonly, 0.5–2.0% lidocaine hydrochloride is used to achieve 60–120 minutes of analgesia, whereas 0.2–0.5% ropivacaine hydrochloride or 0.25–0.5% bupivacaine hydrochloride produce analgesia for 240–360 minutes. Advantages of using regional anesthetic/analgesic techniques in cats include (1) reduction of the required dose of general anesthetic drugs and thus minimal cardiopulmonary depression, (2) complete blockade of sensory and motor nerve fibers, and (3) prevention of the secondary (central) sensitization to pain. Preemptive analgesia theoretically (1) decreases the severity of pain during surgery, (2) reduces drug requirements for pain control, and (3) provides analgesia after surgery.

Topical anesthesia

Local anesthetics, either as lidocaine spray (10%, 100 mg/mL) or lidocaine hydrochloride solution, can be applied topically. One spray delivers 10 mg of lidocaine, which usually is sufficient to desensitize small areas of oral, nasal, and pharyngeal mucous membranes. Administration of 20 mg of lidocaine to the mucous membrane produces surface anesthesia up to 2 mm deep within 2 minutes, which lasts for about 15 minutes. Topical lidocaine (spray or instillation) is useful for minor diagnostic, therapeutic, and surgical procedures (e.g., endoscopy, placement of nasal catheters for tube feeding, foreign-body removal, biopsies, and repair of small mucosal wounds). Instillation of 1.0 mL of lidocaine (20 mg), ropivacaine (2 mg), or bupivacaine (2.5 mg) into the wound of skin incisions or lacerations provides good analgesia in cats (4 kg). These local anesthetics are ineffective when applied topically to intact skin. Sterile lidocaine jelly (2%, 20 mg/mL) provides good analgesia of the urethra during catheter placement, because lidocaine is absorbed across mucous membranes. The eutectic mixture of lidocaine and prilocaine (EMLA cream [lidocaine 2.5% and prilocaine 2.5%]) penetrates the stratum corneum of the skin. Cream is placed on the skin and covered with a clean dressing for at least 20 minutes to facilitate placement of arterial and venous catheters in cats. Proparacaine 0.5%, tetracaine 0.5%, or butacaine 2% can be applied topically to desensitize the cornea for 10–20 minutes. Repeated doses have been reported to prolong anesthesia up to 2 hours without causing harmful effects.

Infiltration anesthesia

Local infiltration is primarily used for repair of superficial lacerations, cutaneous biopsy, and removal of dermal or subcutaneous tumors. Lidocaine hydrochloride (2–5 mg/kg), ropivacaine, or bupivacaine hydrochloride (3 mg/kg) is injected in the form of a subcutaneous bleb, line block, inverted V-block or triangular or rectangular pattern around a small tumor to be surgically removed, using a 25-gauge × 0.6-in. needle or 22-gauge × 1-in. needle. The syringe is aspirated before each injection and great care must be taken to prevent inadvertent IV injection. Sterile saline solution can be used to decrease the concentration and increase the volume of lidocaine (2 mL of a 1% solution instead of 1 mL of a 2% solution) to allow infiltration of a larger lesion. The total dose (20 mg) should be reduced by 30–50% in debilitated cats.

Regional nerve blocks

Regional anesthesia of the face

Commonly used nerve blocks to manage pain during and after surgical and dental procedures are the infraorbital, inferior alveolar, and mental nerves (Figure 10.10). These nerves can be desensitized by injecting 0.1–0.3 mL of either 1.0–2.0% lidocaine, 0.2–0.5% ropivacaine, or 0.25–0.5% bupivacaine hydrochloride solutions, using a 30-gauge × 0.5-in. to 22-gauge × 1-in. needle.

Anesthesia of the maxilla and upper teeth

The upper lip and muzzle, roof of the nasal cavity, soft and hard palates, and teeth in the upper dental arcade are supplied by sensory fibers of the infraorbital nerve. The nerve is blocked at the infraorbital foramen as it emerges from the infraorbital canal, ventral to the eye, approximately 1.0 cm dorsal to the third premolar at the junction of the maxilla

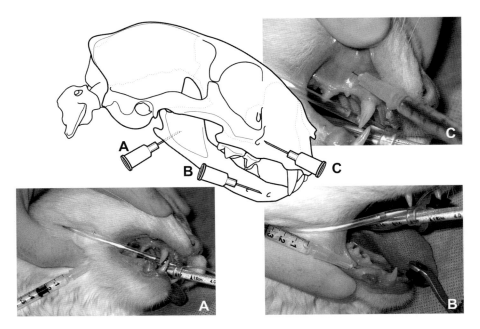

Figure 10.10.　Needle placement for nerve blocks of the head: (A) inferior alveolar (mandibular), (B) mental, and (C) infraorbital.

and zygomatic arch. Improper identification of the infraorbital foramen and branching of a nerve proximal to the region of local anesthetic may cause failure to produce regional anesthesia. The block is facilitated by angling the needle tip slightly medially. The needle is then advanced approximately 0.5 cm into the infraorbital canal, which is not a true canal in cats (Figure 10.10C).

Anesthesia of the mandible and lower teeth

The lower dental arcade, including the molars, canines, and incisors, and the skin and mucosa of the chin and lower lip are supplied by sensory fibers of the mandibular nerve. The nerve can be easily blocked at the point of its entry into the mandibular canal at the mandibular foramen. The needle is inserted percutaneously at the ventromedial aspect of the ramus of the mandible, approximately 1.0 cm rostral to the angular process, and for a depth of 0.5 cm (Figure 10.10A). In an alternative technique, the inferior alveolar nerve can be blocked intraorally, under the buccal fold.

The inferior alveolar nerve branches into the free rostral, middle, and caudal mental nerves, which supply sensory fibers to the lower lip and the medial half of the canine and three incisors. The mental nerve can be blocked at the mental foramina, caudal and ventral to the lower canine (Figure 10.10B). The extremely small size of the mental foramina precludes the insertion of a needle or catheter into the termination of the mandibular canal.

Anesthesia of the limbs

Blockade of the distal branches of the radial, median, and ulnar nerves, blockade of cervical and thoracic nerves (brachial plexus block), and IVRA are cost- and time-effective techniques for providing perioperative anesthesia and managing pain after surgical procedures of the forelimb in cats. In the hind limb, selective blockade of the common peroneal and tibial nerves is easily produced. Injection of the local anesthetic or opioid into the epidural space at the lumbosacral junction provides analgesia of the pelvic limbs and perineum.

Blockade of the radial, ulnar, and median nerves Selective blockade of the distal branches of the radial, ulnar, and median nerves produces brief surgical anesthesia and postoperative analgesia after onychectomy or tenectomy. The nerve blocks are easily performed to supplement anesthesia or provide an alternative to wound irrigation with local anesthetic following onychectomy. The superficial branches of the radial nerve are blocked on the dorsomedial aspect proximal to the carpal joint. The palmar and dorsal cutaneous branches of the ulnar nerve are blocked just proximal and lateral to the accessory carpal bone. The median nerve is blocked proximal to the median carpal pad. A 22-gauge × 1-in. needle can be used, and approximately 0.3 mL of the anesthetic solution is administered subcutaneously at each site (Figure 10.11). In two alternative techniques, the local anesthetic (3 mg/kg body weight) is injected subcutaneously distal to the carpal joint to each of the dorsal and palmar proper digital nerves either as a four-point digital nerve block or as a ring block.

Blockade of the common peroneal and tibial nerves Selective blockade of the distal branches of the common peroneal and tibial nerves produces perioperative and postoperative analgesia in the hind limb for onychectomy or tenectomy. The superficial branches of the common peroneal nerve are easily blocked by subcutaneous infiltration of the local anesthetic on the dorsomedial aspect of the tarsus distal to the tarsal joint. The superficial branches of the tibial nerve are blocked by subcutaneous injection of the local anesthetic ventromedially and distally to the tarsal joint (Figure 10.12).

Brachial plexus block Blockade of the ventral branches of the cervical (C6, C7, and C8) and thoracic (T1) spinal nerves can be used to anesthetize the forelimb and manage pain after surgical repair of the radius and ulna in cats. The procedure is performed in well-sedated or anesthetized cats. A needle (22-gauge × 1 in.) is placed into the axillary space proximal to the shoulder, and approximately 0.5 mL of either 2% lidocaine (10 mg), 0.5% ropivacaine, or 0.5% bupivacaine (2.5 mg) is injected once the needle tip is cranial to the first rib and caudal to the cranial border of the scapula. The same amount of the anesthetic is administered as the needle is withdrawn. The syringe is aspirated prior to each injection to avoid injection into the axillary artery and vein, which are close to the brachial plexus. The brachial plexus should not be blocked bilaterally because of potential bilateral phrenic nerve blockade and subsequent compromised respiratory function.

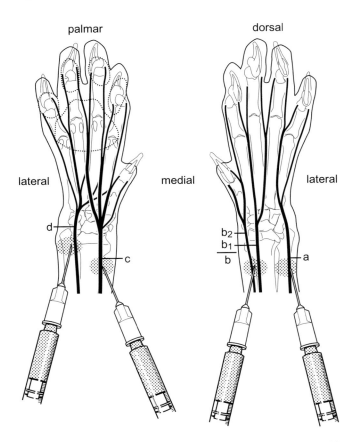

Figure 10.11.   Needle placement for nerve blocks on the foreleg: (a) dorsal branch of ulnar nerve, (b1) lateral branch and (b2) medial branch of superficial branch of radial nerve, (c) median nerve, and (d) palmar branch of the ulnar nerve.

IVRA   First, a 22-gauge × 1-inch IV catheter is inserted into the cephalic vein proximal to the carpus and with the catheter tip pointing distally. Second, an inflatable blood pressure cuff (neonatal no. 2) is placed proximal to the cephalic catheter and is inflated and maintained at 100 mm Hg greater than systolic pressure. Third, a second tourniquet, 6.25 mm rubber tubing, is tied above the elbow and left in place for 20 minutes. Lidocaine (1%, 3 mg/kg) is then injected into the distal cephalic venous catheter to anesthetize the entire limb distal to the tourniquet, as determined by lack of response to toe pinch. After the tourniquet has been removed, analgesia still remains for approximately 20 minutes. The plasma lidocaine concentrations may vary. The reported highest mean lidocaine concentration was 2.8 ± 1.0 mcg/mL after the injection of lidocaine (3 mg/kg) and was 3.1 ± 1.1 mcg/mL after a second injection of lidocaine (3 mg/kg) 20 minutes later. Significant leakage under the tourniquet may occur, as determined by measurable venous plasma lidocaine concentrations (maximum, 4.42 mcg/mL) prior to tourniquet release. Placement of the tourniquet and thus occlusion of blood supply distal to the tourniquet

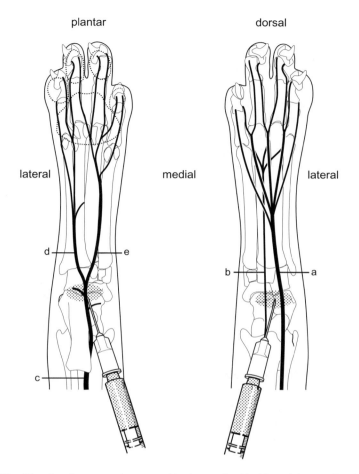

Figure 10.12. Needle placement for nerve blocks on the hind leg: (a) superficial peroneal nerve, (b) deep peroneal nerve, (c) tibial nerve, (d) lateral plantar nerve, and (e) medial plantar nerve.

should be limited to 30 minutes to prevent complications (e.g., lameness or endotoxemia).

Intercostal nerve block

This technique is used to control pain following lateral thoracotomy, rib fractures, or pleural drainage. Two adjacent intercostal nerves, cranial and caudal to the incision site or wound (four sites in total), are blocked (Figure 10.13). A needle (27 gauge × 1 in.) is inserted into the intercostal muscle close to the insertion of the epaxial muscles. The needle is directed dorsomedially and, using caution not to puncture the lung, its tip is walked off the caudal border of the rib. The syringe is aspirated before each injection of anesthetic solution (3 mg/kg body weight), which is equally

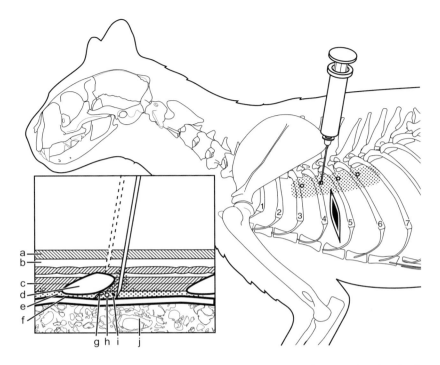

Figure 10.13.   Needle placement for inducing intercostal nerve blocks, showing the lateral aspect and the sagittal section (inset): (a) skin, (b) subcutaneous tissue, (c) intercostal muscles, (d) rib, (e) subcostal space, (f) pleura costalis and fascia, (g) intercostal vein, (h) intercostal artery, (i) intercostal nerve, and (j) lung.

divided among the injection sites. Cats should be observed for development of pneumothorax after the procedure.

Lumbosacral epidural anesthesia

Lumbosacral epidural anesthesia provides a reversible loss of sensation to a reasonably well-defined area of the body caudal to the diaphragm. Epidural injection of a local anesthetic may be used alone in cats that are at high risk of medical complications, that are aged, or that require immediate surgery of the rear quarter. The skin of the lumbosacral area is surgically prepared with an aseptic technique. A needle (22 gauge × 1 inch) is placed into the skin surface at the midline of the lumbosacral space. Except in obese cats, this space can be easily palpated halfway between the dorsoiliac wings and just caudal to the dorsal spinous process of the seventh lumbar vertebra. The needle is pushed ventrocaudally at a 45° angle to the dorsum to avoid pinching the seventh lumbar spinous process (Figure 10.14). Resistance is encountered on reaching the ligamentum flavum. A distinct pop is usually felt when the needle is advanced through this ligament. Needle depth to reach the epidural space may vary from 6 to 25 mm (0.25–1.0 in.), depending

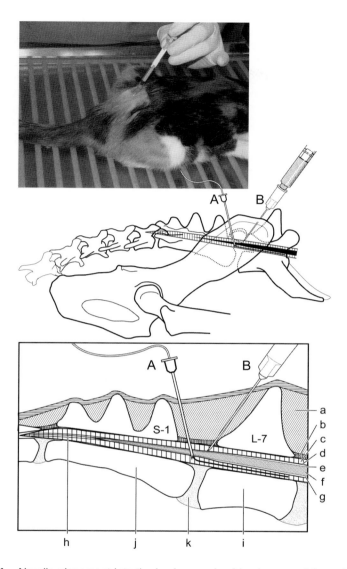

Figure 10.14. Needle placement into the lumbosacral epidural space of the cat (B) and catheter placement for continuous epidural anesthesia by using a local anesthetic and/or analgesia by using an opioid (A). Inset: (a) interspinous ligament, (b) interarcuate ligament (ligamentum flavum), (c) epidural space with fat and connective tissue, (d) dura mater, (e) arachnoid membrane, (f) spinal cord, (g) CSF, (h) cauda equine, (i) seventh lumber (L7) vertebra, (j) first sacral (S1) vertebra, and (k) intervertebral disk.

on the cat's size. Further insertion of the needle will meet resistance, indicating the needle tip has encountered the bony floor of the vertebral canal, and thus necessitates the withdrawal of needle by 1–2 mm. The hub of the needle is observed for blood and CSF. Because the dura sack terminates in the sacral area of cats, CSF may escape from the needle. If CSF is observed or aspirated, either the epidural injection is abandoned or only one-third to one-half of the original calculated dose of the drug is administered. Observation of blood within the needle indicates that the ventral venous sinus has been punctured; therefore, the needle should be removed. Intravascular injection of epidural drugs should be avoided to prevent toxicity. Lidocaine 2%, ropivacaine 0.2%, or bupivacaine 0.25% at the dose of 1.0 mL/4 kg produces analgesia up to the umbilicus. Analgesia duration is at least 1 hour with the use of lidocaine and 4–6 hours with ropivacaine or bupivacaine. When administered at the same dose (1.0 mL/4 kg) subarachnoidally (into the CSF), cranial block may decrease sympathetic activity and cause myocardial depression, hypotension, respiratory insufficiency, respiratory paralysis, and convulsions.

Epidural opioid analgesia

Preservative-free morphine (Astramorph/PF [AstraZeneca Pharmaceuticals LP], 0.5 or 1.0 mg morphine/mL; or Duramorph [Baxter Health Care, Deerfield, IL], 0.5 or 1.0 mg morphine/mL) can be administered through a sterile needle or indwelling epidural catheter into the epidural space to provide intraoperative and postoperative pain control. An aseptic technique, as described for epidural injection of local anesthetic drugs, must be used. In contrast to the administration of a local anesthetic, epidural morphine provides prolonged analgesia (>6 hours) with no effect on motor and sympathetic pathways. The dose of morphine (0.1 mg/kg) must be calculated carefully and the syringe should be aspirated before injection. A cat weighing 4 kg can be administered 0.4 mg morphine, which is 0.8 mL of Astramorph (0.5 mg/mL). If the needle tip has entered the intrathecal (subarachnoid) space, as recognized by free flow of CSF from the needle hub or aspiration by the syringe, the dose is reduced by 50% to 0.2 mg of morphine (0.4 mL of Astramorph). Mild hind-limb ataxia, licking, retching, or vomiting may be observed. Analgesia generally develops first, lasts longer, and is more profound in somatic areas of spinal cord segments, which are presumably exposed to the highest concentration of morphine. The depressant effects of epidural morphine on the hemodynamic and respiratory centers are likely the result of interaction with opioid receptors in the CNS (general analgesia) after diffusion to the brain via the blood and CSF.

Lumbosacral epidural injection of fentanyl (4 mcg/kg) diluted to a total volume of 1 mL with physiological saline reportedly increases the pain threshold of the hind limb for up to 245 minutes. The NMDA receptor antagonistic action of ketamine may be useful in patients with chronic pathological pain states refractory to opioids, anticonvulsants, or antidepressants. However, the safety of neuraxially administered ketamine remains unclear and is not recommended.

Conclusion

Local and regional anesthetic techniques in dogs and cats have been used extensively to relieve the pain related to a variety of medical and surgical procedures. Appropriately selected topical, local, or regional techniques can provide safe, effective, and reliable analgesia with minimal physiological alterations. Similarly, the interpleural administration of local anesthetic drugs or the epidural administration of opioids can provide unparalleled long-term relief of pain while preserving consciousness. Novel techniques for the delivery of analgesics and other therapeutic modalities designed to be used with local anesthetics, opioids, and nonopioid analgesics may greatly facilitate the future management of perioperative pain in companion animals.

Revised from "Local and Regional Anesthetic and Analgesic Techniques: Dogs" and "Local and Regional Anesthetic and Analgesic Techniques: Cats" by Roman T. Skarda and William J. Tranquilli in Lumb and Jones' Veterinary Anesthesia and Analgesia, Fourth Edition.

Chapter 11

Anesthesia for patients with cardiovascular disease

Tamara L. Grubb and Stephen A. Greene

Introduction

The cardiovascular system is comprised of the heart, the vasculature, and the blood. Dysfunction of any or all of these components can occur in patients with cardiovascular disease, disease that secondarily affects the cardiovascular system (e.g., hyperthyroidism), and in patients that are hypovolemic, anemic, or in vasoactive states (e.g., vasodilatory shock). Unfortunately, anesthetic drugs and events (e.g., recumbency, positive pressure ventilation) can exacerbate this dysfunction and contribute to the demise of the patient. Because of the vast number of diseases that affect the cardiovascular system, one anesthetic protocol may not be appropriate for all patients in this category but an understanding of cardiovascular physiology and the cardiovascular effects of the anesthetic drugs will promote appropriate anesthetic protocol selection. Anesthetic considerations for some of the more commonly encountered diseases that affect the cardiovascular system are described in this chapter.

Cardiovascular physiology

In every cell of the body, oxygen is required for normal cellular function and it is delivery of oxygen that drives the cardiovascular system. Regulation of cardiac output, vascular tone, production of red blood cells, and hemoglobin loading and unloading all occur in response to tissue oxygen needs. Sophisticated physiological changes occur in an attempt to regulate these processes, even in the face of progressive cardiac disease.

Most of the changes that occur with cardiac disease, and many of the effects of anesthetic drugs, ultimately affect cardiac output. Cardiac output (Q) is the amount of blood pumped by the left ventricle into the aorta each minute and it is a product of heart rate (HR) and of stroke volume (SV), which is comprised of preload, afterload, and myocardial contractility (inotropy). Most of the drugs associated with sedation and anesthesia cause some degree of dose-dependent cardiovascular depression, which may be manifest as changes in HR, SV, or both.

Essentials of Small Animal Anesthesia and Analgesia, Second Edition. Edited by Kurt A. Grimm, William J. Tranquilli, Leigh A. Lamont.
© 2011 John Wiley & Sons, Inc. Published 2011 by John Wiley & Sons, Inc.

Obviously, since HR is an integral determinant of Q, bradycardia can result in inadequate flow if SV does not increase to compensate for decreased HR. Conversely, tachycardia can be as hazardous as bradycardia, since an increase in HR causes a decrease in diastolic filling time, resulting in a reduction in SV. Also, tachycardia reduces ventricular relaxation time, which decreases the time for myocardial perfusion (which occurs during diastole) and causes an increase in myocardial oxygen consumption. Oxygen debt occurs if oxygen demand is not met by oxygen supply and myocardial ischemia can result. In fact, severe tachycardia in itself (i.e., in the absence of underlying cardiac disease) can result in myocardial ischemia and heart failure.[1]

Preload, or cardiac filling (or venous return), is dictated by blood flow, blood volume, and venous capacitance. Ideally, an appropriate preload volume will fill the ventricle just enough to cause a slight stretch of the myocardium, which will improve contractility and increase SV (due to Starling's law). The volume of venous return is extremely important because: (1) the heart can only eject the amount of blood that is returned to it, making cardiac output highly dependent on preload, and (2) the heart must eject the amount of blood returned to it or congestion will occur. Excessive or even moderate vasodilation causes hypotension and may lead to "pooling" of the blood in the vasculature with minimal cardiac return and inadequate preload. Afterload, or resistance to ejection of blood from the left ventricle, is dictated primarily by arterial tone. The arterial tree must maintain some degree of tone in order to support the flow of blood from the aorta through the vascular tree to the capillaries. However, excessive tone will increase the amount of cardiac work needed to eject blood from the left ventricle and this will decrease cardiac output. Myocardial contractility is impaired by most cardiac diseases and many anesthetic drugs. Clearly, a decrease in myocardial contractility will cause a decrease in cardiac output.

Pharmacology of anesthetic drugs

An overview of the effects of anesthetic drugs on cardiovascular function is listed in Table 11.1.

Sedatives, tranquilizers, and anticholinergics

Excitement, fear, and pain can cause a sympathetic response marked by tachycardia, hypertension, and increased myocardial oxygen consumption, and this response can exacerbate concurrent cardiovascular disease. Thus, most patients with cardiovascular disease should receive a low dose of sedative and analgesic drugs prior to anesthesia. All of the sedatives and tranquilizers listed below are "MAC sparing," meaning that they decrease the minimum alveolar concentration (MAC) of inhalant anesthetic gases required to maintain anesthesia. Because the inhalant gases can cause profound dose-related cardiovascular side effects, decreasing the dose of the inhalant should increase anesthetic safety.

Opioid agonists (e.g., fentanyl, hydromorphone, morphine), agonist-antagonists (e.g., butorphanol), and partial agonists (buprenorphine) causes minimal cardiovascular effects

Table 11.1. Overview of the most common cardiovascular effects of some frequently used anesthetic drugs. Effects are typical of drugs used at clinically relevant dosages

Drug	Heart rate	Heart rhythm	Preload	Afterload	Inotropy	Cardiac output
Acepromazine	↑ or —	—	↓	↓	—	↓ or ↑
Medetomidine and dexmedetomidine	↓↓	+ or —	↑	↑	—	↓
Diazepam and midazolam	—	—	—	— or ↓	—	—
Opioids	— or ↓	—	— or ↓	— or ↓	—	— or ↓
Thiopental	↑	+ or —	↓	↓	↓	↓
Propofol	— or ↓	+ or —	↓	↓	↓	↓
Ketamine and tiletamine	↑	+ or —	↑	↑	↑	↑ or — or ↓
Etomidate	—	—	—	—	—	—
Isoflurane	↓ or ↑	—	↓	↓	↓	↓
Sevoflurane	↓ or —	—	↓	↓	↓	↓

↑, increased; ↓, decreased; —, no change; +, potentially arrhythmogenic.
Source: Adapted from: Muir W.W. Anesthesia of dogs and cats with cardiovascular disease. Part II. *Compend Pract Vet* **20**(4): 473–484, 1998.

when used in low doses and are the mainstay for sedation and analgesia in patients with cardiovascular disease.[2] The opioids do not cause myocardial depression or arrhythmias and cause only a minimal decrease in blood pressure in recumbent patients.[3] In fact, opioids can be cardioprotective and induce pharmacological preconditioning of the myocardium[2] and a slight decrease in afterload.[3] A mild vagally mediated bradycardia can occur after the administration of most opioids.[3] Morphine can cause histamine release and subsequent hypotension, but this effect is associated solely with rapid intravenous (IV) delivery of the drug and is not seen subsequent to intramuscular (IM) injections or IV constant rate infusions (CRIs).[3] Many opioids are also somewhat sedating, especially in dogs. Opioids used alone may not provide adequate sedation in young, healthy patients but are often sufficient for compromised patients. Opioid effects can be reversed with the opioid agonist naloxone, or partially reversed with the opioid agonist-antagonist butorphanol. Reversal of side effects associated with opioid analgesics will also antagonize analgesia.[4] Rapid IV administration of naloxone has been associated with development of cardiac dysrhythmias and even sudden death.[5,6]

The benzodiazepines (e.g., diazepam and midazolam) produce minimal cardiovascular effects. Diazepam produces minimal decreases in systemic blood pressure, cardiac output, and systemic vascular resistance that are similar to that produced by natural sleep.[7] Midazolam produces a greater decrease in systemic blood pressure and increase in HR than diazepam produces, but the effects are short-lived and generally of little clinical significance. Midazolam decreases systemic vascular resistance and this may improve cardiac output in patients with congestive heart failure (CHF).[7] Sedation following the administration of a benzodiazepine alone is generally not adequate for healthy, young animals but is often satisfactory when combined with an opioid for compromised patients. However, the combination of diazepam and fentanyl causes a decrease in systemic vascular resistance and systemic blood pressure that does not occur when fentanyl is used alone.[7] Drug effects can be reversed with the benzodiazepine antagonist, flumazenil.

Acepromazine causes vasodilation secondary to alpha adrenergic blockade. In low doses, this is generally manifest as decreased peripheral resistance or afterload, which allows increased cardiac output without increased cardiac work. Thus, a low dose of acepromazine might be an appropriate tranquilizer choice in a patient with increased afterload and/or mitral valve insufficiency (MVI). However, moderate to high doses of acepromazine will cause a 20–25% decrease in SV, cardiac output, and mean arterial pressure,[8] and these effects can be extremely detrimental in a patient with cardiovascular disease. Acepromazine increases the dose of epinephrine required to induce ventricular arrhythmias, possibly due to alpha$_1$ blockade.[8] Acepromazine does not provide analgesia and is not reversible.

Alpha$_2$ agonists (e.g., medetomidine and dexmedetomidine) cause profound vasoconstriction and increased cardiac work and are thus not appropriate for patients with cardiovascular disease.

Anticholinergics increase HR and myocardial oxygen consumption and can increase the possibility of cardiac arrhythmias and decrease the threshold for ventricular fibrillation. Since patients with cardiovascular disease may not tolerate excessive increases in HR and myocardial oxygen consumption, anticholinergics should not be a routine component of the anesthetic protocol but should be reserved for the treatment of bradycardia that limits cardiac output.

Induction drugs

Etomidate is generally the drug of choice for patients with severe cardiac disease because the drug causes minimal to no changes in myocardial contractility, HR, SV, or cardiac output at clinically relevant dosages.[9] Systemic vascular resistance often decreases, resulting in a decrease in arterial blood pressure. At supraclinical dosages, etomidate is a negative inotrope.[10] Etomidate can produce excitement, muscle twitching, and vocalization but these effects are minimized or eliminated by the administration of a benzodiazepine or acepromazine prior to injection of etomidate.

Ketamine and tiletamine are unique among anesthetic drugs in that they cause an increase in HR, afterload, cardiac output, and arterial blood pressure.[9] These are indirect effects caused by the direct stimulation of the sympathetic nervous system by ketamine and tiletamine. These effects can be beneficial in disease states marked by impaired myocardial contractility (e.g., dilatative cardiomyopathy), hypotension, or bradycardia, but may be detrimental in patients with hypertrophic disease, hypertension, or tachycardia. Ketamine and tiletamine also cause an increase in myocardial oxygen consumption that could precipitate myocardial ischemia.[9] In patients with no sympathetic reserve, as may occur in end-stage cardiac disease, ketamine and tiletamine are unable to improve cardiac function and, in fact, will cause direct myocardial depression.[9] Both the positive and negative effects of these drugs are blunted by the prior administration of tranquilizers (e.g., benzodiazepines, acepromazine), thus improving their safety in patients with cardiac disease.

Propofol causes dose-dependent myocardial depression and hypotension that is comparable to that caused by barbiturates.[9] However, this effect is extremely short-lived and is blunted by the prior administration of sedative drugs with minimal cardiovascular effects, like the opioids and benzodiazepines. Propofol is easily titrated "to effect," thus attenuating the likelihood of overdosage and dose-related side effects. Also, propofol is rapidly cleared from the body by multiple routes, thereby minimizing the duration of anesthesia-induced physiological changes.

Inhalant anesthetics are associated with a moderate to profound dose-dependent decrease in arterial blood pressure that is primarily caused by systemic vasodilation.[9] Thus, high dosages of inhalant gases should usually be avoided in patients with cardiovascular disease. Induction of anesthesia by mask or chamber is often accompanied by stress and struggling with subsequent tachycardia and increased oxygen consumption, which can further exacerbate cardiac disease. The use of inhalant gases alone to induce and maintain anesthesia increases the risk of anesthesia-induced mortality in dogs and cats.[11]

Maintenance drugs

Inhalant anesthetic gases are the drugs of choice for long-term anesthesia; however, as stated, isoflurane, sevoflurane, and desflurane all cause dose-dependent cardiovascular changes and the concentration of the anesthetic must be maintained as low as possible in order to limit hypotension. The use of premedicants, including analgesic drugs, and the use of analgesic drugs during the maintenance phase of anesthesia (e.g., locoregional blockade or CRIs of analgesic drugs) will allow the concentration of inhalant anesthetic gases to remain at a minimum. Although not proven in dogs and cats, sevoflurane may be less likely than isoflurane or desflurane to cause tachycardia and may be preferable in patients prone to myocardial ischemia.[9]

Analgesic drugs

Pain is a stressor that will cause an increase in HR and blood pressure with a subsequent increase in myocardial oxygen consumption. Thus, all attempts should be made to alleviate or eliminate pain in the patient with cardiovascular disease. The positive effects of opioids have already been stated. Local and regional analgesia can be used in patients with cardiovascular disease and may decrease morbidity.[12,13] The nonsteroidal anti-inflammatory drugs (NSAIDs) are appropriate in many patients with cardiovascular disease but NSAIDs can cause or contribute to hypertension and may interfere with diuretic therapy and should not be used in patients with hypertensive disease.[14] Some NSAIDs can contribute to myocardial complications in humans but these are unlikely to occur in dogs and cats due to differences in myocardial perfusion.

Anesthesia overview

Circulation becomes "centralized" in patients with moderate to severe cardiac disease, resulting in greater delivery of blood, and drugs carried by the blood, to the vessel-rich group of tissues, including the brain. However, cardiac output may be decreased in these patients, resulting in slower drug delivery to the brain. Thus, the dosage of anesthetic drugs administered to patients with cardiac disease should be decreased and drugs should be administered slowly and with ample time between doses for delivery to the brain. Furthermore, the cardiovascular effects caused by anesthetic drugs are generally dose dependent and selection of the appropriate dose may be even more important than selection of the appropriate drug.

Monitoring and support of the patient with cardiovascular disease should begin prior to the induction of anesthesia and should continue until the patient is fully recovered from the effects of the anesthetic drugs. Clearly, arterial blood pressure and cardiac rate and rhythm should be monitored in all patients. Support should include the use of IV fluids (including crystalloids, colloids, plasma, packed red cells, and whole blood), antiarrhythmic drugs, and positive inotropic drugs, as appropriate. In most instances, normothermia should be actively and aggressively maintained as hypothermia can have a negative impact on cardiovascular function[15] and shivering can greatly increase metabolic oxygen consumption.[16]

Anesthesia for patients with specific cardiovascular disease

The most commonly encountered cardiovascular diseases in dogs and cats include MVI, dilated cardiomyopathy (DCM), and hypertrophic cardiomyopathy (HCM).

MVI

MVI is the most common cardiac valvular disease in dogs[17] but is uncommon in cats. MVI is usually caused by a progressive degeneration of the atrioventricular valves that allows regurgitant flow of blood into the left atrium during left ventricular systole. Valvular regurgitation causes further pathology, including dilation of the left atrium and eccentric hypertrophy of the left ventricle. Myocardial contractility decreases as the disease worsens. Depending on progression of the disease, patients can present with a wide variety of signs that range from a soft systolic murmur with no signs of cardiac disease to complications from end-stage heart failure.[17]

The anesthetic goals are to maintain adequate HR and myocardial contractility while minimizing afterload. In patients with MVI, a slightly increased HR (not tachycardia) is advantageous since increased ventricular filling and distention may occur when the HR is slow. In a normal ventricle, increased distension is generally met with increased force of contraction. In patients with MVI, increased distension may cause additional enlargement of the AV orifice and further increase of the regurgitant volume. Systemic vascular resistance or afterload should be kept to a minimum in order to promote more flow forward into the systemic vasculature rather than backward through the regurgitant valve.[18] The benzodiazepines or low-dose acepromazine can be used to decrease afterload and opioids should be included to allow a decrease in the MAC of the inhalant drugs. The choice of the opioid will depend on the severity of expected pain from the surgical procedure. Etomidate, propofol, and valium/ketamine are all suitable induction drugs and both isoflurane and sevoflurane are appropriate for maintenance.

Hypotension is common because of the decreased myocardial contractility, and drugs that increase contractility without increasing SVR (e.g., dobutamine) should be utilized, while drugs that promote an increase in vascular resistance (e.g., phenylephrine, ephedrine) are not recommended.[18] Treating hypotension with fluid therapy can be somewhat difficult since adequate preload is necessary for appropriate cardiac output but excessive fluid loading can cause ventricular stretch and increased regurgitant volume.

DCM

DCM is the most common myocardial disease in the dog, with adult medium and large-breed dogs most commonly affected.[19] With the discovery and correction of taurine-deficient diets, DCM has become uncommon in cats. DCM is characterized by cardiac enlargement and impaired systolic function of one or both ventricles (most commonly the left ventricle). A progressive decrease in myocardial contractility with impaired systolic ventricular function occurs in patients with DCM and the clinical presentation is highly variable depending on the stage of the disease.

Measures of pump function such as ejection fraction, fractional shortening, rate of ejection, and rate of ventricular pressure development are all reduced, while end-diastolic ventricular volume is increased.[18] Ventricular relaxation is also impaired. Contractility, SV, and cardiac output continue to decline as the disease progresses, and mitral and tricuspid valve insufficiency, ventricular arrhythmias, and/or atrial fibrillation occur in a significant number of patients. Patients with advanced DCM are at high risk for anesthetic complications and stabilization prior to anesthesia is critical. The anesthetic goals are to maintain or improve contractility (e.g., with positive inotropic drugs) and to avoid drugs that increase afterload.[18]

Opioids should be used as premedicants, and an induction of either IV fentanyl or a benzodiazepine followed in 1–2 minutes with etomidate to effect is the induction protocol of choice. The same premedicants followed by low-dose ketamine is the second choice as ketamine may cause some improvement in cardiac function through stimulation of the sympathetic nervous system. A low dose of propofol is also acceptable in patients with mild to moderate disease. Either isoflurane or sevoflurane can be used during maintenance but maintaining the patient at the lowest possible dose of inhalant is imperative. Thus, additional analgesia will almost certainly be required during maintenance.

IV fluids should be administered intraoperatively but fluid balance can be difficult to achieve in advanced stages of the disease. Adequate circulation and appropriate preload volume is critical since an adequate preload is necessary to compensate for decreased pump function. Yet, since pump function is poor, the heart cannot eject excess fluid load and the volume of fluids should be low to prevent overhydration. Also, poor pump function means that increased afterload can severely limit cardiac output so vasoconstrictive drugs should be avoided. Hypotension can be treated with drugs that have a primary inotropic function, like dobutamine.

HCM

HCM is the most commonly diagnosed myocardial disease in cats but is uncommon in dogs.[20] This disease is characterized by concentric hypertrophy of the ventricles (primarily the left ventricle) with small ventricular chamber size. Atrial enlargement may also occur. The cardiac chambers become stiff, resulting in increased pressure for any given volume during diastolic filling and this will eventually lead to CHF with pulmonary edema and pleural effusion. Myocardial oxygen delivery is often inadequate in patients with HCM since the large myocardial mass consumes a significant amount of oxygen and blood supply to all parts of the muscle may not be adequate. Tachycardia in HCM patients can further tax myocardial oxygen supplies and can cause decompensation and overt cardiac failure. Coronary circulation to the thickened myocardium decreases, predisposing the patient to myocardial ischemia. Thromboembolism may develop. Myocardial relaxation is impaired but contractility is normal. The clinical presentation is highly variable depending on the stage of the disease, and the prognosis of severe HCM is poor and sudden death is not uncommon.

In patients with HCM, myocardial contractility or pump function is adequate but decreased cardiac output and perfusion occur because of inadequate diastolic ventricular volume secondary to the decreased ventricular chamber size. A slightly decreased HR is generally beneficial in these patients. Anesthetic goals include prevention of tachycardia, which will decrease ventricular filling time and increase cardiac work, and prevention of increases in myocardial contractility.[18] Thus, drugs that increase rate or force of contraction (e.g., anticholinergics, ketamine, dobutamine, dopamine) are not generally used.[18] Also, vasodilation (e.g., as occurs with acepromazine, propofol and the inhalant gases) may cause marked hypotension because of a limited ability of the heart to increase SV.

Opioids should be used as premedicants and an induction of either IV fentanyl or a benzodiazepine followed in 1–2 minutes with etomidate to effect is the induction protocol of choice. A benzodiazepine followed by propofol is also acceptable and a benzodiazepine with ketamine can be used in patients with mild disease. Either isoflurane or sevoflurane can be used during maintenance but maintaining the patient at the lowest possible dose of inhalant is imperative. Thus, additional analgesia will almost certainly be required during maintenance.

Hypotension is difficult to treat in patients with HCM. Appropriate (but judicious) fluid therapy both before and during anesthetic drug administration is required for adequate preload. Hypotension that is unresponsive to fluid therapy may be treated with a CRI of phenylephrine,[18] which will promote adequate filling but is not ideal in that the drug will also increase afterload and decrease tissue perfusion.

Revised from "Cardiovascular Disease" by Ralph C. Harvey and Stephen J. Ettinger in Lumb and Jones' Veterinary Anesthesia and Analgesia, Fourth Edition.

References

1. Calò L., De Ruvo E., Sette A., et al. Tachycardia-induced cardiomyopathy: mechanisms of heart failure and clinical implications. *J Cardiovasc Med* **8**(3): 138–143, 2007.

2. Bovill J.G. Intravenous anesthesia for the patient with left ventricular dysfunction. *Semin Cardiothorac Vasc Anesth* **10**(1): 43–48, 2006.

3. Gutstein H.B., Akil H. Opioid analgesics . In: *Goodman & Gilman's The Pharmacological Basis of Therapeutics*, 10th ed. J.G. Hardman and L.E. Limbird, eds. New York: McGraw-Hill, 2001, pp 569–620.

4. Copland V.S., Haskins S.C., Patz J. Naloxone reversal of oxymorphone effects in dogs. *Am J Vet Res* **50**: 1854–1858, 1989.

5. Michealis L.L., Hickey P.R., Clark T.A., et al. Ventricular irritability associated with the use of naloxone hydrochloride. *Ann Thorac Surg* **18**: 608–614, 1974.

6. Andree R.A. Sudden death following naloxone administration. *Anesth Analg* **59**: 782–784, 1980.

7. Stoelting R.K. Benzodiazepines. In: *Pharmacology and Physiology in Anesthetic Practice*, 4th ed. R.K. Stoelting, ed. Philadelphia, PA: Lippincott, Williams & Wilkins, 2006, pp 140–154.

8. Lemke K.A. Anticholinergics and sedatives. In: *Lumb & Jones' Veterinary Anesthesia and Analgesia*, 4th ed. W.J. Tranquilli, J.C. Thurmon, and K.A. Grimm, eds. Ames, IA: Blackwell Publishing, 2007, pp 203–239.

9. Evers A.S., Crowder C.M. General anesthestics. In: *Goodman & Gilman's The Pharmacological Basis of Therapeutics*, 10th ed. J.G. Hardman and L.E. Limbird, eds. New York: McGraw-Hill, 2001, pp 337–366.

10. Stoelting R.K. Nonbarbiturate intravenous anesthetic drugs. In: *Pharmacology and Physiology in Anesthetic Practice*, 4th ed. R.K. Stoelting, ed. Philadelphia, PA: Lippincott, Williams & Wilkins, 2006, pp 155–178.

11. Brodbelt D.C., Blissitt K.J., Hammond R.A., et al. The risk of death: the confidential enquiry into perioperative small animal fatalities. *Vet Anaesth Analg* **35**(5): 365–373, 2008.

12. Hahnenkamp K., Herroeder S., Hollmann M.W. Regional anaesthesia, local anaesthetics and the surgical stress response. *Best Pract Res Clin Anaesthesiol* **18**(3): 509–527, 2004.

13. Thompson J.S. The role of epidural analgesia and anesthesia in surgical outcomes. *Adv Surg* **36**: 297–307, 2002.

14. Basile J.N., Bloch M.J. Identifying and managing factors that interfere with or worsen blood pressure control. *Postgrad Med* **122**(2): 35–48, 2010.

15. Lenhardt R. The effect of anesthesia on body temperature control. *Front Biosci* **2**: 1145–1154, 2010.

16. Guffin A., Girard D., Kaplan J.A. Shivering following cardiac surgery: hemodynamic changes and reversal. *J Cardiothorac Anesth* **1**(1): 24–28, 1987.

17. Haggerstron J., Kvart C., Pedersen H.D. Acquired valvular disease. In: *Textbook of Veterinary Internal Medicine*. S.J. Ettinger and E.C. Feldman, eds. St. Louis, MO: Elsevier, 2005, pp 1022–1039.

18. McMurphy R. Cardiovascular system. In: *Textbook of Small Animal Surgery*. D. Slatter, ed. Philadelphia, PA: WB Saunders, 2003, pp 2572–2578.

19. Meurs K.M. Myocardial disease: canine. In: *Textbook of Veterinary Internal Medicine*. S.J. Ettinger and E.C. Feldman, eds. St. Louis, MO: Elsevier, 2005, pp 1320–1327.

20. MacDonald K. Myocardial disease: feline. In: *Textbook of Veterinary Internal Medicine*. S.J. Ettinger and E.C. Feldman, eds. St. Louis, MO: Elsevier, 2005, pp 1328–1341.

Chapter 12

Anesthesia for patients with respiratory disease and/or airway compromise

Tamara L. Grubb and Stephen A. Greene

Introduction

Because the airway extends from the oral or nasal cavity to the alveoli, airway compromise or respiratory disease has numerous manifestations. Complications can be encountered in both the upper and lower airways and can encompass a vast range of problems, including laryngeal paralysis, collapsing trachea, pneumonia, pulmonary edema, pneumothorax, intrathoracic masses, and diaphragmatic hernias. Anesthesia can cause further complications since anesthetic drugs and equipment can exacerbate, or even cause, airway difficulties and respiratory compromise. When anesthetizing patients with respiratory disease or airway compromise the choice of anesthetic drugs is not necessarily dictated by the presence of the respiratory condition, but rather by the overall health of the patient and the risks to be managed. The choice of anesthetic technique (e.g., method of induction, method of intubation, use of positive pressure ventilation, etc.), on the other hand, is often the critical component of a successful outcome. Patient monitoring and support are critical and should be directed toward normalizing respiratory function and supporting the job of the respiratory system, which is to deliver oxygen (O_2) to, and remove carbon dioxide (CO_2) from, cells throughout the body.

Physiology of the respiratory system

Control of respiratory function includes an integrated series of complex feedback loops made up of sensors, controllers, and effectors. Dysfunction of any one of these components can lead to impaired respiratory system function.[1] The end result of this concert of sensors, controllers, and effectors is regulation of alveolar ventilation (V_A), which is the volume of inhaled gas that reaches the alveoli and participates in gas exchange. V_A is often reported as minute ventilation (V_E) which is the volume of inhaled gas participating in gas exchange multiplied by the respiratory rate. V_A is determined by the ratio of the tidal volume (V_T), or the amount of fresh gas inhaled and exhaled with each normal breath, to the dead space volume (V_D), or the amount of inhaled fresh gas that does not

Essentials of Small Animal Anesthesia and Analgesia, Second Edition. Edited by Kurt A. Grimm, William J. Tranquilli, Leigh A. Lamont.
© 2011 John Wiley & Sons, Inc. Published 2011 by John Wiley & Sons, Inc.

participate in gas exchange. Physiological dead space (V_D) is the volume of gas ventilating alveoli that are not perfused, (ventilation/perfusion [V/Q] mismatch; alveolar dead space), combined with the amount of gas ventilating the conducting airways (nasal passages, nasopharynx, larynx, trachea, and bronchi; anatomical dead space). Anesthetic drugs and equipment and the events of anesthesia can increase V_D and decrease V_T, thereby contributing to hypoventilation, which is defined simply as inadequate gas exchange or inadequate V_A.

Hypoventilation results in hypercarbia (partial pressure of arterial CO_2 [$PaCO_2$] > 45–55 mm Hg), and when severe, hypoxemia (partial pressure of arterial O_2 [PaO_2] < 60 mm Hg; partial pressure of arterial oxygen–hemoglobin saturation [SaO2] < 90%). Because CO_2 is extremely soluble and crosses the alveolar–arterial interface easily, CO_2 that arrives at ventilated alveoli is readily delivered to the airway and exhaled. In fact, $PaCO_2$, and thus, P_ACO_2 (the partial pressure of CO_2 in the alveoli), is related (but inversely) to V_A. Most anesthetic drugs blunt the ventilatory response initiated by rising CO_2 concentrations.

Hypoxemia, on the other hand, is not always caused by hypoventilation. Hypoxemia can also be caused by ventilation/perfusion (V/Q) mismatch, inadequate fraction of inspired oxygen (F_IO_2), diffusion impairment, and true anatomic shunt (Table 12.1). Two calculations used to determine the severity of hypoxemia, the alveolar–arterial oxygen difference ([A − a]DO_2) and the partial pressure of arterial oxygen to the percent fraction of inspired oxygen ratio (PaO_2/FiO_2) are presented in Table 12.2.

Pharmacology of anesthetic drugs

Most anesthetic drugs produce some degree of respiratory depression. The degree of dysfunction is generally dose dependent and normally manageable when dosed appropriately in healthy patients. However, the degree of dysfunction may be significant in patients with preexisting disease or pathology of the respiratory or nervous system and cautious dosing and careful monitoring of the patient are imperative.

Sedatives and tranquilizers

Sedatives and tranquilizers are routinely used in patients with airway dysfunction, particularly upper airway dysfunction, to manage respiratory distress that can occur with excitement, anxiety, or pain. Commonly used sedatives include the phenothiazine derivatives (acepromazine), the benzodiazepines (diazepam and midazolam), and the opioids (morphine, hydromorphone, oxymorphone, fentanyl, methadone, butorphanol, buprenorphine, nalbuphine, etc.). Occasionally, the alpha$_2$ adrenergic agonists (xylazine, medetomidine, and dexmedetomidine) are appropriate for patients with airway disease. The phenothiazine derivatives cause minimal respiratory dysfunction when used alone but can exacerbate respiratory depressant effects caused by other drugs.[2] Acepromazine at low dosages causes a decrease in respiratory rate with a compensatory increase in V_T, resulting in no changes in $PaCO_2$, pH, PaO_2, or SpO_2.[3] Because acepromazine produces mild sedation and has a fairly long duration of action, it is often used to calm anxious patients and is often appropriate for patients with airway disease/dysfunction. However,

Table 12.1. The five causes of hypoxemia, contributing factors, and response to supplemental oxygen therapy

Cause of hypoxemia	Contributing factor	Response to supplemental oxygen and further diagnostics
Hypoventilation	Inadequate alveolar ventilation (V_A). Diagnosed by concurrent hypercarbia.	PaO_2 will increase. Greatest increase will occur with increased V_A. (A – a)DO2 is normal.
Ventilation/perfusion (V/Q) mismatch also called physiological shunt	Any cause of pulmonary atelectasis: dorsal recumbency, GI distension, and pregnancy all cause compression atelectasis; ventilation with 100% oxygen can cause absorption atelectasis; other causes include pneumothorax and external compression of the thorax.	PaO_2 will increase by varying degrees, depending on the magnitude of the mismatch. (A – a)DO2 is high. $PaCO_2$ is normal.
Decreased FiO_2	Primarily occurs only with supplementation of gases other than oxygen (e.g., supplementation with nitrous oxide) or with interruption of oxygen supply when increased FiO2 is expected. $PaCO_2$ may be low due to hypoxemic drive.	PaO_2 will increase. Greatest increase will occur when "offending" gas is discontinued and the patient is allowed to breathe an increased FiO2. (A – a)DO2 is normal.
Diffusion abnormalities	Rarely a cause of hypoxemia in our patients, since red blood cells (RBCs) spend a large portion of time at the alveolar–arterial interface. However, could occur with any disease of this interface, for example, pulmonary edema or fibrosis.	PaO_2 will increase. (A – a)DO2 is normal or increased. $PaCO_2$ is normal.
True anatomical shunt	Any anomaly that causes blood to be shunted from the right side of the heart into the systemic circulation, bypassing the lungs. Patent ductus arteriosus (PDA), tetralogy of Fallot, intrapulmonary shunts.	No change in PaO2 because the blood does not flow through the pulmonary circulation and thus cannot participate in gas exchange. (A – a)DO2 is high. $PaCO_2$ is normal.

acepromazine is a muscle relaxant and relaxation of the muscles in the pharyngeal region can lead to further airway dysfunction. Acepromazine is not reversible and does not provide analgesia.

The benzodiazepines (midazolam and diazepam) cause minimal to no respiratory depression[4] and are also appropriate for patients with airway disease/dysfunction. As with acepromazine, the benzodiazepines can cause relaxation of muscles of the upper airway, but this is generally minimal. The benzodiazepines used alone rarely provide adequate sedation in distressed patients; thus, benzodiazepines are often combined with

Table 12.2. Calculations used to determine the severity of hypoxemia, the alveolar–arterial oxygen difference ($[A - a]DO_2$) and the oxygen partial pressure/fraction of inspired oxygen ratio (PaO_2/FiO_2)

Formula	Alveolar–arterial oxygen difference, $(A - a)DO_2$; also called alveolar–arterial gradient; also described as $P(A - a)O_2$	Oxygen partial pressure/fraction inspired oxygen ratio, PaO_2/FiO_2
Components of the formula	Alveolar oxygen (P_AO_2) equation: $P_AO_2 = ([\text{atmospheric pressure} - \text{water vapor pressure}] \times \text{fraction inspired oxygen}) - \text{AlveolarCO}_2{}^a/0.8{}^b$ PaO_2 is measured using an arterial blood gas.	PaO_2 is measured using an arterial blood gas. FiO_2 is measured or assumed (e.g., assumed to be 0.21 if a patient is breathing room air at sea level).
Values at sea level in patient with normal lung function and hemoglobin concentration breathing FiO2 of 21%.	$P_AO_2 = ([760\,\text{mmHg} - 47\,\text{mmHg}] \times 0.21) - 40/0.8 = 100\,\text{mmHg}$ $PaO_2 = 95\,\text{mmHg}$ $P_AO_2 - PaO_2 = 100 - 95 = 5\,\text{mmHg}$ Normal values = 0–10 mmHg is considered normal; 10–20 is considered mild gas exchange impairment; 20–30 is moderate impairment; and >30 is severe.	$PaO_2 = 95\,\text{mmHg}$ $FiO_2 = 0.21$ $PaO_2/FiO_2 = 452$ Normal values = 400–500 (300–400 may indicate insignificant changes); <250 = severe gas exchange impairment.
Advantages	Includes values for CO_2, which can contribute significantly to alveolar oxygen concentrations (i.e., high $PACO_2$ is likely to cause low P_AO_2).	Easy to calculate. Can be used to estimate dysfunction at any FiO_2; thus, patients on supplemental oxygen (or under anesthesia) DO NOT need to be disconnected from oxygen to assess pulmonary function.
Disadvantages	A bit cumbersome to calculate. Does not work for patients on high FiO_2.	Not as accurate as $(A - a)DO_2$ because the formula does not include values for CO_2.

[a] Because CO_2 is highly diffusible, $PaCO_2$ is used to estimate P_ACO_2.

[b] 0.8 is the respiratory quotient, which is the ratio of carbon dioxide production (VCO_2) to oxygen consumption (VO_2).

a member of the opioid class. Flumazenil can be used to reverse the effects of the benzodiazepines.

If the patient is extremely fractious, a low dose of an alpha$_2$ adrenergic agonist, like medetomidine or dexmedetomidine, can be used. However, because of the potential for profound sedation, vomiting, relaxation of the musculature of the upper airway, and decreased respiratory rate and central respiratory drive,[5] the patient should not be left unobserved following the administration of an alpha$_2$ adrenergic agonist and the anesthetist should be prepared for immediate intubation or reversal of the effects of drug (e.g., atipamezole) in the event of profound cardiovascular or respiratory decompensation. Alpha$_2$ adrenergic agonists provide analgesia as well as sedation.

Opioid-mediated respiratory depression is a major concern in human patients but only a minor concern in most veterinary patients since dogs and cats do not seem to be as sensitive to the respiratory depressant effects of the opioids. However, opioids do cause some dose-dependent, centrally mediated respiratory depression, and this is exacerbated by the concurrent use of other drugs that depress ventilatory function, like the inhalant anesthetic drugs. Because opioids provide sedation and analgesia, they are often the best choice for patients that need both calming and pain relief. Also, the opioids are reversible (e.g., with naloxone) and their effects can be eliminated if the patient has an adverse, or excessively profound or prolonged, reaction. Reversal of side effects associated with opioid analgesics with naloxone will also antagonize analgesia.[6] Rapid intravenous (IV) administration of naloxone has been associated with the development of cardiac dysrhythmias and even sudden death.[7,8] Butorphanol is an agonist-antagonist and can be used to antagonize respiratory depression mediated at the mu receptors while maintaining some analgesic action at the kappa receptors.[9] Nalbuphine[10] and buprenorphine can also be used to reduce, but not eliminate, the effects of mu opioid agonists.

Induction drugs

Propofol is a rapidly acting injectable anesthetic drug that causes respiratory depression through suppression of the central respiratory neuronal network that is marked by a decrease in both V_T and respiratory rate.[11] Propofol can also cause suppression of the ventilatory response to carbon dioxide and hypoxemia.[11] Propofol can also produce apnea after bolus administration and this effect is related to both dose and the speed of injection of the drug, with faster injection rates associated with a greater incidence of apnea.[12]

The dissociative anesthetics (ketamine and tiletamine) do not alter the response to CO_2 and may actually cause an increase in respiratory rate for 2–3 minutes after IV injection. However, they can exacerbate respiratory dysfunction caused by other drugs.[11] Rapid injection or excessive dosing of ketamine or tiletamine can cause apnea, but more commonly an apneustic breathing pattern (pause at the end of inspiration instead of at the end of expiration) is observed.

Etomidate can produce mild dose-dependent respiratory depression marked by decreased V_T that is generally offset by increased respiratory rate.[11] Although apnea following administration of etomidate can occur, the effects are short lived (3–5 minutes) and alleviated by limiting the rate of administration.

Maintenance drugs

The inhalant anesthetic gases isoflurane, sevoflurane, and desflurane are respiratory depressants that cause dose-dependent alteration of the (1) pattern of breathing, (2) depth of ventilation (V_T), (3) ventilatory response to arterial hypoxemia, and (4) airway resistance.[13] During inhalant anesthesia an increase in respiratory rate may occur but not to the degree adequate to compensate for the decrease in V_T. Inhalant anesthetic drugs cause a dose-dependent increase in the set point at which arterial carbon dioxide drives spontaneous ventilation, resulting in a delayed response (altered apneic threshold) and a decreased response (altered carbon dioxide responsiveness) to increases in arterial carbon dioxide.[13] Inhaled anesthetics also depress the ventilatory response to hypoxemia.

Analgesic drugs

Adequate pain management in patients with respiratory disease or airway compromise is essential in the prevention of further respiratory dysfunction. Intermittent boluses of opioids (e.g., fentanyl, hydromorphone, or morphine) are appropriate, but a constant rate infusion (CRI) can provide a more consistent level of analgesia. Fentanyl, administered at either 5 or 10 mcg/kg/h, has been shown to not significantly change the respiration rate or have a clinically relevant effect on SpO_2 in dogs.[14] However, careful monitoring of ventilation and availability of respiratory supportive measures (e.g., oxygen, endotracheal [ET] tube, etc.) should be considered. Morphine or hydromorphone would also be appropriate for an infusion, and combinations of opioids with drugs like lidocaine and/or ketamine provide multimodal analgesia and may be more effective than single-drug administration in many patients.

Local anesthetic drugs are an excellent addition to any analgesic protocol since they not only provide immediate pain relief but also may decrease the incidence of central sensitization (i.e., windup). Nonsteroidal anti-inflammatory drugs may be utilized when appropriate since the pain from surgery is primarily from inflammation.

Anesthesia for patients with specific respiratory disease or airway compromise

Patients with compromised airways may present for surgery of the respiratory system (e.g., arytenoid cartilage lateralization or removal of a consolidated lung lobe) or may present for surgery of other organ systems with airway compromise as a complication (e.g., dental prophylaxis in a patient with collapsing trachea or removal of an intestinal foreign body in a patient with aspiration pneumonia). Regardless of the reason for presentation, the patient should be carefully evaluated before induction of anesthesia. The location, extent, and severity of the problem should be assessed and the degree of respiratory dysfunction should be determined. Along with a routine physical exam, the evaluation should include any specific tests (e.g., thoracic radiographs, bronchoscopy, arterial blood gases, etc.) necessary to fully define the extent of the pathology.

During evaluation the patient should be handled quietly and carefully to avoid stress-induced tachypnea with subsequent increased work of breathing and possible further respiratory dysfunction. Many patients that breathe with difficulty can have elevated body temperatures that may result in further increases in respiratory effort. Tranquilization is often necessary to keep the patient calm and analgesia is required for any painful patients.

   Oxygen should be administered to all patients with respiratory disease during handling and during preparation for anesthesia. Hypoxemia can occur rapidly regardless of the location of the airway dysfunction. However, preoxygenation may delay desaturation.[15]

Anesthesia for patients with upper airway dysfunction

Patients in this category include those with laryngeal paralysis, laryngeal/pharyngeal tumors, airway trauma, cervical tracheal collapse, and upper airway foreign bodies. Other potential complications include diseases that cause external compression of the airway like enlarged pharyngeal lymph nodes or grossly enlarged thyroid glands. Brachycephalic breeds, like bulldogs and pugs, often have a plethora of abnormalities that can lead to upper airway obstruction. Brachycephalic syndrome includes elongated soft palate, everted laryngeal saccules, hypoplastic trachea, and stenotic nares.

   The induction and recovery phases of anesthesia can be associated with significant risk in patients with upper airway dysfunction but the maintenance phase is straightforward since the airway is controlled during maintenance. However, upper airway dysfunction can develop in the maintenance period if the ET tube becomes dislodged (e.g., during patient repositioning for surgery, radiology, or dentistry), plugged (i.e., by blood or mucous) or kinked, or if the ET tube cuff is grossly overinflated, leading to collapse of the lumen of the tube.[16]

Preanesthetic preparation

Patients presenting for surgery of the upper airway generally present with airway narrowing and/or airway dysfunction and are often at risk for total airway obstruction. In addition to the anatomic narrowing of the airway, a variety of factors can cause a physiological narrowing of the airway. Increased respiratory drive, which can be caused by a multitude of factors including pain, excitement, hyperthermia, exercise, hypoxia, and hypercarbia, causes an increase in respiratory effort, which, in turn, causes greater negative pressure in upper airway. This negative pressure pulls the structures of the pharynx into the airway and causes an upper airway collapse. Judicious dosages of sedatives and analgesic drugs may allow the patient to breathe slower and deeper, which alleviates or even eliminates excitement or anxiety-induced increased work of breathing and the resultant exacerbation of negative pressures. Opioids alone are often adequate for sedation in dogs, but panting may occur following some opioids (e.g., hydromorphone). Also in dogs, a combination of acepromazine and buprenorphine has been shown to cause minimal respiratory effects and better sedation than acepromazine used alone.[17] Midazolam or diazepam can also be combined with buprenorphine or butorphanol for mild to moderate sedation that is reversible. Mu agonist opioids (e.g., morphine or hydromorphone) can be used in cases that are in moderate to severe pain and where vomiting is not problematic. Protocols for cats are similar to those used in dogs but opioids may cause excitement and are almost always used in conjunction with a sedative.

In some instances, laryngeal function needs to be evaluated prior to intubation. Small boluses of propofol (2–4 mg/kg) are generally used. The use of 0.2 mg/kg IV diazepam or midazolam just before the propofol boluses will decrease the amount of propofol needed to complete the exam but may interfere with laryngeal function. Thiopental is also useful and both propofol and thiopental are more effective than ketamine/diazepam for upper airway exams.[18] The patient should be intubated immediately after the examination has concluded.

The use of anticholinergics in the preoperative period is controversial. Laryngeal manipulation can cause vagally mediated bradycardia and brachycephalic breeds tend to have high resting vagal tone. Thus, anticholinergics are often used in brachycephalic breeds and other patients with upper airway disease. The use of anticholinergics as antisialagogues and to decrease respiratory tract secretions is generally not recommended, although excessive secretion production may create an exception to this rule.

Induction

If tolerated, the patient should be preoxygenated while the sedatives are taking effect. During this time, an IV catheter should be placed. Following adequate sedation, the patient should be rapidly induced to anesthesia and immediately intubated. Any of the fast-acting injectable induction drugs are appropriate (e.g., propofol, thiopental, or ketamine/diazepam). Induction with inhalant anesthetic gases is too slow to ensure expedient control of the airway without undue stress and is not generally acceptable in patients with airway compromise.

Intubation

The rapid establishment of an airway in all patients, and especially in patients with upper airway disease, is critical. Because intubation needs to occur as rapidly and as smoothly as possible, preparation for intubation is imperative. ET tubes of several different sizes, a laryngoscope, stylet (especially when intubating cats), and tracheostomy kit should all be readily available. The ET tubes should be measured to ensure that they are long enough to bypass any upper airway obstruction but not so long that the tip of the tube could end up in a bronchus.

In all patients, the larynx should be visualized at intubation and the ET tube should be observed passing between the arytenoids. Laryngospasm, which will impede successful intubation, occurs most frequently in cats, swine, rabbits, and primates, but has also been observed in dogs and horses.[1] Laryngospasm may be triggered by touching the larynx during a light plane of anesthesia. Topical application of a local anesthetic such as lidocaine is recommended prior to tracheal intubation in species prone to laryngospasm (e.g., cats) to minimize tactile stimulation-induced laryngospasm. Small boluses of additional propofol (1–2 mg/kg) may also be used to improve laryngeal relaxation and facilitate intubation. However, propofol is a potent respiratory depressant and this technique should be quickly followed by proper placement of the ET tube.

Once intubated, the ET tube cuff should be carefully inflated. To prevent damage to the trachea, patients should be disconnected from the breathing tubes if they are moved or repositioned. Damage from an overinflated cuff or from cuff rotation can cause post-operative tracheal constriction or laceration. This is one of the most common causes of iatrogenic postanesthetic upper airway dysfunction in cats.[19]

Maintenance

Once the patient with upper airway dysfunction is intubated, the patient can be allowed to breathe spontaneously as long as adequate gas exchange occurs. If the ET tube does not extend past the obstruction (e.g., intrathoracic tracheal collapse), ventilatory support will be necessary, and this is discussed in the next section. Appropriate monitoring and support of the patient are critical. If the patient must be extubated during the operative procedure (e.g., for evaluation of airway diameter following an arytenoid cartilage lateralization), dosages of injectable induction drugs, a laryngoscope, a variety of ET tubes (in case the first one can't be reinserted), and a stylet must be readily available. If the patient cannot be intubated because of the location of the surgical repair, anesthesia can be maintained with injectable anesthesia. A CRI of propofol (0.1–0.4 mg/kg/min) with intermittent boluses (1–2 mcg/kg) of fentanyl or a concurrent infusion of fentanyl (0.02–0.1 mcg/kg/min) and supplemental oxygen is an effective means of providing total IV anesthesia.

Recovery

A low-stress recovery is essential in patients with upper airway dysfunction. Excitement and pain, with subsequent increased ventilation and increased peak inspiratory pressure, can cause airway edema and obstruction. Thus, patients should be adequately sedated (e.g., acepromazine) and should be administered analgesics (e.g., opioids) as needed. The patient should remain intubated for as long as it will tolerate the ET tube (if orotracheally intubated) or as long as the upper airway might reobstruct (if intubated through a tracheostomy site). The administration of a single dose of short-acting corticosteroids is often recommended to alleviate or attenuate obstruction of the airway from postoperative swelling. If upper airway edema is present, a diuretic (e.g., 0.5–1.0 mg/kg IV furosemide) can be administered in addition to the corticosteroids. Administration of phenylephrine nasal drops will counteract nasal passage hyperemia or edema. Because of the presence of redundant tissue in the pharynx, most brachycephalic breeds (e.g., bulldog, pug, and Shar Pei) benefit from having the anesthetist hold the dog's tongue and/or extend its neck immediately after extubation of the trachea.[16] In all instances, reobstruction should be anticipated and the anesthesiologist should be prepared to reanesthetize and reintubate the patient or perform a tracheostomy. Thus, injectable anesthetic drugs, a laryngoscope, a variety of ET tubes, and a tracheostomy kit should be readily available.

Dogs with upper airway obstruction can develop life-threatening pulmonary edema.[20] Pulmonary edema formation after airway obstruction is probably multifactorial, so treatment is symptomatic. Oxygen supplementation to maintain SpO_2 greater than 90%, diuretics, and corticosteroids can be used to treat pulmonary edema.

The effects of opioids can be reversed if the patient is having an exaggerated response to these drugs in recovery. However, painful or distressed animals may experience more respiratory difficulty following extubation, so the benefits of opioid reversal should be carefully weighed against the potential complications of the increased pain and stress that may accompany reversal (i.e., increased upper airway pressure secondary to pain-induced increased respiratory drive). Monitoring and oxygen supplementation should continue until the patient is ventilating normally.

Anesthesia for patients with lower airway dysfunction and/or intrathoracic surgery

Patients with pulmonary dysfunction may lack the ability to expand their lungs properly (extrapulmonary disease) and/or may have impairment of oxygen and carbon dioxide transfer across the alveolar membranes (intrapulmonary disease). Examples of extrapulmonary disease include diaphragmatic hernia, pneumothorax, chylothorax, hemothorax, pyothorax, intrathoracic masses, flail chest, and any condition that restricts chest wall expansion (e.g., fractured ribs) or impairs diaphragmatic movement (e.g., obesity, pregnancy or gastrointestinal [GI] distention). Examples of intrapulmonary disease include asthma, chronic obstructive pulmonary disease (COPD), pneumonia, pulmonary edema, intrapulmonary hemorrhage (contusions), atelectasis, or consolidated lung lobes. Patients that have normal lower airway function that must undergo thoracic surgery are also included in this category and include patients with intrathoracic collapsing trachea/bronchi or patients needing intrathoracic cardiovascular surgery.

Patients with lower airway dysfunction may present with, or develop, metabolic derangements including acid–base imbalance (due to hypercarbia) and hypoxemia. These conditions are likely to develop even in patients with normal lung function if the surgical procedure requires an open thorax. Patients may be an emergency if they present with, or develop, a tension pneumothorax, which requires immediate thoracocentesis.

Premedicants

In all patients, fear, pain, and excitement can cause an increased oxygen demand that will result in an increased respiratory drive. If oxygen demand is not met by oxygen delivery, oxygen debt, or hypoxemia with resultant tissue hypoxia, occurs. Pulmonary disease may limit the patient's ability to oxygenate so oxygen debt is likely if patients with lower airway disease experience fear, pain, or excitement. Sedation and analgesia allow slower, deeper breathing with no increase in oxygen demand. Acepromazine, the benzodiazepines, and most members of the opioid class (at low dosages) are generally good choices for sedation. If the patient is extremely obtunded, sedation may be precluded but opioids should be part of the anesthetic protocol as a means to provide analgesia and to lower the dosages of induction and maintenance drugs.

The use of anticholinergics is, again, controversial, although both atropine and glycopyrrolate do have a bronchodilating effect. Bronchodilation occurs due to antagonism of acetylcholine effects on airway smooth muscle and the effects are most prominent in large and medium-sized airways. This effect leads to lowered airway resistance, but also to increased anatomical dead space.[21] The possible beneficial effects of bronchodilation should be weighed against the detrimental effects of tachycardia and inspissation of secretions. Anticholinergics change secretory composition from a watery fluid to a thick mucous. This mucous may not be adequately cleared by the mucociliary system and may remain in the respiratory tree, where it can promote bacterial growth.

Induction

Any of the rapidly acting injectable anesthetic agents are acceptable choices for induction of anesthesia. Both ketamine and propofol have mild bronchodilating effects and may reduce bronchospasm in asthmatic patients.[22] Propofol may be the best choice since it produces anesthesia very quickly and can easily be titrated to effect. Although propofol produces apnea similar to that produced by barbiturates, the effects of propofol are quickly dissipated, allowing ventilation to rapidly return to normal. Etomidate and tiletamine/ zolazepam are also appropriate induction drugs for patients with lower airway disease.

Maintenance

Inhalant anesthesia with controlled ventilation is generally the safest method for anesthetic maintenance of patients with lower airway disease. Inhalant gases have a nonspecific bronchodilating effect. This is especially beneficial in patients who have reactive and/or constricted airways (e.g., cats with asthma) and in those who may undergo surgery that requires direct manipulation of the airways (e.g., lung lobectomy). Inhalant anesthetic gases are potent respiratory depressants and will cause a dose-dependent decrease in V_A and impaired ventilatory response to hypercarbia and hypoxemia. Thus, excessive anesthetic depth must be avoided. Appropriate analgesia will allow a decrease in inhalant gas requirements.

Mechanical ventilation

Intermittent positive pressure ventilation (IPPV) is generally recommended in patients with lower airway disease in order to maximize alveolar function. IPPV is mandatory in patients with an open thorax. IPPV should be instituted at 10–15 breaths per minute, a V_T of 10–15 mL/kg, and a peak inspiratory pressure of 10–20 cm H_2O. Appropriate ventilator settings can be determined by monitoring end-tidal carbon dioxide ($ETCO_2$) (the goal is to maintain $ETCO_2$ between 35 and 55 mm Hg). Positive end-expiratory pressure (PEEP) is occasionally necessary to maintain adequate gas exchange, especially in patients with an open thorax. A PEEP of 5–10 cm H_2O is often effective in maintaining adequate PaO_2. However, inappropriate use of IPPV and PEEP (i.e., excessive airway pressures) may cause decreased venous return and decreased cardiac output. This is more of a concern in hypovolemic patients, and appropriate fluid loading can attenuate the negative cardiovascular effects of mechanical ventilation. If a positive-pressure ventilator is not available, a staff member should be dedicated to maintaining ventilation in the patient by manual intermittent squeezing of the breathing circuit reservoir bag.

Recovery

Patients recovering from thoracic surgery are at high risk for development of postoperative pulmonary complications, including atelectasis and/or pneumonia. The duration of surgery should be kept as short as possible since duration of surgery is highly correlated with postoperative dysfunction with surgeries of 1, 2, 4, and greater than 4 hours, causing postoperative complications in 4%, 23%, 38%, and 73% (respectively) of patients.[23]

Provision of adequate postoperative analgesia is beneficial for return of normal ventilatory function. Pain associated with breathing can cause splinting or tensing of the abdomen, active exhalation, and failure to cough. These actions intensify respiratory dysfunction by promoting retention of secretions, airway closure, and atelectasis. Following thoracotomy, intraoperative blockade of the intercostal muscles[24] with local anesthetic drugs may provide analgesia for 60–360 (depending on the local anesthetic drug used) minutes postoperatively. Infusion of local anesthetics directly into a chest will also provide some degree of analgesia but fluid and blood in the chest will dilute the agents and decrease their efficacy; the patient may need to lie with the surgery site dependent (this may be uncomfortable for the patient) so that the local anesthetic comes in contact with the incision and large volumes of anesthetic agent may be necessary in order to cover adequate surface area. Constant IV infusions of opioids, ketamine, and/ or lidocaine are easy to use and will also provide effective analgesia. The administration of opioids through epidural catheters that are advanced into the thoracic region is a pain relief technique commonly used in human beings but not commonly used in veterinary patients. Morphine epidurals are effective for the relief of thoracic pain in dogs and should be considered as an analgesic option.[25]

Monitoring and support of both respiratory and cardiovascular function should continue well into the recovery period. Support should include administration of oxygen, maintenance of circulating fluid volume through the administration of IV fluids, and normalization of electrolyte and acid–base status. Following thoracotomy, a chest drain should be maintained until negative pressure can be consistently achieved with minimal to no aspiration of air, blood, or fluid.

Revised from "Pulmonary Disease" by Robert R. Paddleford and Stephen A. Greene in Lumb and Jones' Veterinary Anesthesia and Analgesia, Fourth Edition.

References

1. Paddleford R.R., Greene S.A. Pulmonary disease. In: *Lumb & Jones Veterinary Anesthesia*, 4th ed. W.J. Tranquilli, J.C. Thurmon, and K.A. Grimm, eds. Ames, IA: Wiley-Blackwell, 2007, pp 899–903.
2. Baldessarini R.J., Tarazi F.I. Drugs and the treatment of psychiatric disorders. In: *Goodman & Gilman's the Pharmacological Basis of Therapeutics*, 10th ed. J.G. Hardman and L.E. Limbird, eds. New York: McGraw-Hill, 2001, pp 485–520.
3. Popovic N.A., Mullane J.F., Yhap E.O. Effects of acetylpromazine maleate on certain cardio-respiratory responses in dogs. *Am J Vet Res* **33**: 1819–1824, 1972.
4. Haskins S.C., Farver T.B., Patz J.D. Cardiovascular changes in dogs given diazepam and diazepam-ketamine. *Am J Vet Res* **17**: 795–798, 1986.
5. Lerche P., Muir W.W. Effect of medetomidine on breathing and inspiratory neuromuscular drive in conscious dogs. *Am J Vet Res* **65**(6): 720–724, 2004.

6. Copland V.S., Haskins S.C., Patz J. Naloxone reversal of oxymorphone effects in dogs. *Am J Vet Res* **50**: 1854–1858, 1989.
7. Michealis L.L., Hickey P.R., Clark T.A., et al. Ventricular irritability associated with the use of naloxone hydrochloride. *Ann Thorac Surg* **18**: 608–614, 1974.
8. Andree R.A. Sudden death following naloxone administration. *Anesth Analg* **59**: 782–784, 1980.
9. McCrackin M.A., Harvey R.C., Sackman J.E., et al. Butorphanol tartrate for partial reversal of oxymorphone-induced postoperative respiratory depression in the dog. *Vet Surg* **23**: 67–74, 1994.
10. Jacobson J.D., McGrath C.J., Smith E.P. Cardiorespiratory effects of four opioid-tranquilizer combinations in dogs. *Vet Surg* **3**(4): 299–306, 1994.
11. Stoelting R.K. Nonbarbiturate induction drugs. In: *Pharmacology and Physiology in Anesthetic Practice*, 3rd ed. R.K. Stoelting, ed. Philadelphia, PA: Lippincott, Williams & Wilkins, 1999, pp 140–157.
12. Musk G.C., Pang D.S., Beths T., et al. Target-controlled infusion of propofol in dogs-evaluation of four targets for induction of anaesthesia. *Vet Rec* **157**(24): 766–770, 2005.
13. Stoelting R.K. Inhaled anesthetics. In: *Pharmacology and Physiology in Anesthetic Practice*, 3rd ed. R.K. Stoelting, ed. Philadelphia, PA: Lippincott, Williams & Wilkins, 1999, pp 36–76.
14. Lemmens S., Stienen P.J., Jaramillo L.G., et al. The cardiorespiratory effects of a fentanyl infusion following acepromazine and glycopyrrolate in dogs. *Tijdschr Diergeneeskd* **133**(21): 888–895, 2008.
15. McNally E.M., Robertson S.A., Pablo L.S. Comparison of time to desaturation between preoxygenated and nonpreoxygenated dogs following sedation with acepromazine maleate and morphine and induction of anesthesia with propofol. *Am J Vet Res* **70**(11): 1333–1338, 2009.
16. Greene S.A., Harvey R.C. Airway Disease. In: *Lumb & Jones Veterinary Anesthesia*, 4th ed. W.J. Tranquilli, J.C. Thurmon, and K.A. Grimm, eds. Ames, IA: Wiley-Blackwell, 2007, pp 937–943.
17. Stepien R.L., Bonagura J.D., Bednarski R.M., et al. Cardiorespiratory effects of acepromazine maleate and buprenorphine hydrochloride in clinically normal dogs. *Am J Vet Res* **56**(1): 78–84, 1995.
18. Gross M.E., Dodam J.R., Pope E.R., et al. A comparison of thiopental, propofol, and diazepam-ketamine anesthesia for evaluation of laryngeal function in dogs premedicated with butorphanol-glycopyrrolate. *J Am Anim Hosp* **38**(6): 503–506, 2002.
19. Mitchell S.L., McCarthy R., Rudloff E., et al. Tracheal rupture associated with intubation in cats: 20 cases (1996–1998). *J Am Vet Med Assoc* **216**(10): 1592–1595, 2000.
20. Kerr L.Y. Pulmonary edema secondary to upper airway obstruction in the dog: a review of nine cases. *J Am Anim Hosp Assoc* **25**: 207–212, 1989.
21. Gotta A.W., Ray C., Sullivan C.A., et al. Anatomical dead space and airway resistance after glycopyrrolate or atropine premedication. *Can J Anesth* **28**(1): 51–54, 1981.
22. Burburan S.M., Xisto D.G., Rocco P.R. Anaesthetic management in asthma. *Minerva Anestesiol* **73**(6): 357–365, 2007.
23. Kroenke K., Lawrence V.A., Theroux J.F., et al. Operative risk in patients with severe obstructive disease. *Arch Intern Med* **152**(5): 967–971, 1992.
24. Skarda R.T., Tranquilli W.J. Local and regional anesthetic and analgesic techniques: dogs. In: *Lumb & Jones Veterinary Anesthesia*, 4th ed. W.J. Tranquilli, J.C. Thurmon, and K.A. Grimm, eds. Ames, IA: Wiley-Blackwell, 2007, pp 561–595.
25. Pascoe P.J., Dyson D.H. Analgesia after lateral thoracotomy in dogs. Epidural morphine vs intercostal bupivacaine. *Vet Surg* **22**(2): 141–147, 1993.

Chapter 13

Anesthesia for patients with neurological disease

Stephen A. Greene and Tamara L. Grubb

Introduction

Dogs and cats frequently require anesthesia for diagnostic evaluation or surgical correction of neurological disorders. Diagnostic procedures that require either general anesthesia or heavy sedation include electroencephalography (EEG), imaging techniques, and other electrodiagnostic tests. Veterinary neurosurgical anesthesia is more often required in patients with spinal cord rather than intracranial disorders. A frequently performed neurosurgical procedure in veterinary medicine is involved in treatment of intervertebral disk disease. However, the increased use of advanced imaging techniques, such as computed tomography and magnetic resonance imaging (MRI), has led to a greater frequency of intracranial operative procedures in dogs and cats. In animals with neurological disease, consideration of the dynamics of intracranial pressure (ICP), cerebral blood flow (CBF), and cerebrospinal fluid (CSF) production and flow is important in preventing patient morbidity or death. Matching appropriate CBF with cerebral metabolism is critical for optimal homeostasis of the animal with neurological disease. Recognition of the effects of drugs, physiological responses during anesthesia, and therapeutic interventions on CBF is essential in meeting the demands of the patient with intracranial disease.

Physiology

In normal awake animals, blood supply to the central nervous system (CNS) is controlled by autoregulatory mechanisms. Alteration in CBF can result from a variety of changes in arterial oxygenation, carbon dioxide partial pressure, mean arterial pressure (MAP), and venous outflow. The brain and spinal cord are protected by encasement within the bony skull and vertebral column. Increases in blood flow within the noncompliant cranial vault cause an increase in the intracranial volume.[1-3] Once increases in CBF cause the intracranial volume to exceed the limits of effective compliance, ICP increases sharply. When clinical findings suggest ICP is already increased by intracranial masses, trauma, or derangement of autoregulation, extreme care is required, because slight changes in

Essentials of Small Animal Anesthesia and Analgesia, Second Edition. Edited by Kurt A. Grimm, William J. Tranquilli, Leigh A. Lamont.
© 2011 John Wiley & Sons, Inc. Published 2011 by John Wiley & Sons, Inc.

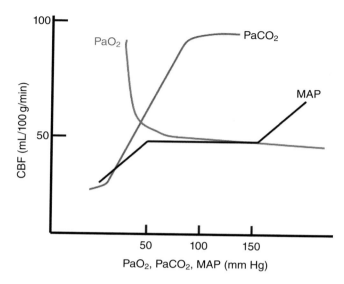

Figure 13.1. Effects on cerebral blood flow (CBF) caused by independent changes in PaO_2, $PaCO_2$, and mean arterial pressure (MAP).

intracranial volume greatly increase ICP.[2] Significant ICP increases may lead to cerebral ischemia and brain herniation.[1]

Autoregulation of CBF

Autoregulation of brain blood flow is usually very effective in a systemic mean arterial blood pressure range of approximately 50–150 mm Hg. Within this range of blood pressure, many factors—including intracranial tumors, hypercapnia, severe hypoxia, and many anesthetics—interfere with autoregulation and cause changes in ICP (Figure 13.1).[1,4,5] Blood vessels in the brain supplying diseased or neoplastic tissues may be fully dilated and unaffected by normal autoregulation mechanisms.

The CNS depression of general anesthesia is usually accompanied by a decrease in cerebral metabolic rate (CMR) and cerebral metabolic requirement for oxygen ($CMRO_2$). This decrease in oxygen requirement is thought to be protective in the possible event of relative ischemia during anesthesia and neurosurgery. There are conflicting reports on the efficacy of various anesthetics in reducing $CMRO_2$, just as there are with regard to the relative effects of the anesthetics on CBF and ICP. Isoflurane, sevoflurane, etomidate, and the barbiturates are generally recognized as contributing substantially to the reduction of $CMRO_2$, affording some cerebral protection.[5]

In patients with preexisting elevated ICP, further increases can be caused by gravitational or positional interference with drainage of venous blood from the head. Obstruction by occlusion of jugular veins through surgical positioning of the head, use of a neck leash, or venous occlusion to obtain blood samples or placement of jugular vein catheters can rapidly cause dangerous increases in ICP.[6] For intracranial neurosurgery, a slight elevation of the head above the level of the heart (with the neck in a neutral position) will facilitate venous drainage, lowering ICP. Extreme elevation is avoided to minimize the risk of venous air embolization.[3]

Only at very low arterial oxygen tensions does the CBF change in response to oxygen partial pressure. When arterial oxygen partial pressure (PaO_2) decreases below a threshold of 50 mm Hg, CBF increases (Figure 13.1). The relationship between arterial carbon dioxide partial pressure ($PaCO_2$) and CBF, on the other hand, is linear. CBF increases by about 2 mL/min/100 g of brain tissue for every 1-mm Hg increase in arterial carbon dioxide over the range of $PaCO_2$ from 20 to 80 mm Hg.[7] Hyperventilation has been used extensively in neuroanesthesia to reduce CBF (via cerebral vasoconstriction). This maneuver decreases tissue bulk, facilitating intracranial surgery. Although quite effective, this technique is somewhat controversial in some situations, because a potential exists for the diversion of remaining blood flow preferentially to diseased tissues lacking autoregulation at the expense of normal brain tissue.[8] Deliberate hyperventilation to decrease ICP may be risky when mean arterial blood pressure is reduced to less than 50 mm Hg. The ensuing ischemia could be deleterious to normal brain tissues if a "steal" of CBF diverts remaining blood flow.[8,9] The rapid and substantial reduction in CBF and ICP achieved by hyperventilation makes it a valuable tool for the immediate reduction in brain bulk to facilitate intracranial surgery and to reduce acute brain swelling.

Although controversial, restriction of intravenous fluids to only that volume necessary to maintain adequate circulating volume and cardiac output is usually recommended in neurosurgical patients with increased ICP.[10,11] Excessive fluid volume has been associated with increased central venous pressure, decreased venous outflow, and increased risk of compounding cerebral edema. Diuretic therapy is frequently indicated in the medical management of patients with intracranial masses and elevated ICP or cerebral edema.[6] Dextrose administration is also somewhat controversial and must be individualized to the situation. Hyperglycemia is associated with adverse outcome in animals with cerebral ischemia, and cerebral edema can be exacerbated by administration of isotonic dextrose. However, intravenous dextrose administration decreases the incidence of seizures in patients after metrizamide myelography and is indicated in hypoglycemic seizures or hypoglycemic coma.[1,12,13]

Glucocorticoids are effective in the treatment of some forms of cerebral edema and have been shown to be effective in reducing the increased ICP that is caused by brain tumors and hydrocephalus. Glucocorticoid therapy may be considered in the management of patients with cerebral edema associated with primary or metastatic brain neoplasia. Since dexamethasone administration has been shown to reduce the rate of CSF formation in dogs, steroid administration may be of some value in the preanesthetic management of hydrocephalic patients considered at risk of further increases in ICP.[14,15] Corticosteroids are now known to be contraindicated in cases of CNS trauma.

Pharmacology

Sedatives, tranquilizers, and analgesics

For many years, the suspected increased seizure activity associated with administration of the phenothiazine (e.g., acepromazine) and possibly butyrophenone (e.g., droperidol) tranquilizers contraindicated their use in seizure-prone patients and in patients for diagnostic EEG.[16] A more recent retrospective study indicates that acepromazine does not potentiate seizure activity.[17] Control of seizures with benzodiazepine tranquilizers (e.g., diazepam or midazolam) is desirable in the management of seizure-prone patients but can obscure characteristic patterns in diagnostic EEGs. In addition, benzodiazepines appear to decrease CBF and ICP.[18]

Evidence for or against the use of alpha$_2$ adrenergic agonists in dogs and cats with neurological disease is scant. Medetomidine administered to isoflurane-anesthetized dogs had no effect on ICP measured using a fiberoptic transducer, whereas antagonism of medetomidine by using atipamezole was associated with a dramatic transient increase in ICP.[19] Dexmedetomidine, the pharmacologically active stereoisomer of medetomidine, decreased CBF in both halothane- and isoflurane-anesthetized dogs.[20,21] The alpha$_2$ agonists appear to be rational choices to provide sedation for examination or as a preanesthetic medication for patients with neurological disease.

Opioids or neuroleptanalgesic combinations are sometimes used in anesthetic management of patients with increased ICP. The direct effects of opioids on CBF and ICP are minimal. However, opioids may indirectly increase CSF pressure and should be used cautiously in patients with cerebral trauma or space-occupying tumors. Increases in pressure within the cranium may aggravate the underlying condition.

The elevation in CSF pressure is caused by accumulation of carbon dioxide, which in turn is caused by opioid-induced hypoventilation. If a patient is ventilated to prevent hypercapnia, the increase in CSF pressure does not occur when opioids are administered.[22] When opioids are used in these cases, the respiratory status must be assessed through arterial blood gas analysis or end-tidal carbon dioxide levels, and when necessary, the patient should be ventilated to prevent hypercapnia. The judicious use of opioids for pain management in the postoperative period often does not cause as much respiratory depression as does pain itself.[23]

Injectable anesthetics

Ketamine can dramatically increase both CMR and CBF. Telazol® (tiletamine and zolazepam; Pfizer Animal Health, New York) is typically placed in the same category as ketamine; however, studies on CBF and ICP as specifically affected by Telazol are lacking. Combination of ketamine with a γ-aminobutyric acid (GABA) agonist has been shown to ameliorate the effect of ketamine on ICP in dogs.[24,25] Whether this is the case for Telazol remains to be proven. In a clinical setting under controlled ventilation, ketamine administration with a GABA agonist and without nitrous oxide has been safely used in neurologically impaired patients.[26] Administration of etomidate is associated with regional reductions in blood flow, but this has been associated with exacerbation of ischemic brain injury in human patients.[27] Thiobarbiturates, etomidate, and propofol all decrease CMR and CBF, effectively maintaining the coupling between flow and metabolism. Propofol infusion combined with infusion of a short-acting opioid such as fentanyl or remifentanil is a popular anesthetic protocol for neurological patients and provides an effective alternative to the subsequent maintenance of anesthesia using inhalants.

Neuromuscular blocking agents

The effect of neuromuscular blocking agents (NMBAs) on ICP will depend on the agent used: most of the nondepolarizing NMBAs such as atracurium, vecuronium, mivacurium, or pancuronium have no significant effect. Agents that are associated with histamine release (e.g., d-tubocurarine) may increase the ICP. Succinylcholine is associated with a direct increase in ICP and should generally be avoided in patients with raised ICP.

Inhalants

All modern volatile anesthetics suppress CMR and, with the exception of halothane, can produce burst suppression of the electroencephalogram. At that depth of anesthesia, CMR is reduced by about 60%. Volatile anesthetics have dose-dependent effects on CBF. In doses lower than the minimal alveolar concentration (MAC), CBF is not significantly altered compared to awake. (The MAC is the lowest end-tidal concentration of inhalant that prevents purposeful movement in 50% of a population.) Beyond doses of 1 MAC, direct cerebral vasodilation results in an increase in CBF and cerebral blood volume. Nitrous oxide has minimal direct effect on ICP when used at concentrations of 50–70% in oxygen. However, nitrous oxide will equilibrate with confined gas spaces and can dramatically increase volume and pressure in these circumstances (e.g., pneumoencephalopathy).

Cardiovascular supportive drugs

Systemic vasodilators (e.g., nitroglycerin, nitroprusside, hydralazine, calcium channel blockers) vasodilate the cerebral circulation and can, depending on MAP, increase CBF (Table 13.1). Vasopressors such as phenylephrine, norepinephrine, ephedrine, and dopamine do not have significant direct effects on the cerebral circulation. Their effect on CBF is dependent on their effect on systemic blood pressure. When MAP is below the

Table 13.1.　Drug effects on CBF and ICP

Increase	Decrease	Minimal or no effect
Nitroprusside	Benzodiazepines	Phenylephrine
Nitroglycerin	Opioids	Norepinephrine
Hydralazine	Thiobarbiturates	Dopamine
Calcium channel blockers	Propofol	Ephedrine
d-Tubocurarine	Etomidate	Acepromazine
Succinylcholine		Dexmedetomidine
Inhalant > 1.0 × MAC		Nitrous oxide
Ketamine		Inhalant < 1.0 × MAC
Atipamezole		Atracurium
		Mivacurium
		Pancuronium
		Vecuronium

MAC, minimal alveolar concentration.

lower limit of autoregulation, vasopressors increase systemic pressure and thereby increase CBF. If systemic pressure is within the limits of autoregulation, vasopressor-induced increases in systemic pressure have little effect on CBF.

Anesthetic management of specific neurological problems

MRI

Anesthetic concerns during MRI examination center on the potentially dangerous environment of a strong magnetic field.[28] Ferromagnetic projectiles have had serious, even lethal, consequences in MRI suites. Anesthetic management of animals undergoing MRI exam can most simply be accomplished by means of injectable agents.[29–31] Inhalant anesthetics have been used in MRI suites by distancing the vital ferromagnetic components of the anesthesia machine from the magnetic field. Use of an extended nonrebreathing circuit, such as the Bain circuit, has been described.[32] One drawback of this technique is the higher fresh gas flow rates required for larger animals. Another modification of anesthetic technique for MRI involves the use of extended rebreathing hoses with the anesthetic machine placed near the magnet, yet just beyond the critical point of magnetic attraction. For equine MRI, a large animal machine suitable for delivering inhalant anesthetics to horses can be used in this manner. There is anecdotal evidence that prolonged exposure (more than 2 hours) in a 3–5-gauss magnetic field begins to affect vaporizer (Isotec; Datex-Ohmeda, Helsinki, Finland) output such that higher vaporizer settings are required to maintain adequate anesthesia. In human patients, this effect has been reported for Fortec vaporizers (Cyprane, Keighley, UK).[33] Although many vaporizers are mainly constructed from nonferrous materials, many do contain components affected by magnetic fields.[34]

Anesthesia in MRI suites can be monitored by using MRI-compatible equipment to measure the electrocardiograph, blood pressure, pulse oximetry, and airway gases.[35] Less expensive alternatives include use of remotely placed monitors with specialized cabling designed to avoid interference with the magnetic field and induction of electric currents leading to burns. Simple systems can be used to measure direct arterial blood pressure, such as the aneroid manometer placed beyond the magnetic field or several feet of extension tubing placed between the transducer and patient. Some dampening and degradation of the arterial pulse wave may occur, but often direct measurement of arterial blood pressure is invaluable to assure maintenance of adequate cerebral perfusion pressure.

Because the magnetic fields vary considerably among various MRI units in clinical practice, consultation with a knowledgeable biomedical engineer is advised prior to implementing a monitoring system or novel means of anesthetic delivery.

Myelography and intervertebral disk disease

For the relatively common surgical procedures to decompress cervical or thoracolumbar intervertebral disk herniation, anesthetic management should address (1) protection from possible seizures and other potential complications associated with administration of myelographic contrast agents, (2) perioperative pain relief, (3) maintenance of adequate spontaneous ventilation, and (4) management of concurrent disorders such as urinary incontinence or other factors predisposing patients to adverse recovery.

Radiographic contrast myelography is sometimes performed in the immediate preoperative period to localize the lesion(s) and to identify the proper site(s) for surgical decompression. As this procedure is often performed during the same anesthetic period, patient management is designed to optimize conditions for both the diagnostic (radiographic) and the therapeutic (surgical) procedures. Dural puncture for sampling of CSF and/or for administration of myelographic contrast agent requires a depth of anesthesia at less than a surgical plane but adequate to prevent patient movement with subsequent trauma.

The incidence of seizure activity and the other potential adverse side effects of myelography appears to be greatly reduced with use of newer contrast agents such as iopamidol and iohexol rather than metrizamide.[36,37] Hyperflexion of the cervical spine for cisternal CSF collection and for cervical administration of myelographic contrast can easily kink most endotracheal tubes, causing airway obstruction. Endotracheal tubes that are armored or contain spiral wire are quite resistant to kinking. Metal or other radiopaque reinforcement in the armored tubes makes them unsuitable for use in cervical and cranial radiographic studies. Close attention to adequacy of the airway and spontaneous ventilation is of paramount importance when flexing the neck.

Intracranial masses and elevated ICP

Patients with intracranial masses, dysfunctional CBF autoregulation, and/or increased ICP are at risk of rapid decompensation under anesthesia. Preoperative assessment should include measurement of arterial blood pressure, because many patients with elevated ICP will have an accompanying increase in systemic arterial blood pressure (Cushing's response). Systemic hypertension is an attempt to compensate and maintain adequate cerebral perfusion pressure. If MAP is significantly elevated prior to drug administration, arterial blood pressure should not be allowed to drop to normally acceptable levels under anesthesia (e.g., a MAP of 60 mm Hg), because cerebral ischemia can result despite an acceptable mean blood pressure.

Manual or mechanical positive pressure ventilation should be immediately available and instituted at induction. Mechanical ventilation should be continued until extubation. In some cases, allowing $PaCO_2$ to rise in order to stimulate spontaneous ventilation, before the respiratory depressant effects of the anesthetics wane, may cause serious elevations in ICP and possibly herniation of the brain. Anesthetic monitoring should address the physiological variables associated with altered ICP. Venous and arterial blood pressures and airway or arterial sampling for carbon dioxide analysis should be included, if possible. Intravenous mannitol (0.5–1.0 g/kg IV slowly) may be useful to reduce ICP before, during, or after anesthesia. Optimal anesthetic management can substantially improve patient status and the outcome of intracranial surgical procedures.

Management of seizures in the perianesthetic period

CMR may be dramatically increased during seizure activity. Therefore, patients with neurological impairment should be critically evaluated to prevent drug-induced seizures during the perianesthetic period. Traditionally, drugs with side effects that may include seizure activity (e.g., ketamine, methohexital) are avoided. Chlorpromazine, when combined with intermittent light stimulation, has been associated with lowered seizure threshold in Beagle dogs.[38] However, a retrospective study found no association between clinical administration of acepromazine in 36 dogs with seizure history and incidence of seizures.[17] In addition, in dogs with active seizures, acepromazine was associated with decreased seizure activity or prevention of short-term recurrence. Another retrospective study of 31 dogs with a history of seizures found no correlation between acepromazine administration in a clinical setting and recurrence of seizure activity.[39] Thus, there appears to be a relevant basis for judicious use of acepromazine in dogs with a seizure history.

Anesthesia for electrodiagnostic techniques

In veterinary medicine, clinical electrodiagnostic techniques are used to record potentials from muscle, peripheral nerves, spinal cord, brain stem, cortex, and retina. Even during those procedures in which the stimulus is innocuous, artifacts caused by movement may render the technique ineffective. Therefore, many of these procedures must be performed in anesthetized or tranquilized animals producing less stress while insuring a minimum of recording artifacts.

Electroencephalogram and bispectral index

Anesthetic effects on the electroencephalogram (EEG) depend on the anesthetic type and depth of anesthesia. Anesthesia initially causes an increase in the voltage and a decrease in the frequency of cortical potentials when compared with the record of an awake, alert dog. Spikes and spindles may also riddle the EEG of lightly anesthetized dogs and cats.[40,41] As anesthesia deepens, the overall voltage begins to diminish. A dose–response decrease in cerebral oxygen consumption ($CMRO_2$) accompanies the use of isoflurane in dogs and causes the EEG to become isoelectric at an end-expired concentration of 3%.[42] The same type of cortical alteration in electrical activity, sometimes referred to as burst suppression, has been reported in swine but may occur in other species as well.[43] Dose-dependent CNS depression of EEG activity by most anesthetics is characteristic and has led to the development of EEG-based anesthetic monitoring techniques.[44]

Notable exceptions to the general rule that anesthetics decrease EEG activity include the dissociative anesthetics and the volatile anesthetic enflurane. Further, alterations in normal $PaCO_2$ are associated with significant changes in the quantitative EEG of dogs during halothane anesthesia.[45] Monitoring CNS depression by using EEG during anesthesia has been the focus of study for decades. However, direct interpretation of the EEG has not proven adequately reliable or time responsive for use in operative circumstances. Processed EEG monitoring has evolved as a way to provide immediate feedback to anesthetists in regard to patients' CNS activity. Spectral edge frequency, total power, beta/delta frequency ratios, and other specific parameters derived from computer-processed EEG have been correlated to varying degrees with anesthetic depth, but interpretation can vary depending on the selection of anesthetic agents.

Intraoperative EEG processing has been developed with significant improvement in reliability. For example, the bispectral index (BIS) monitor is a proprietary device that provides information related to anesthetic depth and is readily interpreted. In addition, the BIS has proven to be reliable as an indicator of anesthetic depth in people given a variety of anesthetic agents and adjuncts.[46,47] The BIS is a unitless number between 0 and 100 derived from the processed EEG.[48] People undergoing surgery are typically maintained at a depth of anesthesia that yields a BIS value between 40 and 60, which reliably prevents intraoperative awareness.[49–53]

In animals, several reports have evaluated the use of BIS as an indicator of anesthetic depth. In dogs, isoflurane and sevoflurane anesthetic depth has been correlated to BIS.[54–56] Anesthetized cats had a nonlinear relationship of BIS with increasing multiples of sevoflurane minimum alveolar concentration.[57] The change in BIS values following stimulation in isoflurane-anesthetized cats provided a useful measure of anesthetic depth.[58] Use of BIS in veterinary medicine has been reviewed.[59]

Nerve-conduction studies

Nerve-conduction velocity has been successfully recorded in dogs while using a variety of anesthetic protocols. Because these procedures have not been done in unanesthetized animals, the effects of anesthetics on these procedures are largely unknown.

Evoked potentials may be altered by anesthetic agents, depending on the specific location of signal generators. Generally, cortical potentials are more likely to be affected than brain stem potentials. Various anesthetics and adjunctive drugs used in the perianesthetic period may affect latencies of evoked potentials. These effects appear to be specific to the particular drug and species.

Revised from "Neurological Disease" by Ralph C. Harvey, Stephen A. Greene, and William B. Thomas in Lumb and Jones' Veterinary Anesthesia and Analgesia, Fourth Edition.

References

1. Shapiro H.H. Neurosurgical anesthesia and intracranial hypertension. In: *Anesthesia*, 2nd ed. R.D. Miller, ed. New York: Churchill Livingstone, 1986, pp 1563–1620.
2. Stoelting R.K. *Pharmacology and Physiology in Anesthetic Practice*. Philadelphia, PA: JB Lippincott, 1987.
3. van Poznak A. Special consideration for veterinary neuroanesthesia. In: *Principles and Practice of Veterinary Anesthesia*. C.E. Short, ed. Baltimore, MD: Williams and Wilkins, 1987, pp 177–183.
4. Hansen T.D., Warner D.S., Vust L.H., et al. Regional distribution of cerebral blood flow with halothane and isoflurane. *Anesthesiology* **69**: 332–337, 1988.
5. Osborn I. Choice of neuroanesthetic technique. *Anesthesiol Clin North America* **5**: 531–540, 1987.

6. Dayrell-Hart B., Klide A.M. Intracranial dysfunctions: stupor and coma. *Vet Clin North Am Small Anim Pract* **19**: 1209–1222, 1989.

7. Grubb R.L., Raichle M.E., Eichling J.O., et al. The effects of changes in PaCO2 on cerebral blood volume, blood flow, and vascular mean transit time. *Stroke* **5**: 530–539, 1974.

8. Cottrell J.E. Deliberate hypotension. Annual Refresher Course Lectures, American Society of Anesthesiologists, sect 245, 1989:1.

9. Harp J.R., Wollman H. Cerebral metabolic effects of hyperventilation and deliberate hypotension. *Br J Anaesth* **45**: 256–262, 1973.

10. Frost E.A.M. Central nervous system trauma. *Anesthesiol Clin North America* **5**: 565–585, 1987.

11. Hirshfeld A. Fluid and electrolyte management in neurosurgical patients. *Anesthesiol Clin North America* **5**: 491–505, 1987.

12. Gilroy B.A. Neuroanesthesiology. In: *Textbook of Small Animal Surgery*. D. Slatter, ed. Philadelphia, PA: WB Saunders, 1985, pp 2643–2650.

13. Gray P.R., Lowrie C.T., Wetmore L.A. Effect of intravenous administration of dextrose or lactated Ringer's solution on seizure development in dogs after cervical myelography with metrizamide. *Am J Vet Res* **48**: 1600–1602, 1987.

14. Franklin R.T. The use of glucocorticoids in treating cerebral edema. *Compend Contin Educ Pract Vet* **6**: 442–448, 1984.

15. Sato O., Hara M., Asai T., et al. The effect of dexamethasone phosphate on the production rate of cerebrospinal fluid in the spinal subarachnoid space of dogs. *J Neurosurg* **39**: 480–484, 1973.

16. Gleed R.D. Tranquilizers and sedative. In: *Principles and Practice of Veterinary Anesthesia*. C.E. Short, ed. Baltimore, MD: Williams and Wilkins, 1987, pp 16–28.

17. Tobias K.M., Marioni-Henry K., Wagner R.A. A retrospective study on the use of acepromazine maleate in dogs with seizures. *J Am Anim Hosp Assoc* **42**: 283–289, 2006.

18. Nugent M., Artru A.A., Michnfelder J.D. Cerebral metabolic, vascular and protective effects of midazolam maleate. *Anesthesiology* **56**: 172–176, 1982.

19. Keegan R.D., Greene S.A., Bagley R.S., et al. Effects of medetomidine administration on intracranial pressure and cardiovascular variables of isoflurane-anesthetized dogs. *Am J Vet Res* **56**: 193–198, 1995.

20. Karlsson B., Forsman M., Roald O., et al. Effect of dexmedetomidine, a selective and potent alpha 2-agonist, on cerebral blood flow and oxygen consumption during halothane anesthesia in dogs. *Anesth Analg* **71**: 125–129, 1990.

21. Zornow M.H., Fleischer J.E., Scheller M.S., et al. Dexmedetomidine, an alpha-2 adrenergic agonist, decreases cerebral blood flow in the isoflurane-anesthetized dog. *Anesth Analg* **70**: 624–630, 1990.

22. Marsh M.L., Marshall L.F., Shapiro H.M. Neurosurgical intensive care. *Anesthesiology* **47**: 149–163, 1977.

23. Bonica J.J., ed. *The Management of Pain*, 2nd ed. Philadelphia, PA: Lea and Febiger, 1990.

24. Artru A.A., Katz R.A. Cerebral blood volume and CSF pressure following administration of ketamine in dogs: modification by pre-or posttreatment with hypocapnia or diazepam. *J Neurosurg Anesthesiol* **1**: 8–15, 1989.

25. Strebel S., Kaufmann M., Maitre L., et al. Effects of ketamine on cerebral blood flow velocity in humans: influence of pretreatment with midazolam or esmolol. *Anaesthesia* **50**: 223–228, 1995.

26. Himmelseher S., Durieux M.E. Revising a dogma: ketamine for patients with neurological injury? *Anesth Analg* **101**: 524–534, 2005.

27. Patel P.M., Drummond J.C. Cerebral physiology and the effects of anesthetic drugs. In: *Miller's Anesthesia, Vol. 1*, 7th ed. R.D. Miller, ed. Philadelphia, PA: Churchill-Livingstone, 2009, pp 594–674.

28. Smith J.A. Hazards, safety and anesthetic considerations for MRI. *Top Companion Anim Med* **25**(2): 98–106, 2010.

29. Chaffin M.K., Walker M.A., McArthur N.H., et al. Magnetic resonance imaging of the brain of normal neonatal foals. *Vet Radiol Ultrasound* **38**: 102–111, 1997.

30. Lukasik V.M., Gillies R.J. Animal anaesthesia for in-vivo magnetic resonance. *NMR Biomed* **16**: 459–467, 2003.

31. Willis C.K., Quinn R.P., McDonnell W.M., et al. Functional MRI as a tool to assess vision in dogs: the optimal anesthetic. *Vet Ophthalmol* **4**: 243–253, 2001.

32. Young A.E., Brown P.N., Zorab J.S. Anaesthesia for children and infants undergoing magnetic resonance imaging: a prospective study. *Eur J Anaesthesiol* **13**: 400–403, 1996.

33. Kross J., Drummond J.C. Successful use of a Fortec II vaporizer in the MRI suite: a case report with observations regarding magnetic field-induced vaporizer aberrancy. *Can J Anaesth* **38**: 1065–1069, 1991.

34. Zimmer C., Janssen M.N., Treschan J.A., et al. Near-miss accident during magnetic resonance imaging by a "flying sevoflurane vaporizer" due to ferromagnetism undetectable by handheld magnet. *Anesthesiology* **100**: 1329–1330, 2004.

35. Shelley K., Shelley S., Bell C. Monitoring in unusual environments. In: *Clinical Monitoring*. C.L. Lake, R.L. Hines, and C.D. Blitt, eds. Philadelphia, PA: WB Saunders, 2001, pp 524–538.

36. Wheeler S.J., Davies J.V. Iohexol myelography in the dog and cat: a series of one hundred cases and a comparison with metrizamide and iopamidol. *J Small Anim Pract* **26**: 247–256, 1985.

37. Cox F.H. The use of iopamidol for myelography in dogs: a study of twenty-seven cases. *J Small Anim Pract* **27**: 159–165, 1986.

38. Redman H.C., Wilson G.L., Hogan J.E. Effect of chlorpromazine combined with intermittent light stimulation on the electroencephalogram and clinical response of the Beagle dog. *Am J Vet Res* **34**: 929–936, 1973.

39. McConnell J., Kirby R., Rudloff E. Administration of acepromazine maleate to 31 dogs with a history of seizures. *J Vet Emerg Crit Care* **17**: 262–267, 2007.

40. Klemm W.R. Subjective and quantitative analyses of the electroencephalogram of anesthetized normal dogs: control data for clinical diagnosis. *Am J Vet Res* **29**: 1267–1277, 1968.

41. Klemm W.R., Mallo G.L. Clinical electroencephalography in anesthetized small animals. *J Am Vet Med Assoc* **148**: 1038–1042, 1976.

42. Newberg L.A., Milde J.H., Michenfelder J.D. The cerebral metabolic effects of isoflurane at and above concentrations that suppress cortical electrical activity. *Anesthesiology* **39**: 23–28, 1983.

43. Rampil I.J., Weiskopf R.B., Brown J.G., et al. I653 and isoflurane produce similar dose-related changes in the electroencephalogram of pigs. *Anesthesiology* **69**: 298–302, 1988.

44. Goodrich J.T. Electrophysiologic measurements: intraoperative evoked potential monitoring. *Anesthesiol Clin North Am* **5**: 477–489, 1987.

45. Smith L.J., Greene S.A., Moore M.P., et al. Effects of altered arterial carbon dioxide tension on quantitative EEG in halothane-anesthetized dogs. *Am J Vet Res* **55**: 467–471, 1994.

46. Sebel P.S., Lang E., Rampil I.J., et al. A multicenter study of bispectral electroencephalogram analysis for monitoring anesthetic effect. *Anesth Analg* **84**: 891–899, 1997.

47. Takkallapalli R., Mehta M., DeLima L., et al. Bispectral index: can it predict arousal from noxious stimuli during general anesthesia? *Anesth Analg* **88**(Suppl 2): S58, 1998.

48. Rampil I.J. A primer for EEG signal processing in anesthesia. *Anesthesiology* **89**: 980–1002, 1998.
49. Katoh T., Suzuki A., Ikeda K. Electroencephalographic derivatives as a tool for predicting the depth of sedation and anesthesia induced by sevoflurane. *Anesthesiology* **88**: 642–650, 1998.
50. Rosow C., Manberg P.J. Bispectal index monitoring. *Anesthesiol Clin North America* **16**: 89–107, 1998.
51. Billard V., Gambus P.L., Chamoun N., et al. A comparison of spectral edge, delta power, and bispectral index as EEG measures of alfentanil, propofol, and midazolam drug effect. *Clin Pharmacol Ther* **61**: 45–58, 1997.
52. Sleigh J., Andrzejowski J., Steyn-Ross A., et al. The bispectral index: a measure of depth of sleep? *Anesth Analg* **88**: 659–661, 1999.
53. Kearse L.A., Rosow C., Zaslavsky A., et al. Bispectral analysis of the EEG predicts conscious processing of information during propofol sedation hypnosis. *Anesthesiology* **88**: 25–34, 1998.
54. Greene S.A., Tranquilli W.J., Benson G.J., et al. Effect of medetomidine on bispectal index measurements in dogs during anesthesia with isoflurane. *Am J Vet Res* **64**: 316–320, 2003.
55. Greene S.A., Benson G.J., Tranquilli W.J., et al. Relationship of canine bispectral index to multiples of sevoflurane minimal alveolar concentration, using patch or subdermal electrodes. *Comp Med* **52**: 424–428, 2002.
56. Carrasco-Jimenez M.S., Cancho M.F.M., Lima J.R., et al. Relationship between a proprietary index, bispectral index, and hemodynamic variables as a means for evaluating depth of anesthesia in dogs anesthetized with sevoflurane. *Am J Vet Res* **65**: 1128–1135, 2004.
57. Lamont L.A., Greene S.A., Grimm K.A., et al. Relationship of bispectral index to minimum alveolar concentration multiples of sevoflurane in cats. *Am J Vet Res* **65**: 93–98, 2004.
58. March P.A., Muir W.W. Use of bispectral index as a monitor of anesthetic depth in cats anesthetized with isoflurane. *Am J Vet Res* **64**: 1534–1541, 2003.
59. March P.A., Muir W.W. Bispectral analysis of the electroencephalogram: a review of its development and use in anesthesia. *Vet Anaesth Analg* **32**: 241–255, 2005.

Chapter 14

Anesthesia for small animal patients with renal disease

Stuart Clark-Price

Introduction

As the science of veterinary medicine advances life-prolonging therapies, clinicians will be exposed to increasing numbers of older patients that will require care. Along with the advancing age of the patients, the prevalence of diseases associated with advanced age will increase. The kidney is an organ commonly associated with disease (i.e., chronic kidney disease) in geriatric patients. In fact, up to 20% of cats will be affected with chronic kidney disease during their lifetime.[1]

In cats greater than 15 years of age, 31% have evidence of renal disease.[1] Although the total prevalence of renal disease in dogs is less than cats, advanced age plays a role in this species as well. Of dogs with renal failure, 45% are older than 10 years of age.[2] It is therefore reasonable to assume that a veterinary practitioner will anesthetize animals with renal diseases in the regular course of daily practice. It is imperative that the veterinarian providing anesthesia have an understanding of renal physiology, renal pathophysiology, and the effects of sedative, analgesic, and anesthetic drugs on the kidney.

Renal physiology

The kidneys have three primary functions: filtration, reabsorption, and secretion. To accomplish these functions, they receive about 25% of the cardiac output. The renal tubules and collecting ducts reabsorb up to 99% of filtered solutes, indicating that the total filtration volume is much greater than daily urine production. Neurohumoral substances and physiological factors that affect reabsorption of the filtered water and sodium include aldosterone, antidiuretic hormone (ADH), arterial blood pressure (ABP), atrial natriuretic factor, catecholamines, prostaglandins, renin-angiotensin, and stress.

Renal blood flow (RBF) is regulated by extrinsic nervous and hormonal control and by intrinsic autoregulation. Renal vasculature is highly innervated by sympathetic constrictor fibers originating in the spinal cord segments between T4 and L1. The kidneys lack sympathetic vasodilating fibers and parasympathetic innervation. Intrinsic

Essentials of Small Animal Anesthesia and Analgesia, Second Edition. Edited by Kurt A. Grimm, William J. Tranquilli, Leigh A. Lamont.
© 2011 John Wiley & Sons, Inc. Published 2011 by John Wiley & Sons, Inc.

autoregulation of RBF is demonstrated by a constant flow when mean ABP ranges from 80 to 180 mm Hg. When the mean ABP is between 80 and 180 mm Hg, the kidney can control blood flow by altering resistance in the glomerular afferent arterioles. Although the exact mechanism of renal autoregulation is not known, the significance of this phenomenon relates to protection of glomerular capillaries during hypertension and preservation of renal function during hypotension. However, even within the range of blood pressure described for function of renal autoregulation, extrinsic forces (e.g., neural, hormonal, and pharmacological) and intrinsic forces (e.g., renal insufficiency/failure) may cause alterations in RBF and glomerular filtration rate (GFR).

Catecholamines are the major hormonal regulators of RBF. Epinephrine and norepinephrine cause dose-dependent changes in RBF and the GFR. Low doses increase ABP and decrease RBF with no net change in the GFR. Higher doses cause decreased RBF and GFR. The renal vascular anatomy is unique in its distribution to cortical and medullary zones. Because of this vascular dichotomy, local tissue ischemia and hypoxia may occur even though total organ blood flow is normal. Oxygen delivery to the kidney is complex, and selective regional hypoxia is a possible source of renal injury during renal hypoperfusion. Experimental evidence indicates that the medullary thick ascending limb of Henle's loop, because of its high metabolic rate associated with active transport of electrolytes, is selectively vulnerable to hypoxic injury.[3]

Renal pathophysiology

The pathophysiology of the kidney can be divided into acute and chronic renal failure. Acute renal failure is determined by a rapid onset of a decrease in GFR over a period of hours to days that manifests as an inability to excrete wastes (i.e., blood urea nitrogen [BUN] and creatinine) and maintain fluid and electrolyte homeostasis.[4] Failure of the sodium–potassium ATPase pump in the renal tubules during acute tubular necrosis is the most common cause of acute renal failure with interstitial nephritis and acute glomerulonephritis comprising the other causes.[5] Acute renal failure can be further classified into prerenal azotemia, intrinsic renal failure, and postrenal obstructive nephropathy.[5] A thorough history, signalment, physical exam, serum chemistry panel, and urinalysis can be used to help differentiate between the three classes and direct treatments.

Chronic renal failure can be defined as the progressive loss of nephron function and decreased GFR over a prolonged period of time.[4] Only when 60% or greater of the total number of nephrons become nonfunctional will clinical and/or laboratory signs of renal insufficiency become evident. At this point, the remaining functional renal mass is no longer able to appropriately eliminate waste, and nitrogenous compounds accumulate. The ability to concentrate filtrate and conserve free water is lost and patients may enter a state of hypovolemia. Additionally, the ability to balance electrolytes may be lost with derangements, eventually becoming severe enough to threaten physiological function of other organ systems (i.e., cardiovascular).

Patients with chronic renal failure may be anemic because of bone marrow suppression, chronic gastrointestinal tract blood loss, reduced red blood cell life span, and decreased secretion of enzymes that are responsible for the formation of erythropoietin with a resulting understimulation of bone marrow. In response to anemia, the cardiovascular system may become hyperdynamic in an attempt to maintain oxygen delivery. Chronic renal disease may therefore be associated with hypertension and increased cardiac output but reduced cardiac reserve.

Anesthetic effects on renal function

Effects of anesthetics on RBF can be summarized with the following generalization: All anesthetics are likely to decrease the rate of glomerular filtration. Anesthetics may directly affect RBF, or they may indirectly alter renal function via changes in cardiovascular and/or neuroendocrine activity. Most anesthetics decrease the GFR as a consequence of decreased RBF (Table 14.1). Anesthetics that cause catecholamine release (e.g., ketamine, tiletamine, and nitrous oxide) have variable effects on RBF.

Sedative and analgesic drugs have varying effects on RBF and GFR and generally relate to individual drug effects on cardiac output and vasomotor tone. Phenothiazine tranquilizers (e.g., acepromazine) produce dose-dependent hypotension through blockade of vascular alpha adrenergic receptors. Phenothiazines also antagonize dopamine receptors. Dopamine receptor blockade by acepromazine premedication may prevent dopamine-induced increases in RBF during surgery. However, RBF and GFR do not change significantly even in the face of mild hypotension and may impart protection of renal function after low-dose acepromazine administration.[6] The use of opioids in patients with renal disease has been recommended.[7] Opioids will provide sedation and analgesia to patients with minimal impact on cardiac output and thus RBF.[8] However, clinicians should be cognizant of the fact that opioids can cause urine retention when administered systemically or as an epidural injection. Alpha$_2$ agonist drugs such as dexmedetomidine and xylazine are well known to have significant dose-dependent depressant effects on heart rate and cardiac output, and increase systemic vascular resistance. Additionally, alpha$_2$ agonist drugs have a diuretic effect through antidiuretic antagonism and can increase urine volume that may be detrimental in patients with postrenal urinary tract

Table 14.1. Effects of anesthetics on renal blood flow (RBF) and glomerular filtration rate (GFR)

Drug	RBF	GFR
Isoflurane	Slight decrease	Decrease
Sevoflurane	Slight decrease	Decrease
Thiopental	No change	No change or slight decrease
Ketamine	Increase	Decrease or no change
Propofol	No change	No change
Etomidate	No change	No change

Source: Adapted from Greene S.A., Grauer G.F. 2007. Renal disease. In: *Lumb and Jones' Veterinary Anesthesia and Analgesia*, 4th ed. W.J. Tranquilli, J.C. Thurmon, and K.A. Grimm, eds. Ames, IA: Blackwell, pp. 915–919.

obstruction.[9] It has been recommended that use of this class of drugs should be avoided in patients with renal disease.[7]

Injectable anesthetic agents can also have an effect on renal parameters. Thiobarbiturates increase systemic vascular resistance but decrease renal vascular resistance with no net change in RBF. In contrast, ketamine increases RBF and renal vascular resistance.[10] However, ketamine administration may result in uneven distribution of blood flow within the kidney. Ketamine is also partially dependent on renal excretion in cats and therefore should be avoided, or used carefully in cats with renal insufficiency.[11] Propofol at moderate to low doses has minimal effect on RBF and GFR and is often used for induction of anesthesia in renal patients.[12,13] Etomidate is an anesthetic agent known for its minimal effects on heart rate, blood pressure, and cardiac output. Etomidate has also been shown to have no significant effect on renal function and urine output in anesthetized rats.[14]

Inhalant anesthetics cause systemic hypotension, especially during excessive depth, which can result in renal ischemia. This is a result of one of the major side effects of potent volatile anesthetics, peripheral vasodilation. Inhalant anesthetics also depress myocardial contractility and cardiac output in a dose-dependent manner. Concurrently, inhalation anesthetics tend to decrease RBF and GFR in a dose-dependent manner as well. Light planes of inhalation anesthesia preserve renal autoregulation of blood flow, whereas deep planes are associated with depression of autoregulation and decreases in RBF. Although isoflurane has little effect on RBF, it decreases GFR and urine output.[15] Sevoflurane, although not well studied, seems to have similar effects on RBF when compared to isoflurane.[16] However, when in contact with carbon dioxide absorbents, sevoflurane degrades to a nephrotoxic substance called compound A. Compound A has been shown to cause permanent damage to the kidneys of rats but has not been shown to cause problems in humans with renal insufficiency or in dogs with normal renal function.[17,18] Desflurane has no effect on RBF at concentrations up to twice the minimal alveolar concentration (MAC); however, it decreases renal vascular resistance at concentrations greater than 1.75 MAC.[19] For most patients, the effects of inhaled anesthetics on renal function are reversed at the termination of anesthesia. Some patients, however, may not regain the ability to regulate urine production for several days.[20] Any patient that demonstrates postanesthetic oliguria should be evaluated immediately for renal insufficiency/failure.

Most anesthetics, whether injectable or inhalant, cause less disruption of renal autoregulation of blood flow at lower doses (lighter anesthetic planes). Renal responses to anesthetics also depend on the preexisting hydration status and quantity of perioperative fluids administered, as well as preexisting renal disease.

Anesthesia and the stress associated with surgery can cause release of aldosterone, vasopressin, renin, and catecholamines. Accordingly, RBF and GFR (and therefore urine production) are generally decreased with surgery in any patient. In fact, in the face of appropriate intravenous (IV) fluid administration during (10 mL/kg/h) anesthesia, dogs with normal kidney function will have urine output less than the usual values of 1–2 mL/kg/h of awake animals.[21] Additionally, these dogs will have evidence of fluid retention that resolves over time after anesthesia. It is therefore recommended to use additional parameters rather than just urine output as an indicator of fluid balance and renal function in anesthetized animals.[21]

Effects of renal disease on anesthesia

Renal insufficiency/failure and azotemia in patients with renal insufficiency can alter the individual patient's response to anesthetic medications. Azotemia can alter the blood–brain barrier, leading to increased drug penetration into the central nervous system. Azotemia can also alter the binding of drugs to carrier proteins and receptors, resulting in increased levels of circulating free drug and an increase or decrease in the expected response of the patient to drug administration. Patients with renal insufficiency/failure may be acidotic, which can lead to increased fractions of unbound injectable drugs in the plasma, thus having a similar effect as azotemia. It may be necessary to decrease the doses of highly protein-bound injectable anesthetics in azotemic and/or acidotic patients.

Serum electrolyte imbalance is common in patients with renal disease. Hyperkalemia may be present in animals with renal insufficiency/failure, obstructed urethra, or rupture of the urinary bladder and can be extremely dangerous. In general, patients presenting for nonemergency anesthesia and surgery should not be anesthetized if they have a serum potassium concentration greater than 5.5 mEq/L. Any patient with a serum potassium concentration greater than 6.0 mEq/L should not be anesthetized until the hyperkalemia can be addressed. Electrocardiographic (ECG) abnormalities are commonly observed with potassium concentrations exceeding 7 mEq/L and during the stress of anesthesia patients with renal disease can quickly elevate their serum potassium concentrations. The resting membrane potential of cardiac muscle depends on the permeability and extracellular concentration of potassium. During hyperkalemia, the membrane's resting potential is raised (partially depolarized), and fewer sodium channels are available to participate in the action potential. As the serum potassium concentration increases, repolarization occurs more rapidly and automaticity, conductivity, contractility, and excitability are decreased. These changes produce the classic ECG appearance of a peaked T wave with a prolonged PR interval progressing to wide QRS complexes and loss of P waves. In cases of prolonged renal disease and chronic hyperkalemia, serum potassium should be lowered gradually to allow intracellular potassium time to reestablish physiological transmembrane concentration gradients. If hyperkalemia is acute or ECG abnormalities are noted, treatment should be initiated prior to induction of anesthesia. The most rapid treatment for the cardiac effects associated with hyperkalemia is 10% calcium chloride (0.1 mg/kg IV). Calcium will increase the membrane's threshold potential, resulting in increased myocardial conduction and contractility. Because increased serum potassium concentration causes the resting potential to be less negative (partially depolarized), the calcium ion-induced increase in threshold potential temporarily restores the normal gradient between resting and threshold potentials. It should be recognized that administration of calcium will not affect the serum potassium concentration, and its effects will therefore be short lived. Regimens to decrease the serum potassium concentration by shifting potassium intracellularly include infusion of 2.5–5% dextrose solutions and, in severe cases, addition of insulin to the dextrose. Often, acidosis is associated with the concurrent increase in serum potassium. Sodium bicarbonate can be administered to enhance hydrogen ion exchange with intracellular potassium. Additionally, during anesthesia, because acidemia favors extracellular movement of potassium and worsens hyperkalemia, intermittent positive pressure ventilation may be required to prevent anesthetic-induced hypercapnia and respiratory acidosis. Patients in renal failure with hypocalcemia are at even greater risk of the arrhythmic effects of hyperkalemia, because hypocalcemia potentiates the myocardial toxicity of hyperkalemia.

Anesthetic management of patients with renal disease

Patients with suspected or known renal disease should have a thorough workup prior to any anesthetic event. This should include a physical exam, complete blood count, serum biochemical profile, and urinalysis. Measurements of the GFR and renal tubular function, such as urine specific gravity and BUN, are not specific for renal disease. Serum creatinine is a more specific indicator of the GFR than BUN because it is influenced by fewer extrarenal variables. Patients with mild renal insufficiency may not have elevated serum creatinine, thus it is important to carefully evaluate other parameters that can be affected. In addition to azotemia, effects of renal system dysfunction can manifest as abnormalities in acid–base balance, electrolyte concentrations (especially potassium), exercise intolerance, hematocrit, hydration status, and urine production. Persistent proteinuria and/or cellular or granular cylinduria may indicate renal damage prior to the onset of renal azotemia.

Preanesthetic stabilization of patients with renal disease may be more critical to a successful outcome than the specific anesthetic drugs selected. By and large, the most important parameter for a patient with renal disease is hydration status and circulating blood volume. Maintaining RBF and GFR through adequate hydration will reduce the likelihood of further renal injury and preserve renal function.[22] Hydration has been shown to be effective in the treatment of renal injury and is a good strategy to prevent the progression of renal insufficiency to frank renal failure.[22] A patient can be admitted 12–24 hours prior to anesthesia and administered IV fluids to achieve hydration and diuresis. When renal function is questioned, the urinary bladder can be catheterized and urine production monitored via a closed, sterile urine collection system. Urine production is an indirect measure of renal perfusion, and normal urine output for awake dogs is 0.5–2.0 mL/kg/h. Animals administered high rates of IV fluids should have urine outputs similar to the amount of fluids administered. Fluid therapy prior to anesthesia can also be used to correct electrolyte and acid–base imbalances. Anemic patients undergoing anesthesia should have a red blood cell transfusion if the hematocrit is less than 18% (cats) or 20% (dogs).

Once the patient is stabilized, anesthesia can be performed. Anesthetic and analgesic drugs that have minimal effects on cardiac output, blood pressure, and perfusion are recommended.[7] Premedication can be achieved with an opioid/benzodiazepine combination and induction of anesthesia can be accomplished with propofol, thiopental, etomidate, diazepam–ketamine, or diazepam–opioid combinations (Table 14.2). It is important to remember that all of these anesthetic drugs can cause some degree of reduced RBF and/or GFR and that using these drugs to effect is recommended. Anesthesia can be maintained with either isoflurane or sevoflurane.

Continuing IV fluid therapy throughout the anesthetic period is recommended to maintain fluid volume and hydration. Initially, a rate of up to 20 mL/kg for the first hour

Table 14.2. Example of an anesthetic plan for patients with renal disease

Premedication:		
Opioid of choice		
Butorphanol	0.2–0.4 mg/kg	Intramuscular
Hydromorphone	0.1 mg/kg	Intramuscular
Morphine	0.1 mg/kg (cats)	Intramuscular
	0.25 mg/kg (dogs)	Intramuscular
Midazolam[a]	0.2–0.4 mg/kg	Intramuscular
Induction:		
Propofol	4 mg/kg (to effect)	IV
Etomidate	2 mg/kg (to effect)	IV
Maintenance:		
Isoflurane	1–2% (to effect)	Inhalation
Sevoflurane	2–3% (to effect)	Inhalation
Supportive treatments:		
Lactated Ringer's solution	10–20 mL/kg for first hour, 10 mL/kg/h thereafter	
Mannitol (20% solution)	Loading dose 500 mg/kg IV	
	Infusion 1 mg/kg/min	

[a] In healthy cats, midazolam may elicit aggressive behavior and can be removed from plan.

can be provided and thereafter a rate of 10/mL/kg/h can be used. Lower fluid rates can be used if the patient has hypoproteinemia, severe anemia, or cardiovascular disease. The choice of IV fluid is based on the animal's electrolyte and acid–base status. In general, animals with mild to moderate renal insufficiency/failure that are well prepared for surgery or anesthesia are given lactated Ringer's solution. If there is potential for urinary tract obstruction or the patient is anuric, IV fluids should be used cautiously to prevent fluid overload until the obstruction can be addressed.

Vigilant monitoring of a patient's vital signs will help the anesthetist to identify hypotension, arrhythmias, hypoxemia, or hypoventilation that could negatively impact renal function. Continuous electrocardiography (ECG) can detect changes in cardiac electrical activity that can be associated with electrolyte abnormalities such as hyperkalemia. ABP should be measured to detect systemic hypotension and decreased renal perfusion pressure. Mean ABP should be maintained above 70–80 mm Hg, and in some cases higher if preanesthetic hypertension was present. Pulse oximetry (SpO_2) can be used to rapidly detect hemoglobin desaturation and alert the anesthetist to the potential for a decrease in tissue oxygen delivery. Continuous end-tidal carbon dioxide ($ETCO_2$) measurement can be used to detect hypoventilation and the need for assisted ventilation. Excessive arterial carbon dioxide can lead to acidemia, which can worsen renal disease. Periodic arterial blood gas analysis can be useful for following trends in pH, oxygen content, and electrolytes. Finally, central venous pressure (CVP) can be measured via a jugular catheter as an indirect measurement of blood volume to evaluate the rate of IV fluid administration. Normal CVP should be between 3 and 5 cm H_2O. If the CVP rises to more than 10 cm H_2O, fluid administration should be slowed or stopped. If the CVP falls in response to the fluids being stopped, they may be resumed at a slower rate. An elevated CVP of more than 10 cm H_2O suggests inadequate myocardial function or volume overload.

Adjunctive treatments for patients with renal disease

During the perianesthetic period, pharmacological manipulation of cardiovascular and renal physiology may be beneficial in renal disease patients. Dopamine infusions (1–10 mcg/kg/min) have long been considered useful in improving myocardial function and cardiac output. In human patients with renal disease, renal doses of dopamine (2 mcg/kg/min) have been shown to increase urinary output but does not improve overall outcome when compared to IV fluid therapy.[23] In dogs, low doses (1–3 mcg/kg/min) are used to promote RBF and GFR, but studies showing benefit are lacking. Controversy exists as to the use of dopamine to improve renal function in cats. Questions remain as to whether or not cats have appropriate dopamine receptors in their kidneys and low-dose dopamine has not been shown to have a diuretic effect in cats.[24] Doses of dopamine above approximately 10 mcg/kg/min may cause α-adrenergic renal vasoconstriction and decreased RBF and should be avoided.

Furosemide has also been investigated as to its use during anesthesia in patients with renal dysfunction. As a loop diuretic, furosemide decreases the metabolic activity of the renal tubules; however, furosemide infusion has been shown to result in elevated creatinine levels in anesthetized human patients and its use is not recommended.[23,25]

The osmotic diuretic mannitol has many potentially beneficial effects on the kidney. Mannitol is freely filtered and non-reabsorbed by the kidney and therefore acts as an osmotic agent in the renal tubules as well as in the systemic circulation. Administration of mannitol can induce renal arteriole dilation, decrease vascular resistance and blood viscosity, and scavenge oxygen free radicals.[26] RBF in cats may be improved by administering an IV loading dose of mannitol (500 mg/kg) and continuing a constant rate infusion (1 mg/kg/min) during the anesthetic period.[27] The author uses mannitol infusions in both cats and dogs with known or suspected renal impairment during anesthesia.

Fenoldopam is a dopamine receptor agonist at the DA_1 receptor that has renal vasodilating properties. Fenoldopam has no effect on DA_2 or alpha receptors that can cause vasoconstriction and result in decreased RBF and GFR. In fact, fenoldopam increases RBF and may assist in preserving renal function. Fenoldopam has been shown to decrease creatinine and improve renal function at a dose of 0.1 mcg/kg/min when compared to dopamine infusion and may be effective in decreasing renal hypoperfusion.[28]

Postanesthetic care of any patient that has had a procedure associated with a painful condition should be treated with analgesic medications. In renal patients, analgesic drugs, including nonsteroidal anti-inflammatory drugs (NSAIDs), that are potentially nephrotoxic should be avoided. Pain can usually be managed with opioid analgesics.

Management of patients with post-renal disease

Patients with urethral obstruction often present with metabolic derangements. These include hyperkalemia, azotemia, acidosis, and hyperphosphatemia. Cats may also develop hyperglycemia, hypocalcemia, and hyponatremia. If the disease condition included rupture of the urinary bladder, the animal may develop more severe electrolyte abnormalities and acidosis. In these cases, potassium enters the abdominal cavity from the ruptured bladder and is reabsorbed into the circulation, causing an increased serum potassium concentration. It is important to recognize that acute urethral obstruction and ruptured bladder are medical emergencies and that any metabolic abnormalities should be evaluated and addressed prior to anesthesia and surgical correction. Hyperkalemia is the primary concern in most cases of urethral obstruction, and an electrocardiogram assessment is warranted. Treatment of hyperkalemia has been discussed earlier.

In animals with urethral obstruction, fine-needle centesis of the urinary bladder may be performed prior to anesthesia, although bladder injury is a potential concern. In animals with uroperitoneum, abdominocentesis can be performed. Removal of urine can help reduce the potassium load and relieve patient discomfort. Once the patient is stabilized, anesthesia can be induced by the previously described techniques. IV ketamine with a benzodiazepine has been used in obstructed cats even though active metabolites of the drug are excreted by the kidney. The rationale is that, once the obstruction is relieved, excretion of the anesthetic will proceed normally. However, cats with a long-term urethral obstruction may develop metabolic disturbances and renal insufficiency such that elimination of drugs is slowed even after the obstruction has been removed. As with other patients with renal disease, IV fluid therapy should be continued throughout the anesthetic period and into the postanesthetic period until ongoing acid–base and electrolyte disturbances are corrected.

Revised from "Renal Disease" by Stephen A. Greene and Gregory F. Grauer in Lumb and Jones' Veterinary Anesthesia and Analgesia, **Fourth Edition.**

References

1. Boyd L.M., Langston C., Thompson K., et al. Survival in cats with naturally occurring chronic kidney disease (2000–2002). *J Vet Intern Med* **22**: 1111–1117, 2008.
2. Polzin D.J., Osborne C.A., Jacob F., et al. Chronic renal failure. In: *Textbook of Veterinary Internal Medicine*, 5th ed. S.J. Ettinger and E.C. Feldman, eds. Philadelphia, PA: W.B. Saunders Company, 2000, pp 1634–1662.
3. Brezis M., Rosen S. Hypoxia of the renal medulla: its implications for disease. *N Engl J Med* **332**(10): 647–655, 1995.
4. Stoelting R.K., Hillier S.C. Kidneys. In: *Pharmacology & Physiology in Anesthetic Practice*, 4th ed. Philadelphia, PA: Lippincott Williams & Wilkins, 2006, pp 817–830.
5. Thadhani R., Pascual M., Bonventre J.V. Acute renal failure. *N Engl J Med* **334**: 1448–1460, 1996.
6. Bostrom I., Nyman G., Kampa N., et al. Effects of acepromazine on renal function in anesthetized dogs. *Am J Vet Res* **64**(5): 590–598, 2003.
7. Weil A.B. Anesthesia for patients with renal/hepatic disease. *Top Companion Anim Med* **25**(2): 87–91, 2010.
8. Lamont L.A., Mathews K.A. Opioids, nonsteroidal anti-inflammatories, and analgesic adjuvants. In: *Lumb & Jones' Veterinary Anesthesia and Analgesia*, 4th ed. W.J. Tranquilli, J.C. Thurmon, and K.A. Grimm, eds. Ames, IA: Blackwell Publishing, 2007, pp 241–271.
9. Saleh N., Aoki M., Shimada T., et al. Renal effects of medetomidine in isoflurane-anesthetized dogs with special reference to its diuretic action. *J Vet Med Sci* **67**(5): 461–465, 2005.

10. Priano L.L. Alteration of renal hemodynamics by thiopental, diazepam, and ketamine in conscious dogs. *Anesth Analg* **61**(10): 853–862, 1982.
11. Flecknell P.A. Injectable anaesthetics. In: *Anaesthesia of the Cat.* L.W. Hall and P.M. Taylor, eds. London, UK: Bailliere Tindall, 1994, pp 129–156.
12. Wouters P.F., Van de Velde M.A., Marcus M.A., et al. Hemodynamic changes during induction of anesthesia with eltanolone and propofol in dogs. *Anesth Analg* **81**(1): 125–131, 1995.
13. Shiga Y., Minami K., Uezono Y., et al. Effects of the intravenously administered anaesthetics ketamine, propofol, and thiamylal on the cortical renal blood flow in rats. *Pharmacology* **68**(1): 17–23, 2003.
14. Petersen J.S., Shalmi M., Christensen S., et al. Comparison of the renal effects of six sedating agents in rats. *Physiol Behav* **60**(3): 759–765, 1996.
15. Gelman S., Fowler K.C., Smith L.R. Regional blood flow during isoflurane and halothane anesthesia. *Anesth Analg* **63**(6): 557–565, 1984.
16. Bernard J.M., Doursout M.F., Wouters P., et al. Effects of sevoflurane and soflurane on hepatic circulation in the chronically instrumented dog. *Anesthesiology* **77**(3): 541–545, 1992.
17. Conzen P.F., Kharasch E.D., Czerner S.F.A., et al. Low-flow sevoflurane compared with low-flow isoflurane anesthesia in patients with stable renal insufficiency. *Anesthesiology* **97**: 578–584, 2002.
18. Sun L., Suzuki Y., Takata M., et al. Repeated low-flow sevoflurane anesthesia: effects on hepatic and renal function in beagles. *Masui* **46**(3): 351–357, 1997.
19. Merin R.G., Bernard J.M., Doursout M.F., et al. Comparison of the effects of isoflurane and desflurane on cardiovascular dynamics and regional blood flow in the chronically instrumented dog. *Anesthesiology* **74**(3): 568–574, 1991.
20. Hayes M.A., Goldenberg I.S. Renal effects of anesthesia and operation mediated by endocrines. *Anesthesiology* **24**: 487–499, 1963.
21. Boscan P., Pypendop B.H., Siao D.T., et al. Fluid balance, glomerular filtration rate, and urine output in dogs anesthetized for an orthopedic surgical procedure. *AJVR* **71**(5): 501–507, 2010.
22. Wagener G., Brentjens T.E. Anesthetic concerns in patients presenting with renal failure. *Anesthesiol Clin* **28**: 39–54, 2010.
23. Lassnigg A., Donner E., Grubhofer G., et al. Lack of renoprotective effects of dopamine and furosemide during cardiac surgery. *J Am Soc Nephrol* **11**: 97–104, 2000.
24. Wohl J.S., Schwartz D.D., Flournoy S. et al. Renal hemodynamic and diuretic effects of low-dosage dopamine in anesthetized cats. *J Vet Emerg Crit Care* **17**(1): 45–52, 2007.
25. Cowgill L.D., Elliott D.A. Acute renal failure. In: *Textbook of Veterinary Internal Medicine*, 5th ed. S.J. Ettinger and E.C. Feldman, eds. Philadelphia, PA: WB Saunders Co., 2000, pp 1615–1633.
26. Ho K.M., Power B.M. Benefits and risks of furosemide in acute kidney injury. *Anaesthesia* **65**: 283–293, 2010.
27. McClellan J.M., Goldstein R.E., Erb H.N., et al. Effects of administration of fluids and diuretics on glomerular filtration rate, renal blood flow, and urine output in healthy awake cats. *AJVR* **67**(4): 715–722, 2006.
28. Brienza N., Malcangi V., Dalfino L., et al. A comparison between fenoldopam and low-dose dopamine in early renal dysfunction of critically ill patients. *Crit Care Med* **34**(3): 707–714, 2006.

Chapter 15

Anesthesia for patients with liver disease

Fernando Garcia

Anatomy and physiology

The liver has four primary functions: (1) synthesis of proteins, (2) detoxification of waste products, (3) biotransformation of drugs, and (4) storage of glycogen. The liver has a dual blood supply with approximately 70% derived from the hepatic portal vein and the remaining 30% coming from the hepatic artery. It is important to realize that only the hepatic arterial blood is well oxygenated and it is responsible for about 50% of the oxygen delivered to the liver.

Any factor that decreases systemic arterial blood pressure (ABP) and/or cardiac output will result in decreased portal vein flow. In normal, conscious patients this is partially compensated for by increased hepatic arterial flow. In anesthetized animals or animals with liver disease, though, this autoregulatory mechanism is lost and the risk of ischemia is increased.

Total hepatic blood flow is determined by hepatic perfusion pressure (mean arterial or portal venous pressure minus hepatic venous pressure) and splanchnic vascular resistance. Decreases in the former or increases in the latter will reduce hepatic blood flow. Positive pressure ventilation of the lungs, congestive heart failure, and fluid overload can all decrease hepatic perfusion pressure by increasing central venous and hepatic venous pressures. Activation of the sympathetic nervous system due to pain, hypoxemia, or surgical stress will increase splanchnic vascular resistance.

The anesthetist must also be aware that some hepatobiliary diseases have breed predispositions. Portosystemic vascular abnormalities, for example, are common in certain small purebreds, especially Maltese terriers, miniature Schnauzers, and Yorkshire terriers.

Animals with hepatic insufficiency may present with a variety of clinical signs including depression, anorexia, weight loss, icterus, ascites, hepatic encephalopathy (HE), and seizures. However, the liver has a great reserve capacity and these signs may be absent even in the face of significant hepatic disease. Only with exhaustion of hepatic functional reserve do clinical signs become evident. Consequently, a lack of clinical signs cannot be interpreted as absence of hepatic disease.

Essentials of Small Animal Anesthesia and Analgesia, Second Edition. Edited by Kurt A. Grimm, William J. Tranquilli, Leigh A. Lamont.
© 2011 John Wiley & Sons, Inc. Published 2011 by John Wiley & Sons, Inc.

Serum hepatocellular enzyme concentrations, such as alanine aminotransferase (ALT), aspartate aminotransferase (AST), alkaline phosphatase (ALP), and γ-glutamyl transpeptidase (GGT) are commonly elevated with hepatobiliary disease. Elevation of these enzymes, although highly sensitive to hepatic damage, is not specific to liver insufficiency or even primary liver disease. Also, in chronic liver disease where hepatic tissue can be largely replaced by fibrosis, liver enzymes might be normal or only slightly elevated. Substrate metabolism tests such as pre- and postprandial bile acids or the elimination of indocyanine green are better indicators of hepatic function. Low serum values of albumin, glucose, and urea nitrogen are usually present in liver dysfunction but are not pathognomonic for liver disease.

A large array of coagulation proteins are produced by the liver and can also be diminished. A coagulation profile should be performed to aid in prediction of possible surgical complications in all patients that have suspected coagulopathy or hepatopathy. Blood typing and plasma and blood crossmatching are recommended before anesthesia if the coagulation profile is abnormal or if liver surgery is planned. Prolongation of prothrombin time (PT) and activated partial thromboplastin time (aPTT) do not necessarily give a diagnosis of active hemorrhage unless clinical signs such as anemia, petechiation, and prolonged bleeding from venous puncture are also present. Fresh frozen plasma can be used to supplement coagulation factors in these patients. Whole blood can be used; however, it should be reserved for anemic patients.

The liver synthesizes several plasma proteins and detoxifies ammonia, the major byproduct of protein metabolism. Albumin is exclusively produced in the liver. Because the liver normally produces albumin at only a third of its capacity, hypoalbuminemia is seen only in severe cases of hepatic disease and portosystemic shunting. Glomerular disease, protein-losing enteropathies, and hemorrhage are other nonhepatic causes of hypoalbuminemia to consider. Albumin is of great importance in the equilibrium of Starling forces due to exertion of colloidal osmotic pressure in the vascular bed. Also, albumin is a common binding site for anesthetic drugs, and therefore alterations in its plasma concentration can, in theory, affect the volume of distribution and half-life elimination of these drugs.

The liver plays an important role in glucose homeostasis. Patients with portosystemic shunts or acute hepatic failure are often hypoglycemic. Mechanisms of hypoglycemia in hepatic dysfunction include one or a combination of the following: decreased gluconeogenesis, decreased glycogen stores, and diminished response to glucagon. Monitoring and maintenance of normoglycemia should be a priority during anesthesia. Dextrose solutions (1–5%) can be given in combination with other isotonic crystalloids during surgery as needed to maintain normoglycemia. During anesthesia, fluid therapy is indicated to counteract relative hypovolemia secondary to anesthetic-induced vasodilation and to replenish fluid losses associated with respiration and surgical exposure of tissues. The use of hypotonic fluids (such as 5% dextrose) alone is not appropriate for this purpose, as they will precipitate a shift in free water from the plasma to the interstitium after rapid breakdown of the dextrose molecule. Consequently, an isotonic crystalloid with or without a colloid is recommended for intraoperative fluid therapy.

Drugs and the liver

Sedatives

Animals with primary liver disease that require anesthesia are often obtunded to some degree. Therefore, most patients require minimal sedation depending on the procedure to be performed. Frequently, the administration of an opioid is enough to provide adequate sedation. Hydromorphone, oxymorphone, and methadone are full agonist opioids that provide good sedation and analgesia for diagnostic or surgical treatments in patients with hepatic disease. Compared to morphine, they present some potential advantages as they are not associated with elevations in plasma histamine concentrations and decreased blood pressure after intravenous administration.[1-3] A decrease in systemic vascular resistance could possibly translate into a decrease in hepatic blood flow and subsequently decreased drug elimination capacity.[4] Opioids with short elimination half-lives such as fentanyl and remifentanil can also be used as constant rate infusions in these patients. Care should be taken, however, because the context-sensitive half-life of most opioids used in constant rate infusions will be longer compared to normal patients.[5] Remifentanil is unique in that it is metabolized by plasma esterases and shows no accumulation after constant rate infusion in humans.[6]

Most of the drugs used for their sedative properties in veterinary medicine can be categorized into one of three groups: phenothiazines, benzodiazepines, and alpha$_2$ adrenergic agonists. Acepromazine is the most commonly used phenothiazine and has sedative and anxiolytic effects in dogs and cats. Acepromazine is not always contraindicated in patients with liver disease but judicious assessment of the patient is necessary. Acepromazine causes vasodilation due to its antagonistic effect at alpha adrenergic receptors.[7,8] Although acepromazine vasodilation may be beneficial to increase renal blood flow in anesthetized dogs, data are not available regarding its effects on hepatic blood flow.[9] When a patient is hypoalbuminemic, intravascular colloidal osmotic pressure is diminished and hypovolemia and hypotension can be present even before sedation. In these cases, a combination of colloid (e.g., Hetastarch) and crystalloid fluid therapy may be necessary if acepromazine is to be used. Also, acepromazine in combination with atropine is known to affect platelet aggregation in dogs for a couple of hours after administration and should be avoided if coagulation abnormalities are present.[10]

Advanced liver disease may result in HE due to accumulation of ammonium, mercaptans, and endogenous benzodiazepinic compounds.[11,12] In humans, the benzodiazepine antagonist flumazenil is often used to minimize clinical signs associated with HE.[13] The use of benzodiazepines in veterinary patients presenting with HE is controversial, as these patients may exhibit increased sensitivity to these drugs, resulting in aggravation of HE.[14] However, in the absence of HE, benzodiazepines can be used safely in patients with liver disease. Sedation is generally obtained with a combination of diazepam or midazolam and an opioid. Unwanted effects can be reversed by flumazenil. In human patients, increased sensitivity to benzodiazepines and prolongation of effect is possible,[15,16] so conservative dosing may be prudent in dogs and cats with liver disease.

Dexmedetomidine provides excellent sedative and analgesic effects yet may be associated with significant cardiovascular depression characterized by decreases in cardiac output of up to 50%.[17,18] Despite this, hepatic blood flow is unchanged in normal dogs after intravenous administration of up to 10 mcg/kg based on the radioactive microsphere method.[19] While it appears that hepatic blood flow is reasonably well preserved during sedation with medetomidine or dexmedetomidine, these drugs have also been shown to decrease hepatic enzyme activity *in vitro*. In this regard, though, it is likely that their sparing effects on doses of other anesthetic agents may be more clinically relevant than any direct effects on liver metabolic capacity.[20] In some cases, alpha$_2$ agonist administration may cause excessive sedation and central nervous system depression in an animal that is already obtunded as a result of hepatic disease; however, reversal with specific antagonists could be a major advantage. Sedative selection should be based on anticipated sedation requirements.

Analgesics

Opioids are the mainstay of analgesia during anesthesia and most induce few adverse cardiovascular effects. However, both morphine and meperidine are associated with significant release of histamine when given rapidly intravenously.[1–3] Histamine release may cause hypotension and therefore reduce hepatic blood flow. In humans, morphine also causes spasm of the common bile duct by constriction of the sphincter of Oddi, which increases the size and pressure in the gallbladder. This effect has not been demonstrated or observed in veterinary medicine.[21]

Most opioids are biotransformed in the liver by oxidation or glucuronidation, and some are converted into active metabolites. Since patients with liver dysfunction may take longer to metabolize these drugs, their effects could last significantly longer than in a healthy patient.[22,23] Frequent assessments of analgesia are required to determine appropriate administration intervals. Sufentanil, alfentanil, fentanyl, and remifentanil are short-acting opioids with pharmacokinetics that are minimally affected by liver disease.[22,24] Remifentanil, in particular, is rapidly hydrolyzed by plasma esterases, resulting in a high clearance and rapid elimination. The context-sensitive half-life seems to be independent of the dose or duration of infusions in human subjects with varying degrees of liver dysfunction.[22,25,26]

Nonsteroidal anti-inflammatory drugs (NSAIDs) are commonly used for acute and chronic pain management in dogs and cats. All NSAIDs have the potential to cause hepatic injury, either intrinsically (as is usually the case with aspirin and acetaminophen) or idiosyncratically (as tends to be the case with other NSAIDs, including the COX-2 selective agents). Idiosyncratic toxic reactions are rare, unpredictable, and not related to dose. Though carprofen was initially thought to be unique in its propensity to cause acute, idiosyncratic hepatotoxicosis, any NSAID has this potential. Clinical signs include inappetence, vomiting, and icterus associated with elevations in serum hepatic enzymes and bilirubin. Any unexplained increase in these biochemical parameters after initiation of NSAID therapy should be investigated. Since there have been no large-scale prospective studies to evaluate the effects of NSAIDs on hepatic structure and function in animals with preexisting liver disease, it is unknown whether or not this practice is safe.

In addition, NSAIDs may also impair coagulation by affecting platelet aggregation and clot formation. In dogs with osteoarthritis, platelet aggregation decreased after aspirin or carprofen administration while it did not change after meloxicam or deracoxib.

Thromboelastography testing in these dogs showed decreased clot strength after carprofen but increased strength after deracoxib.[27] Due to the potential for adverse effects, the administration of NSAIDs to patients with hepatic dysfunction, especially those with coagulopathies, should be avoided or very closely monitored.

Injectable anesthetics

While there are numerous studies evaluating the effects of inhalant anesthetics on hepatic function and blood flow, there are relatively few regarding the impact of injectable anesthetics. Studies comparing the effects of ketamine, thiopental, and etomidate on canine hepatic blood flow suggest ketamine causes a more modest decrease in comparison to the others.[28,29] Propofol has been shown to maintain hepatic blood flow via arterial vasodilation in dogs and thiopental appears to have similar effects.[30,31]

As a general rule, most agents have minimal effects on hepatic blood flow if systemic ABP is maintained within normal limits. Propofol is a phenolic compound in an aqueous emulsion that provides rapid onset of action and short emergence times due to its rapid redistribution and elimination. Propofol clearance exceeds hepatic blood flow, suggesting an extrahepatic site of metabolism and making it a good choice for patients with liver disease.[32] Caution is warranted, however, due to its cardiovascular depressant and systemic vasodilatory effects.[33]

Thiopental is an ultrashort-acting barbiturate with a very quick onset of effect. It is heavily metabolized by the liver, has several active metabolites, and its administration results in increased liver enzyme activity.[34,35] Although termination of its anesthetic effects results from redistribution to nontarget tissues, suggesting it may be acceptable to use as a single bolus for induction, it is probably best avoided to minimize the metabolic load placed on the liver.

Etomidate has been shown to cause minimal cardiovascular effects when compared to propofol in canine anesthetic inductions.[33] Etomidate is an imidazole compound in a propylene glycol-based vehicle. Propylene glycol is a hyperosmolar molecule and may cause erythrocyte rupture.[36] Because some patients presenting with hepatobiliary disease may have bilirubinemia and icterus due to biliary obstruction or decreased hepatic conjugation, the hemolysis caused by etomidate could potentially further overload the liver. While hemolysis does not appear to be significant in normal dogs after a single bolus,[37] the clinical consequences in animals with liver disease have not been studied. Overall, etomidate seems to be a good induction agent for the liver patient due to its minimal cardiovascular effects, which preserve systemic and hepatic blood flow.

Dissociative anesthetics such as ketamine and tiletamine (Telazol®, Pfizer Animal Health, New York) are reasonable choices for induction of anesthesia in patients with hepatic disease. However, the coadministration of a benzodiazepine may result in prolonged effects in animals with impaired hepatic function. In dogs and cats, dissociative anesthetics are largely metabolized by the liver but, if used for induction only, the termination of effect will be fairly quick due to redistribution of the drug to muscle and fat.[38] Dissociative anesthetics decrease the seizure threshold in dogs and cats and may promote seizure activity. They should be avoided in animals with a recent history of seizures or HE.

Inhalants

Hepatic blood flow is variably affected by inhalant anesthetics. In general, inhalants impair autoregulatory mechanisms (i.e., increased hepatic arterial flow in response to decreased portal venous flow) that would otherwise maintain total hepatic blood flow. Studies have shown that isoflurane, sevoflurane, and desflurane better maintain total hepatic blood flow, oxygen supply, and delivery/consumption ratios compared to halothane or enflurane.[39] While sevoflurane and desflurane appear to have the least effect on hepatic blood flow,[40] it is important to note that, among the commonly used agents (isoflurane, sevoflurane, and desflurane), the effect is dose dependent. Consequently, efforts to reduce the dose administered will have a significantly greater impact than choice of anesthetic per se.

Neuromuscular blockers

The disposition of neuromuscular blocking drugs (NMBs) may be affected by liver disease. Vecuronium, rocuronium, and mivacurium all have increased volumes of distribution, prolonged elimination half-lives, and prolonged durations of effect.[41–43] Atracurium and cisatracurium undergo liver-independent elimination (by nonspecific ester hydrolysis or Hofmann elimination) and have similar pharmacokinetics and pharmacodynamics in both healthy and liver-diseased patients.[44–46]

Anesthesia for specific procedures

Liver disease can have a significant impact on drug pharmacokinetics and pharmacodynamics depending on which hepatic functions are altered and the degree of insufficiency. Alterations in protein binding due to decreased production of binding proteins (e.g., albumin and alpha$_1$ acid glycoprotein) and/or third spacing (e.g., ascites) will alter the volume of distribution and half-life of drugs. Furthermore, the metabolism of these drugs may also be altered by decreased hepatic functional capacity and greater tissue deposition, potentially increasing their duration of action. It is important to realize that hepatic blood flow is a key limiting factor in metabolism, especially for drugs with large extraction ratios. Obviously, decreased functional hepatic mass also plays a role but a drug will only be metabolized if blood carries it to the liver. Consequently, maintenance of normal systemic ABP and vascular volume are important for these patients. The use of colloids in conjunction with crystalloids may be necessary to increase colloidal osmotic pressure in hypoproteinemic animals. Hypoglycemia is commonly seen in hepatic patients and blood glucose should be measured perioperatively and, when necessary, dextrose infused to maintain normoglycemia.

Liver biopsy or excision

Liver biopsies may be necessary to diagnose hepatic disease. Samples can be obtained by ultrasound-guided TruCut needles, laparoscopy, and laparotomy. Also, laparoscopy and laparotomy can be used for the excision of abscesses and neoplasias. Knowledge of the specific implications of each technique can help the anesthetist prevent, anticipate, and resolve possible problems that may emerge during the procedure.

Ultrasound-guided biopsy

TruCut biopsies can sometimes be accomplished with sedation alone. For this technique the patient needs to lie still and not react to puncture. There is a chance that bleeding will occur so the technique is not advisable in animals with coagulopathy. The patient's clinical signs and laboratory results, in addition to its demeanor and mentation, will determine drug and dose selection. Benzodiazepines are often used in critically ill patients due to their minimal cardiovascular effects, rapid elimination, and potential reversibility. Administration of midazolam (0.2–0.5 mg/kg, intramuscularly [IM]) in combination with an opioid is frequently adequate to facilitate ultrasound-guided biopsies in mildly to severely obtunded patients. The opioids most commonly used in these combinations are butorphanol (0.2–0.4 mg/kg), methadone (0.3–0.5 mg/kg), hydromorphone (0.05–0.2 mg/kg), and oxymorphone (0.05–0.2 mg/kg). Although usually unnecessary, flumazenil can be administered to reverse the sedative effects of benzodiazepines. In hepatic insufficiency, opioids often cause more pronounced sedation and side effects than in the healthy patient. For this reason, in the absence of pain, naloxone is administered to improve mentation and ventilation when sedation is no longer required or desirable. Even when only sedated, monitoring of the compromised patient is extremely important. Because of the variable degree of hepatic dysfunction and accompanying changes in pharmacokinetics, drug effects can be unpredictable. Pulse oximetry combined with evaluation of respiratory rate, pulse quality, capillary refill time, and mucous membrane color should be considered minimal monitoring standards during these procedures. ABP monitoring can be helpful to guide the initial choices of crystalloid and/or colloid fluid therapy. Oxygen supplementation may be advisable.

Laparoscopy

Laparoscopy is a less invasive alternative to laparotomy and is commonly used for liver biopsies and staging of liver neoplasia. Besides the obvious possibility of bleeding and difficulty in achieving hemostasis, especially in the presence of coagulopathies, this procedure introduces a new set of problems related to insufflation of gases into the abdomen that must be addressed. The infusion of carbon dioxide to improve visualization will decrease venous return and ventilation. The former is caused by the increase in intra-abdominal pressure by the pneumoperitoneum. The latter is caused by absorption of infused CO_2 in combination with cranial displacement of the diaphragm due to increased abdominal pressure. The compression on the diaphragm will make it more difficult for the spontaneously breathing animal to ventilate and will decrease pulmonary functional residual capacity. The sum of these cardiopulmonary effects will also alter ventilation and perfusion relationships. Therefore, intermittent positive pressure ventilation (IPPV) is required to maintain adequate oxygenation and ventilation. IPPV can be achieved manually or by using a mechanical ventilator. The anesthetist should also monitor the intra-abdominal pressure, which should range from 10 to 16 mm Hg, as this can also significantly affect cardiac output.[47] Monitoring of ABP is important as an indirect predictor of tissue perfusion and assessment of the effect of intra-abdominal pressure on venous return. A reversed Trendelenburg position (i.e., with the head higher than the abdomen) can help to minimize the effect of CO_2 infusion on ventilation. Arterial blood gases are useful to evaluate patient ventilation and oxygenation status. Capnography, although helpful, can be misleading because the difference between end-tidal carbon dioxide ($ETCO_2$) and $PaCO_2$ can be significantly increased by ventilation/perfusion mismatching in some of these patients.

Laparotomy

Laparotomy is the most traditional approach for liver biopsies, abscesses, and neoplasia excisions. Besides concerns already mentioned for hepatic patients in particular, including hypoglycemia, hypoproteinemia, coagulopathies, and decreased drug metabolism, universal complications associated with any general anesthetic episode must also be taken in consideration. Hypothermia and hypoventilation are common in these cases and should be monitored and addressed by appropriate use of active warming devices and IPPV, respectively.

Portosystemic shunts

Portosystemic shunts are defined as anomalous vessels that allow blood flowing from the stomach, intestines, pancreas, and spleen to gain access to the central circulation without first passing through the liver. The blood bypassing the liver allows substances normally metabolized there (e.g., ammonia, mercaptans, short-chain fatty acids, etc.) to accumulate in the systemic circulation. Because blood flow to the liver is decreased, hepatotropic substances are not delivered and the liver fails to develop normally. Therefore, any and all of the key hepatic functions may be decreased as with any other form of liver disease. Portosystemic shunt patients may present with hypoglycemia, hypoalbuminemia, coagulopathies, and altered pharmacokinetics and pharmacodynamics of substances metabolized and excreted by the liver. HE and seizures may also be seen in these cases. Flumazenil has been used to improve mental status in humans with HE due to the possible involvement of intrinsic benzodiazepine-like compounds in this syndrome. Whether similar improvements occur in veterinary HE patients with flumazenil administration has not been verified.

Interventional radiology

This technique uses fluoroscopy to guide an intravenous catheter to the site where an anomalous vessel joins the systemic circulation. An auto-expandable stent is placed in the caudal vena cava next to the anomaly insertion. This stent will prevent the thrombotic coils deployed into the shunt vessel from becoming lost in the systemic circulation if they dislodge.[48] The challenge for the anesthetist is to ensure complete immobilization of the patient at the critical stage of stent placement. During general anesthesia, an NMB can be administered to facilitate this if mechanical ventilation is available. Atracurium and cisatracurium can be used in boluses or constant rate infusions to maintain paralysis. In some situations, the surgeon may require an inspiratory hold to decrease patient abdominal movement during critical periods (e.g., measuring the anomalous vessel and placement of the stent). Hypothermia is a common problem and the use of a radiolucent heating pad is essential. Monitoring of cardiovascular (ABP and central venous pressure [CVP]) and respiratory parameters (ETCO$_2$ and SpO$_2$) is essential. Invasive ABP monitoring is ideal, but not mandatory, and CVP can be measured by connecting a sterile electronic transducer to the jugular catheter used by the surgeon to place the stent. The CVP will help assess patient blood volume and guide fluid therapy. As in other hepatic patients, colloidal and inotropic support may be needed. The anesthetist should be sure to restore vascular volume with crystalloids and colloids before inotropic administration. Dopamine (3–12 mcg/kg/min) and dobutamine (2–10 mcg/kg/min) are the most commonly used inotropes in veterinary medicine and can be used in these patients. Caution should be used as these drugs can cause cardiac arrhythmias.

Neuromuscular blockade should be terminated as soon as it is no longer necessary. Patients should be monitored for re-curarization. Reversal of nondepolarizing NMBs with an acetylcholinesterase inhibitor (e.g., neostigmine) is indicated even though spontaneous ventilatory efforts may be observed.

Laparotomy

All of the same concerns described for liver biopsies apply here. In addition, hemorrhage is a potential risk especially during intrahepatic shunt repair. Decreases in venous return should be monitored by the anesthetist (using CVP or by evaluating the character of the ABP waveform), as inadvertent compression of the abdominal vena cava by the surgeon is possible. Effective communication between the anesthetist and surgeon is extremely important.

Revised from "Hepatic Disease" by Stephen A. Greene and Steven L. Marks in Lumb and Jones' Veterinary Anesthesia and Analgesia, Fourth Edition.

References

1. Guedes A.G., Papich M.G., Rude E.P., et al. Comparison of plasma histamine levels after intravenous administration of hydromorphone and morphine in dogs. *J Vet Pharmacol Ther* **30**(6): 516–522, 2007.
2. Robinson E.P., Faggella A.M., Henry D.P., et al. Comparison of histamine release induced by morphine and oxymorphone administration in dogs. *Am J Vet Res* **49**(10): 1699–1701, 1988.
3. Thompson W.L., Walton R.P. Elevation of plasma histamine levels in the dog following administration of muscle relaxants, opiates and macromolecular polymers. *J Pharmacol Exp Ther* **143**: 131–136, 1964.

4. Lagerkranser M., Andreen M., Irestedt L. Central and splanchnic haemodynamics in the dog during controlled hypotension with sodium nitroprusside. *Acta Anaesthesiol Scand* **28**(1): 81–86, 1984.

5. Höhne C., Donaubauer B., Kaisers U. Opioids during anesthesia in liver and renal failure. *Anaesthesist* **53**(3): 291–303, 2004.

6. Dershwitz M., Hoke J.F., Rosow C.E., et al. Pharmacokinetics and pharmacodynamics of remifentanil in volunteer subjects with severe liver disease. *Anesthesiology* **84**(4): 812–820, 1996.

7. Ludders J.W., Reitan J.A., Martucci R., et al. Blood pressure response to phenylephrine infusion in halothane-anesthetized dogs given acetylpromazine maleate. *Am J Vet Res* **44**(6): 996–999, 1983.

8. Hitt M.E., Hanna P., Singh A. Percutaneous transabdominal hepatic needle biopsies in dogs. *Am J Vet Res* **53**(5): 785–787, 1992.

9. Boström I., Nyman G., Kampa N., et al. Effects of acepromazine on renal function in anesthetized dogs. *Am J Vet Res* **64**(5): 590–598, 2003.

10. Barr S.C., Ludders J.W., Looney A.L., et al. Platelet aggregation in dogs after sedation with acepromazine and atropine and during subsequent general anesthesia and surgery. *Am J Vet Res* **53**(11): 2067–2070, 1992.

11. Aronson L.R., Gacad R.C., Kaminsky-Russ K., et al. Endogenous benzodiazepine activity in the peripheral and portal blood of dogs with congenital portosystemic shunts. *Vet Surg* **26**: 189, 1997.

12. Maddison J.E. Newest insights into hepatic encephalopathy. *Eur J Compar Gastroenterol* **5**: 17, 2000.

13. Als-Nielsen B., Gluud L.L., Gluud C. Benzodiazepine receptor antagonists for hepatic encephalopathy. *Cochrane Database Syst Rev* (2): CD002798, 2004.

14. Jones E.A., Yurdaydin C., Basile A.S. The role of endogenous benzodiazepines in hepatic encephalopathy: animal studies. *Alcohol Alcohol Suppl* **2**: 175–180, 1993.

15. Nishiyama T., Hirasaki A., Toda N., et al. Pharmacokinetics of midazolam in patients with liver damage for hepatectomy. *Masui* **42**(6): 871–875, 1993.

16. Bozkurt P., Kaya G., Süzer O., et al. Diazepam serum concentration-sedative effect relationship in patients with liver disease. *Middle East J Anesthesiol* **13**(4): 405–413, 1996.

17. Kuo W.C., Keegan R.D. Comparative cardiovascular, analgesic, and sedative effects of medetomidine, medetomidine-hydromorphone, and medetomidine-butorphanol in dogs. *Am J Vet Res* **65**(7): 931–937, 2004.

18. Flacke W.E., Flacke J.W., Bloor B.C., et al. Effects of dexmedetomidine on systemic and coronary hemodynamics in the anesthetized dog. *J Cardiothorac Vasc Anesth* **7**(1): 41–49, 1993.

19. Lawrence C.J., Prinzen F.W., de Lange S. The effect of dexmedetomidine on nutrient organ blood flow. *Anesth Analg* **83**(6): 1160, 1996.

20. Baratta M.T., Zaya M.J., White J.A., et al. Canine CYP2B11 metabolizes and is inhibited by anesthetic agents often co-administered in dogs. *J Vet Pharmacol Ther* **33**(1): 50–55, 2010.

21. Flancbaum L., Alden S.M., Trooskin S.Z. Use of cholescintigraphy with morphine in critically ill patients with suspected cholecystitis. *Surgery* **106**(4): 668–673; discussion 673–4. 1989.

22. Tegeder I., Lotsch J., Geisslinger G. Pharmacokinetics of opioids in liver disease. *Clin Pharmacokinet* **37**(1): 17–40, 1999.

23. Bower S., Sear J.W., Roy R.C. Effects of different hepatic pathologies on disposition of alfentanil in anesthetized patients. *Br J Anaesth* **68**(5): 462–465, 1992.

24. Chauvin M., Ferrier C., Haberer J.P., et al. Sufentanil pharmacokinetics in patients with cirrhosis. *Anesth Analg* **68**(1): 1–4, 1989.

25. Navapurkar V.U., Archer S., Gupta S.K., et al. Metabolism of remifentanil during liver transplantation. *Br J Anaesth* **81**: 881–886, 1998.

26. Dershwitz M., Hoke J.F., Rosow C.E., et al. Pharmacokinetics and pharmacodynamics of remifentanil in volunteer subjects with severe liver disease. *Anesthesiology* **84**: 812–820, 1996.

27. Brainard B.M., Meredith C.P., Callan M.B., et al. Changes in platelet function, hemostasis, and prostaglandin expression after treatment with nonsteroidal anti-inflammatory drugs with various cyclooxygenase selectivities in dogs. *Am J Vet Res* **68**(3): 251–257, 2007.

28. Thomson I.A., Fitch W., Hughes R.L., et al. Effects of certain I.V. anaesthetics on liver blood flow and hepatic oxygen consumption in the greyhound. *Br J Anaesth* **58**: 69–80, 1986.

29. Thomson I.A., Fitch W., Campbell D., et al. Effects of ketamine on liver blood flow and hepatic oxygen consumption: studies in the anaesthetized greyhound. *Acta Anaesthesiol Scand* **32**: 10–14, 1988.

30. Wouters P.F., Van de Velde M.A., Marcus M.A.E., et al. Hemodynamic changes during induction of anesthesia with eltanolone and propofol in dogs. *Anesth Analg* **81**: 125–131, 1995.

31. Haberer J.P., Audibert G., Saunier C.G., et al. Effect of propofol and thiopentone on regional blood flow in brain and peripheral tissues during normoxia and hypoxia in the dog. *Clin Physiol* **13**(2): 197–207, 1993.

32. Zoran D.L., Riedesel D.H., Dyer D.C. Pharmacokinetics of propofol in mixed breed dogs and greyhounds. *Am J Vet Res* **54**: 755, 1993.

33. Sams L., Braun C., Allman D., et al. A comparison of the effects of propofol and etomidate on the induction of anesthesia and on cardiopulmonary parameters in dogs. *Vet Anaesth Analg* **35**(6): 488–494, 2008.

34. Taylor J.D., Richards R.K., Tabern D.L. Metabolism of S35 thiopental (pentothal): chemical and paper chromatographic studies of S35 excretion by the rat and monkey. *J Pharmacol Exp Ther* **104**: 93, 1952.

35. Sams R.A., Muir W.W. Effects of phenobarbital on thiopental pharmacokinetics in greyhounds. *Am J Vet Res* **49**(2): 245–249, 1988.

36. Nebauer A.E., Doenicke A., Hoernecke R., et al. Does etomidate cause haemolysis? *Br J Anaesth* **69**(1): 58–60, 1992.

37. Ko J.C.H., Thurmon J.C., Benson G.J., et al. Acute haemolysis associated with etomidate-propylene glycol infusion in dogs. *J Vet Anaesth* **20**: 92, 1993.

38. Kaka J.S., Hayton W.L. Pharmacokinetics of ketamine and two metabolites in the dog. *J Pharmacokinet Biopharm* **8**(2): 193–202, 1980.

39. Frink E.J., Morgan S.E., Coetzee A., et al. The effects of sevoflurane, halothane, enflurane, and isoflurane on hepatic blood flow and oxygenation in chronically instrumented greyhound dogs. *Anesthesiology* **76**: 85–90, 1992.

40. Hartman J.C., Pagel P.S., Proctor L.T., et al. Influence of desflurane, isoflurane and halothane on regional tissue perfusion in dogs. *Can J Anaesth* **39**: 877–887, 1992.

41. Van Miert M.M., Eastwood N.B., Boyd A.H., et al. The pharmacokinetics and pharmacodynamics of rocuronium in patients with hepatic cirrhosis. *Br J Pharmacol* **44**(2): 139–144, 1997.

42. Lebrault C., Berger J.L., D'Hollander A.A., et al. Pharmacokinetics and pharmacodynamics of vecuronium (ORG NC 45)in patients with cirrhosis. *Anesthesiology* **62**: 601–605, 1985.

43. Devlin J.C., Head-Rapson A.G., Parker C.J. Pharmacodynamics of mivacurium chloride in patients with hepatic cirrhosis. *Br J Anaesth* **71**: 227–231, 1993.

44. De Wolf A.M., Freeman J.A., Scott V.L., et al. Pharmacokinetics and pharmacodynamics of cisatracurium in patients with end-stage liver disease undergoing liver transplantation. *Br J Anaesth* **76**: 624–628, 1996.

45. Ward S., Neill E.A. Pharmacokinetics of atracurium in acute hepatic failure (with acute renal failure). *Br J Anaesth* **55**: 1169–1172, 1983.
46. Kisor D.F., Schmith V.D. Clinical pharmacokinetic of cisatracurium besylate. *Clin Pharmacokinet* **36**: 27–40, 1999.
47. Mayhew P.D. Advanced Laparoscopic Procedures (Hepatobiliary, Endocrine) in Dogs and Cats. *Vet Clin North Am Small Anim Pract* **39**(5): 925–939, 2009.
48. Bussadori R., Bussadori C., Millán L., et al. Transvenous coil embolisation for the treatment of single congenital portosystemic shunts in six dogs. *Vet J* **176**(2): 221–226. Epub 2007 Apr 26, 2008.

Chapter 16

Anesthesia for patients with gastrointestinal disease

Jennifer G. Adams

Conditions associated with the oral cavity and pharynx

Patients with trauma, swelling and/or edema, or space-occupying masses of the pharynx, oral cavity, and sometimes the head and neck frequently require general anesthesia. These patients are often difficult to intubate to secure and maintain a patent airway. (Figure 16.1) Fractures of the mandible, maxilla, or temporomandibular joint may not permit examination to determine the range motion of the jaw. Masticatory myositis may prevent opening of the mouth even when the patient is anesthetized. Intubation via a tracheostomy may be necessary in these patients. Although lesions of the tongue are usually readily seen, problems at the base of the tongue or in the back of the pharynx may not be realized until the patient is sedated or ready to be intubated. Some patients may not allow any examination of the oral cavity without sedation, so the nature of the problem may be completely unknown. General anesthesia without a secure airway may result in aspiration, which can be fatal. Evaluation of available diagnostic imaging prior to the procedure is valuable to determine the type and severity of the lesions present. These can help determine the extent of difficulty that may be expected with intubation and the potential for airway compromise following extubation. Preparation for placement of a tracheostomy tube should be performed prior to induction in cases where there is high suspicion that oral intubation may not be possible. Preoxygenation using a face mask with the flow meter set at 5 L/min will prolong the time until hypoxemia develops, and should be utilized in all patients in this category.

Intramuscular (IM) or subcutaneous (SC) administration of alpha$_2$ agonists or μ agonist opioids in dogs or cats may cause emesis. Dogs and cats with oral or pharyngeal masses are at high risk for aspiration pneumonia, so the use of medetomidine, dexmedetomidine, morphine, and other drugs that commonly induce emesis should be avoided. In dogs, a combination of IM acepromazine (0.02–0.05 mg/kg) and IM or intravenous (IV) hydromorphone (0.05–0.2 mg/kg) will induce a neuroleptanalgesic state with sufficient muscle relaxation to enable examination of the mouth and jaw. If the animal's laryngeal function or its ability to open its mouth is questionable, IV fentanyl (0.005 mg/kg) should be substituted for hydromorphone because there is a risk of vomiting associated with

Essentials of Small Animal Anesthesia and Analgesia, Second Edition. Edited by Kurt A. Grimm, William J. Tranquilli, Leigh A. Lamont.
© 2011 John Wiley & Sons, Inc. Published 2011 by John Wiley & Sons, Inc.

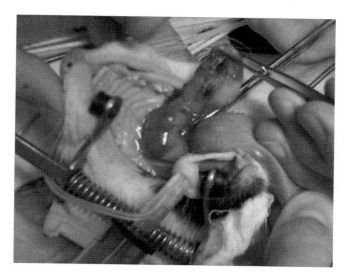

Figure 16.1. Example of a difficult intubation from a large mass that completely obstructed the nasal passages and partially obstructed the pharynx in a cat. Reprinted from Byron J.K., Shadwick S.R., Bennett A.R. 2010. Megaesophagus in a 6-month-old cat secondary to a nasopharyngeal polyp. *J Feline Med Surg*, **12**: 322–324, with permission from Elsevier and Dr. Julie Byron.

hydromorphone administration. Older or debilitated patients may respond well to midazolam (0.2 mg/kg) in combination with butorphanol (0.2–0.3 mg/kg), both given IM or IV. If the patient is amenable, placement of an IV catheter before premedication is useful to allow titration of drugs IV. Premedication with an anticholinergic agent is recommended to avoid opioid-induced bradycardia. An anticholinergic will also decrease salivation, which may be helpful in patients with oral or pharyngeal lesions.

In cats, a low dose of ketamine (4 mg/kg IM) combined with acepromazine (0.05 mg/kg IM) usually enables examination of the oral cavity. An anticholinergic should also be given when ketamine is used to prevent salivation. If an IV catheter is in place, very low doses of propofol (1 mg/kg) or alfaxalone (0.5–1 mg/kg in dogs; 1–2 mg/kg in cats) can be used following premedication in dogs and cats to deepen sedation if needed. When induction agents are used even at low doses, attention to anesthetic depth is paramount, as intubation may be needed in some patients.

Patients with gastrointestinal (GI) disease are at risk for airway compromise (see Table 16.1) and should be observed at all times following premedication and in recovery. Supplies for reintubation should be available in case airway obstruction occurs following extubation. Sedation alone may result in airway compromise, especially when lesions extend into the nasal passage(s). Swelling or edema associated with surgical manipulation or positioning may result in airway compromise that is not apparent until the patient is extubated. Keeping the patient in sternal recumbency and the mouth open in such patients will usually improve the volume of air flow. These patients should remain intubated until conscious, swallowing well, and able to remain in sternal recumbency without assistance. Pulse oximetry is very helpful to evaluate oxygenation in

Table 16.1. Anesthetic concerns/complications during GI procedures

Oral and pharyngeal lesions	Exploratory laparotomy
Regurgitation, aspiration	Hypoventilation
Unknown lesions	Anesthetic drug effects
Airway compromise	Distention of GIT
Tracheostomy	Presence of mass, fluid, blood
Megaesophagus	Hypotension
GER	Anesthetic drug effects
Regurgitation, aspiration	Patient status
Hypothermia	Sepsis, inflammation
Endoscopy	Distention of GIT
Hypoventilation	Presence of masses
Distention of GIT	Manipulation of masses, GIT
Hypothermia	Cardiac arrhythmia
Dislodgement of ET tube	GDV
Pneumothorax	Splenic mass
Pneumomediastinum	Hemorrhage
Pneumoperitoneum	Abdominal mass
Work in dark	Traumatic injury
GER	Hypothermia
Pancreatitis	Exposure of abdominalorgans
Concurrent diseases	Effects of anesthesia on thermoregulation
+/– peritonitis, sepsis	Environment
Very painful	Access to patient can be difficult
Obesity	GER
Preop exam difficult	
Hypoventilation	
Drug levels may vary	
Concurrent disease(s)	

recovery. For comparison, oxygen saturation should be measured in recovery after anesthesia has been discontinued but while the patient is still on oxygen, after the patient has been breathing room air for 5 minutes, and after extubation. Extubation should not be performed unless an $SpO_2 \geq 95\%$ (or a $PaO_2 > 80\,mmHg$) can be maintained. If the patient is breathing well, but remains hypoxemic, oxygen supplementation is necessary. If needed, opioids and benzodiazepenes can be reversed with naloxone or flumazenil, respectively.

Conditions associated with the gastrointestinal tract

Megaesophagus

Megaesophagus is rare in cats but not uncommon in dogs. The most common cause in cats is dysautonomia, an acquired malfunction of the autonomic ganglia that leads to GI dysfunction. Congenital idiopathic megaesophagus is reported in both dogs and a few cats. It is presumed to be caused by a sensory defect in the vagal innervation, such that peristalsis of the esophagus does not occur because dilation from a food bolus is not detected.

Acquired megaesophagus can be caused by mechanical obstruction. Vascular ring anomaly, esophageal stricture, hiatal hernia, tumor, granuloma, and foreign bodies can result in irreversible dilation of the esophagus proximal to the lesion. Idiopathic mega-esophagus is the most common cause of the acquired form in adult dogs, where loss of normal esophageal motility eventually results in esophageal dilation. Some cases of acquired megaesophagus are secondary to or associated with other disease conditions. Peripheral neuropathy, laryngeal paralysis, acquired myasthenia gravis, severe esopha-gitis, and lead poisoning, lupus myositis, and chronic or recurrent gastric dilatation with or without volvulus were associated with an increased risk of megaesophagus in a ret-rospective study of 44 dogs. Hypothyroidism was not associated with megaesophagus in these dogs.[1]

Patients with megaesophagus may be anesthetized for diagnosis or treatment such as endoscopy, electromyography, nerve conduction velocity, muscle and nerve biopsy, computed tomography for mass lesions, bougienage, removal of foreign body or vas-cular ring anomaly, and so on. The megaesophagus may also be a concurrent disease in patients anesthetized for unrelated procedures. Patients with myasthenia gravis may be more sensitive to neuromuscular relaxants. Gastroesophageal reflux (GER), regur-gitation, and aspiration are the primary concerns when anesthetizing patients with megaesophagus. Since the dilation of the esophagus is often tortuous, prolonged fasting is not likely to eliminate all the contents; in fact, increased GER has been seen with long fasting times in normal dogs.[2] Some patients with chronic disease may be thin or debilitated due to malnutrition, and some may be dehydrated if unable to retain ade-quate fluid intake. Many have aspiration pneumonia and will be susceptible to hypox-emia during anesthesia and recovery. Patients with megaesophagus should be stabilized prior to anesthesia with IV fluid therapy and appropriate treatment for pneumonia. A dedicated anesthetist is very important in patients with megaesophagus, as constant monitoring for leakage of esophageal contents into the pharynx is necessary throughout the anesthetic episode and recovery. Sternal recumbency and elevation of the head and neck may decrease the incidence of regurgitation. If regurgitation occurs, the head should be immediately lowered to allow drainage and prevent aspiration. Preoxygen-ation is recommended especially for patients with pneumonia. IV premedication, rapid IV induction, and intubation are necessary to secure a protected airway as quickly as possible. Examination of the pharynx for debris should be performed in recovery prior to extubation. Oxygenation should be evaluated throughout anesthesia and recovery. The patient should be kept intubated as long as possible; extubation should be per-formed with the cuff inflated. Anesthetic drugs should be chosen based on the patient's status with IV premedication preferred. Choices are similar to those for endoscopy as described below.

GI endoscopy

Many procedures for diagnosis and treatment of GI disease are now often performed using flexible or rigid endoscopy. Endoscopy is performed under general anesthesia for a variety of procedures, including examination and/or biopsy of the intestinal lining, biopsy of masses, removal of foreign bodies or polyps, treatment of esophageal strictures

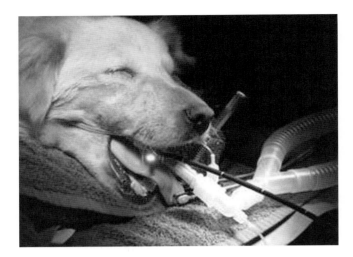

Figure 16.2. Adult dog anesthetized for upper GI endoscopy. Courtesy of Dr. Jeannette Cremer.

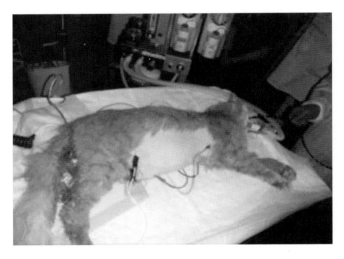

Figure 16.3. Cat anesthetized for endoscopic placement of a feeding tube. Courtesy of Dr. Christina Braun.

with bougienage or balloon dilation, and placement of feeding tubes. Patients are usually in lateral or sternal recumbency so ventilation and access to the patient is better than when in dorsal recumbency (Figures 16.2 and 16.3). Often, the procedure is performed in partial darkness; some sort of light source should be available for the anesthetist. Endoscopic examination involves distention of the gastrointestinal tract (GIT) via the instillation of air so that lesions of the mucosal layer are easily viewed. Distension of the stomach occurs, sometimes significant enough to affect ventilation and venous return to the heart. The distension can also be painful, especially when esophageal strictures are present. Patients anesthetized for bougienage or balloon dilation of the esophagus may require additional analgesic therapy during this part of the procedure.

Gastric distention must be monitored closely; excessive air should be removed as needed. The stomach should be emptied of air at the end of the procedure. Fluid and gastric contents often leak into the oral cavity during endoscopy; the pharynx should be thoroughly examined and cleaned. The security of the endotracheal (ET) tube should be checked regularly, as dislodgement can occur during passage of the endoscope or feeding tube. This can be avoided by marking the tube in some fashion when it is properly positioned so that any slippage can be quickly identified. Using pieces of plastic IV fluid tubing to secure the ET tube during endoscopy may also help avoid dislodgement, since ET tubes slip easily when gauze strips get wet. Supplies for reintubation should be readily available, including extra IV anesthetic, gauze sponges, and long forceps to clean the pharynx. Pneumothorax and/or pneumoperitoneum can result when the esophagus or stomach is distended from tearing or rupture of preexisting pathology or during removal of foreign bodies, and may not be realized until difficulty with ventilation or a fall in cardiac output develops. Pulse oximetry is useful to identify decreasing oxygen saturation that is seen with this complication. The swallowing reflex is difficult to abolish under general anesthesia and can affect retroflex endoscopic examination of lesions in the caudal choanal area of the nasopharynx. Bilateral maxillary nerve block with a short acting local anesthetic such as lidocaine may facilitate retroflex examination with the endoscope.[3]

Patients in good condition can be anesthetized for endoscopy as for most elective procedures. If vomiting is a significant part of the primary disease, drugs that cause emesis such as alpha$_2$ agonists (medetomidine and dexmedetomidine) and the μ agonist opioids hydromorphone or morphine can be avoided in favor of butorphanol. IM administration of acepromazine 15 minutes prior to administration of a μ agonist opioid decreases the incidence of vomiting; however, this antiemetic effect is not 100% reliable.[4] Although most of the commonly used opioids have been used for endoscopy in small animals, a side effect of opioids is increased tension of sphincters in the GIT. Passage of the endoscope through the pyloric sphincter could therefore be affected by the use of opioids. Two studies have looked at this effect of opioids in small animals. Morphine in combination with atropine was associated with some difficulty passing the endoscope into the duodenum in dogs. Glycopyrrolate combined with morphine and either atropine or glycopyrrolate combined with meperidine were not different from saline.[5] Premedication of cats using hydromorphone, hydromorphone and glycopyrrolate, medetomidine, or butorphanol administered IM did not interfere with passage of the endoscope.[6] It is not known if hydromorphone in dogs could interfere with endoscopy; however, reversal can be accomplished with butorphanol or naloxone if needed. Buprenorphine has a long duration and is difficult to reverse and has not been studied; its effects on endoscopy are unknown. Induction drugs should be chosen based on patient status; halothane, isoflurane, or sevoflurane are suitable for endoscopy. Nitrous oxide should not be used for endoscopy since it diffuses readily into the intestinal lumen; it would cause further GI distention and pollution of the environment.

Patients that require endoscopy for intestinal biopsy, esophageal stricture, or feeding tube placement may be quite debilitated and/or hypoproteinemic (Figure 16.4). They are

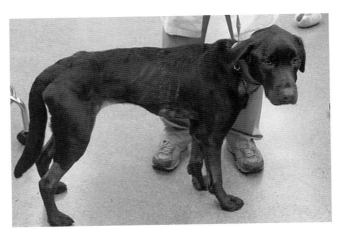

Figure 16.4. Debilitated dog with an esophagitis and stricture following a previous exploratory laparotomy to be anesthetized for bougienage of the esophagus. Courtesy of Jennifer Adams, DVM.

often more sensitive to effects of anesthetic drugs because of decreased protein binding and lack of body mass for redistribution of drugs. Combinations of shorter acting, reversible sedatives such as midazolam and butorphanol are useful for debilitated patients requiring endoscopy. Thiopental should be avoided for induction. Propofol or midazolam/ketamine can be used for induction, at lower doses, to effect, for intubation. Isoflurane or sevoflurane are preferred for maintenance. Low infusion rates of a colloid (1–2 mL/kg/h) with no or a very low (<5 mL/kg/h) infusion rate of crystalloid solution to replace standard IV infusion therapy can be helpful to avoid hypotension and hemodilution.

During general anesthesia for esophageal foreign bodies (+/– endoscopy), relaxation of the striated muscular layer of the esophagus may aid in removal of the obstruction with less damage to the mucosal layer. Skeletal muscle relaxation is increased at deeper planes of anesthesia and can be further enhanced by administration of a neuromuscular blocker (NMB). In cats, the proximal two-thirds of the esophagus have a striated muscle layer, whereas in dogs, the entire esophagus contains striated muscle.[7] A depolarizing muscle relaxant such as succinylcholine should not be used since it initially causes contraction of skeletal muscle and results in damage to the esophagus. Administration of a short-acting nondepolarizing NMB agent—for example, atracurium, 0.1–0.2 mg/kg IV—may facilitate endoscopic or surgical access to the foreign body. Administration of NMBs must always be accompanied by tracheal intubation and support of ventilation. Although rare, histamine release may occur following administration of atracurium. Bronchoconstriction and vasodilation may follow, causing hypoxemia and hypotension, respectively. Antihistamine and/or bronchodilator therapy may counteract these effects; however, slow IV administration should prevent or reduce histamine release. Atracurium breaks down spontaneously in the plasma and is metabolized by plasma esterases. The duration of neuromuscular block usually lasts 20–35 minutes but can be extended by alkalosis and hypothermia, which slow the elimination of the drug.

Anesthetic considerations for colonoscopy depend primarily on the patient's condition since interference is not expected with the airway, and sphincters are not present in the colon. GI hemorrhage is often a preexisting problem in these patients and some will be anemic. Distention is not generally as severe as that seen in upper GI endoscopy, but can sometimes cause discomfort. Excessive hemorrhage and colonic perforation have been reported, but are rare complications of colonoscopy.[8] Some patients will be subjected to both upper and lower GI endoscopy; considerations as described above will apply to these patients as well.

Exploratory laparotomy

Exploratory laparotomy (EL) always requires general anesthesia with variable levels of anesthetic management depending on the specific problem and the patient status. It is both a diagnostic and therapeutic procedure for many diseases of the GIT, and is one of the most challenging types of cases for both surgeon and anesthetist. The preanesthetic status of these patients varies from healthy with no apparent systemic abnormalities to those with life-threatening conditions. Some problems may not be apparent until a diagnosis is made during surgery. A wide spectrum of potential anesthetic and surgical problems should be anticipated and prepared for prior to anesthesia. General considerations for EL will be discussed first followed by concerns specific to some of the more common disease conditions seen.

Many anesthetic considerations are similar because of the positioning, the surgical techniques utilized, and patient status. Dorsal recumbency is required for an EL, and is associated with several potential anesthetic problems or complications. Ventilation is compromised in dorsal recumbency compared to lateral or sternal since the abdominal organs lie against the diaphragm. This can be further exacerbated when abdominal distention is present from excessive abdominal fluid or hemorrhage, distention of the GIT, or large masses. Hypoventilation can result in hypoxemia, hypercarbia, and inadequate anesthetic depth in some patients. Manual or mechanical ventilation is necessary in these patients. Postoperative pulmonary complications are common in patients who have undergone a laparotomy, especially when vomiting, regurgitation, or peritonitis is present. Mortality is greater in patients that develop pulmonary complications.[9] Hypotension is more common in dorsal recumbency than sternal or lateral, and can be exacerbated by the patient's status, positive pressure ventilation, and surgical manipulation of abdominal organs or masses. Rolling into dorsal recumbency can result in a precipitous drop in blood pressure, especially in large dogs and when abdominal distention is present. Clinical signs of anesthetic depth and blood pressure should be checked immediately upon repositioning and again within a few minutes to detect hypotension. Intravascular access and anesthetic monitoring is more difficult once patients are positioned in dorsal recumbency. Placement of an extra peripheral venous catheter or a central venous catheter in some cases prior to or following induction should be considered in those patients where numerous IV therapies may be required. (Figure 16.5) Monitoring equipment should be secured carefully to the patient and all wires, probes, and tubing should be safely positioned before the surgical drapes are applied. Access to the mucous membranes and the eyes for monitoring of anesthetic depth should be ensured. Exposure of abdominal organs, in addition to thermoregulatory dysfunction, is caused by anesthetic drugs. Prolonged recovery, cardiac arrhythmia, and

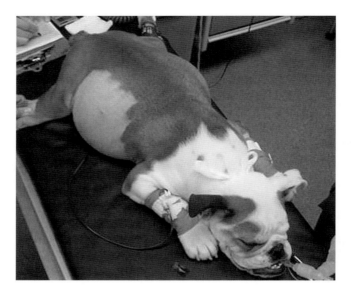

Figure 16.5. Bulldog with abdominal distention caused by a large splenic mass following induction of anesthesia. He is receiving a blood transfusion during preparation for an EL to remove the mass. Courtesy of Jennifer Adams, DVM.

increased incidence of wound infection are associated with significant hypothermia. GER is seen more often in intra-abdominal procedures.[10] Surprisingly, the incidence of GER has not been associated with positioning, in spite of the finding that the lower esophageal pressure was decreased in dorsal recumbency versus other positions. As previously mentioned, GER increases the risk of aspiration pneumonia, postanesthetic esophagitis, and esophageal stricture.[10,11] During anesthesia, the head should be positioned to direct drainage of reflux fluid away from the head while still allowing access to the eyes for monitoring. The pharynx should be examined and cleared of any reflux fluid or debris prior to recovery. Lavage of the distal esophagus with tap water and instillation of dilute bicarbonate following lavage has been suggested for patients with extensive regurgitation; however, this may not always prevent repeat episodes of GER or the development of esophagitis and/or esophageal stricture.[12] Prophylactic therapy with antacids and prokinetic agents is not always successful in prevention of GER and esophagitis. However, a recent study showed that the incidence of GER was decreased in patients given omeprazole 4 hours prior to anesthesia.[13] In recovery, patients with GER should be positioned in sternal recumbency with the head elevated and supported and should not be extubated until a vigorous swallow reflex is present. The ET tube should be removed with the cuff still partially inflated to help remove any gastric contents that may be present in the proximal trachea. Signs of esophageal dysfunction postoperatively include coughing, salivation, dysphagia, difficulty swallowing, and retching, regurgitation, vomiting, and/or anorexia in spite of continued interest in food, and should be treated aggressively to prevent further damage.

Anesthetic protocol for elective laparotomy

The plan for an EL will vary primarily with the patient's systemic condition. Some of these patients are quite healthy and may not need much intervention except for increased use of analgesics, since a very large ventral midline abdominal incision is usually necessary. Other patients may be severely ill and require a laparotomy as a life-saving intervention. Some patients may have preexisting organ dysfunction that may or may not be the reason for the EL. Ketamine should be avoided in patients with renal azotemia, especially in cats. Thiopental should not be used in debilitated patients, or those with liver disease. It should also be avoided in sighthounds and very thin animals. Both thiopental and propofol will sensitize the myocardium to arrhythmias and alternatives should be considered in patients with preexisting dysrhythmias, cardiac disease, or when arrhythmias are highly likely such as gastric dilatation-volvulus (GDV) or splenic masses. Propofol and alfaxalone, and tiletamine/zolazepam are acceptable in healthy patients with a known diagnosis, but should be avoided in debilitated animals. Etomidate is useful for patients with preexisting cardiac dysfunction. A dose of midazolam or diazepam, 0.2 mg/kg, just prior to injection of etomidate will improve muscle relaxation and make intubation easier. Inhalant induction is not recommended for patients with GI disease, especially those with emesis. Premedication with a benzodiazepine and an opioid are generally preferred for EL. Midazolam or diazepam with hydromorphone, oxymorphone, or fentanyl can be titrated IV to effect. Induction drugs can be avoided entirely in compromised patients by titrating doses of the benzodiazepine/opioid combination until intubation is possible. Alternatively, a low dose of ketamine will usually allow intubation following premedication. Fentanyl can be continued as an infusion following induction.

Isoflurane, sevoflurane, or desflurane are preferred for maintenance of anesthesia for EL over halothane as the latter sensitizes the myocardium to arrhythmias and decreases tissue blood flow to a greater degree. Nitrous oxide is not recommended for use in laparotomy as it will diffuse into the GIT, causing distention. The cardiovascular and respiratory effects of all the inhalants are more pronounced in debilitated patients; hypotension and hypoventilation are often seen. Sick patients frequently require much lower levels of inhalant to remain anesthetized. The vaporizer setting should be kept as low as possible to avoid hypotension. If anesthetic depth is inadequate, additional sedatives or analgesics may be given intermittently or given as constant rate infusions (CRIs). Continuous infusion provides a more constant level of sedation and analgesia and is a very effective method to reduce the level of inhalant anesthetic required in both healthy and sick patients. The CRIs are kept at a constant rate, and the inhalant setting can be manipulated to adjust anesthetic depth and minimize cardiovascular effects. Morphine or fentanyl, lidocaine, and/or ketamine can be given as CRIs in dogs; lidocaine is not currently recommended for cats. If hypotension persists (mean arterial blood pressure <65 mm Hg or systolic pressure <90 mm Hg), supportive therapy with inotropes such as dobutamine and/or dopamine are useful to increase cardiac output. Vasopressors may be necessary when vasodilation is a significant cause of hypotension. Ephedrine can be given as a bolus, and is only effective for mild decreases in blood pressure. Phenylephrine, norepinephrine, vasopressin, and epinephrine are usually given as infusions. These drugs are potent vasoconstrictors and should be used at the lowest effective dose possible. In patients without coagulopathy or skin disease in the lumbosacral area, epidural analgesia with morphine is also useful for intra- and postoperative pain management.

Monitoring should be vigilant and continuous throughout anesthesia and recovery, and should include clinical signs of anesthetic depth, heart and respiratory rate, mucous membrane color and capillary refill time, temperature, blood pressure, and electrocardiography. Pulse oximetry and capnography are very useful to evaluate ventilation and gas exchange.

Gastric dilatation and volvulus

The GDV syndrome is a life-threatening GI disease seen most often in adult large or giant breed dogs, especially those with a deep-chested conformation. However, it has been seen in a few small dogs and puppies, and even three cats that also had diaphragmatic hernias.[14,15] Mortality rates of 40–60%[15] and 33.3%[16] seen in the 1980s and earlier have improved but are still somewhat variable. More recent retrospective studies have reported rates of 16.2%,[17] 26.8%,[18] and 10%.[19] Improvement in mortality is likely associated with attention to immediate fluid resuscitation, decompression of the stomach, and early surgical intervention. Mortality has been associated with the extent of damage to the stomach and surrounding organs, the presence of cardiac arrhythmia pre- or postoperatively, both hypo- and hyperthermia at presentation, the development of postoperative acute renal failure, hypotension at any time during hospitalization, and increased time from onset to presentation or surgery as well as increased time from presentation to surgery.[14,17–20] Reperfusion injury has also been implicated as a factor associated with mortality from GDV.[21]

GDV is always an emergency, as compromise of blood flow to the stomach and surrounding organs and obstruction of the caudal vena cava and portal vein greatly decrease venous return to the heart, resulting in severe hypovolemic shock. Distention of the stomach also restricts ventilation from pressure on the diaphragm. Early clinical signs include restlessness and anxiety, followed by salivation, vomiting and/or retching, and distention of the stomach. Eventually depression, weakness, and dyspnea develop if distention is not relieved. The vomiting, salivation, and gastric sequestration of hydrogen and chloride ions initially cause metabolic alkalosis. Later in the course of the disease, metabolic acidosis arises, secondary to the effects of ischemia with increased lactate production and the release of inflammatory mediators. Endotoxemia can also develop from damage to the portal system. Reperfusion injury also occurs when ischemia is reversed by therapy.

IV fluid therapy and gastric decompression should be initiated as quickly as possible. Blood samples for baseline information should include packed cell volume (PCV), total solids (TS), electrolytes, creatinine, and acid–base status. A clotting profile and venous lactate are useful to evaluate prognosis as gastric necrosis is likely present when more than one hemostatic test is abnormal and when lactate is greatly elevated at presentation and fails to decrease significantly with resuscitation.[22–24] Radiography to distinguish between dilatation and dilatation-volvulus should be delayed until cardiovascular resuscitation is completed or well underway. Anesthetic personnel, equipment, and supplies should be made ready prior to arrival of a GDV so that surgical intervention can be attempted as soon as possible. Standard emergent therapy has been to give shock doses (80–90 mL/kg) of crystalloid solution via at least two large-bore catheters, using the cephalic, saphenous, and/or jugular veins. This is still a useful therapy, however faster and possibly more effective resuscitation can be achieved with the addition of small volumes of hypertonic saline (HS) 7.5% at 2–4 mL/kg over 15 minutes, or colloids such as Hetastarch at 10 mL/kg over 30 minutes. Alternatively, a colloid and HS can be combined and given at 4–6 mL/kg. Crystalloid solutions remain in the vasculature for less than an hour, eventually ending up in the interstitial tissue, and may result in tissue edema. Colloids are more effective and efficient as they expand vascular volume to a greater degree using a much lower dose, and redistribute to the interstitial tissue to a lesser degree than crystalloid fluids.[25] The use of HS and colloids has been shown to improve cardiovascular status in both experimental and clinical cases of GDV.[26,27]

Electrocardiography should be performed soon following presentation as cardiac arrhythmias are often seen with GDV, and should be identified and treated prior to induction of anesthesia. They are usually ventricular in origin, but atrial fibrillation and sinus tachycardia are also seen.[28] In some cases, antiarrhythmic agents may not be necessary; correction of hypovolemia, hypoxemia, hypercarbia, acid–base, and/or electrolyte abnormalities may resolve the arrhythmia. Treatment of ventricular tachycardia is necessary when extrasystoles are numerous or multifocal, when the sustained rate is very high (>160/min), when extrasystoles are very early such that an R on T phenomenon may occur, and always when hemodynamic status is affected by the arrhythmia. Lidocaine is given slowly IV at 2–4 mg/kg bolus followed by an infusion at 25–100 mcg/kg/min.[29] Postoperative treatment of cardiac arrhythmias may also be necessary.

Gastric lavage is sometimes necessary during correction of a GDV. Considerations for this procedure are similar to those during upper GI endoscopy, as dislodgement of the ET tube and leakage of gastric contents into the pharynx can occur.

As previously described, acid–base and electrolyte abnormalities generally reflect the stage of the disease. Initially, alkalosis and hypokalemia may be present secondary to vomiting and gastric sequestration. With progression, acidosis may be seen due to the development of hypovolemia and tissue damage. However, pH can be difficult to predict as concurrent alkalosis and acidosis can result in a pH in the normal range. Serial evaluation of blood gases (or bicarbonate or TCO_2), PCV, electrolytes, and TS is warranted. Fluid resuscitation should resolve the metabolic acidosis; correction of the volvulus is necessary for complete resolution. Blood pressure should also be measured at presentation and throughout the perioperative period. If hypotension exists following fluid resuscitation, inotropes and/or vasopressor therapy may be necessary to restore mean arterial blood pressure to >65 mmHg or systolic pressure to ≥90 mmHg. Therapy to prevent reperfusion injury may be useful in dogs with GDV. Adequate oxygen delivery via treatment of hypovolemia and hypotension and avoidance of hypoxemia are the primary concerns. In spite of much research devoted to the effects of ischemia reperfusion injury and its prevention or treatment, few therapies have been included in clinical practice. Avoidance of hyperoxia may be useful since greater damage has been seen following reperfusion in patients maintained at higher than normal PaO_2 levels. Inhibition of

oxygen radical formation with antioxidants and iron-chelating drugs such as deferox-
amine has shown to reduce reperfusion injury in dogs with GDV.[21,30]

Hemoabdomen

Hemorrhage into the peritoneal cavity can be spontaneous from an abdominal lesion or
associated with trauma. Abdominal disease of the larger parenchymal organs such as the
liver or spleen can result in hyperplasia or the formation of masses. These lesions often
result in hemorrhage that can be life threatening. Vascular damage may also occur in
addition to bleeding from parenchymal tissues. Masses in the small and large intestine
can also cause vascular damage and hemorrhage, but this is less common and usually
not as severe. Hemorrhage from GIT lesions is more often intraluminal and presents as
chronic anemia with or without melena or hematochezia. Traumatic injury can involve
organs, vasculature, and the abdominal wall as well. Specific concerns for patients with
hemoabdomen are the severity of hypovolemia and anemia, the speed of ongoing blood
loss, and any organ dysfunction that may be present. Ideally, the patient should be stabilized as much as possible prior to surgery; however, there is a difference of opinion as
to how much volume replacement should be performed prior to surgery. Some surgeons
prefer to replace much of the blood lost after the source of the hemorrhage is stopped.
However, unstable patients will not tolerate cardiovascular effects of general anesthesia.
It is not necessary to correct the entire red blood cell (RBC) deficit preoperatively;
however, the patient should be treated to achieve normovolemia and a PCV ≥30% in
dogs or 20% in cats, as oxygen delivery is usually adequate above these levels. TS or
total protein levels should be maintained at greater than 4–4.5 g/dL. Serial PCV and TS
can be helpful in determining the efficacy of therapy and the speed of blood loss, realizing that hemodilution will be present and that colloids will interfere with refractometer
readings. Blood pressure, heart rate (HR), pulse pressure, mucous membrane color, and
the direct blood pressure waveform are also useful parameters to help evaluate the cardiovascular status in response to blood loss. However, there is no absolute method to
determine blood loss. The volume of prior and ongoing blood loss must be estimated
and replaced before hypovolemia affects the cardiovascular system. Monitoring blood
loss can be difficult; techniques include weighing bloody sponges and towels, tracking
the volume of lavage used, and the volume of blood and fluid collected in suction bottles.
Crystalloids can be used to replace blood loss; however, the volume required is several
multiples of the volume lost. Colloids are a better replacement for blood loss and can be
given at closer to a 1:1 ratio if PCV and protein levels are adequate. Amounts greater
than 20% of the patient's total blood volume must be replaced with whole blood, plasma
or colloid and packed RBCs, or an RBC substitute such as Oxyglobin® (OPK Biotech
LLC., Cambridge, MA) to ensure adequate oxygen delivery.

   Arrhythmias are often seen with splenic masses, usually ventricular tachycardias and
most often in dogs. The cause is uncertain and they can be difficult to eliminate until the
mass is removed. Predisposing factors such as hypovolemia, hypotension, hypoxemia,
hypercarbia, and electrolyte abnormalities should be treated first. Specific antiarrhythmic
therapy for ventricular tachycardia is needed when HR is very high or the patient is
compromised by the dysrhythmias, when multifocal ectopic foci exist, or when extremely

early premature contractions are seen such that the "R on T" phenomenon. Lidocaine is most often used. A bolus followed by a CRI can be useful for arrhythmias and as an adjunct to anesthesia since the inhalant anesthetic can be decreased to 30–50% in some patients. Lidocaine should be used judiciously in cats since they are more sensitive to its toxic effects. Alternatively, procainamide or a beta blocker can be used in cats.

Anesthetic considerations for intestinal obstruction or foreign body removal, biopsy or removal of abdominal masses, and colectomy are similar to those of the general EL discussed above. Hemorrhage is most often associated with removal of large abdominal masses as discussed above; however, it may also occur when extensive adhesions or fibrous tissue are part of intestinal lesions. Foreign body removal and other lesions of the small or large intestine may be straightforward. The duration may be long as meticulous dissection of lesions and resection and anastamoses of the GIT may be required. Patients with prior leakage of intestinal contents or bile will have peritonitis and may be septic. These patients can be very challenging to anesthetize as they are much more sensitive to the cardiovascular and sedative effects of anesthetic drugs, especially inhalants. Bile peritonitis can be very severe as bile can be septic and bile acids cause direct tissue damage. Sepsis results in severe cardiovascular changes such that hypotension is common, can be severe, and is sometimes difficult to treat.

Disorders of the pancreas

Acute pancreatitis in dogs is associated with lethargy, vomiting, anorexia, and abdominal pain that can be severe. Clinical signs in cats are often more nonspecific such as lethargy and inappetance. Vomiting is seen in some cats, but much less often than in dogs. Cats also do not exhibit signs of abdominal pain as consistently as dogs. The diagnosis of acute pancreatitis is often difficult to make antemortem, especially in cats. Serum levels of amylase and lipase are no longer considered useful in the diagnosis because they may be elevated with other disease conditions and may even be normal in some patients with confirmed pancreatitis. Measurement of species-specific pancreatic lipase immunoreactivity (PLI) has been found to be more sensitive and specific for pancreatic disease in both dogs and cats (canine PLI [cPLI] or feline PLI [fPLI]). Ultrasound examination is also very useful, especially in dogs. Currently, diagnosis of pancreatitis in dogs and cats relies on clinical signs, PLI measurement, ultrasound, and response to treatment.[31–33] Pancreatitis can occur following abdominal surgery in humans,[34] and has been seen concurrently in dogs with other diseases such as diabetes mellitus, hyperadrenocorticism, renal failure, neoplasia, congestive heart failure, or autoimmune disorders.[35] Iatrogenic pancreatitis has been induced by drugs, including corticosteroids, nonsteroidal anti-inflammatory agents, organophosphates, thiazide diuretics, sulfonamides, tetracycline, azothioprine, furosemide, and estrogen.[36] Thus, it is likely that animals with acute pancreatitis are often anesthetized for reasons unrelated to diagnosis or treatment of pancreatitis.

Most cases of pancreatitis in small animals are idiopathic or unidentified. Pancreatic edema secondary to inflammation is thought to be the cause of mild cases. Medical management of acute pancreatitis is attempted first and is usually successful. IV fluid therapy, withholding of food and water per os, and pain management is the basis of medical therapy. Fresh frozen plasma has also been advocated for management of pancreatitis to provide replacement of alpha$_2$ macroglobulin and when coagulopathy is present. More severe cases involve suppuration and/or necrosis of the pancreas, sometimes with abscess formation. Damage to the pancreas liberates digestive enzymes, which results in autodigestion of the pancreas itself and surrounding tissues. Local peritonitis develops, which in some cases may cause severe systemic disease with activation of the systemic inflammatory response syndrome.

Surgical therapy may be indicated in cases with acute necrotizing pancreatitis, pancreatic abscess, bile duct obstruction, evidence of infection or mass formation, and in those who fail to response to medical therapy. Endoscopic, surgical, or laparoscopic techniques may also be performed in patients with pancreatitis to place enterostomy tubes for enteral nutrition.

The choice of anesthetics for use in a patient with pancreatitis is often based on other complicating factors identified for the patient. Some patients may be severely compromised at presentation, but surgical intervention is usually performed only after stabilization and usually only when medical therapy has failed. IV administered alpha$_2$ adrenergic agents cause hyperglycemia from inhibition of insulin release from beta cells in the islets of Langerhans of the pancreas. This effect has been observed with xylazine, medetomidine, and dexmedetomidine in both dogs and cats.[37–39] It is unknown whether the alpha$_2$ adrenergic effects on the pancreas are of clinical significance in patients with pancreatitis. However, a conservative approach to anesthetic management of these patients avoids the use of alpha$_2$ agonists. Many opioids are known to stimulate contraction of the Sphincter of Oddi and increase the pressure in the bile duct. Despite these concerns, since the pain of pancreatitis can be quite severe, the contraction of the sphincter has already occurred, and opioids provide the best analgesia, they have become the mainstay of analgesic therapy in both humans and animals.[33,40,41] In patients without coagulopathy or skin disease, epidural administration of morphine provides pain relief with fewer side effects and can be used in addition to IV administration of other μ agonist opioids. Interpleural block with local anesthetic can also provide pain relief.

There is no clear best choice for induction of anesthesia for patients with pancreatitis. Propofol has been associated with the development of pancreatitis in humans[42]; however, this has not been seen in dogs or cats. In fact, a report of the use of propofol in 44 cats with primary hepatic lipidosis showed no signs of pancreatic disease.[43] Halothane would not be the inhalant of choice in compromised patients, those with concurrent liver disease, or those with cardiac dysrhythmias. Maintenance of anesthesia with isoflurane or sevoflurane is preferred in such cases. During surgery, the anesthetist should provide vigilant monitoring of anesthetic depth, maintain adequate vascular volume, and prevent hypotension.

Obesity

Obesity is becoming more prevalent in companion animals, similar to the situation in humans at this time. Two recent studies identified 34% of 21,754 adult dogs[44] and 35% of 8159 adult cats[45] from veterinary practices from all over the United States as

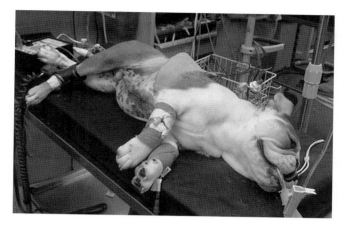

Figure 16.6. Same bulldog in recovery after removal of a splenic mass. Note the two IV catheters placed in the cephalic veins, and an arterial catheter in the dorsal pedal artery of the right rear leg. Direct blood pressure monitoring, pulse oximetry, and end-tidal gas analysis was performed during anesthesia. Pulse oximetry and indirect blood pressure monitoring with a Doppler are continued in recovery. Courtesy of Jennifer Adams, DVM.

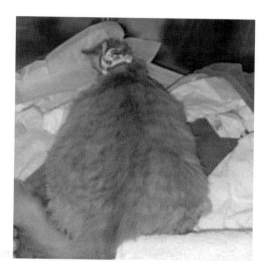

Figure 16.7. Obese cat following placement of a feeding tube. Courtesy of Dr. Christina Braun.

overweight or obese (Figure 16.7) Adipose tissue is metabolically active and is associated with numerous disease states. Effects can be seen directly from the mechanical presence of fat tissue, and from endocrine and/or inflammatory effects of substances produced by adipose cells.[46,47] Obesity in dogs has been associated with metabolic disorders, endocrinopathies, cardiorespiratory diseases, orthopedic disorders, neoplasia, urogenital disorders, and other functional problems. Obese cats are more likely to have endocrine disease,

Table 16.2. Increased incidence or risk of diseases associated with obesity in dogs and cats

Dogs	Cats
Metabolic Hyperlipidemia/dyslipidemia Insulin resistance Glucose intolerance Metabolic syndrome	Hepatic lipidosis
Endocrine Hyperadrenocorticism Diabetes mellitus Insulinoma Hypopituitarism Hypothalamic lesions	Diabetes mellitus
Cardiorespiratory Tracheal collapse Brachycephalic syndrome Laryngeal paralysis Obesity hypoventilation syndrome Portal vein thrombosis	Obesity hypoventilation syndrome
Orthopedic Osteoarthritis Humeral condylar fractures Cranial cruciate ligament rupture Intervertebral disk disease	Lameness
Urogenital Urethral sphincter incompetence Urolithiasis (calcium oxalate) Transitional cell carcinoma Dystocia	Urinary tract disease
Gastrointestinal Pancreatitis	Increased oral cavity and GI disease
Neoplasia Mammary Transitional cell carcinoma	Increased risk various cancers
Miscellaneous/functional problems Exercise intolerance Heat intolerance Heat stroke Decreased immune function Increased anesthetic risk Decreased lifespan	Skin disorders Increased anesthetic risk

Source: Adapted from German et al. 2010,[47] Lund et al. 2006,[44] Lund et al. 2005.[45]

hepatic lipidosis, urinary tract disease, lameness, and increased incidence of GI, oral cavity, and skin disease (Table 16.2). Obese patients therefore often have underlying physiological problems in addition to the condition for which anesthesia is required. If they are anorexic from their primary disease, they may also have secondary hepatic lipidosis with subsequent liver dysfunction. Evaluation of obese animals for presence of pancreatitis, diabetes mellitus, hepatic insufficiency, or cardiac disease should be included in the diagnostic workup. An obese animal's veins may be more difficult to locate and catheterize. Auscultation of the heart and lungs may also be more difficult in these patients. Additional diagnostics such as thoracic radiographs, electrocardiography, and in some cases, echocardiography should be performed if there is a suggestion of cardio-pulmonary dysfunction.

Premedicants and induction drugs should be selected based on the patient's status, keeping in mind that the pharmacokinetic behavior of anesthetic drugs is affected by the presence of a large fat depot. The volume of distribution and the elimination half-life of many drugs differ in obese patients. Dosages of drugs calculated on actual body weight can result in overdose in obese patients since the blood supply to fat is poor compared to other tissues. However, obese patients also have an increased blood volume that effectively results in a lower peak plasma concentration of drugs injected IV. Repeated IV injection or continuous infusion of drugs that are lipid soluble can result in a pro-longed effect as drug is gradually released from the fat depot. Specific pharmacokinetic studies of some anesthetic drugs performed in obese patients are available for humans, but not companion animals. Propofol behaves similarly in obese and normal weight humans. Neuromuscular blocking agents that do not rely on hepatic elimination such as atracurium are dosed similarly as well. Thiopental has prolonged effects in obese patients since it is very lipid soluble.[48] In general, IM doses of sedatives can be based on total body weight, and IV dosing should be based on ideal weight. Deposition into actual muscle tissue can be a problem in severely obese patients. The efficacy of premedication given should be considered to determine how much induction drug will be needed. A range should be used, beginning at the low end and giving incremental IV doses to enable intubation. Crystalloid fluid therapy, even when given at standard infusion rates to anes-thetized patients of normal body weights, has been shown to result in pulmonary com-plications and tissue edema. IV fluid rates should be calculated at the ideal body weight for obese patients to avoid fluid overload, especially in cats. Regional anesthesia, espe-cially epidurals, may be more difficult in obese patients as landmarks are harder to find. Obese animals anesthetized with halothane will have a longer recovery time than other patients because of significant sequestration of the anesthetic in fat. Isoflurane and sevo-flurane are more desirable inhalation anesthetics for obese animals because of their minimal biotransformation and low tissue solubility.

Perioperative hypoxemia due to the obesity hypoventilation (or Pickwickian) syn-drome is a common feature of obesity in humans and is markedly worsened by anesthe-sia. Decreased compliance is caused by the presence of fat in the thorax and abdomen, and from increased pulmonary blood volume in obese patients.[48] Excursion of the dia-phragm is also limited by the increased weight of the abdominal contents and decreases the functional residual capacity (FRC). The combination of decreased compliance and FRC results in hypoventilation. Hypoventilation is worse under anesthesia, especially in dorsal recumbency, as muscle relaxation, craniad displacement of the diaphragm, and the weight of abdominal contents cause atelectasis. The increased mass of the pharyngeal tissues and tongue may lead to upper airway obstruction after premedication with tran-quilizers or during induction of anesthesia. Obese patients given sedatives or tranquilizers prior to anesthesia should be continuously observed for airway obstruction. Preoxygen-ation is recommended since FRC decreases further with induction. Rapid control of the airway at induction and positive pressure ventilation during anesthesia are recommended.

The respiratory depression caused by opioids may be more significant in obese patients. Any edema or swelling that develops in the oral or pharyngeal area during anesthesia can add to potential airway compromise in recovery. During recovery from anesthesia, obese patients should be kept intubated until they will no longer tolerate the ET tube. Obese animals must regain normal muscle function to maintain an adequate tidal volume and a patent airway after extubation. Oxygenation should be evaluated and supplemental oxygen given to those patients who cannot maintain an SaO_2 or SpO_2 of 95% or greater.

Revised from "Gastrointestinal Disease" by Stephen A. Greene and Steven L. Marks in Lumb and Jones' Veterinary Anesthesia and Analgesia, Fourth Edition.

References

1. Gaynor A.R., Shofer F.S., Washabau R.J. Risk factors for acquired megaesophagus in dogs. *J Am Vet Med Assoc* **211**(11): 1406–1412, 1997.
2. Galatos A., Raptopoulos D. Gastro-oesophageal reflux during anaesthesia in the dog: the effect of preoperative fasting and premedication. *Vet Rec* **137**(19): 479–483, 1995.
3. Cremer J., Sum S.O., Braun C., et al. Assessment of maxillary and infraorbital nerve blockade for rhinoscopy in sevoflurane anesthetized dogs. Proceedings of the Association of Veterinary Anesthetists Autumn Meeting, September 2–4, Santorini, Greece, 2010, p. 52.
4. Valverde A., Cantwell S., Hernández J., et al. Effects of acepromazine on the incidence of vomiting associated with opioid administration in dogs. *Vet Anaesth Analg* **31**(1): 40–45, 2004.
5. Donaldson L.L., Leib M.S., Boyd C., et al. Effect of preanesthetic medication on ease of endoscopic intubation of the duodenum in anesthetized dogs. *Am J Vet Res* **54**(9): 1489–1495, 1993.
6. Smith A.A., Posner L.P., Goldstein R.E., et al. Evaluation of the effects of premedication on gastroduodenoscopy in cats. *J Am Vet Med Assoc* **225**: 540–544, 2004.
7. Nickel R., Schummer A., Seiferle E., et al. *The Viscera of the Domestic Animals*. New York: Springer-Verlag, 1973.
8. Leib M.S., Baechtel M.S., Monroe W.E. Complications associated with 355 flexible colonoscopic procedures in dogs. *J Vet Int Med* **18**: 642–646, 2004.
9. Alwood A.J., Brainard B.M., LaFond E., et al. Postoperative pulmonary complications in dogs undergoing laparotomy: frequency, characterization and disease-related risk factors. *J Vet Emerg Crit Care* **16**(3): 176–183, 2006.
10. Galatos A., Raptopoulos D. Gastro-oesophageal reflux during anaesthesia in the dog: the effect of age, positioning and type of surgical procedure. *Vet Rec* **137**(20): 513–516, 1995.
11. Wilson D.V., Walshaw R. Postanesthetic esophageal dysfunction in 13 dogs. *J Am Anim Hosp Assoc* **40**: 455–460, 2004.
12. Wilson D.V., Evans A.T. The effect of topical treatment on esophageal pH during acid reflux in dogs. *Vet Anaesth Analg* **34**: 339–343, 2007.
13. Panti A., Bennett R.C., Corletto F., et al. The effect of omeprazole on oesophageal pH in dogs during anaesthesia. *J Small Anim Pract* **50**(10): 540–544, 2009.
14. Glickman L., Glickman N.W., Perez C.M. Analysis of risk factors for gastric dilatation and dilatation-volvulus in dogs. *J Am Vet Med Assoc* **204**(9): 1463–1471, 1994.
15. Formaggini L., Schmidt K., Lorenzi D. Gastric dilatation-volvulus associated with diaphragmatic hernia in three cats: clinical presentation, surgical treatment and presumptive aetiology. *J Feline Med Surg* **10**: 198–201, 2008.

16. Friskies Petcare Division of the Carnation Company Canine bloat panel offers research and treatment recommendations. *Friskies Res Dig* **24**(2): 1–7, 1988.
17. Beck J., Staatz A., Pelsue D., et al. Risk factors associated with short-term outcome and development of perioperative complications in dogs undergoing surgery because of gastric dilatation-volvulus: 166 cases (1992–2003). *J Am Vet Med Assoc* **229**(12): 1934–1939, 2006.
18. Buber T., Saragusty J., Ranen E., et al. Evaluation of lidocaine treatment and risk factors for death associated with gastric dilatation and volvulus in dogs: 112 cases (1997–2005). *J Am Vet Med Assoc* **230**(9): 1334–1339, 2007.
19. Mackenzie G., Barnhart M., Kennedy S., et al. A retrospective study of factors influencing survival following surgery for gastric dilatation-volvulus syndrome in 306 dogs. *J Am Anim Hosp Assoc* **46**: 97–102, 2010.
20. Brourman J., Schertel E., Allen D., et al. Factors associated with perioperative mortality in dogs with surgically managed gastric dilatation-volvulus: 137 cases (1988–1993). *J Am Vet Med Assoc* **208**(11): 1855–1858, 1996.
21. Lantz G.C., Badylak S.F., Hiles M.C., et al. Treatment of reperfusion injury in dogs with experimentally induced GDV. *Am J Vet Res* **53**(9): 1594–1598, 1992.
22. Millis D.L., Hauptman J.G., Fulton R.B. Jr. Abnormal hemostatic profiles and gastric necrosis in canine GDV. *Vet Surg* **22**(2): 93–97, 1993.
23. de Papp E., Drobatz K.J., Hughes D. Plasma lactate concentration as a predictor of gastric necrosis and survival among dogs with GDV: 102 cases (1995–1998). *J Am Vet Med Assoc* **215**(1): 49–52, 1999.
24. Zacher L.A., Berg J., Shaw S.P., et al. Association between outcome and changes in plasma lactate concentration during presurgical treatment in dogs with GDV: 64 cases (2002–2008). *J Am Vet Med Assoc* **236**(8): 892–897, 2010.
25. Aldrich J. Shock fluids and fluid challenge. In: *Small Animal Critical Care Medicine*. D.C. Silverstein and K. Hopper, eds. St. Louis, MO: Saunders Elsevier, 2009, pp 276–280.
26. Allen D.A., Schertel E.R., Muir W.W. 3rd, et al. Hypertonic saline/dextran resuscitation of dogs with experimentally induced GDV shock. *Am J Vet Res* **52**(1): 92–96, 1991.
27. Schertel E.R., Allen D.A., Muir W.W., et al. Evaluation of a hypertonic saline-dextran solution for treatment of dogs with shock induced by GDV. *J Am Vet Med Assoc* **210**(2): 226–230, 1997.
28. Muir W.W., Lipowitz A.J. Cardiac dysrhythmias associated with gastric dilatation-volvulus in the dog. *J Am Anim Hosp Assoc* **172**(6): 683–689, 1978.
29. Cole S., Drobatz K. Chapter 18: emergency management and critical care. In: *Manual of Canine and Feline Cardiology*, 4th ed. L.P. Tilley, F.W.K. Smith, Jr., M.A. Oyama, and M.M. Sleeper, eds. St. Louis, MO: Saunders Elsevier, 2008, p 352.
30. Badylak S.F., Lantz G.C., Jeffries M. Prevention of reperfusion injury in surgically induced GDV in dogs. *Am J Vet Res* **51**(2): 294–299, 1990.
31. Thompson L.J., Seshadri R., Raffe M.R. Characteristics and outcomes in surgical management of severe acute pancreatitis: 37 dogs. (2001–2007). *J Vet Emerg Crit Care* **19**(2): 165–173, 2009.
32. Son T.T., Thompson L., Serrano S., et al. Surgical intervention in the management of severe acute pancreatitis in cats: 8 cases (2003–2007). *J Vet Emerg Crit Care* **20**(4): 426–435, 2010.
33. Gaynor A.R. Chapter 124: acute pancreatitis. In: *Small Animal Critical Care Medicine*. D.C. Silverstein and K. Hopper, eds. St. Louis, MO: Saunders Elsevier, 2009, pp 537–542.
34. Estabrook S.G., Levine E.G., Bernstein L.H. Gastrointestinal crises in intensive care. *Anesthesiol Clin North America* **9**: 367, 1991.
35. Cook A.K., Breitschwerdt E.B., Levine J.F., et al. Risk factors associated with acute pancreatitis in dogs: 101 cases (1985–1990). *J Am Vet Med Assoc* **203**(5): 673–679, 1993.

36. Bunch S.E. The exocrine pancreas. In: *Small Animal Internal Medicine*, 3rd ed. R.W. Nelson and C.G. Couto, eds. St Louis, MO: CV Mosby, 2003, p 552.

37. Ambrisko T.D., Hikasa Y. Neurohormonal and metabolic effects of medetomidine compared with xylazine in beagle dogs. *Can J Vet Res* **66**: 42–49, 2002.

38. Kanda T., Hikasa Y. Neurohormonal and metabolic effects of medetomidine compared with xylazine in healthy cats. *Can J Vet Res* **72**: 278–286, 2008.

39. Dexdomitor package insert. Available at http://www.dexdomitorusa.com/pdf/DEXDOMITOR_PI_21308.pdf.

40. Thompson D.R. Narcotic analgesic effects on the sphincter of Oddi: a review of the data and therapeutic implications in treating pancreatitis. *Am J Gastroenterol* **96**(4): 1266–1272, 2001.

41. Toouli J. Sphincter of Oddi: function, dysfunction, and its management. *J Gastroenterol Hepatol* **24**(S3): S57–S62, 2009.

42. Devlin J.W., Lau A.K., Tanios M.A. Propofol-associated hypertriglyceridemia and pancreatitis in the intensive care unit: an analysis of frequency and risk factors. *Pharmacotherapy* **25**(10): 1348–1352, 2005.

43. Posner L.P., Asakawa M., Erb H.N. Use of propofol for anesthesia in cats with primary hepatic lipidosis: 44 cases (1995–2004). *J Am Vet Med Assoc* **232**: 1841–1843, 2008.

44. Lund E.M., Armstrong P.J., Kirk C.A., et al. Prevalence and risk factors for obesity in adult dogs from private US veterinary practices. *Int J Appl Res Vet Med* **4**(2): 177–188, 2006.

45. Lund E.M., Armstrong P.J., Kirk C.A., et al. Prevalence and risk factors for obesity in adult cats from private US veterinary practices. *Int J Appl Res Vet Med* **3**(2): 88–96, 2005.

46. Radin M.J., Sharkey L.C., Holycross B.J. Adipokines: a review of biological and analytical principles and an update in dogs, cats, and horses. *Vet Clin Pathol* **38**(2): 136–156, 2009.

47. German A.J., Ryan V.H., German A.C. Obesity, its associated disorders and the role of inflammatory adipokines in companion animals. *Vet J* **185**: 4–9, 2010.

48. Ogunnaike B.O., Whitten C.W. Chapter 36: anesthesia and obesity. In: *Clinical Anesthesia*, 5th ed. P.G. Barash, B.F. Cullen, and R.K. Stoelting, eds. Philadelphia, PA: Lippincott Williams, and Wilkins, 2005, pp 1040–1045.

Chapter 17

Anesthesia for patients with endocrine disorders

Stephen A. Greene and Tamara L. Grubb

Disorders of the adrenal gland

Adrenal insufficiency

Disease that results in insufficient adrenal hormone production (i.e., hypoadrenocorticism or Addison's disease) may adversely affect the condition of the patient and overall anesthetic risk. The main risks are associated with electrolyte abnormalities and impaired stress response-associated compensatory mechanisms.

The primary function of the mineralocorticoid aldosterone is to stimulate absorption of sodium ions in the distal renal tubules and to promote potassium excretion. Aldosterone deficiency may thereby result in hyponatremia and hyperkalemia. Hyponatremia with concurrent water loss can produce lethargy, nausea, decreased cardiac output, hypovolemia, hypotension, and/or impaired renal perfusion. Hyperkalemia may result in muscle weakness, decreased cardiac conduction, and excitability and bradycardia. Hyperkalemia greater than 5.5 mEq/L should be addressed prior to anesthesia whenever possible. Dextrose administration, alkalinization of plasma (to drive potassium back into the cells), and/or insulin administration may be effective for treatment of hyperkalemia. For severe hyperkalemia affecting cardiac conduction, calcium gluconate (0.3 mL/kg) may be administered intravenously (IV) slowly using a 10% solution (which provides 9.3 mg Ca^{2+}/mL or 0.47 mEq/mL) to provide immediate relief from the electrical conduction abnormalities associated with hyperkalemia. Calcium therapy is effective in this instance by raising the threshold potential for depolarization to compensate for the raised resting potential associated with hyperkalemia.

A patient with hypoadrenocorticism should be stabilized prior to anesthesia. The treatment objectives are: (1) to correct the dehydration and treat hypovolemic shock if present, (2) to support renal function, (3) to correct electrolyte imbalances, and (4) to supply glucocorticoids. In an Addisonian crisis, priorities are to correct the patient's pH, hypotension, hyponatremia, hyperkalemia, hypoglycemia, and electrocardiographic dysrhythmias.[1]

Essentials of Small Animal Anesthesia and Analgesia, Second Edition. Edited by Kurt A. Grimm, William J. Tranquilli, Leigh A. Lamont.
© 2011 John Wiley & Sons, Inc. Published 2011 by John Wiley & Sons, Inc.

Cortisol depletion impairs renal excretion of water and energy metabolism, decreases stress tolerance, and can cause anorexia, vomiting, and/or diarrhea. Addisonian patients have decreased stress tolerance, thus their anesthetic management involves glucocorticoid supplementation and IV fluid volume replacement. Use of the anesthetic etomidate is associated with a 2–3-hour depletion of glucocorticoids following a single injection, and should be avoided in Addisonian patients. A balanced electrolyte solution should be administered intraoperatively at a rate of 10–20 mL/kg/h.

Hyperadrenocorticism

Hyperadrenocorticism (Cushing's disease) is a common endocrine disease and presents fewer challenges for successful anesthetic care than does hypoadrenocorticism. Patients with hyperadrenocorticism will be predisposed to infection and poor wound healing. There is increased risk of pulmonary thrombosis in the perianesthetic period. Due to the aforementioned reduction in endogenous corticosteroid release associated with etomidate injection, this anesthetic may be suitable for the patient with Cushing's disease.[2] Propofol is another option for induction of anesthesia due to its potent vasodilating effect on peripheral vasculature.

Blood pressure monitoring and support are important for patients with hyperadrenocorticism because they are prone to hypertension. Preanesthetic evaluation should include baseline arterial blood pressure measurement. Chronic preexisting hypertension may predispose the anesthetized patient to greater risk during periods of anesthetic-related hypotension due to downregulation of vascular control.[3]

Many patients with hyperadrenocorticism have a large pendulous abdomen, which can impair ventilation during anesthesia. Monitoring ventilation with end-tidal carbon dioxide, pulse oximetry, and/or arterial blood gas analysis is warranted.

Pheochromocytoma

Animals with a functional tumor of the adrenal gland producing excessive catecholamines represent a high-risk group for anesthesia. Pheochromocytoma may be suspected in middle-aged dogs with a history of acute collapse, panting, tachycardia, and restlessness. Hypertension and tachycardia are of primary concern and should be evaluated prior to administration of anesthetic premedications. Premedication with acepromazine (0.05 mg/kg, up to a maximum of 1 or 2 mg per dog) may be helpful for lowering arterial blood pressure, as is the use of other alpha antagonist medications such as phenoxybenzamine (0.25 mg/kg) or phentolamine (loading dose 0.05–0.1 mg/kg followed by infusion at 10 mcg/kg/min). Blood pressure should be monitored during anesthesia. Nitroprusside infusion (1–5 mcg/kg/min) or magnesium sulfate (40 mg/kg IV bolus followed by infusion at 15 mg/kg/h) may be effective for treatment of surgical-induced periods of extreme hypertension.[4] Following surgical removal of a pheochromocytoma, exogenous catecholamine support for blood pressure should be available (e.g., dobutamine or dopamine infusion) as blood pressure and cardiac output can fall precipitously.

Disorders of the pancreas

Diabetes mellitus

Insulin is essential for normal cellular metabolism and function. The effects of insulin on normal cellular function include: (1) inhibition of glycogenolysis, (2) inhibition of gluconeogenesis, (3) inhibition of lipolysis, (4) stimulation of glucose uptake into cells, (5) stimulation of potassium transport into cells, and (6) suppression of ketogenesis. Lipolysis is inhibited with a resultant accumulation of ketone bodies, causing osmotic diuresis and metabolic acidosis. Prolonged hyperglycemia and ketonemia can lead to: (1) metabolic acidosis, (2) dehydration, (3) circulatory collapse, (4) renal failure, and/or (5) coma and death.

Diabetes mellitus should be suspected in any patient with the following clinical signs: (1) a recent history of polyuria, polydipsia, weight loss, or rapid onset of cataracts; (2) dehydration, weakness, collapse, mental dullness, hepatomegaly, and/or muscle wasting; and/or (3) increased rate and depth of respiration and breath with a sweet acetone odor.[5] Severe metabolic acidosis (a pH of less than 7.1) should be treated with sodium bicarbonate to return pH to at least 7.2.

A patient with diabetes mellitus should be stabilized and regulated prior to anesthesia. Anesthesia should be delayed in patients with serum glucose concentration >300 mg/dL when practical to do so. Ideal anesthetic management of a diabetic involves proper patient preparation and use of antagonizable or short-acting agents such that recovery time can be minimized. Drugs that can be antagonized (opioids and benzodiazepine tranquilizers) or are readily eliminated from the patient (propofol, etomidate, and inhalant anesthetics) should be considered. In normal animals, alpha$_2$ adrenoceptor agonists (xylazine, dexmedetomidine) decrease pancreatic release of insulin, resulting in hyperglycemia. The impact of alpha$_2$ adrenoceptor agonists in patients with diabetes mellitus has not been determined in a clinical setting. Therefore, most clinicians avoid the use of these agents in diabetic patients. The clinician should attempt to get the patient awake as soon as possible so the animal can resume its normal feeding schedule. The procedure should be scheduled early in the morning after the administration of one-half the patient's normal dose of insulin. Preoperative and serial intraoperative and postoperative blood glucose levels should be determined. Ideally, the blood glucose should be maintained between 150 and 250 mg/dL. During the procedure, 2.5–5% dextrose in a balanced electrolyte solution should be administered to prevent hypoglycemia when blood glucose trends downward.

Diabetes insipidus

While not a disorder of the pancreas, diabetes insipidus does mimic the clinical sign of polyuria seen with diabetes mellitus. Polyuria resulting from vasopressin deficiency is characterized by dilute urine in spite of a strong stimulus for vasopressin secretion. There is an absence of renal disease and a rise in urine osmolality can be documented following administration of vasopressin. When presented for anesthesia, the patient with diabetes insipidus is predisposed to water and electrolyte abnormalities. Thus, the serum sodium, chloride, and potassium concentrations should be determined. Hypernatremia is likely to occur in this condition and should be corrected slowly in cases with chronic elevation. This may be accomplished by judicious free water administration using 5% dextrose in water. Desmopressin has been used to treat diabetes insipidus and may prevent hypernatremia. Cases of surgical hypophysectomy given desmopressin have been reported to become hypernatremic despite prophylaxis.[6] It is theorized that fluid administration and water intake in the postoperative period may have resulted in insufficient compensation for hypercortisolism-induced vasopressin resistance.

Insulinoma

Malignant proliferation of beta-cells in the pancreas leads to excessive insulin secretion and hypoglycemia. Animals with insulinoma may receive medical therapies or ultimately, surgical excision of the tumor. Medical therapy may be directed toward destruction of the beta cells using streptozocin. Administration of corticosteroids, diazoxide, somatostatin analogues (e.g., octreotide), and dietary management are used to mitigate the hypoglycemia. During anesthesia of the patient with insulinoma, serum glucose should be monitored and glucose-containing fluids should be administered IV as needed. Dextrose solutions (2.5% or 5%) may be used for IV bolus or continuous infusion. Following surgical excision of an insulinoma, the animal should be monitored closely for signs of pancreatitis. Approximately 10% of dogs will develop diabetes mellitus following surgical excision of an insulinoma.

Disorders of the parathyroid

Hyperparathyroidism occurs with much greater frequency than hypoparathyroidism. Middle-aged dogs that present with polyuria/polydipsia and have hypercalcemia may be hyperparathyroid, a condition that appears overrepresented by the Keeshond breed. Three other commonly diagnosed conditions that should also be considered on the differential list are lymphosarcoma, hypoadrenocorticism, and chronic renal failure. Preanesthetic considerations for these patients should focus on assessment and correction of significant electrolyte abnormalities and hydration status. During surgical excision of parathyroid tumors, aggressive treatment of hypercalcemia is not warranted and efforts should be directed toward the management of fluid therapy to correct dehydration using physiological saline solution. Potassium supplementation may be required as well. Following adequate hydration of the patient, diuretic therapy with furosemide (2–4 mg/kg IV) for enhancing calciuresis may be initiated. When possible, at least one normal parathyroid gland will be left *in situ* during tumor excision and this will prevent permanent hypoparathyroidism. A transient hypocalcemia may develop following tumor excision if the normal glands have suffered atrophy due to chronic parathyroid hormone suppression. This scenario is more likely when the presurgical serum calcium concentration is greater than 15 mg/dL.[7] Postoperative administration of vitamin D may help to avoid hypocalcemic-induced tetany.

Hypoparathyroidism occurs with less specificity in signalment compared to hyperparathyroidism. Hypocalcemic animals with abrupt onset of neurological or neuromuscular abnormalities that seem to become worse with exercise may be hypoparathyroid. Differential diagnosis of hypocalcemia includes hypoparathyroidism, renal failure, ethylene glycol toxicosis, acute pancreatitis, eclampsia, anticonvulsant therapy, and hypoalbuminemia. In dogs with naturally occurring hypoparathyroidism, 80% were observed to have grand mal convulsions. Thus, perianesthetic management of the hypoparathyroid patient may include administration of diazepam. Treatment of hypocalcemia with 10% calcium gluconate (1 mL/kg, slowly, IV) is preferred over calcium chloride due to the potential for the latter to cause extravascular tissue sloughing.

Disorders of the thyroid

Hypothyroidism is a common disorder among dogs and very rare in cats. Decreased secretion of thyroxine (T_4) and triiodothyronine (T_3) may result from dysfunction within the thyroid, lack of thyrotropin-releasing hormone by the hypothalamus, or lack of thyroid-stimulating hormone (TSH) from the pituitary (secondary hypothyroidism). Canine thyroiditis is generally thought to be an autoimmune disorder of middle-aged dogs, but can occur at any age. Clinical presentation is fairly nonspecific and includes low metabolic rate, lethargy, mental dullness, weight gain, and cold intolerance. Slow recovery from general anesthesia can often be related to hypothyroidism. Laryngeal paralysis, megaesophagus, and, rarely, seizure activity may be associated with hypothyroidism. Sinus bradycardia, low QRS amplitude, inverted T waves, and decreased left ventricular function have been observed in hypothyroid dogs.[8] While there is no specific anesthetic protocol directed to animals with hypothyroidism, use of drugs that are readily antagonizable or that normally undergo rapid metabolism and elimination are logical choices. Cardiovascular support to maintain normal blood pressure during anesthesia is also warranted. Since obesity may be associated with hypothyroidism, close attention should be given to ventilatory function during anesthesia. Mechanical ventilation may be required to maintain normocapnia. Hypothyroid patients may be prone to developing hypothermia while anesthetized and therefore core body temperature should also be monitored.

Hyperthyroidism is commonly diagnosed in both dogs and cats. Clinical findings include weight loss, increased appetite, polyuria/polydipsia, hyperactivity, and tachycardia. Presence of a cardiac murmur may also be noted. Congestive heart failure and hypertrophic cardiomyopathy are sometimes associated with hyperthyroidism in cats.[9] One or more liver enzymes (alanine transaminase, alkaline phosphatase, lactate dehydrogenase, and aspartate transaminase) are frequently elevated in cats with hyperthyroidism, although this finding is usually of minor consequence in terms of anesthetic management. The primary goal during anesthetic management of the hyperthyroid patient is to avoid exacerbation of the tachycardia associated with this hypermetabolic state, especially in the face of cardiac dysfunction. Alpha$_2$ adrenoceptor agonists and anticholinergic agents are avoided while opioids are often included as premedications in these patients. Induction of anesthesia is accomplished using propofol or, when congestive heart failure or cardiomyopathy is suspected, etomidate. Ketamine (including the combination of diazepam and ketamine) and Telazol® (tiletamine and zolazepam; Pfizer

Animal Health, New York) are usually avoided in order to minimize drug-related increases in heart rate. The electrocardiograph and arterial blood pressure should be monitored during anesthesia. Hypercapnia (as a consequence of hypoventilation) should be prevented by supporting ventilation as guided by end-tidal or arterial carbon dioxide tensions determined using capnography or blood gas analysis, respectively. Tachycardia may be treated during anesthesia using propranolol (0.05 mg/kg IV), esmolol (100–200 mcg/kg IV), or lidocaine (0.25–0.5 mg/kg IV).

Revised from "Endocrine Disease" by Ralph C. Harvey and Michael Schaer in Lumb and Jones' Veterinary Anesthesia and Analgesia, Fourth Edition.

References

1. Harvey R.C., Schaer M. Anesthesia for the patient with endocrine disease. In: *Lumb and Jones' Veterinary Anesthesia*, 4th ed. W.J. Tranquilli, J.C. Thurmon, and K.A. Grimm, eds. Ames, IA: Blackwell, 2007, pp 933–936.
2. Smith J.A. Endocrine disease. In: *Veterinary Anesthesia and Pain Management Secrets*. S.A. Greene, ed. Philadelphia, PA: Hanley and Belfus, 2002, pp 197–200.
3. Melian C., Perez-Alenz M.D., Peterson M.E. Hyperadrenocorticism in dogs. In: *Textbook of Veterinary Internal Medicine*, 7th ed. S.J. Ettinger and E.C. Feldman, eds. St. Louis, MO: Elsevier, 2010, pp 1816–1847.
4. Herrera M., Nelson R.W. Pheochromocytoma. In: *Textbook of Veterinary Internal Medicine*, 7th ed. S.J. Ettinger and E.C. Feldman, eds. St. Louis, MO: Elsevier, 2010, pp 1865–1871.
5. Nelson R.W. Canine diabetes mellitus. In: *Textbook of Veterinary Internal Medicine*, 7th ed. S.J. Ettinger and E.C. Feldman, eds. St. Louis, MO: Elsevier, 2010, pp 1782–1796.
6. Rijnberk A. Diabetes insipidus. In: *Textbook of Veterinary Internal Medicine*, 7th ed. S.J. Ettinger and E.C. Feldman, eds. St. Louis, MO: Elsevier, 2010, pp 1716–1722.
7. Feldman E.C. Disorders of the parathyroid glands. In: *Textbook of Veterinary Internal Medicine*, 7th ed. S.J. Ettinger and E.C. Feldman, eds. St. Louis, MO: Elsevier, 2010, pp 1722–1751.
8. Scott-Moncrieff J.C.R. Hypothyroidism. In: *Textbook of Veterinary Internal Medicine*, 7th ed. S.J. Ettinger and E.C. Feldman, eds. St. Louis, MO: Elsevier, 2010, pp 1751–1761.
9. Mooney C.T. Hyperthyroidism. In: *Textbook of Veterinary Internal Medicine*, 7th ed. S.J. Ettinger and E.C. Feldman, eds. St. Louis, MO: Elsevier, 2010, pp 1761–1779.

Chapter 18

Anesthetic considerations for special procedures

Marjorie E. Gross, Elizabeth A. Giuliano, Marc R. Raffe, Rachael E. Carpenter, Gwendolyn L. Carroll, David D. Martin, Sandra Manfra Marretta, Glenn R. Pettifer, Tamara L. Grubb, Elizabeth M. Hardie, Victoria M. Lukasik, Janyce L. Cornick-Seahorn, Jennifer B. Grimm, and Steven L. Marks

Ocular patients

General considerations

Development of an appropriate anesthetic and pain management plan for any ocular patient requires knowledge of not only the patient's physical status and the ophthalmic procedure to be performed, but also familiarity with ocular physiology and medications administered for ophthalmic purposes.

Ocular and periocular structures are often neglected during anesthetic induction. Positioning of hands and equipment relative to the eyes should be noted during induction, especially when dealing with severely compromised globes with the potential to rupture. Mask induction may not be an option if the mask rubs or puts pressure on the eye, and patient struggling during induction with a face mask may increase intraocular pressure (IOP) or potentiate eye rupture. Providing analgesia is particularly important in patients with substantial discomfort from ophthalmic disease. It is imperative that the use of analgesic and preanesthetic drugs that are associated with vomiting be avoided in cases where brief increases in IOP (e.g., corneal laceration) may cause rupture of the eye. These patients may also be more inclined to struggle when restrained, which may result in increased IOP and additional damage to the globe.

Protection of the dependent, nonaffected eye should also be considered during patient positioning. In unilateral procedures, corneal protection of the unoperated eye may be

Essentials of Small Animal Anesthesia and Analgesia, Second Edition. Edited by Kurt A. Grimm, William J. Tranquilli, Leigh A. Lamont.

provided by application of corneal lubrication with or without a temporary tarsorrhaphy. Positioning of the patient's head and application of any topical ophthalmic preparations should be coordinated between the anesthesia personnel and ophthalmologist to ensure the best possible surgical outcome when both eyes are to be operated on. Resting the periocular region of the dependent eye on a soft padded eye ring or "doughnut" may help protect the eye from corneal abrasion and external globe compression that may result in hypotony.

Laryngeal stimulation should be minimized at induction and endotracheal intubation accomplished as smoothly as possible to avoid any possible increases in IOP. Lidocaine applied topically to the larynx or administered intravenously (IV) may be helpful in suppressing the cough reflex. The occurrence of increases in IOP during endotracheal intubation has not been clearly established in dogs and cats.

Positioning for the ophthalmic procedure may render ocular patients less accessible for anesthetic monitoring, and maintaining an appropriate level of anesthesia may be difficult. Eye reflexes, jaw tone, and oral mucous membranes cannot be routinely monitored although the ophthalmologist may be able to provide information about eye position and movements. Once the head has been surgically draped the airway also becomes inaccessible. A guarded (i.e., wire-reinforced) endotracheal tube is recommended to prevent unobserved kinking and occlusion of the airway during surgical positioning. Capnography is very useful for detection of an obstructed airway or inadvertent disconnection from the anesthetic delivery system. Similarly, pulse oximetry may help detect desaturation should the endotracheal tube become kinked or the delivery system disconnected. However, the pulse oximeter probe may have to be placed somewhere other than the tongue to prevent movement by the ophthalmologist interfering with its function. Since many ocular patients benefit from or require mechanical ventilation, capnometry is particularly useful to ensure maintenance of normocapnia.

Monitoring heart rate (HR) and arterial blood pressure (ABP) are crucial in ocular patients when opportunities to directly visualize the patient are limited. This is even more important when neuromuscular blocking agents (NMBs) have been included in the anesthetic protocol, as assessment of anesthetic depth becomes more challenging in this setting. Increased ABP or HR may indicate an inadequate plane of anesthesia or the need for additional analgesics. Conversely, precipitous decreases in HR or ABP may indicate an excessive plane of anesthesia or initiation of the oculocardiac reflex (OCR). Increased respiration rate may also be indicative of inadequate anesthesia but such a response will not be evident in mechanically ventilated patients that may or may not be paralyzed.

Tear production decreases substantially within 30–60 minutes of the onset of general anesthesia, with or without preemptive administration of atropine, and this may persist for up to 24 hours after the anesthetic procedure. Consequently, corneal lubrication every 90 minutes during general anesthesia is recommended.

Transient lens opacification may occur in mice, rats, and hamsters during prolonged sedation or anesthesia. The opacification is believed to be caused by lack of blinking and subsequent evaporation of fluids from the shallow anterior chamber, which then resolves upon awakening.

If intraocular surgery is planned or globe rupture has occurred, application of topical ophthalmic medications including lubricants should be restricted to aqueous-based formulations. Petroleum-based ointments that gain access to intraocular structures may cause severe uveitis and further compromise vision and ocular comfort. Taping the palpebrae closed or performing a partial temporary tarsorrhaphy are additional techniques for protecting the globe and keeping it moist.

A smooth anesthetic recovery including appropriate analgesia and prevention of self-trauma is the primary postoperative management goal. For patients who have undergone intraocular surgery periods of excitement, incoordination, coughing, gagging, or retching are particularly undesirable. Recovery should be in a quiet, dimly lit enclosure where external stimuli will be kept to a minimum. Patients can be kept comfortable and quiet by appropriate analgesia and sedation, although gentle physical restraint or words of reassurance while holding some small patients may be more effective. Elizabethan collars for small patients and padded helmets or protective eyecups for large patients may help protect their eyes but may not be well tolerated by some. Recovery cages should have extraneous structures such as feed-bowl rings removed to prevent eye trauma during recovery.

Ocular physiological considerations

Selection of an anesthetic protocol for intraocular surgery should include consideration of its effects on IOP, pupil size, and globe position. Success of an ophthalmic procedure may depend on control of IOP before, during, and after the procedure. The overall effect of most anesthetics is to decrease IOP. This reduction may be attributable to a combination of factors, including depression of diencephalic centers regulating IOP, increased aqueous outflow, decreased venous and ABPs, and relaxation of extraocular musculature.

Pupil size is controlled by iris smooth muscle that is controlled primarily by the autonomic nervous system. Parasympathetic stimulation of the iris constrictor muscle results in miosis (pupillary constriction), while sympathetic stimulation of the iris dilator muscle results in mydriasis (pupillary dilation). Pupil size is of greatest concern in cataract removal surgery, which requires the pupil to be widely dilated and the eye immobilized. Most anesthetic or sedative agents, with the exception of ketamine, will cause miosis. Opioids have variable effects on pupil size depending on the species. In cats they tend to cause mydriasis, while in dogs they tend to cause miosis. Prostaglandins, histamines, and other mediators of inflammation may also contribute to miosis, and antiprostaglandins and antihistamines are often administered prior to intraocular surgery. Any sympathomimetic, cholinergic, or anticholinergic drug applied topically to the eye also has the potential to affect pupil size. It has been suggested that mydriasis is more difficult to achieve *after* the onset of sedation or anesthesia, whereas mydriasis achieved prior to anesthetic induction or sedation is usually unaffected by the miotic properties of anesthetics and sedatives.

Globe motion during general anesthesia is not unusual. For corneal or intraocular surgery, any motion of the globe is undesirable. Excessive manual traction to maintain a stable globe position may cause expulsion of intraocular contents or initiation of the OCR. In addition, palpebral eye reflexes that may be evident at lighter planes of anesthesia may also interfere with procedures. Paralysis with NMBs or retrobulbar regional anesthesia during general anesthesia should eliminate ocular reflexes and enable positioning of the globe without excessive manual traction.

Cardiovascular physiological considerations

Many ocular patients are geriatric and the reader is referred to a subsequent section in this chapter for a discussion of anesthesia in geriatric dogs and cats. The depth of anesthesia required for adequate depression of ocular reflexes and globe motion necessary for intraocular surgery often results in pronounced hypotension and may represent additional risk for geriatric patients. This can often be managed intraoperatively by the use of NMBs, controlled ventilation, inotropic drugs, and adequate patient monitoring.

The OCR is a trigeminovagal (cranial nerves V and X) reflex that may be induced by pressure or traction on the eyeball, ocular trauma or pain, or orbital hematoma. Initiation of the reflex manifests as cardiac arrhythmias, which may include bradycardia, nodal rhythms, ectopic beats, ventricular fibrillation, or asystole. Although the OCR occurs most commonly during ocular surgery, it may also occur during nonocular surgery when pressure is placed on the eyeball. It has been suggested that the more acute the onset and the more sustained the pressure or traction, the more likely the OCR is to occur. Hypercapnea may significantly increase the incidence of bradycardia associated with the OCR.

Preemptive intramuscular anticholinergic administration during the preanesthetic period does not necessarily prevent occurrence of the OCR during general anesthesia. Additionally, use of antimuscarinics in patients with glaucoma may exacerbate intraocular hypertension. Treatment of the OCR should begin with discontinuing stimulation. If bradycardia persists, treatment with atropine (0.02 mg/kg IV) or injection of lidocaine into the eye muscles to prevent transmission along the afferent limb of the reflex may be effective. Precautions against initiation of the OCR should include assuring an adequate depth of anesthesia, maintaining normocapnia, and minimizing aggressive surgical manipulations.

Ophthalmic medications

Eye drops and ointments are concentrated medications that may cause systemic side effects especially when administered to very small patients. Systemic effects may be minimized by diluting topical medications and limiting their frequency of application. For a summary of commonly used topical ophthalmic medications that may impact anesthetic management, please refer to Table 18.1.

Anesthetic and sedative agents in ocular patients

Commonly used anesthetic and sedative agents may induce ocular side effects and impact the outcome of ocular procedures. For a summary of commonly used anesthetic and sedative agents and their ocular effects, please refer to Table 18.2.

Analgesic agents in ocular patients

Ocular and periocular structures are richly innervated and highly sensitive. Symptoms of ocular pain include blepharospasm, photophobia, ocular discharge, rubbing of the eyes, and avoidance behavior. A variety of topical and systemic drug therapies are

Table 18.1. Ophthalmic medications with potential systemic side effects commonly used in dogs and cats presenting for ocular surgery

Drug	Class	Ophthalmic indications	Potential side effects
Pilocarpine	Direct-acting cholinergic agonist	Glaucoma—↓ IOP by ↑ aqueous outflow	Bradycardia, AV block
Echothiophate, isoflurophate	Indirect-acting cholinergic agonist (anticholinesterase)	Glaucoma—↓ IOP by ↑ aqueous outflow	Bradycardia, AV block
Epinephrine, dipivefrine	Nonselective adrenergic agonist	Glaucoma—↓ IOP by ↑ aqueous outflow	Tachycardia, hypertension, dysrhythmias
Phenylephrine	Alpha adrenergic agonist	Precataract surgery or uveitis—mydriasis	Hypertension, reflex bradycardia
Timolol	Nonselective beta-adrenergic antagonist	Glaucoma—↓ IOP by ↓ aqueous production	Hypotension, bradycardia
Methazolamide	Carbonic anhydrase inhibitor	Glaucoma—↓ IOP by ↓ aqueous production	Metabolic acidosis, hyperchloremia, hypokalemia
Predisolone acetate, dexamethasone, hydrocortisone acetate	Corticosteroid	Uveitis, epischleritis, allergic conjunctivits, and so on.	Adrenocortical suppression with long-term treatment
Mannitol[a], glycerin[b]	Osmotic agent	Glaucoma—↓ IOP by ↑ aqueous outflow	↑ CVP, ↑ serum osmolality, pulmonary edema

[a] Administered intravenously.
[b] Administered orally.
IOP, intraocular pressure.

currently available to address pain management adequately in ophthalmic patients. For a summary of commonly used analgesics and their ocular effects, please refer to Table 18.3.

Local and regional anesthesia in ocular patients

Local or regional anesthesia may be adequate for less invasive procedures or may be included as part of a balanced general anesthetic protocol. Topical anesthesia for diagnostic and therapeutic procedures in veterinary ocular patients usually requires accompanying sedation to gain cooperation of the patient.

Local anesthetics applied topically are readily absorbed through mucous membranes. Systemic toxicosis is possible, though unlikely, but judicious administration in small patients is recommended. Topical anesthetics can be irritating and cause transient conjunctival hyperemia as well as damage corneal epithelium, delay corneal wound healing, and mask signs of disease or discomfort. It is recommended, therefore, that topical

Table 18.2. Ocular effects of anesthetics, sedatives, and anticholinergics

Drug	Class	Comments regarding use in ophthalmic patients
Isoflurane Sevoflurane	Inhalant	• Dose-dependent ↓ IOP if normocapnia maintained • Use as part of a balanced protocol to ensure smooth recovery and positive ocular outcome • No arrhythmogenic potentiation with topical epinephrine administration
Nitrous oxide	Inhalant	• Contraindicated with intraocular injection of gas/air into a closed eye (gas expansion may ↑ IOP); discontinue nitrous for >15–20 minutes prior to air injection
Thiopental	Injectable anesthetic	• ↓ IOP in normal and glaucomatous eyes
Propofol	Injectable anesthetic	• ↓ IOP in normal and glaucomatous eyes
Etomidate	Injectable anesthetic	• ↓ IOP directly but associated myoclonus may lead to ↑ IOP; therefore, coadminister with a benzodiazepine in patients with potential for globe rupture
Ketamine	Dissociative anesthetic	• May ↑ IOP even when coadministered with benzodiazepines; therefore, avoid in patients with potential for globe rupture • May induce nystagmus → problematic in certain ocular procedures • Palpebrae remain open → predisposes to corneal drying • Pupils dilate and palpebral and corneal reflexes persist • Recoveries may be rough if not modified with other drugs
Telazol®	Dissociative/ benzodiazepine	• Similar to ketamine
Atropine Glycopyrrolate	Anticholinergic	• May prevent the OCR or counteract bradycardia associated with administration of other vagotonic agents such as opioids • May make cannulation of the parotid duct more challenging in parotid duct transposition surgery • Potential for systemic anticholinergics to induce cycloplegia and mydriasis and ↑ IOP is unclear; glycopyrrolate may be less likely to induce ocular effects compared to atropine due to decreased penetration of end organs
Dexmedetomidine Medetomidine	Alpha$_2$ agonist	• Topical administration causes mydriasis and ↓ IOP in cats and rabbits • Systemic administration causes miosis and no change in IOP in dogs (miosis *not* evident with tropicamide pretreatment) • May be useful for postoperative sedation to ensure a smooth recovery

Table 18.2. (*Continued*)

Drug	Class	Comments regarding use in ophthalmic patients
Diazepam Midazolam	Benzodiazepine	• ↓ IOP • Conflicting evidence regarding ability to counteract ↑ IOP associated with ketamine administration
Acepromazine	Phenothiazine	• Antiemetic effects may be useful in ocular patients • May be useful for postoperative sedation to ensure a smooth recovery

IOP, intraocular pressure.

Table 18.3. Ocular effects of selected analgesics

Drug	Class	Comments regarding use in ophthalmic patients
Morphine Hydromorphone Oxymorphone Fentanyl Butophanol Buprenorphine	Opioid	• Morphine ↓ IOP (other opioids assumed to have similar effects) • May induce emesis, which ↑ IOP; may need to delay administration until the patient is anesthetized if globe rupture is a concern • Induce vagotonic effects that may cause bradycardia and/or contribute to the OCR • Morphine causes miosis in dogs and mydriasis in cats (other opioids assumed to have similar effects) • Topical morphine (1%) reduces corneal pain in dogs with ulcers
Carprofen Meloxicam Deracoxib Firocoxib Tepoxalin Flunixin	Nonsteroidal anti-inflammatory	• Appear to be effective for pain associated with corneal inflammation, uveitis, and other ocular pathology • Prevent intraoperative miosis • Used systemically and topically (topical application results in systemic absorption through nasal mucosa, therefore must coordinate systemic and topical use to avoid toxicity) • Topical use associated with irritation of conjunctiva, corneal cytopathy, ↓ aqueous outflow
Lidocaine	Local anesthetic	• IV constant rate infusion provides comparable analgesia to morphine constant rate infusion for intraocular surgery in dogs

IOP, intraocular pressure.

anesthetics be reserved for diagnostic rather than therapeutic purposes. Tear production and the blink reflex will be reduced after topical anesthetic administration, necessitating the application of ocular lubricant to protect the cornea after completion of the diagnostic procedure.

Topical administration of 1% morphine sulfate solution appears to provide local analgesia in dogs with corneal ulcers. The antinociceptive effect is possibly a result of interaction with mu opioid receptors, which have been identified in small numbers in normal canine corneas, and delta opioid receptors, which have been identified in the corneal epithelium and stroma of dogs. In contrast with the local anesthetics, this local analgesic effect is produced without delaying corneal wound healing or causing any discernible tissue damage.

Neuromuscular blockade for ophthalmic surgery

Paralysis of extraocular muscles relaxes the eye and allows the globe to roll centrally and proptose slightly. These effects greatly facilitate positioning of the globe for ophthalmic surgery, eliminating the need for significant surgical manipulation to obtain proper globe positioning and decreasing the potential for initiating the OCR. Mechanical ventilation is indicated for patients receiving neuromuscular blockers during general anesthesia to maintain normocapnia.

Depolarizing NMBs, such as succinylcholine, tend to increase IOP just prior to paralysis, while nondepolarizing NMBs, such as pancuronim, vecuronium, atracurium, and cisatracurium, do not appear to have this effect.

In glaucoma patients receiving treatment with an indirect-acting cholinergic agent (i.e., anticholinesterase), metabolism of succinylcholine may be delayed and paralysis induced by this NMB may be prolonged. It has been recommended that indirect-acting cholinergic drugs be discontinued 2–4 weeks prior to neuromuscular blockade with succinylcholine, although normal levels of plasma pseudocholinesterase activity may not be totally restored for 4–6 weeks.

While depolarizing NMBs are not reversible, the effects of nondepolarizing NMBs may be reversed with anticholinesterases such as neostigmine and edrophonium. Anticholinesterase administration is not associated with increased IOP. An anticholinergic (atropine or glycopyrrolate) is commonly administered prior to the anticholinesterase to prevent profound bradycardia. Alternatively, the use a nondepolarizing NMB with a shorter duration of action, such as atracurium or cisatracurium, may be indicated to avoid the need for reversal. Reversal of neuromuscular blockade should be complete to prevent hypoventilation, struggling during recovery, self-trauma, and increases in IOP.

Electroretinography and anesthesia

Electroretinography (ERG) is used primarily as a diagnostic test for progressive retinal atrophy or other degenerative retinal disorders, and to assess retinal integrity in dogs where ophthalmoscopic evaluation of the fundus is not possible prior to cataract surgery. Complete ocular akinesia is preferred for diagnostic ERG, which requires general anesthesia and possibly neuromuscular blockade. The ERG requires dark adaptation of the patient and is performed in the dark, which makes anesthetic monitoring a challenge. Inhalant agents depress the ERG in dogs but the results are considered useful as long as the ERG for the patient and the control animal are generated under identical anesthetic conditions. No single anesthetic protocol has been established for performance of ERGs, although propofol induction with isoflurane maintenance has been used successfully in dogs. Sedation with dexmedetomidine and an opioid such as butorphanol or nalbuphine, and a cooperative patient may prove adequate for a semiquantitative ERG as is typically performed for preoperative screening of cataract patients.

Cesarean section patients

General considerations

The ideal anesthetic protocol for cesarean section would provide adequate hypnosis, analgesia, and muscle relaxation for optimal operating conditions without adversely impacting either mother or fetus. Because the physicochemical properties that allow sedative, anesthetic, and analgesic drugs to cross the blood–brain barrier also enable their placental transfer, it is not possible to selectively anesthetize the mother. Agents that affect the maternal central nervous system (CNS) will also produce fetal effects, resulting in fetal depression and potentially decreased viability. In many cases, cesarean section is an emergency procedure where the physical condition of the mother and fetus is less than optimal, making anesthetic management even more challenging.

Selection of an anesthetic plan for cesarean section should take into account the safety of the mother and fetus, provision of adequate patient comfort, and the veterinarian's familiarity with the anesthetic technique. Factors in decision making include considerations of the physiological alterations induced by pregnancy and labor, the pharmacology of selected drugs and their direct and indirect effects on the fetus/neonate, the benefits and risks of the techniques chosen, and the risk of procedure-related complications associated with anesthetic management. Regardless of the anesthetic technique used, surgical expediency is crucial to decrease maternal recumbency time and fetal drug absorption. With prolonged uterine isolation prior to fetal delivery, placental perfusion decreases, resulting in fetal hypoxemia, acidosis, and distress.

Physiological alterations induced by pregnancy

Metabolic demands of gestation and parturition are met by altered physiological function. Although little work has been done in dogs and cats specifically, it is reasonable to extrapolate from other species. A summary of the major cardiovascular, pulmonary, gastrointestinal, and hepatorenal alterations induced by pregnancy is provided in Table 18.4.

Uterine blood flow during pregnancy

Maintaining stable uteroplacental circulation is important to fetal and maternal homeostasis and neonatal survival. Uterine blood flow is directly proportional to

Table 18.4.   Physiological alterations induced by pregnancy

Cardiovascular	Pulmonary
↑ HR	↑ MV
↑ stroke volume	↑ oxygen consumption
↑ CO	o arterial pH
↓ vascular resistance	o PaO_2
↑ blood volume	↓ $PaCO_2$
↑ plasma volume	o total lung and vital capacity
↓ PCV, hemoglobin	↓ FRC
↓ plasma protein	↓ pulmonary resistance
o ABP	o lung compliance
o CVP (↑ during labor)	
Gastrointestinal	**Hepatorenal**
↑ gastric emptying	↑ liver serum enzyme concentrations
↑ gastric pressure	↑ sulfobromophthalein sodium retention
↓ gastric motility	o bilirubin concentration
↓ pH of gastric secretions	↓ plasma cholinesterase
↑ gastric chloride ion and enzyme concentration	↑ renal blood flow
	↑ glomerular filtration rate

CVP, central venous pressure; o, no change; PaO_2, arterial partial pressure of oxygen; $PaCO_2$, arterial partial pressure of carbon dioxide. See text for definitions of other abbreviations.

systemic perfusion pressure and inversely proportional to myometrial vascular resistance. Placental blood flow is mainly dependent on uteroplacental perfusion pressure but placental vessels have rudimentary mechanisms for changing vascular resistance. Obstetric anesthesia may decrease uterine and placental blood flow and thereby contribute to reduced fetal viability. In addition, uterine vascular resistance is indirectly increased by uterine contractions and hypertonia (oxytocic response). Decreased placental blood flow may occur with hypovolemia, anesthetic-induced cardiovascular depression, or sympathetic blockade producing reduced uterine perfusion pressure. Uterine vasoconstriction is induced by endogenous sympathetic discharge or by exogenous sympathomimetic drugs having alpha₁ adrenergic effects (epinephrine, norepinephrine, methoxamine, phenylephrine, or metaraminol). Every effort should be made to avoid or minimize hypotension induced by anesthetic agents and increased uterine tone induced by ecbolic agents.

Impact of physiological changes on anesthetic management

Parturients are at greater anesthetic risk than are healthy nonparturient patients because of pregnancy-associated physiological alterations and the often emergent nature of the surgery. Cardiac reserve diminishes during pregnancy and high-risk patients can suffer acute cardiac decompensation or failure. The use of ecbolic agents during or after parturition can also adversely affect cardiovascular function. Oxytocin in large or repeated doses induces peripheral vasodilation and hypotension, which can adversely affect both mother and fetus through decreased tissue perfusion.

Because functional residual capacity (FRC) is decreased, anesthetic-induced hypoventilation will induce hypoxemia and hypercapnia more readily in pregnant patients. Hypoxemia is further exacerbated by increased oxygen consumption during labor. Preoxygenation prior to anesthetic induction will increase oxygen reserve and is advisable if the patient is tolerant.

Inhalant induction occurs more rapidly due to increased alveolar ventilation and decreased FRC in the parturient. Additionally, increased progesterone and endorphin levels in the CNS decrease anesthetic requirements (i.e., the minimum alveolar anesthetic concentration is reduced). Thus, anesthetic induction may be extremely rapid, requiring as little as one-fourth to one-fifth the time required for nonpregnant patients, so care must be taken to prevent volatile agent overdose. Local anesthetic requirements are also decreased in the parturient.

As a result of altered gastric function, the risk of regurgitation (both active and passive) and aspiration is greater in parturients. Because increased gastric acidity and decreased gastric muscular tone may be present, metoclopramide and an H_2 antagonist drug (cimetidine, ranitidine, or famotidine) may be administered as part of the preanesthetic medication. Frequently, patients presented for cesarean section have been fed or the time of the last feeding is unknown. Parturients should be regarded as having a full stomach and anesthesia techniques should be selected that produce rapid airway control to prevent aspiration of foreign material. Incidence of vomiting is increased by hypotension, hypoxia, and toxic reactions to local anesthetics. Smooth induction of general anesthesia and prevention of hypotension during epidural anesthesia will decrease the incidence of vomiting. Because silent regurgitation can occur when intragastric pressure is high, a cuffed endotracheal tube is preferred for airway management. Atropine administration may increase gastroesophageal sphincter tone and help to prevent regurgitation, but it may also inhibit the actions of metoclopramide to increase gastric motility and emptying by sensitizing gastric smooth muscle to acetylcholine.

Decreased plasma cholinesterase levels may lead to prolonged action of succinylcholine in pregnant patients, particularly if they have been exposed recently to organophosphate parasiticides in flea collars or dips. Normal or slightly elevated blood urea nitrogen or creatinine levels may indicate renal pathology or compromise in parturient patients. It would appear wise in such patients to avoid the use of drugs with known nephrotoxic potential, such as methoxyflurane, aminoglycoside antibiotics, and nonsteroidal anti-inflammatory drugs (NSAIDs).

Placental transfer of drugs

The placenta is highly permeable to anesthetic drugs. The physiochemical properties that make a molecule a good anesthetic drug also enable rapid transfer across the uteroplacental interface. Anesthetic drugs administered to the mother cross the placenta and induce fetal effects proportionate to those observed in the mother. Placental transfer of drugs can occur by several mechanisms, but by far the most important is simple diffusion.

Diffusion across the placenta is determined by molecular weight (MW), the degree to which the drug is bound to maternal plasma proteins, lipid solubility, and degree of ionization. Drugs with low MW (<500 daltons), a low degree of protein binding, high lipid solubility, and poor ionization diffuse rapidly across the placenta. Most anesthetics and anesthetic adjuncts fit into this category. The muscle relaxant drugs are an exception and are generally regarded as having minimal placental transfer and negligible fetal effects. The placenta does not appear to metabolize anesthetics or anesthetic adjuncts.

The degree to which a drug is ionized is determined by its pK_a and the pH of the fluid compartment. Drugs that are weak acids will be less ionized as pH decreases. For example, thiopental is a weak acid with a pK_a of 7.6. In acidemic patients (pH < 7.4), a greater proportion of the administered dose is in the nonionized (nonprotein-bound) form. Consequently, acidemia tends to decrease the required anesthetic dose of thiopental and other barbiturates. Weakly basic drugs such as opioids and local anesthetics are more highly ionized at pH values less than their pK_a. Thus, a greater fraction will be protein bound in acidemic states, which may potentially increase dose requirements. Because fetal pH is 0.1 pH unit less than that of the mother, weakly basic drugs (i.e., opioids, local anesthetics) are found in higher concentrations in fetal tissues and plasma compared to those of the mother because of ion trapping.

Fetal pharmacokinetics

Fetal drug concentrations are affected by redistribution, metabolism, and protein binding. The drug concentration in the umbilical vein is greater than drug exposure to fetal organs (brain, heart, and other vital organs). As much as 85% of umbilical venous blood initially passes through the fetal liver, where drug may be sequestered or metabolized. In addition, umbilical venous blood containing the drug enters the inferior vena cava via the ductus venosus and mixes with the drug-free blood returning from the lower extremities and pelvic viscera. Therefore, the fetal circulation buffers fetal tissues from sudden high drug concentrations. Binding of drug to fetal proteins may also reduce bioavailability. Fetal drug metabolism is not efficient, as microsomal enzyme systems have not reached full capacity in the fetus. Drug concentration and effects in the fetus can be considerably greater and last longer than in the mother. Fetal drug toxicity can be enhanced by fetal or maternal metabolism to more toxic metabolites and by drug interactions.

The administration of a fixed dose of a drug with rapidly decreasing plasma concentration (such as thiopental, propofol, or succinylcholine) briefly exposes the fetus and placenta to a high maternal blood drug concentration. This is in contrast to the sustained maternal blood levels of drugs administered by continuous infusion or inhalation, which result in continuous placental transfer of drug to the fetus.

Anesthetic drugs in the cesarean section patient

Anesthetic drugs and techniques should be carefully chosen and properly administered to minimize maternal depression and risk and to maximize neonatal vigor and viability. No agent should be used unless distinctly indicated. A brief overview of anesthetic drug classes in periparturient anesthesia follows. Please refer to Table 18.5 for a summary of drugs used in the perianesthetic period and their effects in the cesarean section patient.

Table 18.5. Effects of anesthetic agents in cesarean section patients

Drug	Class	Comments regarding use in cesarean section patients
Atropine Glycopyrrolate	Anticholinergic	• Recommended in most to counteract ↑ vagal tone associated with uterine traction • May ↓ incidence of emesis? • ↑ gastric pH → may reduce severity of aspiration pneumonia if it occurs • Glycopyrrolate does not readily cross the placenta → fewer fetal effects compared to atropine
Acepromazine	Phenothiazine	• Induces significant maternal and fetal neurobehavioral depression • Long lasting and not reversible • Contraindicated for routine use
Medetomidine Dexmedetomidine	Alpha$_2$ agonist	• Induces significant maternal and fetal circulatory and neurobehavioral depression • Contraindicated for routine use
Diazepam Midazolam	Benzodiazepine	• Induce neonatal depression • Neonatal effects may be dose dependent but safe doses have not been determined for use in dogs and cats • Reversible (in mother and/or neonate) with flumazenil • Not recommended for routine use
Morphine Hydromorphone Oxymorphone Fentanyl Butorphanol Buprenorphine	Opioid	• Induce neonatal respiratory and neurobehavioral depression • Fetus may require 2–6 days to eliminate • May cause maternal emesis if given in the preanesthetic period (especially morphine) • Reversible in neonate with naloxone given sublingually but renarcotization may require redosing
Thiopental	Thiobarbiturate	• Rapid induction in the mother • Rapidly cleared from neonatal circulation • Neonatal suckling activity may be decreased post-thiopental
Propofol	Isopropylphenol	• Rapid, smooth induction in the mother • Rapidly cleared from neonatal circulation • Associated with ↑ puppy vigor, vocalization, and survival postsurgery • Injectable drug of choice for induction of anesthesia
Etomidate	Carboxylated imidazole	• Rapid induction but myoclonus is possible • Rapidly cleared from neonatal circulation
Alphaxalone-CD	Steroid	• Rapid, smooth induction in the mother • Appears promising but limited data in this patient population
Ketamine	Dissociative	• ↑ puppy risk → respiratory depression, apnea, ↓ vocalization, ↑ mortality at birth • Not recommended for routine use
Telazol®	Dissociative/ benzodiazepine	• Limited data available in this patient population • Not recommended for routine use

(Continued)

Table 18.5.   *(Continued)*

Drug	Class	Comments regarding use in cesarean section patients
Isoflurane Sevoflurane Desflurane	Inhalant	• Dose-dependent maternal and fetal depression • Rapid inductions and recoveries • Drugs of choice for maintenance of anesthesia • Suitable for induction of anesthesia in selected patients
Nitrous oxide	Inhalant	• Potential adjunct to volatile inhalants • Minimal neonatal depression and no neonatal diffusion hypoxia if administered at concentrations <60%
Succinylcholine Mivacurium Vecuronium Atracurium	Muscle relaxant (short to intermediate acting)	• Minimal placental transfer → minimal neonatal effects • May be useful adjunct in a balanced anesthetic protocol • Avoid long-acting agents such as pancuronium
Lidocaine Bupivacaine Mepivacaine Ropivacaine	Local anesthetic	• Minimal neonatal effects when appropriate doses used for epidural administration • Sympathetic blockade may cause maternal hypotension → uterine hypoperfusion if not treated

General anesthesia for cesarean section

Cesarean section anesthesia can be accomplished either by regional or general anesthesia. Advantages of general anesthesia include speed and ease of induction, reliability, reproducibility, monitoring, and control. General anesthesia provides optimum operating conditions by providing a relaxed immobile patient. Tracheal intubation ensures control of the maternal airway, thereby preventing aspiration of vomitus or regurgitated gastric contents. In addition, it provides a route for maternal oxygen administration, thereby improving fetal oxygenation. When general anesthesia is administered properly, maternal cardiopulmonary function is well maintained.

General anesthesia may be more appropriate than regional anesthesia in selected clinical situations. These include maternal hypovolemia; prolonged dystocia, in which the mother is exhausted and the fetus is severely stressed; maternal cardiac disease or failure; morbid obesity, cases in which the mother is aggressive or fractious; and in brachycephalic dogs with upper airway obstruction. Finally, most veterinarians are more confident of their ability to induce general anesthesia safely than to use regional anesthesia techniques in dogs and cats.

General anesthesia does have certain disadvantages. It will likely produce greater neonatal depression than will regional anesthesia. Inadequate anesthetic plane causes maternal catecholamine release, which may result in hypertension and decreased uteroplacental perfusion, leading to both maternal and fetal stress and deterioration of cardiopulmonary function. Loss of airway protective reflexes following anesthetic induction

Table 18.6.   Selected general anesthetic techniques for elective and emergency cesarean section patients

Protocol	Comments
• ± Anticholinergic • Propofol IV to effect for induction • Endotracheal intubation • Inhalant for maintenance • Opioid IV following fetal removal • ± Single-dose NSAID (depending on maternal risk factors) following fetal removal	Suitable for elective cesarean sections
• ± Anticholinergic • Fentanyl (0.003–0.005 mg/kg IV) • Propofol IV to effect for induction • Endotracheal intubation • Inhalant for maintenance • Additional opioid (because of fentanyl's short duration) following fetal removal • ±Single-dose NSAID (depending on maternal risk factors) following fetal removal • Treat neonates with Naloxone	Suitable for elective or emergency cesarean sections
• Inhalant induction via face mask • Endotracheal intubation • Inhalant for maintenance • Opioid following fetal removal • ±Single-dose NSAID (depending on maternal risk factors) following fetal removal	Suitable for emergency cesarean sections

may produce aspiration and airway management challenges when the trachea is not properly intubated. Several selected general anesthetic protocols for canine and feline cesarean section patients are provided in Table 18.6.

Maternal oxygen administration can significantly increase fetal oxygen content and can result in more vigorous neonates. Consequently, it is recommended for all cesarean section patients. Maternal tidal volume and minute ventilation (MV) must be critically evaluated during the anesthetic period to avoid either hypoventilation or hyperventilation. The total effect of carbon dioxide on the fetus is not clear, but passive hyperventilation of the dam causes hypocapnia with decreased uterine artery blood flow. This decreased placental perfusion causes fetal hypoxia, hypercapnia, and acidosis. With adequate arterial oxygenation, a modest increase in arterial partial pressure of carbon dioxide ($PaCO_2$) is well tolerated by the fetus. Adequacy of ventilation and oxygenation may be assessed by observing the rate of respiration, excursion of the chest wall and/or reservoir bag, and the color of mucous membranes. Capnometry and pulse oximtery are particularly useful pieces of monitoring equipment.

Regional anesthesia for cesarean section

This is a well-established technique for cesarean section in some species but is used less frequently in dogs and cats. Because there is a decreased dose requirement and enhanced distribution of local anesthetic agents during gestation and parturition, the dose of local anesthetic for epidural or spinal anesthesia can be reduced by approximately one-third in parturients. Regional anesthesia (epidural or subarachnoid) has the advantages of technique simplicity, minimal exposure of the fetus to drugs, less intraoperative bleeding, and, because the mother remains awake, minimal risk of aspiration. In addition, muscle relaxation and analgesia are optimal. In dogs, the subarachnoid space usually terminates at the level of the sixth lumbar vertebra, thereby reducing the risk of subarachnoid (true spinal) injection of the local anesthetic agent. In cats, the termination is variably between L7 and midsacrum, making subarachnoid injection a greater possibility.

Epidural anesthesia has been successfully used in dogs and cats for cesarean section anesthesia. Traditionally, a short-acting local anesthetic (2% lidocaine or mepivacaine) is administered at a dose of 1 mL per 3.25–4.5 kg of body weight into the epidural space to provide surgical site anesthesia. Alternatively, a 1:1 volumetric mixture of lidocaine and bupivacaine can be administered to extend the duration of surgical anesthesia and pain management into the early recovery period. This may be supplemented with epidural opioids and alpha$_2$ adrenergic agonists.

Disadvantages of epidural or subarachnoid anesthesia include hypotension secondary to sympathetic blockade. Hypotension induced by epidural anesthesia can be managed with IV fluid and/or catecholamine administration. An isotonic crystalloid solution can be administered at approximately 20 mL/kg over 15–20 minutes to maintain ABP. When hypotension is severe, ephedrine may be administered (0.05–0.15 mg/kg IV). Ephedrine is considered the catecholamine of choice in this setting as it induces minimal effects on uterine blood flow and perfusion. Nausea and vomiting may also occur during the procedure and are usually associated with hypotension or visceral manipulation. Because the dam remains conscious, the forelimbs and head often move and gentle restraint is necessary. This precludes the use of a regional anesthetic technique in highly excited or fractious patients.

Care of newborns

Following delivery, the newborn's head is cleared of membranes and the oropharynx of fluid. The umbilical vessels should be milked toward the fetus to empty them of blood, clamped approximately 2–5 cm from the body wall, and severed from the placenta. Neonates can then be gently rubbed with a towel to dry them and stimulate breathing. Vigorous motion should be avoided because amniotic fluid is readily absorbed in the lungs and contributes to distribution of pulmonary surfactant in the alveoli. The head and neck should be supported to avoid whiplash and prevent injury.

Flow-by oxygen administration in the vicinity of the muzzle is helpful to increase HR and oxygen delivery to tissues in distressed, exhausted neonates. Reversal of opioids by sublingual administration of 1–2 drops naloxone is warranted in cases where opioids were administered as part of the general anesthesia technique. An oral dose of 2.5% dextrose (0.1–0.5 mL) is helpful to improve energy substrates required to initiate breathing in stressed neonates. Finally, maintaining warmth is vital because hypothermia can occur rapidly after birth.

A small IV catheter may be used to intubate and support oxygen delivery in neonates that do not spontaneously initiate breathing, and breathing can be artificially supported by using a syringe and three-way valve attached to an oxygen source. As a final measure, doxapram can be used to stimulate breathing in neonates. In pups, a dosage of 1–5 mg (approximately 1–5 drops from a 20–22-gauge needle) is topically administered to the oral mucosa or injected intramuscularly or subcutaneously. In kittens, the dosage is 1–2 mg (1–2 drops). Airways must be clear before doxapram administration. External thoracic compressions may be warranted if HR is slow and does not respond to other supportive measures. A rapid physical examination checking for genetic defects (cleft palate, chest wall deformity, or abdominal wall fusion) is also important to determine viability.

After completion of surgery and recovery from anesthesia, the young can be introduced to their mother. If introduction is delayed, the neonates should be exposed briefly to the mother to provide colostrum and then kept in a warm environment until anesthesia recovery is complete to avoid accidental crushing. If regional anesthesia was used, neonates can be placed with their mother as soon as the surgery is complete.

Pain management

This represents a challenge in cesarean section patients because of concerns regarding transfer of analgesic drugs into milk and its impact on neonates. While data specific to dogs and cats are not available, it appears that short-term perioperative administration of postoperative opioids and NSAIDs is not associated with significant adverse effects in newborns.

Trauma and critically ill patients

General considerations

Anesthetic management in the traumatized or critically ill patient requires advanced planning, an ordered protocol, and efficient use of time and resources. A team approach to patient management in the emergency room, where each team member has specific preassigned duties, ensures rapid evaluation and treatment. The patient's airway, breathing, circulatory, and neurological status must be assessed immediately upon arrival and reassessed frequently during the initial treatment period.

The initial physical examination must include, at a minimum, evaluation of respiratory rate and effort, HR and rhythm, pulse quality, capillary refill time (CRT), mucous membrane color, ABP, core body temperature, CNS function, and pain. A minimum panel of standard patient-side laboratory tests should be run, typically including assessment of packed cell volume (PCV), total solids (TS), blood urea nitrogen or creatinine, blood glucose, lactate, electrolytes, blood gas analysis or total carbon dioxide, activated clotting time, and urine specific gravity. Other diagnostic procedures including imaging, electrocardiographic (ECG) evaluation, and extended laboratory testing should be completed as indicated.

Severely traumatized or critically ill patients commonly develop serious complications within the first few days of presentation. Such complications may not be directly related to the initial insult but reflect overall tissue destruction, immune suppression, and metabolic imbalances. Critically ill patients are particularly prone to developing some form of shock, which is broadly defined as a generalized state of inadequate *effective* tissue perfusion.

When anesthetizing critically ill patients, the primary goal is to optimize tissue perfusion and oxygen delivery to vital organs while simultaneously ensuring a level of CNS depression resulting in unconsciousness, analgesia, and muscle relaxation. The ultimate goal should be optimal physiological function rather than restoration of measured hemodynamic parameters to "normal." In fact, values considered normal for healthy anesthetized patients are associated with higher rates of mortality in high-risk patients. In humans, survivability is associated with cardiac indexes 50% higher and blood volumes greater than 100% higher than normal at the end of surgery.

Traumatized or critically ill patients are at increased risk of cardiopulmonary collapse. Common causes of acute circulatory failure include severe myocardial ischemia, malignant dysrhythmias, hypoxemia associated with severe lung injury or airway obstruction, hemorrhagic shock, acid–base or electrolyte abnormalities, and profound vasovagal responses.

Shock

The shock syndrome is commonly subcategorized into three distinct phases. The compensatory phase occurs early in the time course when the endogenous response is adequate to stabilize hemodynamic parameters. Modest increases in HR and respiratory rate may be noted but ABP and lactate levels remain within normal limits. Because clinical signs are not dramatic, this phase of shock may go unrecognized. The reversible or early decompensatory phase occurs when endogenous mechanisms of compensation are inadequate and hypotension, tachycardia, hypothermia, altered mentation, and lactic acidosis are documented. By definition, this stage remains amenable to intervention and treatment. The irreversible or terminal decompensatory phase is when prolonged tissue hypoxia results in permanent microvascular and organ damage. The sympathetic and neurohormonal response is exhausted and resuscitation during this phase will be ineffective.

There are numerous systems for classifying types of shock based on pathophysiology and more than one type may develop from a single etiology (Table 18.7). As a general rule, anesthesia should not be undertaken until vital organ functions have been assessed and stabilized. If the patient is in shock, the etiology should be determined and corrective measures initiated before anesthesia. A brief discussion of the most common clinical forms of shock in dogs and cats is presented below.

Systemic inflammatory response syndrome and septic shock

Systemic inflammatory response syndrome (SIRS) is a term applied to widespread inflammatory and immune activity occurring in response to sepsis or severe tissue trauma, injury, or necrosis. Criteria for diagnosis of SIRS in dogs and cats based on the

Table 18.7. Classification system for different types of shock

Hypovolemic	Cardiogenic	Obstructive	Distributive
Hemorrhage: • External • Gastrointestinal • Retroperitoneal • Intra-abdominal	Myopathic: • Cardiomyopathy • Myocarditis • Myocardial contusions • Myocardial depression (sepsis)	Vena caval obstruction: • Gastric dilatation-volvulus • Neoplasia	Sepsis or inflammatory toxic shock

Nonhemorrhage fluid depletion:
• External
  – Dehydration
  – Vomiting
  – Diarrhea
• Interstitial redistribution
• Cavitary effusion
	Mechanical:
	• Valve failure
	• Myocardial hypertrophy
	• Ventricular septal defect
		Increased intrathoracic pressure:
		• Tension pneumothorax
		• Positive pressure ventilation
		• Asthma
			Anaphylactic/anaplhyactoid

Venodilation:
• Sepsis
• Anaphylaxis
• Toxins
	Dysrhythmic:
	• Bradycardia
	  – Sinus
	  – AV block
	• Tachycardia
	  – Supraventricular
	  – Ventricular
		Decreased cardiac compliance:
		• Cardiac tamponade
		• Constrictive pericarditis
			Endocrinologic:
			• Adrenal crisis

		Increased ventricular afterload:
		• Right side
		  – Pulmonary embolus
		  – Pulmonary hypertension
		• Left side
		  – Aortic thromboembolism
			Neurogenic:
			• Spinal injury

presence of various key clinical signs have been proposed and are presented in Table 18.8.

Sepsis is a term used to describe patients meeting criteria for SIRS that also have proven microbial infections. Septic shock describes the syndrome of cardiovascular dysfunction and compromised tissue perfusion that accompanies sepsis.

Classic early signs of SIRS and septic shock include brick-red mucous membranes, rapid CRT, tachycardia, bounding pulses, normal or low ABP, hyperpnea, and hyperthermia. In cats, normothermia or hypothermia may be observed at this stage and bradycardia is not uncommon. This may represent a true difference in the way cats respond to sepsis or may reflect the fact that they tend to be referred for treatment at a later stage. The later phase of SIRS and septic shock is characterized by weak pulses, prolonged CRT,

Table 18.8.   Proposed definitions of systemic inflammatory response syndrome (SIRS)[a] in dogs and cats

Clinical parameter	Dogs	Cats
HR (beats per minute)	>120	<140 or >225
Respiratory rate (breaths per minute) or Ventilation ($PaCO_2$ in mm Hg)	>20 or <32 mm Hg	>40 or <28 mm Hg
Body temperature	>39.7°C or <37.8°C	>39.7°C or <37°C
Neutrophils ×10⁹/L	>180,000, <5,000, or >10% immature (band) forms	>190,000 or <5,000, or >10% immature (band) forms

[a] SIRS can be diagnosed if there is reason to suspect the presence of an inflammatory process in combination with two or more of above criteria.
$PaCO_2$, arterial partial pressure of carbon dioxide.

cyanotic, dusky pink, gray, or pale mucous membranes, and cool extremities. If oxygen delivery to tissues is chronically impaired, SIRS can lead to a phenomenon known as multiple organ dysfunction syndrome (MODS). Successful management of animals with SIRS and septic shock depends on anticipation, not reaction. Appropriate antibiotic administration, aggressive cardiopulmonary support, and intensive monitoring of susceptible organs must be undertaken early.

Hemorrhagic shock

Clinical signs of hemorrhagic shock in acutely traumatized patients depend on the magnitude of blood loss. In dogs (blood volume approximately 90 mL/kg) and cats (blood volume approximately 60 mL/kg), hemorrhage may be classified as (1) mild, <10–15% blood volume loss; (2) moderate, 20–25% blood volume loss; (3) severe, 25–35% blood volume loss; and (4) immediately life-threatening, 35–50% blood volume loss. Please refer to Table 18.9 for a summary of clinical signs according to these categories. Note that with significant blood loss, ABP may remain normal to increased.

The source of hemorrhage and concurrent injuries must also be taken into account, as these will impact volume resuscitation strategies. When external (i.e., compressible) hemorrhage is identified, immediate compression of the hemorrhagic site is indicated. With compressible hemorrhage, once pressure has been applied and the hemorrhage stopped, fluid resuscitation should be initiated with the goal of restoring an optimal hemodynamic state (Table 18.10).

When hemorrhage is suspected but cannot be readily localized, assume that there is a source causing internal (i.e., noncompressible) hemorrhage until proven otherwise. Aggressive fluid therapy in patients with noncompressible hemorrhage may be harmful and result in increased blood loss and mortality. In patients with noncompressible hemorrhage, even if it is classified as severe or life threatening, only rapid volume resuscitation to an adequate hemodynamic state (Table 18.10) is indicated until hemorrhage is controlled.

Table 18.9. Guidelines for assessing the magnitude of acute hemorrhage in dogs and cats

Mentation and attitude	Mucous membranes	CRT	Pulse	MAP	SAP	Hemorrhage category
Depressed, stuporous	Pale to very pale	Slow	Weak to absent	<60 mm Hg	<90 mm Hg	Life threatening (35–50% loss)
Depressed	Pale	>2 seconds	Weak	<70 mm Hg	<90 mm Hg	Severe (25–35% loss)
Anxious, alert, responsive	Pink to pale pink	2 seconds	Slightly decreased	>70 mm Hg	>90 mm Hg	Moderate (20 to 25% loss)
Alert	Bright pink to pink	<2 seconds	Normal	>70 mm Hg	>100 mm Hg	Mild (<10 to 15% loss)

CRT, capillary refill time; MAP, mean arterial blood pressure; SAP, systolic arterial blood pressure.

Table 18.10. Suggested optimal and adequate hemodynamic end points for volume resuscitation in dogs and cats

End point	Optimal resuscitation	Adequate resuscitation
Mean arterial pressure (mm Hg)	80–100	60–65
Systolic arterial pressure (mm Hg)	100–120	90–95

If pulmonary contusions are noted during the initial assessment, aggressive volume administration may lead to pulmonary edema. Consequently, patients with hemorrhage and pulmonary contusions should be cautiously resuscitated to adequate end points and then reevaluated.

In cases of mild to moderate hemorrhage, aggressive fluid therapy is actually contraindicated, as elevations in ABP may prevent effective clot formation. Conservative therapy with a balanced electrolyte solution (BES) is indicated during the assessment period, and it is imperative to continue to monitor vital signs frequently to confirm that there is no ongoing hemorrhage.

In cases of severe and life-threatening hemorrhage, rapid volume resuscitation to adequate hemodynamic end points is the first priority until hemorrhage is controlled, at which point further stabilization to optimal end points is recommended. A BES should be infused rapidly at 90 mL/kg in dogs and 60 mL/kg in cats until other fluid options can be obtained. With blood volume loss of greater than 25–30%, transfusion of whole blood or packed cells with plasma or colloids is required in addition to crystalloids. Whole blood at approximately 10–20 mL/kg is the treatment of choice. There is no time for a test dose in this situation but blood typing in cats is strongly suggested to determine if type A or B blood should be given. Hypertonic saline may be administered in immediately life-threatening situations while whole blood transfusion is being prepared. If whole blood is not available, packed red blood cells with a crystalloid or colloid should be administered while fresh frozen plasma is thawed. For a summary of available fluid options for treatment of shock syndromes, please refer to Table 18.11. Surgical intervention may be necessary when resuscitative efforts fail to reach the desired end points.

Table 18.11. Fluid options for volume resuscitation in hypovolemic shock

Fluid type	Dosage	Indications and comments
Isotonic crystalloids (BES) • Lactated ringers, Plasmalyte, Normosol, 0.9% NaCl	Dog: 90 mL/kg rapidly Cat: 60 mL/kg rapidly	• Initial volume resuscitation • Interstitial fluid replacement (correction of dehydration) • Often administer 1/4 to 1/3 of dose, reevaluate, and repeat as needed
Hypertonic crystalloids 7% NaCl	Dog: 4–8 mL/kg given at 1 mL/kg/min Cat: 2–4 mL/kg given at 0.5 mL/kg/min	• Initial volume resuscitation in animals with adequate hydration • Initial volume resuscitation in life-threatening hemorrhagic shock while obtaining/preparing whole blood transfusion
Whole blood	Maximum infusion rate is 22 mL/kg/h	• Blood volume loss >25–30% • Can also estimate required volume based on patient and donor PCV if fluid shifts have reduced patient PCV • Patient PCV will *not* reflect magnitude of blood loss in acute hemorrhage
Packed red blood cells	Maximum infusion rate as for whole blood assuming cells have been diluted	• Anemia • In combination with plasma or synthetic colloids for whole blood loss • Can estimate required volume based on patient and donor PCV if fluid shifts have reduced patient PCV • Patient PCV will *not* reflect magnitude of blood loss in acute hemorrhage
Plasma	10–20 mL/kg	• Low oncotic pressure, hemostatic disorders • In combination with packed cells for whole blood loss
Synthetic colloids • Hetastarch, pentastarch, dextran, gelatins	Dog: 10–20 mL/kg Cat: 5–10 mL/kg	• Initial volume resuscitation • Low oncotic pressure • In combination with packed cells for whole blood loss
Hemoglobin-based oxygen-carrying solutions • Oxyglobin® (OPK Bitoech LLC. Cambridge, MA)	Dog: 10–30 mL/kg Cat: 5–15 mL/kg	• Initial volume resuscitation • Low oncotic pressure • Situations where blood products not available

BES, balanced electrolyte solution.

Neurogenic shock

This is a potential sequela to spinal cord injury or blunt trauma that can disrupt the sympathetic nervous system and result in vasodilation, hypotension, and bradycardia. Patients are relatively hypovolemic, as intravascular capacity greatly exceeds intravascular volume and organ perfusion maybe compromised. Hypothermia is common secondary to peripheral vasodilation. Aggressive fluid therapy is required to increase vascular volume and pharmacological support with inotropes (i.e., dobutamine, dopamine, or ephedrine), vasopressors (i.e., phenylephrine, norepinephrine), and possibly anticholinergics (i.e., atropine or glycopyrrolate) are indicated.

Cardiogenic shock

This type of shock occurs when the ability of the heart to maintain cardiac output (CO) is insufficient to meet the body's demand. Circulatory compromise may be caused by any type of acquired or congenital cardiac disease. This is the only type of shock where volume resuscitation is not a primary treatment strategy. Instead, fluid redistribution from the lungs to the circulation, inotropic support, and antiarrhythmic therapy are the cornerstones of treatment.

Supportive therapies for shock

In addition to volume resuscitation as described in the section on hemorrhagic shock, there are a number of other supportive therapies indicated in shock syndromes. Antibiotic therapy is crucial in management of septic shock but will not be discussed here.

Cardiovascular support

If volume resuscitation is not successful in restoring hemodynamic stability, administration of a positive inotropic agent to increase CO, thereby increasing mean arterial blood pressure (MAP) and tissue perfusion is indicated. Note that in order for inotropic drugs to be effective, adequate circulating volume is required. The most commonly used drug for this purpose is the direct-acting (relatively) selective $beta_1$-adrenergic agonist dobutamine. The mixed inotrope and vasopressor dopamine has both direct and indirect actions and is also commonly used at low to intermediate doses to improve CO. In some cases, ephedrine, a noncatecholamine sympathomimetic agent with both direct and indirect actions, may also be used. Ephedrine is the only agent with inotropic effects that is useful when administered as an IV bolus. Please refer to Table 18.12 for a summary of selected inotropes.

In states of refractory hypotension, treatment with a vasopressor may be indicated to increase ABP and maintain blood flow to the heart and brain. The resulting vasoconstriction may sacrifice blood flow to other organ systems (e.g., kidney) so this therapy requires intensive monitoring. Patients with refractory hypotension generally have a poor prognosis for uncomplicated recovery. Commonly used vasopressors include the mixed

Table 18.12.   Selected inotropes for cardiovascular support in dogs and cats

Drug	Adrenergic activity					Indirect NE release	IV dose (mcg/kg/min)	Comments
	α1	α2	β1	β2	DA			
Dobutamine	+/o	+/o	+++	+	o	No	2–15; start low and titrate to effect	• Drug of choice to ↑ CO and ABP • Minimal effects on SVR • Less likely to ↑ HR than dopamine • Less likely to ↑ myocardial oxygen demand than dopamine or epinephrine
Dopamine	++ (high dose)	+	++ (low dose)	+	+++	Yes	2–10; start low and titrate to effect	• Low doses (1–4 mcg/kg/min) → renal, mesenteric, cerebral vasodilation • Intermediate doses (4–10 mcg/kg/min) → β1 stimulation → ↑ CO • High doses (>10 mcg/kg/min) → α stimulation → ↑ SVR
Dopexamine	o	o	o	+++	+++	No	2–20; start low and titrate to effect	• ↑ CO and ↓ SVR • Usually ↑ ABP
Ephedrine	+	+	+	+	o	Yes	0.05–0.2 mg/kg IV bolus; CRI?	• ↑ CO • Variable effects on SVR • Usually ↑ ABP • Effects after IV bolus often transient

DA, dopamine; ABP, arterial blood pressure; CO, cardiac output; HR, heart rate; NE, norepinephrine; SVR, systemic vascular resistance; o, no change/effect.

agents epinephrine and norepinephrine, and the pure pressor agent phenylephrine. At high dose rates, dopamine also induces significant vasoconstriction. Vasopressin (also known as antidiuretic hormone) is a noncatecholamine that acts at V1a receptors on vascular smooth muscle. Patients with vasodilatory shock appear to be extraordinarily sensitive to its pressor effects. Please refer to Table 18.13 for a summary of selected vasopressors.

Table 18.13. Selected vasopressors for cardiovascular support in dogs and cats

Drug	Adrenergic activity					IV dose (mcg/kg/min)	Comments
	α1	α2	β1	β2	DA		
Epinephrine	++	++	+++	+++	o	0.05–0.3; start low and titrate to effect	• ↑ CO and ABP • May cause ventricular fibrillation
Norepinephrine	+++	+++	++	o	o	0.05–0.3; start low and titrate to effect	• ↑ SVR and ABP • May see reflex ↓ HR • Potential ↓ splanchic perfusion
Phenylephrine	+++	+	o	o	o	0.5–3; start low and titrate to effect	• Selectively ↑ SVR • May see reflex ↓ HR and/or bradyarrhythmias
Vasopressin	o	o	o	o	o	0.8 U/kg	• Binds V1a receptors on vascular smooth muscle • Intense ↑ SVR in vasodilated patients • Used in CPCR as an alternative to epinephrine • May also be useful in management of septic and hemorrhagic shock

DA, dopamine; ABP, arterial blood pressure; CO, cardiac output; CPCR, cardiopulmonary-cerebral resuscitation; SVR, systemic vascular resistance; o, no change/effect.

Antiarrhythmic therapy

While any type of cardiac rhythm disturbance may occur in shock syndromes, ventricular dysrhythmias are the most common. Stabilization of fluid and electrolyte balance should be the first priority, but administration of pharmacological agents may be indicated if CO is significantly impaired or potential for progression to fibrillation is high. The sodium channel blockers lidocaine and procainamide are used most frequently to manage ventricular dysrhythmias, while the ultrashort-acting beta-blocker esmolol or the calcium channel blocker diltiazem may be useful for acute management of supraventricular dysrhythmias (Table 18.14).

Bicarbonate therapy

Bicarbonate therapy is no longer routinely recommended in shock patients and treatment should focus on restoration of adequate tissue perfusion, which, in most cases, will reverse the accompanying metabolic acidosis. Based on current recommendations, bicarbonate should only be administered when pH is less than 7.2 and only in amounts necessary to increase it to 7.2. Empirical doses for bicarbonate range from 0.25 to 1 mEq/kg administered IV over 10–15 minutes. It is recommended to start at the lower end of this range and reassess acid–base status before redosing.

Table 18.14.   Selected antiarrhythmics for use in dogs and cats

Drug	IV dose	Indications and comments
Lidocaine	Dog: 2–4 mg/kg bolus followed by 40–80 mcg/kg/min infusion Cat: 0.5–1 mg/kg over 5 minutes	• Class Ib antiarrhythmic • First-line drug for ventricular dysrhythmias
Procainamide	Dog: 3–6 mg/kg bolus followed by 10–40 mcg/kg/minute infusion Cat: ?	• Class Ia antiarrhythmic • For dysrhythmias refractory to lidocaine • Greater negative inotropic effects compared to lidocaine • Associated with higher incidence of hypotension
Esmolol	0.5 mg/kg SLOW IV followed by 50–200 mcg/kg/minute infusion	• Class II antiarrhythmic • For acute supraventricular tachycardia

?, unknown or undetermined.

Analgesia

Opioids are the drugs of choice for shock syndrome patients. Since peripheral perfusion may be compromised, the IV route is recommended for administration. Low doses can be titrated to effect to achieve adequate analgesia without inducing excessive CNS or respiratory depression, though diligent monitoring is still required. Care must also be used when administering drugs that can increase vagal tone in animals with compensatory tachycardia. A direct vagal bradycardia from high doses of drugs like fentanyl may result in rapid decompensation during unreplaced hemorrhage.

For mild to moderate pain, butorphanol or buprenorphine are good options. For moderate to severe pain, hydromorphone, oxymorphone, or fentanyl are recommended. The pure opioid agonists also routinely form the basis of anesthetic protocols for this patient population so they are good choices for initial pain management in animals likely to require surgery. Note that the NSAIDs are contraindicated during the resuscitative phase of shock and should only be administered after stabilization in patients where NSAID-associated risk factors have been ruled out.

Guidelines for anesthetic management

Most classes of anesthetic agents may be used in trauma and critically ill patients; however, dosage requirements are usually reduced.

The preanesthetic period

Trauma and/or critically ill patients should have indwelling IV catheters so administration of all anesthetic and analgesic drugs, including those given in the preanesthetic period, should use the IV route. Multiple IV catheters are often required to deliver anesthetic and analgesic agents, IV fluids, and drugs for hemodynamic support. It is important to anticipate venous access requirements and plan accordingly so that catheters can be placed prior to moving the patient into the operating room.

Anticholinergics are rarely indicated in these patients, as preexisting tachycardia is common, and further increases in myocardial oxygen consumption will be detrimental. One exception may be when high doses of mu agonist opioids such as fentanyl are going to be given intraoperatively as a part of a balanced anesthetic. Sedatives with potential for significant adverse hemodynamic side effects, such as acepromazine and dexmedetomidine, are not indicated in most cases either. In animals that are particularly stressed or anxious, a benzodiazepine such as diazepam or midazolam in combination with an opioid will usually provide an adequate calming effect.

Monitoring of cardiopulmonary function during the preanesthetic and induction periods is indicated if the patient is amenable to instrumentation. Continuous ECG monitoring and frequent assessment of ABP should be performed. In debilitated patients, it may be possible to place an arterial catheter for direct ABP measurement and arterial sampling for blood gas analysis during this time. Preoxygenation using oxygen delivered via a face mask is recommended if the patient will tolerate mask placement.

Patients presenting for emergency surgery are at greater risk of developing postoperative pulmonary complications associated with regurgitation and aspiration of gastric contents. Steps to minimize this risk include administration of an H_2 receptor antagonist (such as ranitidine or famotidine) and/or proton pump inhibitor (such as omeprazole), administration of antiemetics such as maropitant and ondansetron, maintaining the patient in sternal recumbency with the head up during induction, rapid endotracheal intubation and immediate inflation of the cuff, and suction of the oropharynx to clear gastric contents.

Anesthetic induction

While any IV anesthetic agent can be used for induction (unless specifically contraindicated such as ketamine with neurological injury), steps are usually taken to minimize the required dose and therefore reduce potential adverse effects. Low doses of propofol, ketamine, etomidate, or alphaxalone-CD are typically coadministered with an opioid and benzodiazepine to facilitate intubation and transfer to an inhalant anesthetic or opioid-based injectable protocol.

In patients that are depressed or obtunded, the combination of an opioid (hydromorphone, oxymorphone, fentanyl, or remifentanil) and a benzodiazepine (diazepam or midazolam) given in alternating IV increments often results in a smooth induction with minimal depression of CO or blood pressure. Opioid-induced bradycardia may be managed with an anticholinergic if necessary and mechanical ventilation may be indicated to maintain normocapnia, especially in the face of preexisting metabolic acidosis.

While IV inductions are usually preferred because they facilitate rapid control of the airway, mask induction with isoflurane or sevoflurane may be appropriate in selected patients. Remember that high inspired concentrations of inhalant anesthetics will be required for induction and these will induce comparable cardiopulmonary depression to an injectable protocol.

Anesthetic maintenance

Maintenance protocols for this patient population may be inhalant or opioid based. Maintenance with low inspired concentrations of isoflurane, sevoflurane, or desflurane supplemented with opioids, benzodiazepines, ketamine, and/or lidocaine (in dogs only) is a common approach. Alternatively, higher doses of a short-acting opioid (usually fentanyl or remifentanil) given as a continuous rate infusion (CRI) can form the basis of the maintenance protocol. The opioid-based protocols often involve coadministration with one or more of the nonopioid supplemental agents described above. Note that administration of high doses of opioids may induce bradycardia, which is responsive to anticholinergic treatment, and ventilatory depression, which may necessitate mechanical ventilation.

The use of nitrous oxide is contraindicated in patients with pneumothorax, gastric dilatation-volvulus, diaphragmatic hernia, and head and/or ocular trauma due to the potential for expansion of air-containing cavities. Its use also mandates decreasing the inspired oxygen concentration to approximately 30%, which may predispose patients with pulmonary contusions or other lung pathology to development of hypoxemia. Consequently, it should be used cautiously or not at all in this patient population.

Patient monitoring

The importance of intensive patient monitoring during anesthesia cannot be overstated. Assessment of ABP (often direct/invasive), cardiac rhythm, end-tidal carbon dioxide ($ETCO_2$), hemoglobin saturation, airway inhalant and oxygen concentrations, and body temperature are standard. Assessment of arterial oxygen and carbon dioxide tensions (arterial partial pressure of oxygen [PaO_2] and $PaCO_2$, respectively) will provide greater insight into oxygenation and ventilation in patients with gas exchange abnormalities that are inspiring enriched oxygen concentrations than pulse oximetry and capnometry can provide. Central venous pressure (CVP) values may be used as end points during volume resuscitation in profoundly hypovolemic patients and serial CVP assessment is particularly useful if impaired ventricular function is suspected. CO measurement using the lithium dilution method or cardiac function assessment with transesophogeal echocardiography will also provide useful information about global oxygen delivery and may be feasible in some clinical settings.

Fluid therapy and cardiovascular support

In most situations volume resuscitation will have been initiated prior to induction but in many cases fluid deficits will be ongoing and frequent reevaluations and readjustments will be necessary. Once anesthesia has been induced, it becomes impossible to assess the animal's mentation and attitude and the sympathetic nervous system's ability to compensate for volume depletion will be compromised. Serial evaluations of PCV, TS, and lactate often continue throughout the perianesthetic period and are used, along with hemodynamic parameters, to tailor the fluid therapy plan. Other supportive interventions such as administration of inotropic, vasopressor, or antiarrhythmic agents are also commonly indicated and have been discussed previously.

Mechanical ventilation

As stated previously, mechanical ventilation is often indicated in traumatized or critically ill patients to optimize oxygenation and maintain normocapnia. In patients with traumatic brain injury, ventilatory strategies remain controversial. It is understood that decreased cerebral perfusion pressure (CPP) resulting from elevated intracranial pressure (ICP) and/or decreased MAP is associated with poor neurological outcomes. In patients where elevated ICP is due to hypercarbia-induced cerebral vasodilation, mechanical ventilation to restore normocapia is indicated. Indiscriminate use of hyperventilation (i.e., $PaCO_2$ <30 mm Hg) to reduce ICP should be avoided, as it may induce cerebral vasoconstriction and actually reduce CPP.

Patients with thoracic trauma also warrant special consideration with regard to mechanical ventilation during anesthesia. High peak inspired airway pressures have the potential to worsen a preexisting or resolving pneumothorax and may cause rupture of a pulmonary bulla. If positive pressure ventilation is required in such patients, low peak pressures (<12 cm H_2O) should be employed with frequent reevaluation of PaO_2 and $PaCO_2$ values. Thoracocentesis prior to induction of anesthesia is warranted and placement of an indwelling thoracostomy tube is indicated if reaccumulation of air or fluid in the pleural space is anticipated.

Clinical signs associated with the development of tension pneumothorax in an anesthetized patient include marked hypotension, decreased hemoglobin saturation and/or PaO_2, and increased $PaCO_2$. It is important to recognize that $ETCO_2$ as measured by capnometry may not accurately reflect $PaCO_2$ in patients with pneumothorax or other types of pleural space pathology. In fact, abrupt decreases in $ETCO_2$ during anesthesia may be associated with cardiovascular collapse secondary to acute tension pneumothorax and warrant immediate investigation and intervention. In patients ventilated with a volume-preset ventilator, increased peak airway pressures will be noted with acute pneumothorax. In spontaneously breathing patients or patients ventilated with a pressure-preset ventilator, decreased tidal volume will be noted.

Other supportive interventions

Hypothermia should be addressed by using warm-water circulating blankets, forced air warmers, or conductive fabric warmers. Warming IV fluid solutions to 37°C will help maintain body temperature. Note that bradycardia and hypotension become refractory to pharmacological interventions with significant hypothermia, and cardiac dysrhythmias are more likely. Placement of an indwelling urinary catheter and closed collection system allows measurement of urine output and early detection of oliguria in patients with acute renal injury due to direct trauma or hypoperfusion.

Regional anesthesia

Epidural or spinal anesthesia is contraindicated in patients that are septic and/or have a coagulopathy. Administration of a local anesthetic into the epidural or subarachnoid space in hypovolemic patients may induce profound sympathetic blockade and exacerbate hypovolemia. Epidural administration of opioids (0.1 mg/kg of preservative-free morphine) is an effective way to supplement analgesia and is not associated with sympathetic blockade. Other local and regional anesthetic–analgesic techniques such as intercostal nerve blocks and interpleural anesthesia may be useful adjuncts to general anesthesia in traumatized or critically ill patients.

Recovery

Intensive patient monitoring and supportive interventions do not terminate with the end of anesthesia in traumatized and/or critically ill patients. In fact, analysis of perioperative fatalities indicates that the recovery period is associated with a high percentage of the reported deaths. Concerted efforts to optimize fluid and electrolyte balance, cardiopulmonary function, pain management, gastrointestinal and renal function, and nutrition while providing appropriate nursing care will help to ensure the best possible outcome.

Neonatal and geriatric patients

General considerations

In the practice of veterinary anesthesia, neonatal and geriatric animals are a significant proportion of the patient population. Attention to the unique physiology and particular requirements of individuals within either of these age groups will contribute to the provision of safe, effective anesthesia and analgesia.

Physiology of neonatal and pediatric animals

In dogs and cats the neonatal period refers to the first 6 weeks of life and the pediatric period extends from 6 to 12 weeks. Compared to young and middle-aged adults, neonatal and pediatric patients have limited organ reserve capacity and decreased ability to respond to physiological challenges. They also exhibit exaggerated or prolonged effects with administration of sedative and anesthetic drugs in dosages considered appropriate for young adults. This results in increased risk of perianesthetic complications if careful attention to drug selection and vigilant patient monitoring is not paid. A summary of key physiological differences in neonates as they relate to anesthesia is presented in Table 18.15.

Physiology of geriatric animals

The effect of aging on perioperative morbidity is a function of the decreased physiological reserve capacity of various organ systems, resulting in decreased ability to compensate for altered physiology during anesthesia. The effects of disease, stress, lack of exercise, genetics, malnutrition, and environment may hasten these changes. The time course of the aging process varies between organ systems within the same individual

Table 18.15. Key physiological differences in neonates relevant to anesthetic management

Physiological difference	Comments
Hypoalbuminemia	Increased proportion of active drug available for highly protein-bound drugs (thiopental, ketamine, NSAIDs)
Increased blood–brain barrier permeability	Increased percentage of drug reaches CNS
Increased total body water content but fixed, centralized circulating volume	Increased apparent volume of distribution is offset by greater drug delivery to highly perfused tissues (brain)
Low body fat percentage	Decreased capacity for drug redistribution out of CNS
Immature hepatic metabolism	Decreased drug metabolism may prolong duration of effect
Immature GFR	Decreased renal excretion may prolong duration of effect for certain drugs such as diazepam
Increased metabolic rate and oxygen consumption	Increased alveolar ventilation results in more rapid inhalant anesthetic induction
Decreased myocardial contractile tissue and decreased ventricular compliance	CO is largely dependent on HR; cardiac reserve is minimal
Immature sympathetic nervous system	Cardiac reserve is minimal; limited hypotension-induced baroresponse
Potential persistence of fetal cardiopulmonary circulation	Pulmonary overcirculation or cyanosis may result depending on the direction of shunt flow
Impaired ability to excrete fluid and solute load	Predisposed to volume overload
Compliant chest wall	Ventilation is less efficient and work of breathing is increased
Increased MV, MV/FRC ratio, and closing capacity	Pulmonary reserve is minimal; predisposed to hypoxemia
Decreased hematocrit	Minor hemorrhage may adversely impact oxygen delivery
Immature thermoregulatory system, high surface area/mass ratio, and poor vasomotor control	Predisposed to hypothermia

CNS, central nervous system; CO, cardiac output; FRC, function residual capacity; GFR, glomerular filtration rate; MV, minute ventilation; NSAIDs, nonsteroidal anti-inflammatory drugs.

and between individuals. There may be little correlation between chronological and physiological age. For the purposes of this discussion, geriatric animals are considered to be those that have attained 75% of their expected life span. A summary of key physiological changes occurring in geriatric patients as they relate to anesthesia is presented in Table 18.16.

Patient evaluation and preparation

A thorough physical examination including careful auscultation of the heart is an essential component of the preanesthetic assessment. Exercise tolerance may be an important

Table 18.16. Key physiological differences in geriatric patients relevant to anesthetic management

Physiological difference	Comments
Decreased myocardial and arterial compliance	Myocardial atrophy and fibrosis → impaired pump function and CO; Increased resistance to LV output → progressive ventricular hypertrophy → greater dependence on atrial kick and normal sinus rhythm to maintain CO
Decreased beta receptor responsiveness, maximal HR, maximal CO	Limited response to physiological stress
Decreased gas exchange efficiency	Increased ventilation–perfusion mismatch
Decreased vital capacity, increased closing capacity	Pulmonary reserve is minimal; predisposed to hypoxemia
Decreased thoracic compliance and lung elasticity	Increased work of breathing
Increased sympathetic and decreased parasympathetic nervous system activity	Less effective response to acute hemodynamic challenge
Decreased central neurotransmitter activity, loss of functional neurons	Decreased anesthetic requirements
Decreased drug clearance	Effects of anesthetic drugs may be prolonged
Decreased GFR and RBF	Renal ischemia more likely to cause renal failure
Impaired ability to excrete fluid and solute load	Predisposed to volume overload
Decreased hepatic and renal mass	Decreased metabolism and clearance of anesthetics
Decreased skeletal muscle mass, increased body fat percentage, decreased total body water content	Increased plasma drug levels → increased percentage of anesthetic drugs reach CNS
Decreased basal metabolic rate	Predisposed to hypothermia

CNS, central nervous system; CO, cardiac output; GFR, glomerular filtration rate; HR, heart rate; LV, left ventricular; RBF, renal blood flow.

predictor of outcome in geriatric anesthesia and this should be probed during history taking. Significant preexisting abnormalities should be corrected prior to induction as they may be exacerbated by anesthesia. Hydration status should be assessed and fluid requirements carefully calculated. Fluid deficits should be corrected prior to anesthesia whenever possible.

In neonates, minimum preanesthetic laboratory testing should include assessment of PCV or hematocrit, TS or protein, blood urea nitrogen or creatinine, and blood glucose. Other tests should be performed as indicated. In geriatrics, the preanesthetic assessment should include a complete blood count, serum biochemistry profile, electrocardiogram, and urinalysis.

Neonates that are still suckling should not be held off food prior to anesthesia. Pediatric animals that are eating solid food should be denied food for 2–4 hours only prior to anesthesia and should not be denied water at any time. Perioperative blood glucose monitoring can reduce the risk of hypoglycemia and delayed anesthetic recovery or neurological sequela.

The preanesthetic period

Because of the immaturity of the neonatal nervous system, it has been a commonly held theory that neonates are incapable of experiencing pain. However, we now know that neonatal humans and animals do indeed experience pain. In addition, evidence suggests that pain experienced at an extremely young age may actually lead to dynamic changes in nociceptive pathways predisposing to chronic pain conditions later in life. Like many pathologies, pain is easier to prevent than to treat. Regardless of age, every patient anesthetized for a painful procedure should receive appropriate analgesic therapy. As with other drugs, dosages of analgesics should be conservative and patients should be closely monitored for adverse side effects. The opioids are potent analgesics whose effects are reversible, making them excellent choices for analgesia in neonates with immature metabolism or geriatrics with reduced hepatic function. The addition of local or regional anesthetic–analgesic techniques to anesthetic protocols is particularly appropriate in this patient population. The inclusion of such techniques provides supplemental analgesia and reduces the requirement for general anesthetics that may have more profound side effects. NSAIDs may be an option in older pediatric patients or in geriatric patients with competent renal function.

The routine preemptive use of anticholinergics in adult patients is not necessary. However, because CO is largely HR dependent in neonates, preemptive administration of atropine or glycopyrrolate in the preanesthetic period is common practice in these patients. Anticholinergics should also be considered in breeds with high vagal tone (such as brachycephalics) and for surgical procedures that are likely to stimulate a vagal reflex (such as ocular procedures). In geriatric animals, preemptive anticholinergic administration may cause tachycardia and unnecessarily increase myocardial work and oxygen consumption. Consequently, it is recommended to monitor HR closely and treat bradycardia when or if it occurs during the anesthetic period.

Sedation may not be necessary in quiet or debilitated patients. However, sedatives alleviate stress in anxious patients and decrease the dosage of drugs needed for induction and maintenance of anesthesia. The side effects of sedatives should be weighed against the side effects of having to use a larger dose of anesthetic drug. The opioids often provide adequate sedation and have the added advantage of also providing analgesia. The pure agonist opioids such as morphine, hydromorphone, and oxymorphone provide the most profound analgesia but also may cause greater cardiovascular and respiratory depression. Partial agonists (buprenorphine) and agonist-antagonists (butorphanol) provide only mild to moderate analgesia but are associated with few cardiopulmonary side effects. Selection of an appropriate opioid is based on the patient's health status and an understanding of the intended procedure and its associated analgesic requirements.

Benzodiazepines are also useful sedatives–anxiolytics in neonatal or geriatric animals. Although they do not provide analgesia, they are reversible and produce little to no cardiovascular and respiratory depression. Benzodiazepines do not provide consistent or profound sedation and may need to be combined with other sedatives in very active or anxious neonatal or geriatric animals. The judicious use of low doses of the alpha$_2$ adrenergic agonist dexmedetomidine may also be considered for use in certain neonatal or geriatric animals. However, dexmedetomidine produces profound cardiovascular side effects (bradycardia, atrioventricular [AV] conduction block, and increased peripheral vascular resistance) and its use in neonatal or geriatric animals should be confined to those cases where the benefits of its use outweigh the negative side effects associated with its administration. The phenothiazine acepromazine may also be used for sedation of neonates or geriatrics but its cardiovascular effects, particularly hypotension, may be poorly tolerated in this patient population. The vasodilation caused by acepromazine can also contribute to the development of hypothermia. Acepromazine is not reversible and possesses no inherent analgesia.

Anesthetic induction

Anesthesia can be induced by using a variety of injectable anesthetic drugs or by mask delivery of inhaled anesthetics when necessary. Etomidate or propofol may be excellent choices in neonates and geriatrics. Both agents are rapidly eliminated from the body by a variety of routes so that termination of activity does not depend on the functioning of a single organ system. Propofol does produce respiratory and cardiovascular depression and should be titrated carefully to achieve the desired depth of anesthesia. The administration of oxygen by face mask for approximately 5 minutes prior to the induction of anesthesia with propofol will reduce the risk of complications associated with propofol-induced apnea in either neonatal or geriatric animals. Preinduction sedation of animals, particularly with a sedative–analgesic combination, will reduce the dose of etomidate or propofol needed for induction. Ketamine in combination with a benzodiazepine is also a reasonable choice for induction of anesthesia in either neonates or geriatric animals. Ketamine causes only mild respiratory depression and may actually improve cardiovascular function through stimulation of the sympathetic nervous system. Note that this response may be less in neonates because their sympathetic nervous systems remain immature. Ketamine requires either hepatic metabolism or renal clearance for termination of activity so its effects may be prolonged in patients with either immature or failing hepatic and renal systems. Thiopental may be used in low dosages for the induction of anesthesia in neonatal, pediatric, or geriatric animals but remember that the barbiturates are highly protein bound and their termination of activity depends on both redistribution and hepatic metabolism. The response to barbiturates can be both pronounced and prolonged in either neonates or geriatrics with reduced plasma protein concentrations and/or immature or failing hepatic or renal function. The steroid anesthetic alphaxalone-CD may also be appropriate for induction, though data evaluating its use in neonatal or geriatric patients are not yet available.

Inhalant anesthetics may be used for induction as well as maintenance of anesthesia. This method is recommended only in sedated or debilitated patients because the prolonged excitement phase that occurs during induction can be more physiologically detrimental than a carefully titrated dose of an injectable anesthetic. Environmental pollution and personnel exposure are also concerns during mask inductions with inhalant anesthetics. Because anesthesia can be induced with an inhalant agent very rapidly in depressed neonatal and geriatric animals, excessive anesthetic depth may be reached very rapidly. Careful monitoring is mandatory to prevent overdose.

Anesthetic maintenance

Inhalant anesthetics that are minimally metabolized and easily cleared in animals with either immature or reduced hepatic or renal function should be used for maintenance of anesthesia. However, it should be remembered that inhalants cause dose-dependent hypotension, hypoventilation, impaired cardiac contractility, and hypothermia. Because of these side effects, inhalants must be very carefully titrated and vigilant monitoring should be employed to avoid excessive anesthetic depth. The preanesthetic administration of analgesics and sedatives will reduce inhalant anesthetic requirements, thereby decreasing the magnitude of their unwanted side effects. Supplemental analgesics may also be administered during the maintenance phase in longer procedures.

Supportive care

Along with a carefully chosen anesthetic drug protocol and conservative drug dosing, vigilant monitoring and provision of hemodynamic support are imperative when anesthetizing neonatal, pediatric, or geriatric animals. Compared with adults, fluid requirements are greater in neonates because of their higher body surface area, immature renal function (decreased ability to concentrate urine), higher percentage of body water, and higher respiratory rates leading to greater fluid losses. Conversely, overhydration should be avoided because renal clearance may be limited and excessive dilution of serum protein can occur more readily in animals with preexisting hypoalbuminemia. Neonates have minimal stores of hepatic glycogen and are prone to hypoglycemia, so the use of dextrose-containing fluids should be considered. Reassessment of blood glucose levels at recovery is recommended and oral or IV dextrose supplementation may be indicated.

In geriatric patients that have difficulty excreting salt and water loads, aggressive fluid and electrolyte therapy may result in volume overload and possibly congestive heart failure and pulmonary edema. Thus, fluid therapy in geriatric animals during the perianesthetic period should be targeted at correcting specific deficits and maintaining adequate perfusion and oxygen delivery without delivering an excessive electrolyte or fluid load.

Both neonatal and geriatric animals are highly susceptible to hypothermia so every effort should be made to maintain normal body temperature. Hypothermia increases the incidence of adverse myocardial outcomes in high-risk patients, increases the incidence of surgical wound infection, adversely affects antibody- and cell-mediated immune defenses, changes the kinetics and actions of various anesthetic and paralyzing agents, increases thermal discomfort, and is associated with delayed postanesthetic recovery. The attempt of the body to actively rewarm itself is not benign and shivering may cause a tremendous increase in oxygen consumption (200–300%). This increased oxygen demand may not be met by an increase in oxygen delivery, particularly in the face of anesthetic-induced hypoventilation.

Diligent monitoring is crucial during the entire anesthetic period and well into recovery. Some commonly monitored indices are different in neonates compared to adults and anesthetists should be familiar with the normal physiological indices in these patients. Generally, neonatal and pediatric animals have a higher HR but lower ABP than adults. The normal HR in conscious neonatal dogs and cats is approximately 200 beats per minute and the respiratory rate is approximately 15–35 breaths per minute. MAP in 1-month-old puppies is only 49 mm Hg.

Key points

Suggested protocols for neonatal dogs and cats include an opioid for premedication combined with a sedative if required. An anticholinergic may be administered at this time if not contraindicated. Anesthesia can be induced with the IV administration of propofol or ketamine–benzodiazepine combinations. In severely compromised animals, anesthesia may be induced with an inhalant anesthetic delivered by face mask. Anesthesia is typically maintained with an inhalant in combination with a local or regional anesthetic technique if indicated.

No one ideal anesthetic protocol exists for all geriatric patients. An understanding of the pathophysiological changes and the alterations in pharmacodynamics and pharmacokinetics that arise in conjunction with aging is necessary when choosing an anesthetic protocol for a geriatric dog or cat. Particular attention to decreased dosage requirements and titration of anesthetics to achieve the CNS depression necessary for a specific surgical procedure is advocated. Whenever possible, local and regional anesthetic techniques should be employed to reduce the required dosage of injectable and inhalant anesthetics. Successful anesthetic management of geriatric animals depends on thorough patient evaluation and assessment, preoperative correction of identified abnormalities, careful titration of anesthetic drugs, vigilant perianesthetic monitoring, and appropriate perianesthetic support.

Dental patients

General considerations

Although sedation and local blocks alone have been advocated by some authors for dental procedures, most procedures are best accomplished under general anesthesia. Quite recently, several individuals have advocated anesthesia-free teeth cleaning. Proponents feel that more clients will pursue teeth cleaning if anesthesia is not used because of the decreased cost and alleviated fears of anesthetic death or complications. Many of the people performing and teaching these procedures are nonveterinarians and a recent decision in a case brought before the Veterinary Medical Board in California has ruled that the procedure amounts to "the practice of veterinary medicine without a license." The American College of Veterinary Dentistry has stated that thorough oral exams and dental radiographs are not possible in an unanesthetized patient and are needed to uncover any hidden dental disease that may be present.

General guidelines for anesthetic management

As is the case with any anesthetic procedure, appropriate premedications and induction agents should be selected based on the requirements of the individual. An IV catheter should be placed to enable administration of fluids and for emergency access if needed. All dental patients should be intubated with a cuffed endotracheal tube immediately after induction to prevent aspiration of water or cleaning solutions during dental procedures. Gauze sponges may be inserted in the pharyngeal area to further prevent aspiration. Packing the pharyngeal area too tightly can impede venous return and result in swelling of the tongue. If pharyngeal packing is used, a systematic method of ensuring that gauze is removed after the procedure prior to recovery from anesthesia is necessary. Dentistry in cats has been associated with tracheal rupture, likely from overinflation of the cuff, contributing to tracheal trauma when the patient is turned from side to side to provide access to both sides of the mouth. In all instances, it is best to disconnect the breathing circuit from the endotracheal tube (after turning off the oxygen flow to minimize waste gas exposure) before repositioning the patient.

Following induction, heart and respiratory rates are assessed and pulse oximetry, capnography, and blood pressure monitoring devices should be applied. Hypothermia is a common perianesthetic complication because anesthetic agents depress thermoregulatory function, which inhibits the normal response to hypothermia, and also cause vasodilation, which further exacerbates the problem. If a patient's attempt to regain body temperature is accompanied by severe shivering, increases in myocardial work and oxygen consumption occur and hypoxia may result. This may be especially important in geriatric animals with significant loss in functional cardiopulmonary reserve. Generally, it is safer to maintain core body temperature during anesthesia than to try to restore normothermia after anesthesia and surgery.

Perioperative pain management

A balanced anesthetic plan for dental patients should include preemptive, intraoperative, and postoperative analgesics. Pain associated with the procedure should be estimated prior to induction of anesthesia. Depending on the degree and magnitude of oral surgery performed, most pain will occur in the first 24–72 hours postoperatively. Some residual discomfort might last longer. Individual patients should be frequently reassessed and treated as needed. Behaviors indicative of pain such as lack of willingness to eat and drink, decreased grooming behaviors, and reduced activity level may be best observed by the owners in the home environment. Analgesics commonly used in managing pain include local anesthetics, opioids, alpha$_2$ agonists, and NSAIDs. Opioids and alpha$_2$ agonists can be used in the immediate pre- and postoperative periods while the patient is hospitalized. Injectable or oral NSAIDs and longer-acting opioid preparations may be used during prolonged convalescence and for take-home medications.

Local and regional anesthesia

Local and regional anesthetic techniques are commonly used in anesthetic and pain management plans for dental patients. Infraorbital, maxillary, mental, and mandibular inferior alveolar nerve blocks may be used before extractions. Caution should be used when blocking the inferior alveolar branch of the mandibular nerve because inadvertent blocking of the lingual nerve may result in desensitization of the tongue and potential self-mutilation upon recovery. The lingual nerve is best avoided by keeping the needle close to the bone of the ventral mandible when performing the intraoral approach to the inferior alveolar branch of the mandibular nerve. For analgesia of the maxillary teeth, care should also be taken to avoid insertion of the needle into the infraorbital canal when performing infraorbital blocks in cats and brachycephalic breed dogs. The canal is extremely short in these animals and insertion of the needle into it may cause ocular damage. As an alternative, infiltration anesthesia can be used where local anesthetic is injected directly into the periodontal ligament and surrounding tissues. This technique is facilitated by small needles and luer lock syringes where high injection pressure can be used to inject into the relatively tight tissue space. It is most effective when performed in areas with thin cortical bone (maxillary teeth and mandibular incisors) and when a small number of teeth need to be desensitized.

When using either lidocaine or bupivacaine it is important to calculate the total dose of local anesthetic that can be safely used to avoid toxicity. Generally, toxic doses of lidocaine are 10 mg/kg in dogs and 6 mg/kg in cats. The toxic doses of bupivacaine are lower and are approximately 3 mg/kg in dogs and 2 mg/kg in cats. Recent reports have examined the usefulness of opioids in extending the analgesia from local anesthetics in regional anesthetic techniques in humans. Both 0.075 mg/kg morphine and 0.003 mg/kg buprenorphine have been shown to double the analgesic duration in humans when combined with either lidocaine or bupivacaine. Mu opioid receptors have been located in human dental pulp, suggesting that local administration of opioids may be beneficial for dental procedures. Little data are available regarding the use of opioids with local analgesics for dental blocks in veterinary patients but it may prove to be a useful local application of this class of analgesics.

Dispensable pain medications

One challenging aspect of pain management for canine and feline dental patients involves identifying strategies for managing ongoing pain in patients after they have been discharged from hospital. At present, oral NSAIDs appear to be the most commonly recommended dispensable medications for short-term treatment of dental pain. When using NSAIDs, appropriate patient selection is important to reduce risks associated with this class of drugs. If additional analgesics are needed, oral opioids (such as butorphanol tablets, codeine tablets, and morphine tablets) are available for combination with an NSAID. The opioid-like oral agent tramadol has demonstrated good analgesic activity for mild to moderate pain. Tramadol is not scheduled and has been shown to be useful for management of postoperative pain in dogs. In addition, there are several commercially available opioid–acetaminophen preparations (such as codeine–acetaminophen or oxycodone–acetaminophen) that may be useful for dental pain management in dogs but are contraindicated for use in cats.

The administration of the parenteral form of buprenorphine given transmucosally has proven to be an efficacious means of providing outpatient analgesia in cats. Cat owners tend to prefer this method of administration, which also increases owner compliance. The short-term transmucosal administration of buprenorphine and an NSAID may provide an effective method of controlling moderate to severe pain in cats after invasive dental manipulation.

Orthopedic patients

General considerations

Veterinarians are asked to assess and treat orthopedic pain almost daily. In many cases, surgical correction of the orthopedic disease is not an option and a treatment plan for managing ongoing chronic pain must be devised. If surgery is indicated, a plan for both anesthesia and pain management must be designed. If trauma is the cause of the orthopedic injury, the anesthetic plan must include assessment and management of shock and injuries to other body systems. Aggressive treatment of pain associated with acute orthopedic injuries will help prevent progression to chronic pain. Once chronic pain is present, sensitization of the CNS may make pain control more difficult. Drug combinations using multiple classes of drugs are often required to obtain adequate pain relief.

Patient evaluation and preparation

Documenting a patient's history helps to determine the chronicity of the orthopedic injury. Acute pain is more likely with traumatic or recent injury and a good response to conventional analgesics at standard doses would be expected. If the injury is more chronic, anatomical and biochemical changes in pain processing may be present and a more complex approach to pain management may be required. Selection of appropriate anesthetic and analgesic drugs is influenced by the animal's general health status and the type of pain present.

A thorough physical examination is mandatory for all patients undergoing anesthesia. If there is a history of trauma or potential trauma, thoracic radiographs (two views minimum) should be performed to identify pneumothorax, pulmonary contusions, or diaphragmatic hernia, even if thoracic auscultation is unremarkable. In young, otherwise healthy orthopedic patients, minimal preanesthetic laboratory screening tests include PCV or hematocrit, TS or protein, blood urea nitrogen or creatinine, and blood glucose. If there is a history of preexisting disease or trauma, or abnormalities are identified on physical examination, further testing including complete blood count, serum biochemical profile, and urinalysis is warranted. Other tests such as ECG, blood gas analysis, hemostatic testing, and endocrine testing should be performed when indicated. As for any patient presenting for anesthesia and surgery, fluid and electrolyte balance should be stabilized prior to induction.

The preanesthetic period

Considerations for selection of preanesthetic medications in orthopedic patients are the same as for other surgical patients. In most young to middle-aged healthy animals, a sedative–analgesic combination is recommended. Commonly used sedatives in dogs and cats include dexmedetomidine, acepromazine, and midazolam. The alpha$_2$ agonist dexmedetomidine has the potential to produce the most intense sedation, but it also associated with the most significant adverse cardiovascular effects, so patient selection is important. The phenothiazine acepromazine induces moderate sedation and hemodynamic side effects and is widely used in dogs and cats. The benzodiazepine midazolam produces minimal sedation but tends to produce a calming effect with minimal adverse side effects in debilitated or geriatric patients.

An opioid should be administered in the preanesthetic period to all patients undergoing orthopedic surgery. A pure agonist such as hydromorphone, oxymorphone, or morphine is recommended for patients experiencing or anticipated to experience moderate to severe perioperative pain. The partial agonist buprenorphine may be effective in the treatment of mild to moderate pain but is usually less effective than the pure agonists for severe pain. The mixed agonist-antagonist butorphanol is usually only effective in patients experiencing mild pain. It is the authors' opinion that butorphanol is not appropriate for managing the pain intensity experienced by most orthopedic patients.

While not routinely necessary, an anticholinergic such as atropine or glycopyrrolate may also be administered to orthopedic patients in the preanesthetic period. This practice is contraindicated in patients with preexisting tachycardia or in patients that may be adversely affected by tachycardia. In most cases, it is appropriate to monitor HR throughout the perianesthetic period and administer an anticholinergic when or if necessary.

In certain patients that are particularly aggressive it may be necessary to include a dissociative agent such as ketamine or Telazol® (tiletamine–zolazepam; Pfizer Animal Health, New York) in the protocol to facilitate safe handling during catheterization and transfer to an inhalant anesthetic.

Anesthetic induction

Induction of general anesthesia in orthopedic patients is best accomplished using injectable drugs administered via an IV catheter. Injectable inductions are preferred because they allow a more rapid loss of consciousness, less patient struggling, earlier control of the airway, and less risk of injury to the patient and staff. Popular drugs for IV induction include propofol, thiopental, and ketamine–diazepam. Induction doses will vary with the general health and age of the patient. Administration of preanesthetic medications can considerably reduce induction dose requirements.

Immediately after induction an endotracheal tube should be placed and the cuff inflated. Avoid overinflation of the endotracheal tube cuff to avoid tracheal crush injury or tracheal rupture. Animals with pulmonary injury caused by trauma can develop pneumothorax as a consequence of positive pressure ventilation (either manual or mechanical) during anesthesia. Development of tension pneumothorax during mechanical ventilation is a life-threatening complication requiring prompt recognition and immediate therapeutic intervention. If pneumothorax has been diagnosed in the preanesthetic period, placement of a thoracostomy tube prior to or immediately following induction may be indicated. Please refer to the sections "Trauma and Critically Ill Patients" and "Selected Diagnostic and Therapeutic Procedures" for more information.

Anesthetic maintenance

Because orthopedic procedures usually last longer than 30–60 minutes, inhalant agents are preferred for anesthetic maintenance. Isoflurane, sevoflurane, or desflurane are all suitable options. Due to the longer duration of the surgical procedure and the potential for significant perioperative pain, supplemental analgesics are often administered during this period.

Supplemental systemic analgesics

Orthopedic pain is typically classified as severe and patients with orthopedic injuries are at risk of developing chronic pain syndromes. Aggressive pain management at the time of initial injury or surgical intervention helps to prevent progression to chronic pain. Chronic pain patients undergoing surgery to correct orthopedic disease may already have sensitized CNSs and may require adjunctive techniques to manage their pain. Please refer to Chapter 4 for a more detailed discussion of chronic pain management.

Techniques used to provide additional systemic analgesia for orthopedic patients include the following: (1) preoperative injection of an NSAID (if not contraindicated), (2) repeated opioid IV bolus injections, (3) opioid IV CRIs, (4) ketamine IV CRIs, (5) lidocaine IV CRIs (in dogs only), and (6) transdermal fentanyl administration. Supplemental systemic analgesics will decrease overall anesthetic requirements and hopefully lessen the incidence and severity of adverse side effects.

Local and regional anesthesia and analgesia

Local and regional anesthetic techniques are often used to inhibit nociceptive input to the CNS during surgical manipulations. Blockade of the infraorbital or maxillary nerve can be performed for procedures involving the maxilla. The mandibular nerve can be blocked for procedures involving the mandible. The foot can be desensitized by several techniques, including a ring block; blocks of the radial, median, and ulnar sensory nerves; and IV regional anesthesia (Bier block). The front limb can be desensitized from the elbow distally by performing a brachial plexus block. When amputating a limb or tail, intraoperative neural injection with a long-acting local anesthetic (such as bupivacaine) should be performed prior to severing the nerves.

Lumbosacral epidural administration of morphine is beneficial for both forelimb and rear limb procedures because it is water soluble and will travel cranially. For hind limb, pelvic, and tail procedures, morphine is usually combined with a long-acting local anesthetic to provide an intense analgesic effect. For more information on local and regional anesthetic–analgesic techniques in dogs and cats please refer to Chapter 10.

Patient monitoring

Monitoring anesthetized orthopedic patients involves the same basic principles as for other patients. If the animal has suffered trauma, additional considerations may be warranted and the reader is referred to the section on anesthesia in trauma and critically ill patients in this chapter.

Supportive care

It is vital to patients undergoing long periods of orthopedic repair that physiological parameters are maintained as close to normal as possible throughout the perianesthetic period. Routine supportive interventions include the following: (1) the use of IV fluids to optimize circulating volume and perfusion, (2) provision of an external heat source to prevent hypothermia, (3) assisted or mechanical ventilation in patients with inadequate spontaneous ventilation, (4) correction of specific physiological derangements, and (5) proper patient positioning in natural anatomical alignment.

Recovery

It is essential to provide adequate pain relief to all orthopedic patients even though they may not show outward signs of pain or distress. Some techniques for providing postoperative analgesia require preoperative and intraoperative planning. Fentanyl patches are best placed before surgery because therapeutic levels of fentanyl will not be present for at least 8–12 hours after placement. Provision of a wound infusion catheter for ongoing administration of local anesthetics into the wound requires placement of the catheter during surgery. Single intra-articular injections of local anesthetics, morphine, and/or ketamine are performed at the conclusion of the surgical procedure. Placement of an epidural catheter for management of severely painful patients is best performed while the animal is still anesthetized.

Patients that are dysphoric at recovery may risk reinjuring the surgical site. They may require sedation to calm them and potentiate analgesic drugs. Acceptable postoperative sedatives include diazepam, midazolam, dexmedetomidine, or acepromazine administered in low IV doses.

Most orthopedic patients require systemic opioid analgesics for at least 24 hours after surgery. Examples of commonly employed opioid regimens include IV CRIs of morphine, hydromorphone, or fentanyl, or periodic IV injections of oxymorphone, hydromorphone, morphine, or buprenorphine. The combination of morphine, lidocaine, and ketamine administered together as an IV CRI provides excellent analgesia in dogs. Wound infusion catheters are also excellent options for provision of analgesia in cats and dogs undergoing major surgery.

Provision of adequate padding, an external heat source, and a quiet environment are all essential for a smooth and uneventful recovery. Monitoring of physiological parameters should continue postoperatively until patients are awake, aware, responsive, and resting quietly.

Most patients should be transitioned to oral analgesic drugs for discharge to the owner's care. Orthopedic patients are typically given analgesics for at least 1 week after surgery and often for much longer periods. If analgesic requirements suddenly change or are prolonged, the surgery site should be reassessed to rule out reinjury, infection, or other surgical complications. Tramadol–NSAID combinations, opioid–NSAID combinations, and NSAIDs alone are all acceptable choices for at-home analgesic therapy. Transmucosal buprenorphine is an excellent option in cats. To maintain patients on individualized, optimal analgesic protocols, it is important to evaluate analgesic needs and patient well-being on a regular basis.

Management of chronic orthopedic pain

Management of chronic orthopedic pain requires a partnership between the veterinarian and the owner. The goal of long-term pain management is to provide the animal with a good quality of life. The owner is relied on to evaluate how well the animal is functioning in its normal daily routine. Weight control and routine controlled exercise including physical rehabilitation are essential elements in the management of orthopedic disease and require an ongoing commitment from the owner. One common strategy for pharmacological management of chronic pain involves a stepwise approach. After establishing a baseline pain-control regimen, additional drugs are added to obtain better analgesia or to manage progressively worsening pain. The owner must assess efficacy at each step using assessments that have been individualized for the specific patient (e.g., Is the animal able to climb the stairs to and from the backyard? Is the animal able to jump up on the couch? etc.). Nonpharmacological approaches to treatment of chronic pain such as rehabilitation therapy, acupuncture, or therapeutic massage require a large time commitment. Engaging the owner as a key player in the treatment and assessment team will help to ensure optimal pain management.

In most instances, NSAIDs are the first-line drugs for treatment of orthopedic pain. Baseline serum chemistry and complete blood count should be determined and urinalysis should be performed when chronic dosing is anticipated or preexisting disease(s) are present. Renal disease, liver disease, hyperadrenocorticism, ongoing corticosteroid therapy, and evidence of gastrointestinal bleeding or occult blood loss are contraindications to initiating NSAID therapy. If there are no contraindications, an NSAID is chosen and a trial period is initiated. If the animal tolerates the NSAID without adverse effects, efficacy is evaluated by the owner. On a population basis, there is no difference in efficacy between different NSAIDS, but in individual patients, efficacy can vary greatly. Adverse events associated with NSAID therapy include inappetence, vomiting and diarrhea, acute idiosyncratic liver toxicity, perforating duodenal ulcer, gastrointestinal hemorrhage, and renal disease. Owners should be adequately informed of potential complications and the owner information handouts provided by pharmaceutical manufacturers should be given to owners when drugs are dispensed.

NSAIDs may be used intermittently in the early stages of orthopedic pain, particularly if a period of sustained activity is anticipated. Once an animal is dependent on NSAIDs to maintain normal daily activities, adjunctive drugs should be considered. Tramadol and acetaminophen or acetaminophen with codeine (dogs only) may be added at this stage. If there are contraindications to NSAID use, adjunctive and opioid drugs become preferred treatments. Nonpharmacological therapy (such as weight control, ongoing rehabilitation therapy and exercise, use of diets or dietary supplements containing anti-inflammatory compounds, and acupuncture) is used to slow the progression of pain and disability. As pain progresses, more potent opioids such as oral morphine or oxycodone are prescribed.

Selected diagnostic and therapeutic procedures

General considerations

Several minimally invasive advanced diagnostic and therapeutic procedures have become more commonly used over the last decade because of increased availability of the technology and expertise in application and interpretation. General anesthesia or sedation is usually required to assure patient immobility during these procedures. These patients will vary greatly in physical status and underlying disease processes so there is no one ideal anesthetic protocol. Because many of the procedures discussed in this chapter are elective, minimally invasive, and of short duration, anesthetic protocols associated with smooth, rapid recoveries are desirable. Perianesthetic considerations are presented for selected minimally invasive diagnostic or therapeutic techniques, including laryngoscopy, bronchoscopy, bone marrow aspiration, thoracic drain placement, and esophagostomy tube placement; for advanced imaging techniques, including computed tomography (CT), magnetic resonance imaging (MRI), and ultrasonography; and for radiation therapy. With a few exceptions, these procedures are considered diagnostic, not life saving, and every effort should be made to minimize potential adverse effects of general anesthesia or sedation.

The approach to anesthetic management should be kept simple and observe the following principles: (1) identify and correct underlying patient problems when possible to minimize anesthetic risk, (2) formulate an anesthetic protocol that will work in the existing environment and that can be readily adapted to each individual patient and disease process, (3) apply effective monitoring tools that will alert the anesthetist to potential problems and ensure that quick and effective corrective measures are taken, and (4) provide appropriate supportive therapy based on the underlying disease and guided by information provided by monitoring devices.

Laryngoscopy and bronchoscopy

Laryngoscopy is used in evaluating laryngeal disease, specifically laryngeal paralysis. Sedation is required to facilitate relaxation of the jaw but must be carefully selected to have a minimal effect on laryngeal function. It can be challenging to keep patients adequately sedated without affecting laryngeal function. The combination of an opioid and benzodiazepine is adequate for most patients. These drugs have the advantage of preserving laryngeal function and being reversible if respiratory distress develops. Challenge with doxapram at 1.0 mg/kg IV to increase respiratory activity may be used if evaluation is hindered by drug-induced respiratory depression.

Bronchoscopy is performed in dogs and cats for evaluation of airway disease and to perform bronchoalveolar lavage. Many of the patients presented for laryngoscopy and bronchoscopy are at increased risk for development of hypoxemia. Preoxygenation should accompany both procedures and the anesthetist should always be prepared to take control of the airway by endotracheal intubation and application of ventilatory support. During bronchoscopy, oxygen may be delivered to smaller patients via an endoscope (working channel). Larger patients may be intubated and connected to oxygen by a breathing system and a Y-piece aperture may be used to pass the endoscope into the trachea. An opioid–benzodiazepine combination for sedation, followed by administration of low-dose propofol to effect, is commonly used to facilitate bronchoscopy.

Thoracic drain placement

Thoracostomy tube placement may be required to manage pleural space disorders such as pneumothorax, pyothorax, and chylothorax. These patients are often considered high risk, especially those with pneumothorax and concurrent pulmonary contusions. In dogs, thoracic drain placement can often be performed using sedation in combination with a local anesthetic technique such as infiltration or intercostal nerve block. In patients in respiratory distress or with hypoxemia, general anesthesia, endotracheal intubation, oxygen delivery, and provision of ventilatory support may be indicated. For cats, general anesthesia is usually preferred. Reversible agents with minimal cardiopulmonary effects, such as the combination of a benzodiazepine with butorphanol or buprenorphine, provide adequate sedation for most patients. For general anesthesia, a rapid sequence induction to gain control of the airway is recommended. Propofol, benzodiazepine–ketamine, or etomidate are good induction choices and are associated with relatively rapid recoveries.

Bone marrow aspiration

This procedure is performed to evaluate bone marrow disease, to stage certain cancer patients, and collection of stem cells for use in treatment of musculoskeletal disease. Protocol selection should be based on the individual patient and take into account the animal's level of activity. Bone marrow aspiration may be performed in dogs with local infiltration alone or in combination with sedation. Uncooperative dogs and the majority of cats may require general anesthesia.

Esophagostomy tube placement

This is used to provide enteral nutrition for both dogs and cats. General anesthesia is required to protect the airway in case of regurgitation and the endotracheal tube facilitates placement of the esophagostomy tube. The aforementioned protocols for thoracostomy tube placement are applicable for this procedure.

For the procedures listed earlier, identification of an individual animal's underlying disease, anticipation of and planning for potential complications, and close monitoring throughout the anesthetic period will help to assure a successful outcome regardless of the anesthetic agents used.

CT and MRI

CT and MRI were first introduced in 1972 and 1980, respectively. Routine clinical use of CT and MRI technology in veterinary medicine has evolved recently as equipment availability and expertise in interpretation have increased. Anesthetic management for CT and MRI presents a unique challenge in that there is no painful stimulation during the anesthetic period, so response to noxious stimuli cannot be used as a method for assessing anesthetic depth. Patient access is usually limited during CT and MRI scanning depending on the unit configuration. Consequently, routine subjective evaluation of the patient's pulse quality and mucous membrane color may not be feasible. With CT, although patient access is usually not problematic, exposure of the anesthetist to radiation is an issue and direct patient assessment while the scan is being performed is discouraged.

Contrast agents for CT and MRI

An additional consideration is the common use of contrast agents for both MRI and CT. While reaction to contrast administration appears to be relatively uncommon in animals, anesthetists must be aware of this potential complication. IV iodinated contrast is often given to patients during a CT scan. These contrast agents consist of meglumine and/or sodium salts of iothalomate or diatrizoate and are ionic and hyperosmolar. Adverse reactions to these contrast agents include hypotension, tachycardia, and depressed ST segments and prolonged Q-T intervals on the ECG. One case of cardiac arrest has been reported in a dog after IV administration of iodinated contrast media. Adverse reactions are usually seen in the first 5–10 minutes following administration and are potentiated by dehydration. Therefore, normal hydration status is essential prior to contrast administration. Humans are at risk for serious reactions if they have any of the following preexisting conditions: diabetes mellitus, renal insufficiency, congestive heart failure, hypovolemia, multiple myeloma, hypertension, or combined hepatic and renal failure. No specific treatment is necessary following a mild reaction to the contrast media, but fluid administration rate should be increased for treatment of mild hypotension and tachycardia. If an anaphylactic reaction does occur, administration of epinephrine, diphenhydramine, and/or corticosteroids is/are indicated. The fluid administration rate for patients with underlying renal disease should be increased to 20 mL/kg/h during the first 30 minutes of anesthesia to promote contrast clearance and to maintain adequate renal perfusion.

All contrast agents used in MRI contain the paramagnetic element gadolinium. These contrast agents present a lower osmotic burden to the patient and smaller volumes are required compared with CT contrast agents. There have been no reported cases of adverse reactions to MRI contrast agents in animals but allergy-type symptoms, hypotension, hypertension, vasodilation, tachycardia, nausea, vomiting, and headache have been reported in humans. An increased administration rate of IV fluids should be used to treat hypotension and tachycardia.

MRI safety considerations

MRI safety is an important concern in anesthesia monitoring because ferromagnetic objects are attracted toward the magnet and projectile-related accidents can occur.

Traditional anesthetic equipment and monitors may be unsafe, may be damaged, may malfunction, or may interfere with image generation when used in the MRI suite. The MRI consists of a strong static magnetic field, gradient magnetic fields, and radiofrequency (RF) fields. Any ferromagnetic object has the potential to be drawn into the bore of the magnet, causing injury to the patient or personnel in the room. The influence of the MRI scanner on equipment depends on the strength of the magnet, proximity to the magnet bore, the amount of ferromagnetic material present, and the design of the circuitry. Also, the RF fields and the applied magnetic gradient fields in the room can affect the function and accuracy of monitoring equipment. Conversely, the monitoring equipment can also alter the quality of the images obtained. Ferromagnetic equipment within the room should be replaced with nonferromagnetic or minimally ferromagnetic metal such as stainless steel, brass, or aluminum. Alternatively, ferromagnetic equipment may be securely anchored to a wall or the floor as far away from the bore of the magnet as possible. Monitoring equipment may be adapted by placing the devices outside of the room and using long connecting wires. If possible, oxygen tanks should be located outside of the MRI suite or tanks made of aluminum should be used.

Several companies sell MRI-compatible anesthesia and monitoring equipment. Keep in mind the definitions of MRI safe and MRI compatible. MRI safe means that the device, when used in the MR environment, has been demonstrated to present no additional risk to the patient or other individual but may affect the quality of the diagnostic information. MRI compatible means that a device is MR safe and, when used in the MR environment, has been demonstrated neither to significantly affect the quality of the diagnostic information nor to have its operations affected by the MR unit. Some companies market their product as MRI compatible but the instruction manuals must be carefully read because there have been several reports of "MRI-compatible" monitoring equipment being propelled into the bore of the magnet. Instructions for such potentially hazardous equipment state that the item must be placed a certain distance away from the magnet. Ideally, equipment should be checked by a biomedical engineer responsible for the area before it is brought into the vicinity of the MRI scanner. Some companies that supply MRI-compatible or MRI-safe anesthetic equipment and monitors are listed in Table 18.17.

Special consideration should also be given to patients with any type of metallic implants such as hemoclips, patent ductus arteriosus (PDA) occlusion coils, or pacemakers. Ferromagnetic hemoclips can dislodge and migrate, causing internal damage. An electrical current can be induced in PDA coils, causing thermal damage, and pacemaker leads or generators can dislodge. The magnetic field may cause the pacemaker generator

Table 18.17. Companies that manufacture MRI-compatible, MRI-safe anesthesia equipment

Smiths Medical Veterinary Division (Surgivet)	http://www.surgivet.com
DRE Medical	http://www.dreveterinary.com
In vivo	http://www.invivoresearch.com
Medrad	http://www.medrad.com
Datex	http://www.datex-ohmeda.com
Nonin	http://www.nonin.com

to malfunction or readjust. An electrical current in the lead wire may produce enough heat to cause injury. If a metallic implant is located in the region that is being imaged, severe image artifacts often occur, resulting in a nondiagnostic study.

One other safety issue that may occur in the MRI suite is magnetic quenching. If the liquid helium that surrounds and cools the superconducting solenoid of the magnet rapidly escapes, it can displace the oxygen in the room, causing hypoxia to the patient and personnel present. Ideally, oxygen sensors should be placed in MRI suites.

Ultrasonography

This imaging modality has been used in veterinary medicine since the late 1970s and has become a routine diagnostic procedure for animals. Most animals tolerate ultrasonographic evaluation without sedation or anesthesia but sedation may be necessary in fractious, aggressive, or painful animals. Ultrasound-guided organ or tissue biopsies are becoming more common as a method for collecting samples less invasively. Dogs and cats usually tolerate the procedure well with sedation and local anesthetic infiltration but general anesthesia may be preferred in some individuals.

Radiation therapy

External beam radiation is used to treat many types of neoplasia in small animals. Treatment usually consists of multiple small doses of radiation daily for a curative intent or larger less frequent doses for pain palliation. Treatment times per dose last from approximately 1 minute up to 7 or 8 minutes. Therefore, patients must remain motionless and require precise positioning. Since most animals receive radiation doses daily and remain in the hospital for up to 4 weeks or go home nightly, a protocol that induces profound sedation or general anesthesia, is convenient to administer, and has a quick recovery time is recommended. During treatment, personnel cannot be present in the therapy room to directly monitor the animal because of radiation safety. Remote monitors or cameras focused on the patient and in-room monitors should be used to assess the patient.

Revised from "Ocular Patients" by Marjorie E. Gross and Elizabeth A. Giuliano; "Anesthetic Management of Cesarean Section Patients" by Marc R. Raffe and Rachael E. Carpenter; "Trauma and Critical Patients" by Gwendolyn L. Carroll and David D. Martin; "Neonatal and Geriatric Patients" by Glenn R. Pettifer and Tamara L. Grubb; "Dental Patients" by Rachael E. Carpenter and Sandra Manfra Marretta; "Orthopedic Patients" by Elizabeth M. Hardie and Victoria M. Lukasik; and "Selected Diagnostic Procedures" by Janyce L. Cornick-Seahorn, Jennifer B. Grimm, and Steven L. Marks in Lumb and Jones' Veterinary Anesthesia and Analgesia, Fourth Edition.

Chapter 19

Anesthetic emergencies and accidents

A. Thomas Evans and Deborah V. Wilson

Introduction

In many veterinary practices, after the induction of anesthesia, no one is assigned the task of anesthetist to monitor anesthesia and be vigilant for untoward events that might result in accidental morbidity and mortality. As with most unwanted events, the anticipation of possible complications and having a plan of action already prepared will facilitate successful resolution of the problem. Since the onset of general anesthesia upsets the physiological equilibrium of patients and can bring them closer to harmful outcomes, preparation to manage these problems is even more critical.

Monitors that display vital parameters such as oxygen saturation of hemoglobin, end-tidal carbon dioxide, blood pressure, and heart rhythm are available to facilitate early detection of critical events such as bradycardia, changes in oxygen availability, and hypoventilation. Veterinarians who vigilantly monitor have a better opportunity to respond quickly to a harmful trend before a disaster occurs.

Anesthetic risk

The risk of death from disease or related surgery is usually greater than the risk of death from anesthesia. However, anesthesia involves the controlled administration of potentially toxic drugs and thus carries a risk of organ dysfunction and damage, delayed recovery, and death. Mistakes are not necessarily reversible, and death can occur suddenly, and often without warning when patients are not appropriately monitored.

The goal of anesthetists should be to manage the risks associated with anesthesia and the perioperative period, affording patients the best chance of a successful outcome. Risk management is a term developed by the insurance industry and adopted by the health-care industry to describe processes used to prevent injury, litigation, and financial loss. The real aim of this process is to use analysis of adverse events to prevent similar injuries to subsequent patients.

Essentials of Small Animal Anesthesia and Analgesia, Second Edition. Edited by Kurt A. Grimm, William J. Tranquilli, Leigh A. Lamont.
© 2011 John Wiley & Sons, Inc. Published 2011 by John Wiley & Sons, Inc.

Risk management starts with an unbiased and nonjudgmental review and analysis of all "critical events" causing real or potential patient harm. The next step is formation or modification of standard operating procedures. For example, in aviation, accident investigation begins with discovery of the facts by an independent board (National Transportation Safety Board) and then analysis and publication of the findings. There is also an anonymous reporting system (Aviation Safety Reporting System) that involves the documentation and analysis of events that were considered hazardous by the participants but did not lead to an accident. These aviation review procedures provide a model for the improvement of anesthesia safety in both human and veterinary medicine. A commitment to the highest quality patient care will ultimately lead to the routine performance of such analyses by medical providers.

Species-related risk

Advances in medical technology and pharmacology, as well as the increase in training of anesthesiologists, veterinarians, and licensed technicians, have done much to decrease the inherent risks associated with anesthesia. The risk of anesthetic-related death in people is estimated at between 1:10,000 and 1:200,000. The rate of anesthetic-related death among dogs and cats anesthetized in private practice has been assessed at approximately 0.1%. When interpreting studies of comparative anesthetic-related morbidity and mortality, it should be remembered that the definitions of the anesthetic period may vary and often include additional surgical and disease risk factors.

High-risk patients

Based on clinical experience, the small animal patients that are associated with a high risk of adverse outcome from anesthesia and surgery include geriatric (especially hyperthyroid) cats; posttrauma cases with pulmonary pathology, hemothorax, or pneumothorax or pulmonary hemorrhage; and cases of acute head trauma and severe intra-abdominal hemorrhage. Patients requiring a high level of care and commitment to achieve a good outcome include neonates; those with low body weight or morbid obesity; and patients undergoing portosystemic shunt occlusion or cardiac, intracranial, or intraocular surgery.

Cardiovascular emergencies

Hemorrhage and fluid loss

Blood loss during surgery may be insidious or obvious. Body fluids may also be lost during surgery to transudation, sequestration, or evaporation. Extravasation of fluid to a nonfunctioning or sequestered edema space is commonly referred to as loss to the third space, the first and second spaces being the intracellular and extracellular spaces. These losses may reduce circulating blood volume significantly. Regardless of cause or route of loss, a decrease in circulating blood volume is not well tolerated by anesthetized patients.

Quantifying blood loss is important but can be difficult, so the severity of hemorrhage is often assessed by its impact on the patient. Severe blood loss causes tachycardia, reduced arterial pressure, pale mucous membranes, decreased pulse pressure, and decreased area under the arterial pulse wave. Packed cell volume decreases only during resuscitation or as fluid shifts into the vascular space, but base deficit increases as changes in bicarbonate and venous pH correlate with blood volume lost. Physiological responses to blood loss may be blunted or masked by anesthetic and anesthetic adjunctive drugs (e.g., alpha$_2$ agonists or high doses of fentanyl), further emphasizing the need for appropriate monitoring for early detection and correction of hypovolemia.

Shed blood can be replaced with crystalloids or colloids (e.g., plasma, hemoglobin-based oxygen-carrying solutions, dextrans, whole blood, or a combination of these solutions). In most situations, hypertonic solutions do not seem to have a distinct advantage over isotonic crystalloid solutions. Crystalloid solutions such as lactated Ringer's, Plasmalyte (Baxter, Deerfield, IL), or Normosol (Hospira, Lake Forest, IL) are usually administered at threefold the volume of shed blood, as a rough guideline for resuscitation. The main advantage of crystalloid solutions is their low cost. Colloid solutions such as whole blood, plasma, hydroxyethyl starch, and hemoglobin-based oxygen carriers can be used as a substitute for crystalloids. Hemoglobin-based oxygen-carrying solutions (e.g., Oxyglobin, OPK Biotech LLC. Cambridge, MA) are relatively expensive, but have a long shelf life and do not require crossmatching. The use of colloids has the advantage of sustaining colloid osmotic pressure while preserving plasma volume, but has the disadvantage of being more expensive than crystalloid solutions.

Acute hemorrhage of greater than 20% of the blood volume or a decline in pack cell volume to less than 20% because of the combined effects of blood loss and crystalloid fluid administration can be treated with an appropriate mass of red blood cells by either transfusion of whole blood or packed red cells. Red blood cells are preferred because of the need for restoring adequate hemoglobin concentrations to carry oxygen to the tissues. Smaller amounts of surgical hemorrhage, not associated with severe decreases in the hemoglobin concentration, can be managed with crystalloids (e.g., lactated Ringer's) or colloids rather than red blood cells.

Cardiac dysrhythmia

Most dysrhythmias are caused by preexisting medical conditions, administration of premedications, anesthesia induction and maintenance agents, and surgical stimulation. Dysrhythmias require treatment if they reduce cardiac output, cause sustained tachycardia, or are likely to initiate dangerous ventricular dysrhythmias.

Canine gastric dilation/volvulus, splenic tumors, or multiple traumas often precipitates dysrhythmias that may require treatment prior to induction of anesthesia. Dysrhythmias following gastric dilation/volvulus presumably have their origin in acid–base imbalance, electrolyte disturbance, myocardial ischemia, circulating cardiac stimulatory substances, and/or autonomic nervous system imbalance. Treatment involves correcting physiological abnormalities and administering lidocaine or procainamide. It is absolutely imperative that ventricular premature contractions (VPCs) be differentiated from ventricular escape beats before administration of antiarrhythmic drugs, because suppression of an escape rhythm can cause immediate asystole and death. If the sinus rate is low, an intravenous atropine injection of 0.02 mg/kg may increase the sinus rate and invoke overdrive suppression, which may inhibit the dysrhythmia. VPCs and ventricular tachycardia resulting from a traumatized myocardium are commonly treated during the perioperative period with lidocaine or procainamide. If possible, surgery should be delayed 2–4 days or until the dysrhythmias have subsided.

Several popular drugs used as preanesthetic medication can predispose patients to conduction abnormalities. Atropine or glycopyrrolate can cause sinus tachycardia and increase myocardial work and oxygen consumption. Phenothiazine tranquilizers reportedly predispose the heart to sinus bradycardia, sinus arrest, and, occasionally, first-degree and second-degree heart block, although it has also been shown to protect against VPCs. Xylazine may cause bradycardia and second-degree atrioventricular blockade and decreases the epinephrine threshold for VPCs. The μ-receptor agonist opioids morphine, hydromorphone, fentanyl, and oxymorphone will also precipitate a slowing of heart rate via increased vagal efferent activity. The anesthesia induction agents thiopental and ketamine have been reported to increase the likelihood of dysrhythmia formation after epinephrine administration during halothane anesthesia. This multidrug interaction has also been described for thiopental and isoflurane.

Other factors responsible for the development of the dysrhythmias during the surgical period include altered arterial carbon dioxide partial pressure ($PaCO_2$), altered PaO_2, altered pH, and autonomic reflexes from surgical manipulation, as well as central nervous system disturbances and cardiac disease. Because most perioperative dysrhythmias do not seriously affect cardiac output, treatment can be discrete. Changing to a different inhalation anesthetic, using intermittent positive pressure ventilation or increasing the depth of anesthesia may eliminate the dysrhythmia. Other treatments for controlling ventricular dysrhythmias include correcting blood gas abnormalities or administering a small quantity of intravenous lidocaine (0.5 mg/kg) or procainamide (1.0 mg/kg).

Allergic reactions

Allergic reactions involving anesthetics are uncommon but could occur after sensitization to a drug. Allergic or anaphylactic reactions are mediated by the immune system. They are more commonly associated with repeated exposure to an allergen, but cross-reactivity may be seen with some preexisting allergies (e.g., allergies to eggs and to egg proteins in propofol). Anaphylactic reactions following thiopental administration have been reported. Intravenous injection of the intravenous contrast agent diatrizoic acid (Hypaque, Amersham Health, Princeton, NJ) has caused tachypnea, bronchoconstriction, and mucoid diarrhea in dogs. Allergic reactions are treated with intravenous fluids, antihistamines, and corticosteroids. Epinephrine should be administered in severe reactions accompanied by severe bronchoconstriction or cardiovascular collapse. Many unexpected responses to anesthetic and anesthetic adjunctive drugs have been labeled as "allergies" by veterinarians; however, proper diagnosis is crucial because it may have serious ramifications for future anesthetic delivery.

Cardiac arrest

Successful treatment of cardiac arrest requires early diagnosis. Because of its high metabolic requirements, the brain is the organ most susceptible to hypoxia or ischemia. Serious brain injury develops after only 4–5 minutes of cardiac arrest. The brain injury can be multifactorial, including the rapid loss of high-energy phosphate compounds during ischemia, cell structural damage during reperfusion, progressive brain hypoperfusion especially in certain areas, and suppression of protein synthesis in selectively vulnerable neurons. Once the diagnosis of cardiac arrest has been confirmed, all efforts must be toward restoration of effective oxygen delivery and reestablishing a heartbeat. Cardiopulmonary resuscitation (CPR) with external cardiac massage appears to be ineffective in protecting the brain from injury and should be only part of the initial resuscitation protocol. If not quickly successful, time should not be wasted with external CPR in lieu of more effective, but more invasive, internal techniques.

Cardiac arrest is diagnosed when some or all the signs listed in Table 19.1 are present. When the heartbeat or peripheral pulse cannot be palpated, the systolic blood pressure is generally less than 50 mm Hg. In this circumstance, the heart may actually have a weak beat, but cardiac output is probably very low and true cardiac arrest imminent. A nonpalpable weak heartbeat along with a regular rhythm has been termed pulseless electrical activity (PEA), formerly known as electrical mechanical dissociation. This type of functional cardiac arrest occurs with anesthesia overdose and from many other causes, such as hypovolemia, acute cardiogenic decompensation, severe acidosis, or hypoxemia. It is important to look for correctable causes of PEA during the first moments of resuscitation to improve the odds of success. Other forms of cardiac arrest include asystole and ventricular fibrillation. The three types of cardiac arrest can be differentiated with an electrocardiogram (ECG) or by direct observation of the heart during thoracic surgery or internal CPR.

Table 19.1. Signs of cardiac arrest

1. No palpable heart beat
2. No palpable pulse
3. Apnea
4. Lack of surgical hemorrhage
5. Cyanosis
6. No muscle tone
7. Dilated pupils (later)

Source: Evans AT, Wilson DV. 2007. Anesthetic emergencies and procedures. In: *Lumb and Jones' Veterinary Anesthesia and Analgesia*, 4th ed. W.J. Tranquilli, J.C. Thurmon, and K.A. Grimm, eds. Ames, IA: Blackwell Publishing, p. 1037.

CPR

When any or all of the signs listed in Table 19.1 are present, the traditional *ABCD* protocol for treatment of cardiac arrest must be started immediately. *A* refers to airway and reminds the resuscitator that a patent airway is a necessity. Endotracheal intubation is the best method of insuring a patent airway. The goal of *B*, breathing, is to supply high concentrations of oxygen to the alveoli and to eliminate carbon dioxide. Intermittent positive pressure ventilation is usually instituted in intubated patients, although when breathing room air and using chest compressions only (no artificial ventilation), dogs have maintained adequate gas exchange and oxygen saturation greater than 90% for longer than 4 minutes. The real value of artificial breathing has been questioned for routine resuscitation in people. The current recommendations for a breathing rate of 10–24 breaths per minute may be too high. Assuming there is enough blood flow to provide a reading and motion artifact does not cause erroneous readings, the pulse oximeter can be useful as a guide to determine respiratory rate. Simply ventilate at a rate that maintains hemoglobin saturation at 90% or higher.

C refers to cardiac massage, which can be either external (thoracic) or internal. External thoracic massage is thought to produce cardiac output by one or a combination of two methods. The thoracic pump theory holds that blood moves out of the thoracic cavity during the compression half of the CPR cycle because of a buildup of internal thoracic pressure (Figure 19.1). This mechanism is thought to occur primarily in animals with a

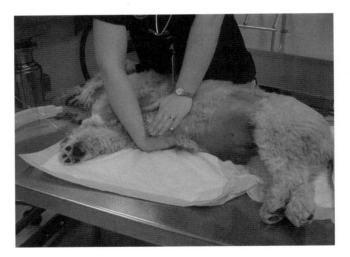

Figure 19.1. External thoracic massage administered to a larger dog that probably derives blood flow primarily from the thoracic pump mechanism. The resuscitator, standing at the dog's back, is applying thoracic compressions over interspace 4 or 5 at the level of the costochondral junction. In larger dogs, the thoracic compressions may not mechanically contact the heart, so all blood flow is derived from increased intrathoracic pressure. The right hand is supplying a counterforce for thoracic compressions with the palm of the left hand. The compression rate for this dog should be from 80 to 100 beats per minute. *Source*: Evans A.T., Wilson D.V. 2007. Anesthetic emergencies and procedures. In: *Lumb and Jones' Veterinary Anesthesia and Analgesia*, 4th ed. W.J. Tranquilli, J.C. Thurmon, and K.A. Grimm, eds. Ames, IA: Blackwell Publishing, p. 1037.

body weight greater than 15–20 kg. Evidence for the thoracic pump theory includes the phenomenon of cough CPR in humans and artificial cough CPR in dogs. The cardiac pump theory explains blood flow in smaller animals or animals with a narrow side-to-side thoracic width and refers to actual mechanical compression of the myocardium by the thoracic wall during CPR systole (Figure 19.2). Blood flow in some patients may be produced by a combination of the cardiac and thoracic pump mechanisms. Whatever the reason for forward blood flow, it appears that external thoracic massage is not very protective of the brain, because CPR performed for more than 3 or 4 minutes is often associated with significant neurological injury. Because traditional external thoracic massage is apparently ineffective in many patients, various maneuvers have been proposed to improve blood flow during CPR. For example, interposed abdominal compression (IAC) involves manually compressing the abdomen in counterpoint to the rhythm of the chest compression. The physiological reason for improvement of blood flow is that compression of the abdominal aorta responds like an intra-aortic balloon pump and that pressure on the abdominal veins primes the right heart and pulmonary vasculature in preparation for the next thoracic compression. This method of augmenting external CPR has been associated with improved survival in people and vital organ perfusion in dogs. Utilization of IAC–CPR in over 100 dog CPR labs as part of a clinical anesthesia rotation demonstrated that venous return and arterial blood pressure improved for about 1 minute, after which hemodynamics began to fail again. Another way of improving blood flow during CPR is to simultaneously ventilate at the time of thoracic compression. Simultaneous ventilation-compression (SVC) CPR has improved carotid blood flow

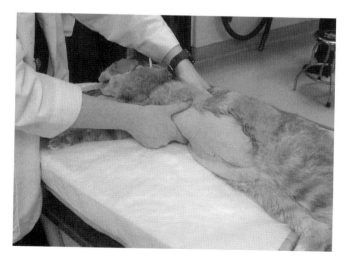

Figure 19.2. External thoracic massage administered to a cat with blood flow derived from the cardiac pump. The thoracic walls contact the heart with each compression. Note that only the thumb and fingers of the right hand compress the thorax, while the left hand stabilizes the cat. The compression rate should be from 100 to 120 beats per minute. *Source*: Evans A.T., Wilson D.V. 2007. Anesthetic emergencies and procedures. In: *Lumb and Jones' Veterinary Anesthesia and Analgesia*, 4th ed. W.J. Tranquilli, J.C. Thurmon, and K.A. Grimm, eds. Ames, IA: Blackwell Publishing, p. 1037.

during resuscitation of animals. Opposing evidence has also been presented that shows that the mitral valve of dogs may actually close in response to rhythmic increases in intrathoracic pressure. Despite this evidence to the contrary, SVC–CPR probably improves blood flow during CPR of large dogs when the thoracic pump is the primary mechanism in generating blood flow.

Open thoracic or internal CPR is more effective at perfusing the heart and brain during the critical beginning minutes of CPR. Higher blood pressure and cardiac output can be achieved with internal CPR. Most veterinary practices are well equipped to perform internal CPR because controlled ventilation and thoracotomy can be performed. The limiting factor in its employment is often the surgical inexperience of the attending veterinarian or the "do not resuscitate" wishes of the animal owner. Although it can be a difficult subject to broach, it is desirable to ascertain prior to the procedure the owner's wishes concerning CPR, in writing, in the event that cardiac arrest should occur during anesthesia and surgery. Valuable time may be lost trying to contact owners. Whichever method of CPR is chosen, there are some guidelines for CPR technique that, when followed, can improve success. The animal should be in right lateral recumbency with the resuscitator standing at its back (Figure 19.1). The thoracic or cardiac compression rate should be from 80 (large dogs) to 120 (cats) per minute. A longer compression time will augment forward blood flow when using the thoracic pump mechanism.

The recommendations for *D*, definitive or drug therapy, start with the immediate use of epinephrine. Epinephrine should be administered early, preferably into a central vein or alternatively into a peripheral vein, intrabronchially, or directly into the chamber of the left ventricle. For intrabronchial administration, use a flexible catheter wedged into a distal bronchus. For intracardiac injection, use a long, 22-gauge needle inserted at the left thoracic fourth or fifth interspace and costochondral junction. For intravenous administration, a dose of 0.05–0.1 mg/kg is used, whereas bronchial administration requires 0.05–0.1 mg/ kg diluted to a 2–3 mL volume with saline. The dose for intracardiac epinephrine is 0.025– 0.05 mg/kg. Even though intracardiac epinephrine seems appealing as a way of efficiently delivering the drug to the heart, the technical difficulty of positioning the needle in the chamber of the left ventricle when the heart cannot be palpated, along with the potential for myocardial or coronary vascular injury, makes this technique the least advantageous. Since the goal of CPR is to revive the heart as soon as possible, early administration of epinephrine is crucial, and it should be given immediately after diagnosis of cardiac arrest.

The use of vasopressin in asystolic cardiac arrest has been recommended as a new standard of care in people. The interest in vasopressin as treatment for cardiac arrest was due to an observation in the early 1990s that endogenous vasopressin levels were greater in survivors of cardiac arrest than in patients that died. The resuscitation success from the injection of vasopressin compared with epinephrine may be because the heart continues to consume oxygen after epinephrine injection (especially with tachycardia that often follows successful epinephrine-assisted resuscitation), whereas vasopressin augments coronary blood flow through an increase in systemic vascular resistance and increased diastolic perfusion pressure without an accompanying tachycardia. In people, epinephrine may be potentially detrimental in early asystolic cardiac arrest because exogenous epinephrine could be expected to potentiate hypoxemia and advancing acidosis, which could further impair the pressor effects of epinephrine. Tracheal administration of vasopressin (1.2 U/kg) in anesthetized dogs has resulted in systolic, diastolic, and mean blood pressure increases that last longer than 1 hour. Although research into the effects of vasopressin in treating cardiac arrest in dogs is scarce, an intravenous dose of 0.8 U/kg has been suggested for treatment of shock-refractory ventricular fibrillation, pulseless ventricular tachycardia, asystole, and PEA.

Lidocaine is used after resuscitation if ventricular dysrhythmias are compromising cardiac output. The use of lidocaine during ventricular fibrillation to improve the results of electrical defibrillation is being reevaluated. Lidocaine is usually given as an intravenous bolus at a dose of 0.5 mg/kg.

Amiodarone has also been recommended for shock-refractory ventricular tachycardia or fibrillation in people. Because of its vasodilatory effects on the coronary circulation, amiodarone (5 mg/kg intravenously) is best administered in combination with epinephrine. Metabolic acidosis from hypoxia and ischemia, and respiratory alkalosis caused by iatrogenic hyperventilation during treatment of cardiac arrest, commonly occur during resuscitation. The immediate use of bicarbonate is controversial, because metabolic acidosis is slow to develop during CPR and is somewhat neutralized by an ensuing respiratory alkalosis. Respiratory alkalosis is caused by external thoracic compression and controlled ventilation during CPR. Sodium bicarbonate (1 mEq/kg) administered after 10 minutes of resuscitation will improve the chance of return of spontaneous circulation and may play a role in mitigating postresuscitation cerebral acidosis. However, bicarbonate administration can result in production of carbon dioxide as metabolic acid is neutralized. Careful monitoring of $PaCO_2$ can be a guide to adequate ventilation postresuscitation to avoid paradoxical cerebral acidosis.

Atropine or glycopyrrolate are important drugs to administer during CPR because reflex bradycardia may have contributed to the initial cardiac arrest. In addition, bradycardia often occurs after a heartbeat has been established. Atropine at 0.02–0.04 mg/kg or glycopyrrolate at a dose of 0.01 mg/kg intravenously will enhance the automaticity and conduction of both sinoatrial and atrioventricular nodes.

In dogs and cats, PEA is apparently more common than ventricular fibrillation. Asystole, observed as a flatline ECG, is the next most common form of cardiac arrest, with ventricular fibrillation the least common. It is fortuitous that ventricular fibrillation is the least common expression of cardiac arrest, because most veterinary practices do not have access to a direct current cardiac defibrillator. If a direct current defibrillator is available, clip the hair from a small area from each side of the thorax. After applying electrode gel to each paddle, firmly apply the paddles to the thorax (Figure 19.3) and administer a shock of approximately 3–5 joules (watts per seconds) per kilogram of body weight. Sequential discharges of increasing energy may be more effective at converting fibrillation. Internal defibrillation requires a smaller electrical discharge: a total of 10–50 joules. Alcohol should not be used for ECG lead placement during CPR because alcohol is highly flammable and may be ignited by a defibrillator.

Internal CPR

After administration of epinephrine, and after attention to airway and breathing of the CPR protocol, begin external thoracic massage. It seems reasonable to start external CPR even though success rates are low with this method. Some animals respond positively to one or two doses of epinephrine and 1 or 2 minutes of external CPR. These appear to

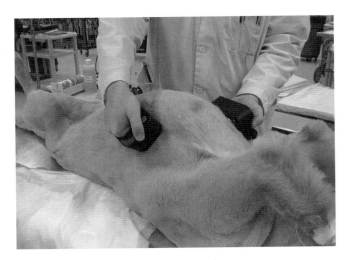

Figure 19.3. Placement of direct-current paddles for defibrillation of the heart during cardiac arrest. An area under the paddles has been shaved and electrode jelly applied to the paddles. Administer a shock of approximately 35 joules per kilogram of body weight. Sequential discharges of increasing energy of 50% at each shock may be more effective at converting fibrillation.
Source: Evans A.T., Wilson D.V. 2007. Anesthetic emergencies and procedures. In: *Lumb and Jones' Veterinary Anesthesia and Analgesia*, 4th ed. W.J. Tranquilli, J.C. Thurmon, and K.A. Grimm, eds. Ames, IA: Blackwell Publishing, p. 1038.

be primarily animals in PEA or asystole. If there is no response after 2 minutes, one should quickly begin the more productive internal CPR technique. Unfortunately, many practitioners may not feel confident about performing a thoracotomy when they have little or no previous experience with this procedure. There is little to lose, however, when a patient is in cardiac arrest and has not responded to initial resuscitation attempts. Emergency thoracotomy can be accomplished quickly in an arrested animal. Clip the hair from the left thorax at the fifth intercostal space. Spray or wipe the area with an antiseptic solution and incise the skin starting 1 in. from the spine to within 1 in. of the sternum. With surgical scissors, continue incision through the various tissue layers, avoiding the internal thoracic artery near the sternum. Bluntly penetrate the pleura, extend the incision, and spread the ribs. If the abdomen is open during surgery, a trans-diaphragmatic approach has been used (especially during diaphragmatic hernia surgery) to reach the heart in a timely manner. Reach into the thorax and begin cardiac massage at a rate of 80–120 compressions per minute. Depending on its size, the heart can be massaged with fingers, one hand, or two hands. Epinephrine can now be easily administered into the left ventricle as required. If the resuscitation is successful and mental alertness improves, the patient can be anesthetized to complete closure of the thoracic incision. The thorax should be flushed with warm, sterile physiological saline and closed in a routine manner. Infection is rare after emergency thoracotomy in people and, from clinical experience, uncommon in dogs. An algorithm for patients with confirmed cardiac arrest is presented in Figure 19.4.

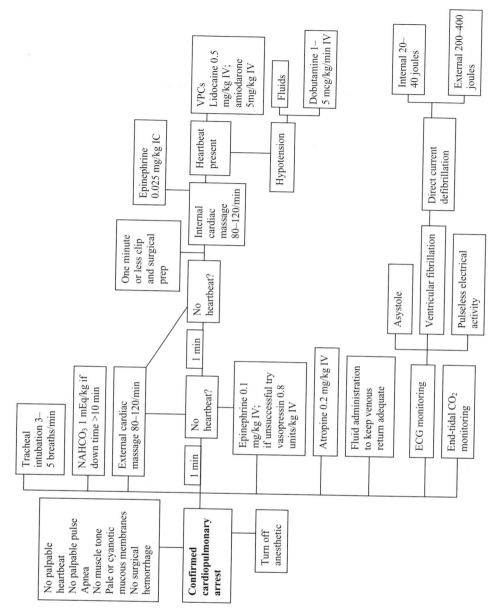

Figure 19.4. An algorithm for cardiopulmonary resuscitation (CPR). This simplified protocol for CPR is used to resuscitate animals that might be able to survive cardiac arrest. Because early restoration of brain perfusion is the most important goal., a quick decision for internal cardiac massage is required. ECG, electrocardiogram; IC, intracardiac; IV, intravenously; NaHCO₃, sodium bicarbonate; VPCs, ventricular premature contractions.
Source: Evans A.T., Wilson D.V. 2007. Anesthetic emergencies and procedures. In: *Lumb and Jones' Veterinary Anesthesia and Analgesia*, 4th ed. W.J. Tranquilli, J.C. Thurmon, and K.A. Grimm, eds. Ames, IA: Blackwell Publishing, p. 1040.

Postresuscitation care

Once there is a return of spontaneous circulation, attention must be directed toward limiting the neurological injury and other sequelae produced by the cardiac arrest. Intensive care must be provided to address blood gas abnormalities, respiratory insufficiency, hypotension, cardiac dysrhythmias, and temperature. Clinical trials in people have demonstrated the neurological benefit of mild therapeutic hypothermia (32–34°C) in survivors of out-of-hospital cardiac arrest. Mild hypothermia should be instituted as soon as possible after resuscitation and maintained for at least 12 hours. Cooling methods that may work in smaller animals involve surface cooling of the head and neck, as well as circulation of cool air over the patient's body. Tympanic membrane temperature can be used as a proxy for brain temperature. Application of mild hypothermia may improve the rather dismal success rate of cardiac and brain resuscitation in animals.

After successful CPR, the use of intravenous antibiotics has been recommended to counter the potential septicemia that can follow ischemic insult of the integrity of the lining of the gastrointestinal tract. Administration of osmotic diuretics such as mannitol (0.5–1.0 g/kg intravenously) after resuscitation has also been recommended to counter cerebral edema secondary to ischemia.

Perivascular injection

Among all of the injectable anesthetics in use today, the perivascular injection of thiopental has likely caused more local tissue damage than all other anesthetics put together, primarily because of its very alkaline pH. It is, however, unusual for a perivascular slough to occur if the concentration of thiopental is 2.5% or less. If thiopental is inadvertently injected, perivascular treatment should consist of infiltration of the area with saline to dilute the thiopental, lidocaine to vasodilate capillaries and increase absorption, and corticosteroids to decrease the inflammatory response. Propofol, ketamine, and etomidate normally do not cause tissue sloughing if accidentally injected perivascularly; however, perivascualar injection may be painful. Many catecholamine solutions, including dopamine, can lead to tissue necrosis after perivascular injection. Intense alpha$_1$ receptor-mediated vasoconstriction is likely the cause.

Respiratory insufficiency

Respiratory depression is defined by an increase in $PaCO_2$, and not by a decrease in respiratory rate alone. It is common for respiratory rate to decrease with a decrease in the level of activity and awareness (e.g., sleep), but tidal volume typically increases to compensate, resulting in no net change in $PaCO_2$. During anesthesia, respiratory insufficiency is common because many factors alter the chemoreceptor responsiveness to carbon dioxide, leading to elevated $PaCO_2$. Causes include the administration of opioids and other sedatives prior to anesthesia, the relative overdose of induction agents, positioning for surgery, respiratory depressant effects of inhalants, surgical trauma, recovery from bronchial alveolar lavage (BAL), and excessive use of opioids during recovery. The use of opioids with or without tranquilizers prior to induction of anesthesia to provide sedation and analgesia often results in a patient being well sedated but with depressed ventilatory drive.

High doses of μ-receptor agonists such as oxymorphone, hydromorphone, and morphine are more likely to produce respiratory depression than is the κ-receptor agonist butorphanol. In addition, the decreased responsiveness to increased carbon dioxide tensions during halothane, isoflurane, or sevoflurane anesthesia tends to cause hypoventilation, although surgical stimulation often overrides some anesthetic-induced loss in respiratory drive. In addition to the depressant effects of inhalants on responsiveness to increased $PaCO_2$, subanesthetic doses depress the peripheral chemoreceptors such that hypoxia does not stimulate a ventilation response. Hypoxia often occurs during recovery from anesthesia after diagnostic BAL. Although BAL with volumes of up to 4L have only transient effects in healthy dogs, BAL can lead to increased morbidity and mortality in dogs and cats with severe respiratory disease. During BAL, supplemental oxygen can be administered by insufflation with a small rubber tube placed in the trachea alongside the bronchoscope. After the procedure, oxygen should be administered by endotracheal tube, mask, or chamber until the pulse oximeter readings remain at 90% saturation or higher while room air is breathed. Airway obstruction may also occur after ear ablation surgery. Soft tissue swelling in the posterior pharynx may be severe enough to require a tracheostomy for relief.

Apnea is common during routine anesthesia. It occurs during induction after the administration of thiobarbiturates or propofol, during maintenance of anesthesia with ketamine, when controlled ventilation is discontinued, excessive accumulation of carbon dioxide, and as a consequence of deeper inhalation anesthesia. Apnea occurring at induction is generally transient and is treated by low frequency intermittent ventilation that is adequate to maintain hemoglobin–oxygen saturation at greater than 90%. Apnea occurring later during anesthesia, especially in spontaneously breathing animals, must be quickly recognized and treated with decreasing anesthetic concentrations and/or high frequency positive-pressure ventilation. Apnea late in anesthesia is usually caused by excessive depression of the respiratory centers of the brain secondary to high anesthetic and/or carbon dioxide concentrations, or because of decompensation associated with severe neurological disease such as hydrocephalus or intracranial neoplasia.

Generally, apnea during induction of anesthesia with thiobarbiturates or propofol is caused by a relative overdose or a fast bolus injection. Ketamine and diazepam in a 1:1 mixture by volume is commonly used for anesthesia in cats. Apnea often occurs, especially when anesthesia is maintained with supplemental isoflurane. This combination of drugs, each of which is a respiratory depressant alone, can induce a persistent respiratory depression. If, in response to respiratory depression, assisted or controlled ventilation is employed, $PaCO_2$ will often be reduced below the arterial or alveolar PCO_2 level at which cats will remain apneic (apneic threshold). Decreased functional residual capacity (FRC) during anesthesia can increase hypoxia by lowering alveolar ventilation/perfusion ratios (V_A/Q) and expanding atelectatic areas. This occurs because the FRC is close to or less than the closing volume (CV) of the lung. The CV is the volume of the lung at which small airways begin to close. When the tidal volume is less than the CV, small airways remain closed throughout the breathing cycle, and atelectasis increases. If the CV of some airways remains within the tidal volume range, then there is some air exchange during inspiration and expiration, though not the normal amount. This partial ventilation decreases the V_A/Q. These lung changes are prevalent in older animals and during anesthesia. Intermittent positive-pressure breathing and positive end-expiratory pressure (PEEP) can be used to diminish the hypoxia that occurs from changes in FRC.

Equipment malfunction

Routine equipment maintenance and leak tests should be used to reduce the chances of anesthesia machine malfunctions. Common equipment malfunctions include channeling of gas flow through the carbon dioxide absorbent canister, sticking of the exhalation check valve in the open position, interruption of oxygen supply, and kinking of the endotracheal tube. All of these equipment malfunctions can be rapidly detected with the routine use of a capnograph and pulse oximeter during inhalant or injectable anesthesia. Channeling occurs when gas flow through the carbon dioxide absorbent canister is uneven, resulting in early termination of carbon dioxide absorption. If the pathway is through the center of the canister, there is not likely to be any observable change in color of the carbon dioxide absorbent, although the end-tidal carbon dioxide monitor should indicate increased rebreathing of exhaled gases (i.e., elevation of inspired carbon dioxide). Another cause of increased rebreathing of exhaled gases involves a malfunction of the exhalation check valve. The accumulation of moisture from humidified exhaled gases condensing on the cooler anesthesia machine parts can cause the check valve to remain in the open position (Figure 19.5). In this situation, patients will rebreathe more exhaled gas and higher levels of carbon dioxide.

The oxygen supply to a patient can be mistakenly interrupted when the oxygen lines have been pressurized before the oxygen cylinder has been turned off. When the oxygen flow meter is turned on again, oxygen flow is initially present, giving the impression the oxygen cylinder is open, but will cease when the oxygen in the lines is exhausted. This is more likely to occur when switching from a central supply of oxygen to smaller oxygen cylinders mounted onto the anesthetic machine.

The endotracheal tube can kink during extreme flexion of the animal's neck during positioning for cerebral spinal fluid tap, cervical spine radiographs, or ophthalmologic procedures. One should always determine patency of the endotracheal tube after extreme flexion of the head and neck. Use of a wire-reinforced endotracheal tube can reduce the incidence of obstruction (Figure 19.6).

Delayed recovery

Occasionally, an animal will fail to recover normally from anesthesia. Common causes of this problem include hypothermia, severe hypercapnea, hypoglycemia, and heavy narcotization. Hypoglycemia has been shown to decrease the minimum alveolar concentration of halothane in rats. Hypoglycemia can be clinically silent in anesthetized

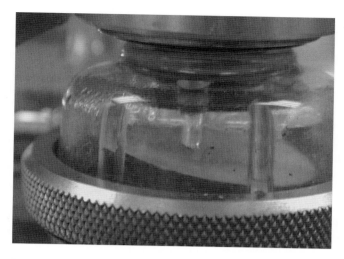

Figure 19.5. Because of condensation of humidified exhaled gases on the dome and valve, this exhalation valve has become lodged in the open position, enabling rebreathing of expired gases. An end-tidal carbon dioxide monitor would detect this equipment problem. *Source*: Evans A.T., Wilson D.V. 2007. Anesthetic emergencies and procedures. In: *Lumb and Jones' Veterinary Anesthesia and Analgesia*, 4th ed. W.J. Tranquilli, J.C. Thurmon, and K.A. Grimm, eds. Ames, IA: Blackwell Publishing, p. 1042.

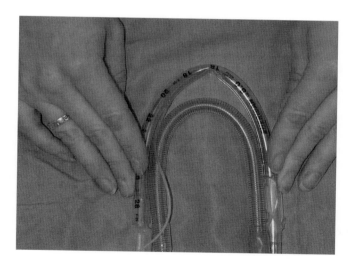

Figure 19.6. The use of a wire-reinforced endotracheal tube will prevent kinking of the tube and obstruction of the airway.
Source: Evans A.T., Wilson D.V. 2007. Anesthetic emergencies and procedures. In: *Lumb and Jones' Veterinary Anesthesia and Analgesia*, 4th ed. W.J. Tranquilli, J.C. Thurmon, and K.A. Grimm, eds. Ames, IA: Blackwell Publishing, p. 1042.

patients, which emphasizes the importance of glucose monitoring in susceptible patients. During anesthesia, signs of sympathetic overactivity or ventricular arrhythmias may be the only detectable evidence of life-threatening hypoglycemia. Patients at high risk of developing hypoglycemia in the perianesthetic period include neonates, very small patients, fasting diabetics treated with their usual insulin dose, and dogs with glucocorticoid deficiency.

Occasionally, coma or blindness can follow anesthetic-related insult to the central nervous system. If persistent neurological deficit follows an apparently uneventful anesthetic procedure, likely causes include hypoxia, severe hypotension, undiagnosed hydrocephalus, other preexisting neurological dysfunction, or an idiosyncratic drug-related response. In these cases, the exact etiology may be harder to determine. Treatment of these patients is primarily supportive, and the prognosis has to be guarded. In cases of anesthesia-related cortical blindness, vision may return as long as 2 weeks later, so cautious optimism is appropriate.

Reports of poor or delayed recoveries from anesthesia are abound in popular canine and feline breed journals, and many breed societies relay stories of anesthetic-related problems. There are indeed situations where breed-specific anatomical or physiological peculiarities or common genetic or congenital diseases may complicate anesthetic management. Also, genetic differences in specific populations of a species or breed can perhaps increase the risk of performing anesthesia in some individual animals. Nevertheless, most animals presented with nonspecific warnings about delayed recovery from anesthesia respond normally to the careful dosing of commonly used anesthetic agents. Inappropriate dosage of anesthetic or inadequate patient monitoring is more likely the common culprit in many cases of reported anesthetic sensitivity.

Gastroesophageal reflux and regurgitation

Reflux of gastric contents into the esophagus has occurred if esophageal pH decreases below 4 (reflux of gastric acid) or above 7.5 (reflux of bile). This reflux is clinically silent and usually acidic. The lower esophageal sphincter is considered to be the primary barrier to the development of this reflux. Lower esophageal sphincter pressure in dogs is decreased with the use of isoflurane, atropine, acepromazine, and xylazine. The effects of many other anesthetic agents on sphincter function have not been determined. Gastroesophageal reflux (GER) reportedly occurs during anesthesia in approximately 17% of dogs receiving thiopental, halothane, and other agents; in 50% of dogs receiving propofol; and in up to 60% of dogs receiving preanesthetic morphine. A 5% incidence of GER has been reported in a population of anesthetized people, which suggests that anesthetic-induced GER occurs less frequently in people than in dogs, even though opioids are commonly used in both species. In some cases, the refluxate is of sufficient volume to reach the pharynx and even drain from the mouth (regurgitation). The incidence of regurgitation is currently estimated at around 0.1% in animals anesthetized at the Michigan State University Veterinary Teaching Hospital. This material may be aspirated into the lungs, leading to pneumonitis, or may cause local irritation of the esophagus as a prelude to the development of ulcerative esophagitis and stricture formation.

Hypothermia

This occurs commonly in anesthetized patients because of depressed thermoregulation, excessive heat loss relative to metabolic production, and mixing of core and peripheral blood by indiscriminant vasodilation. Heat is lost to the environment through convection, conduction, radiation, and evaporation, and occurs more rapidly when body surface is larger relative to body mass. Many anesthetic drugs, including opioids, the inhalant anesthetics, and alpha$_2$ agonists, interfere with thermoregulation and contribute to prolonged postoperative hypothermia. Inhalation anesthetics lower the threshold for response to hypothermia in people to about 34.5°C, and presumably this occurs in animals as well. Anesthetized dogs have been shown to have a decrease in rectal temperature of 1.9°C/h in the first hour of anesthesia. Hypothermia has been associated with pain, suppressed phagocytic activity including decreased migration of polymorphonuclear cells, reduced superoxide anion production, and reduced bacterial killing, and thus may contribute to systemic suppression of immune reactivity in the perioperative period. In a retrospective study of dogs, mild decreases (1°C) in body temperature during surgery were not related to increased risk of incisional infections. Surgical hypothermia can be limited by increasing the ambient temperature, but this is seldom feasible. Circulating warm-water pads, especially applied to the legs, have been shown to help preserve body heat in dogs. Forced-air warming systems currently are the most efficient and effective means of preserving or increasing body heat in anesthetized patients. Humidification and warming of inhaled gas has been shown to be ineffective as a sole means of maintaining core temperature in dogs or cats. The use of uncovered electrical heating pads or hot water bottles is discouraged because of the potential for thermal injury.

Hyperthermia

Drug-induced hyperthermia is rare in the practice of veterinary anesthesia. However, μ-receptor opioid agonists such as hydromorphone and fentanyl have been associated with moderate hyperthermia in some cats. The most commonly used drugs in human practice that can cause hyperthermia include antipsychotic agents, serotonin antagonists, sympathomimetic agents, inhalation anesthetics, and agents with anticholinergic properties. The resultant hyperthermia is frequently accompanied by intense skeletal muscle rigidity (contracture), rhabdomyolysis, and hyperkalemia. Neuroleptic malignant syndrome is a rare but potentially lethal reaction to antipsychotic drugs, including phenothiazines and lithium. Dopaminergic antagonism, a direct myotoxicity, altered thermoregulation, or extrapyramidal hyperactivity are postulated to contribute to the development of this syndrome. It is very possible that this syndrome could even occur in phenothiazine-treated animals placed in a very warm environment.

Malignant hyperthermia is an inherited membrane-linked abnormality (ryanodine receptor mutation) that has been documented in several species, including pigs, dogs, cats, and horses. Susceptible patients should be anesthetized with barbiturates, propofol, opiates, and tranquilizers, and may be pretreated with dantrolene. Avoidance of known triggering agents such as potent inhalation anesthetics, depolarizing muscle relaxants, and stress is advised.

Accidental iatrogenic hyperthermia can develop during warm ambient temperatures, in animals with thick hair coats, and with the use of forced-air warming systems. It is important to monitor body temperature in patients where active heating strategies are being used. Some smaller patients, when treated with forced-air warming on the highest setting (43°C), heat up rapidly. In most situations, iatrogenic hyperthermia subsides rapidly after the heat source is removed.

Injuries

A number of other conditions can lead to injury during anesthesia:

(1) *Swollen feet*   Limbs can be secured by ties placed so tight that they reduce venous drainage.
(2) *Corneal ulcers*   Anesthetics reduce or eliminate the palpebral and corneal reflex and reduce tear formation. Chemical irritants, physical trauma, or drying can lead to ulceration. Artificial tears are important in preventing these problems.
(3) *Tracheal mucosal injury*   Overinflation of the cuff or moving the cuff while it is inflated can cause mucosal injury, tracheal rupture, or tracheal chondromalacia. Tracheal rupture is an uncommon sequela to intubation in cats and can usually be treated medically. When changing patient positions, the endotracheal tube should be disconnected from the Y-adapter, and the patient's head and neck supported to prevent sliding or movement of the endotracheal tube cuff. To prevent pressure-induced mucosal necrosis, it is wise to inflate the cuff of the endotracheal tube only sufficiently to seal a leak at $10–20\,cm\ H_2O$. It is not recommended to simply put "some air" in the cuff without checking its pressure.
(4) *Joint pain*   Older animals with arthritic joints that are placed on their backs for surgery may have joint pain for days following anesthesia.
(5) *Pulmonary barotrauma*   Overinflation of the lungs will damage the pulmonary structures significantly if pressures exceed $30\,cm\ H_2O$. Inadvertently leaving the adjustable pressure-limiting valve (pop-off valve) closed or using the oxygen flush when the patient is on a Bain's system can create pulmonary overpressurization. One simple way to provide protection for the patient if the pop-off valve inadvertently remains in the closed position is to place a commercially available PEEP valve in the breathing circuit.

Epidural analgesia and regional nerve block

The use of the epidural route for delivery of opioids and local anesthetics is becoming increasingly popular, especially with prolonged drug delivery by epidural catheter. There are reports of epidural catheters having been placed and left in dogs for 7 days, with the main complication being catheter dislodgement and local tissue response. Meticulous attention to aseptic technique is essential when drugs or catheters are placed in the epidural space. Epidural abscessation and discospondylitis have been reported following epidural injection. Other complications reported following epidural injection in dogs include urinary retention and prolonged cerebrospinal fluid levels of morphine, myotonus, and pruritus. Subarachnoid injection of preservative-free morphine in a dog caused such severe pruritus and myoclonus that the dog had to be anesthetized for several hours until the reaction resolved.

Regional nerve block has some risk of causing local anesthetic toxicity, although combining local anesthetics with epinephrine (5 mcg/mL) will dramatically reduce this risk. Direct needle trauma to the nerve being blocked can cause a prolonged or permanent neural deficit. Local hemorrhage may result in hematoma formation, but this is generally self-limiting.

Electrolyte abnormalities

Hyperkalemia is one electrolyte abnormality that can be associated with acute death. The causes of rapid-onset hyperkalemia during anesthesia and surgery include transfusion of old stored blood, chronic heparin therapy (dogs), uroperitoneum, and iatrogenic administration (potassium penicillin or potassium chloride). Hyperkalemia produces very characteristic ECG changes. Arrhythmias caused by hyperkalemia can lead to cardiac arrest and may not respond to conventional antiarrhythmic therapies, but do respond to the rapid treatment of hyperkalemia. Aggressive lowering of serum potassium by using furosemide, dextrose, and sodium bicarbonate, and the reversal of hyperkalemic effects on cell membrane potential by calcium administration, can help resolve a hyperkalemic crisis if it occurs during anesthesia.

Hypokalemia caused by hemodilution and decreased intake is the most common cause of postoperative arrhythmias in people. Arrhythmias (ventricular ectopy) associated with this electrolyte disturbance are not commonly observed in other animals.

Revised from "Anesthetic Emergencies and Procedures" by A. Thomas Evans and Deborah V. Wilson in Lumb and Jones' Veterinary Anesthesia and Analgesia, Fourth Edition.

Index

Page numbers followed by an f denote figures, those followed by a t denote tables, and those followed by a b denote boxes.

AAHA pain management standards, 4, 5t
Abdominal (diaphragmatic) breathing pattern, as anesthetic depth indicator, 199
ABP. *See* Arterial blood pressure (ABP)
Absorbents, carbon dioxide, 179–180
Absorption, of local anesthetics, 340–341
Acepromazine
  boxers and, 291
  cardiovascular effects, 380t, 381
  in cesarean section patients, 473t
  described, 44
  in GI endoscopy patients, 439
  hypotension and, 231–232
  in liver disease patients, 424
  in neonatal and geriatric patients, 494
  in neurological disease patients, 407
  ocular effects, 467t
  in orthopedic patients, 500
  preanesthetic use, 279, 282t
  in respiratory disease patients, 388–389, 393, 396
  in rodents and rabbits, 316t
Acetaminophen
  for chronic pain, 154
  codeine combined with, 111
  COX-3 inhibition, 120
  dosage ranges, 126t
  overview of, 127–128
Acetylcholinesterase, 76, 80–81
Acid, defined, 241

Acid-base balance, 240–258
  analysis
    anion gap approach, 251–253, 252t
    base excess approach, 251
    strong ion approach, 253–258, 254t
      base excess modification, 256–257, 256t, 257t
      effective SID modification, 255–256
      SID (strong ion difference), 253–255
      simplifications of, 255
      simplified SIG modification, 257–258
    traditional approach, 247–251, 248t, 249f
      expected compensatory changes, 250t
      limitations of approach, 250–251
      mixed disorders, 250
      simple disorders, 248–249, 249f
  causes of disorders, 248t
  compensatory changes, 249, 249f, 250t
  fluid balance assessment and, 267
  regulation of, 240–247
    chemical buffering, 243–245
      bicarbonate buffer system, 243
      factors influencing intracellular, 244–245
      isohydric principle and, 245
      phosphate buffer system, 244
      protein buffer system, 244
    renal, 245–247

Essentials of Small Animal Anesthesia and Analgesia, Second Edition. Edited by Kurt A. Grimm, William J. Tranquilli, Leigh A. Lamont.
© 2011 John Wiley & Sons, Inc. Published 2011 by John Wiley & Sons, Inc.